Pediatric Diagnostic Labs for Primary Care: An Evidence-based Approach

Rita Marie John

Editor

Pediatric Diagnostic Labs for Primary Care: An Evidence-based Approach

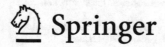 Springer

Editor
Rita Marie John (iD)
School of Nursing
Columbia University
New York, NY, USA

ISBN 978-3-030-90644-3   ISBN 978-3-030-90642-9   (eBook)
https://doi.org/10.1007/978-3-030-90642-9

This Springer imprint is published by the registered company Springer Nature Switzerland AG
The registered company address is: Gewerbestrasse 11, 6330 Cham, Switzerland

Foreword

This book is written for primary care providers who care for children. The book will meet the need of primary care providers to increase their knowledge of diagnostic labs and how to interpret them. While guidelines have been developed to guide clinicians in ordering diagnostic laboratory tests during a well-child visit, the interpretation of diagnostic labs must be organized. The clinician seeing patients who present with various complaints cannot order tests in a disorganized way. The clinician must rule out the worst-case scenarios and consider which diagnostic laboratory tests will provide the best information to determine the diagnosis.

The ordering of diagnostic laboratory tests and their interpretation was not well taught when I became a nurse practitioner in the late 1970s. Today, many programs have limited time to teach all the different tests and interpret them. This book will fill in that gap and update clinicians who were trained several years ago.

Diagnostic laboratory stewardship involves using the right test for the right patient at the right time (Morjaria & Chapin 2020). The tendency to overutilize diagnostic tests has been well documented in multiple studies, with an estimate that one out of five lab tests is unnecessary (Zhi et al. 2013). Clinicians must understand which test will answer their diagnostic questions. It is important to note that 60% to 70% of medical decisions are based on diagnostic laboratory results (Molinaro et al. 2012). Therefore, understanding the limitation of tests is critical to the proper diagnosis.

Parents have access to diagnostic laboratory tests and get very concerned when they see a result flagged with high and low, even when the result is only .1 over or under the normal value. Carefully explaining the interpretation of the result is key to alleviating anxiety and increasing understanding of the result. Ordering more tests when the results are not significant can lead to over-ordering of diagnostic laboratory tests. The clinician must be able to completely understand the results to explain the results to concerned families.

The format of each chapter is designed to address common presenting complaints in the primary care office. The organization is designed so that the laboratory tests follow an explanation of a variety of diagnoses. The book has 12 chapters, and chapters 2 to 12 are divided by systems. Each of the authors has clinical experience in their section and gives insight into the differential diagnosis and the clinical guidelines if the guidelines are available.

The book's first chapter reviews how to interpret laboratory tests and hopefully increases the reader's understanding of what false-negative or false-positive results mean. The molecular panels can be very helpful in diagnosing infectious diseases. Still, the clinician must understand that ordering diagnostic laboratory tests with a low pretest likelihood may cause diagnostic errors. Baird (2019) pointed out that a low pretest likelihood may increase diagnostic mistakes. Newer and more accurate tests have led to a greater ability to diagnose, but not with absolute certainty (Bindraban et al. 2018). Lippi et al. reported that the rate of inappropriate laboratory tests ranges from 23% to 67%. Therefore, understanding pre- and post-test probability will improve the clinician's diagnostic accuracy.

Chapter 2 reviews the care of pregnant adolescents. Frequently, the primary care provider makes the diagnosis of intrauterine pregnancy. The problems of getting the adolescent involved with proper obstetrical care can depend on insurance and local availability. This chapter gives an insight into the management of pregnant adolescents.

Chapter 3 discusses the care of the newborn. It reviews the interpretation of possible laboratory tests that might be ordered and the importance of newborn screening. Congenital infections are discussed in detail, including the new febrile well-appearing newborn guidelines. Chapter 4 focuses on the well-child and the variety of screening tests that are recommended. There is a discussion regarding the pitfalls of drug screening. Chapter 5 discusses point-of-care (POC) testing. This chapter includes information on COVID testing as well as several common POC tests. POC is a rapidly expanding area, and clinicians must be aware of the availability of point-of-care testing so that patient treatment can be expedited.

Chapter 6 discusses pediatric infectious diseases and the variety of available laboratory tests. Children frequently present to the office with a fever, and a knowledge of infectious diseases diagnostic testing can help pinpoint the child's diagnosis. The limitations and pitfalls of the variety of tests are reviewed to aid the clinician in understanding the results.

Clinicians today have the advantage of genetic diagnostic tests to aid them in determining the cause for the presenting complaint. Many clinicians were trained before the advent of the broad variety of diagnostic genetic tests. The diagnostic potential of the newer technology of genetic tests in pediatric patients allows early timely and specific interventions to improve clinical outcomes. Understanding the limitation of these tests can be very helpful.

Chapter 8 reviews a variety of hematological problems. Chapter 8 reviews a systematic approach to the interpretation of the CBC. The clinician orders hematological tests based on the patient's history, the family history, and the physical exam. The child with anemia may have a problem with another system, such as the gastrointestinal, renal, or endocrine system, or have a rheumatological disorder. Chapters 9–12 review these systems. The reader can improve their knowledge of a variety of laboratory tests.

I hope that the reader will review each chapter utilizing the cases to reinforce the readers. There are boxes of key learning throughout each chapter to reinforce the reader's knowledge. There are several questions with rationales at the end of each chapter for review.

References

Baird G. The Choosing Wisely initiative and laboratory test stewardship. Diagnosis. 2019;6(1):15–23.

Bindraban RS, Ten Berg MJ, Naaklgeboren CA, Kramer MHH Vansolinge WW, Nanayakkara PWB. Reducing test utilization in a hospital setting: a narrative review. Ann Lab Med. 2018;38:402–12.

Morjaria S, Chapin KP. Who to test, when and for what? J Molecular Diag. 2020;22:9.

Molinaro RJ, Winkler AM, Kraft CS, Fantz CR, Stowell SR, Ritchie JC, Koch DD, Heron S, Liebzeit J, Santen SA, Guarner J. Teaching laboratory medicine to medical students: implementation and evaluation. Arch Pathol Lab Med. 2012;136(11):1423-9.

Zhi M, Ding EL, Theisen-Toupal, J. Whelan, J. Arnaout R. The landscape of inappropriate laboratory testing: a 15-year meta-analysis. PLoS one. 2013;8:e78962

Acknowledgment

"Sometimes it takes a mountain" is a popular song that speaks clearly to all the people that helped me get this book to publication. First and foremost, I want to acknowledge all my authors who spent hours preparing their chapters. They took time away from their busy lives to write their chapter. I appreciate their dedication and knowledge. I know that every reader will learn something from this book no matter how much experience they have. The authors have clinical expertise that will certainly help the practicing clinician. My sincere thanks to each of them.

I want to acknowledge my husband, who has always supported me in my clinical and academic endeavors. He has been a source of encouragement and support. He understood that this book was one of my career goals. He understood when I was in the office working for hours. I am blessed to have had him in my life for greater than 50 years.

I want to thank my previous editors, who helped me develop chapters for their books. I would specifically like to acknowledge Margaret Brady, who guided me through multiple chapters for Pediatric Primary Care. Chapter writing can be challenging for the novice author, and it takes patience to deal with delays.

I want to thank my students at Columbia and the PNPs that attended my conferences over the past 21 years. Their questions gave me the idea for this book. I learned from students what they needed to know and what I could accomplish during their education. This book is an extension of what I learned from them.

I want to thank my pediatric nurse practitioner and physician colleagues who worked with me along the way. Dr. Susan Margolin, Dr. Chitra Reddy, Dr. Maria Toft, Dr. Geraldine Nelson, and Jeanne Gibian, CPNP, who worked with me at the University of Medicine and Dentistry in Newark, NJ (now Rutgers's Medical School). We would have lively discussions about laboratory test interpretation. Dr. Frank Cunningham and the Newark Beth Israel Pediatric ED physician staff also increased my knowledge of laboratory diagnostic tests. Finally, to the staff at Springfield Pediatric Group, who continued to enhance my knowledge of diagnostic laboratory tests.

Finally, I would like to thank my editor at Springer publishing, Marie-Elia Come-Garry, and my project manager, Smitha Diveshan, for their support and understanding in completing this project. I appreciate their publishing expertise and acknowledgment that the pandemic interfered with the completion of this book.

Contents

1   **Pediatric Diagnostic Lab Tests: An Overview** 1
    Arlene Smaldone and Rita Marie John

2   **Laboratory Screening and Diagnostic Testing
    in Antepartum Care** 29
    Adena Bargad and Hannah VogtSchaller

3   **Care of the Newborn**................................. 67
    Rita Marie John, Ashley N. Gyura, Emily R. Harrison,
    and Bobbie Salveson

4   **The Well Pediatric Primary Care Visit
    and Screening Laboratory Tests** 101
    Rita Marie John

5   **Point-of-Care Testing in Primary Care**..................... 135
    Laura Britton Stace

6   **Care of the Child with an Infectious Disease
    or Immunological Defect** 171
    Ashley N. Gyura and Emily R. Harrison

7   **Genetics and Pediatric Patient**........................... 239
    Rita Marie John and Angela Kenny

8   **Hematology** 263
    Rita Marie John and Caroline Anne Bell

9   **Care of the Child with a Gastrointestinal Disorder**.......... 319
    Anna L. Rundle, Nicole Baron, and Rita Marie John

10   **Care of the Child with a Renal Problem**................... 365
    Deanna Schneider and Clare Cardo McKegney

11   **Care of the Child with a Pediatric Endocrine Disorder** 413
    Rebecca Crespi, Leigh Pughe, and Amy Dowd

12   **Care of the Child with a Possible Rheumatological Disorder**... 461
    Rita Marie John and Kathleen Kenney-Riley

Pediatric Diagnostic Lab Tests: An Overview

1

Arlene Smaldone and Rita Marie John

Learning Objectives

After completing the chapter, the learner should be able to

1. Distinguish differences in pediatric blood sample collection from that of adults and identify the differences in pediatric patients that can affect lab results.
2. Define concepts fundamental to diagnostic testing: disease prevalence, pretest probability, and post-test probability.
3. Interpret characteristics of diagnostic tests: sensitivity, specificity, positive likelihood ratio, and negative likelihood ratio.
4. Summarize the problems of overutilization and underutilization of diagnostic laboratory tests.

1.1 Unique Issues in Pediatric Blood and Urine Collection

Children are not small adults, and this is certainly true when it comes to diagnostic laboratory tests. Not only is the task of obtaining samples for diagnostic testing problematic for our youngest patients and children with chronic health condi-

tions, but the interpretation of the results must sometimes also be age-adjusted to be correctly interpreted. Commercial laboratories vary as to whether they appropriately report the normal age-adjusted ranges for children. Some values, such as total bilirubin levels in newborns, quickly change over a short period. A total bilirubin level considered within the normal range for a 3-day-old infant would indicate a disease state in a 2-week-old infant. Young infants can rapidly change from well to critically ill in a matter of hours, and they have little fat and glycogen reserves. The newborn's body composition is higher in water, making dehydration a real risk if the infant experiences significant GI loss or deficient fluid intake. The newborn kidney has more difficulty compensating for an increased loss of electrolytes.

Some laboratory tests like the tests that comprise the newborn screening panel are used to diagnose rare inborn errors of metabolism, hematological, and endocrine disorders, or vanillylmandelic acid or homovanillic acid is used to diagnose neuroblastoma. Some disorders, like type 2 diabetes, dyslipidemia, and obesity, are far more common in children today. Therefore, the clinician must screen and monitor lipid levels, glucose, and liver function tests in children with obesity. The skillset of the clinician who cares for children must be broad with a solid understanding of the biochemical and hematological changes that occur in children as they grow.

A. Smaldone (✉) · R. M. John
Columbia University School of Nursing,
New York City, New York, USA
e-mail: ams130@columbia.edu

Age-related differences in the interpretation of laboratory results are common. Measurement of alkaline phosphatase (AP), insulin-like growth factor-1 (IGF-1), IGF binding proteins, and neutrophil counts are good examples. AP is primarily expressed in the liver and the bone. Children below the age of 5 years have a significant elevation of the AP, likely due to decreased enzyme clearance. AP concentrations then decline and remain stable until the child enters puberty, when AP levels increase significantly due to bone growth. Neither elevation requires a workup if the elevations are within the normal variation for the child's age (Ridefelt et al. 2014). The levels of insulin-like growth factor-1 (IGF-1) and IGF binding proteins also vary in childhood and are elevated during periods of rapid growth (Blankenstein et al. 2015). The neutrophil count during infancy is markedly lower than during adolescence; the neutrophil count increases throughout early childhood until it reaches adult levels during early adolescence (Segel and Halterman 2008).

1.1.1 Blood Sampling in Pediatric Patients

Infants and young children have a smaller total blood volume. For example, a newborn weighing between 6 and 7 pounds has an average blood volume of approximately 300 ml, whereas a 40- to 45-pound child has a blood volume of 1700 ml. Therefore, blood samples need to be collected and analyzed using pediatric-specific vials to minimize blood loss. Limiting the amount of blood for testing in hospitalized and sick pediatric patients will decrease iatrogenic anemia secondary to frequent blood sampling. The clinician needs to consult with the lab to ensure that vials are used appropriately for the patient's size and the minimum amount of blood that the lab needs to run the requested test. Reduced volume tubes enable the clinician to collect less blood and still have the right amount of tube preservatives required for the test.

1.1.2 Collection of Pediatric Blood and Urine Samples

The methods used to obtain blood include heel or finger stick, venipuncture, and withdrawal of specimens from umbilical or central lines. The method employed will vary according to the age and circumstance of the child. A parent or guardian can soothe the child during the procedure; however, parents or guardians are often not the best people to help restrain them. Adequate teaching about gentle techniques for restraint should be used. Medical restraint is rarely needed in pediatrics. There are times when phlebotomy should not be attempted if the child is too combative and may injure themselves or the phlebotomist. Blood collection via a phlebotomy/heel stick requires meticulous attention to pain reduction by applying a topical anesthetic agent or using techniques such as hypnotism, blowing bubbles, mindfulness, or buzzing or vibrating devices (Gaglani and Gross 2018).

Heel or finger sticks. In children less than 6 months of age, heel sticks can be used, while for infants between 6 months and 1 year, although heel sticks are preferred, obtaining a specimen by finger stick is acceptable. Lancets are specific for each procedure and are not interchangeable; therefore, finger stick lancets should not be used to collect a sample via a heel stick and vice versa. Some heel stick devices have a quick-moving pendulum blade, and its use to obtain a specimen from the finger will cause excessive bleeding. It is important to avoid the bone when puncturing the skin to obtain a specimen, as this can cause osteomyelitis (Yuksel et al. 2007). Before heel stick collection, the heel should be warmed to increase blood flow, and the lateral or medial plantar surface should be used, as seen in Picture 1.1. The use of finger stick or heel collection requires very small collection tubes called bullets. Bullets are associated with a higher rejection rate secondary to hemolysis, especially if the person collecting the sample uses excessive force to squeeze the heel or finger. If the collection is prolonged, clotting is more likely with these tubes.

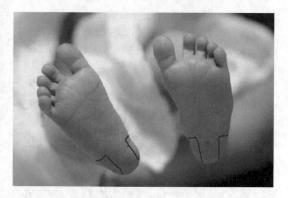

Picture 1.1 Areas for a heel stick. From: https://pixabay.com/photos/baby-feet-new-born-child-newborn-1025398/

Tube order: The tube collection order is important as the additives from one tube can contaminate the subsequent tube. Therefore, when using a needle, butterfly, or transfer device, the order of specimen collection is important. For phlebotomy, blood cultures should be collected first to avoid contamination. Following this, tubes without additives are collected, followed by tubes with weaker anticoagulants (i.e., sodium citrate), and lastly, tubes with stronger anticoagulants (i.e., EDTA).

In contrast, when collecting specimens via a heel or finger stick, the blood starts to clot right away, so anticoagulated tubes should be collected first, and any specimen that can be clotted should be collected last. The clinician must remember that certain anticoagulants such as EDTA can cause platelet clumping (Tan et al. 2016; Fang et al. 2015; Nagler et al. 2014) and, to get an accurate result, a different anticoagulant must be used for the follow-up exam.

Venipuncture. In children between 1 and 2 years, while a finger stick can be used for specimen collection, a venipuncture may be necessary if the quantity of blood required is larger than can be obtained via a finger stick. For children over 2 years of age, venipuncture should be employed to obtain the specimen. A butterfly with a syringe is better in children and adolescents with small veins that may collapse if a transfer device is used. The suction amount can be more precisely controlled using a butterfly and a syringe leading to a successful venipuncture.

Urine collection. In infants, the bladder capacity is smaller and empties within 4 hours. Nitrite-producing bacteria need around 4 h to produce nitrites in the urine during a urinary tract infection. Urinary catheterization is the correct way to collect a specimen for a urine culture in children under 2 years (Jackson 2015). In contrast, a bagged urine sample can be used in pediatric patients who are not toilet trained and over 2 years. A urine collection bag must be put on an infant who has a clean, dry peritoneum. Wringing out a diaper or collecting urine by placing cotton balls in the diaper is never advised. It allows fibers and chemicals to get into the sample, interfering with the test results. It can be very challenging to collect a 24-h urine sample in a young child. A study of 241 adults showed that more than half (51.5%) of 24-h samples were collected incorrectly (Boyd et al. 2018). If a 24-h urine sample is needed, the child's first void of the day is discarded; the 24-h collection period begins after the first void. All urine specimens are collected during the day and night; the 24-h sample concludes with the first void on the second day. Generally, the collection container is kept refrigerated during the collection period. In general, spot urine for creatinine and protein is often done in place of 24-h collections (Kaminska et al. 2020).

1.1.3 Handling and Timing of the Specimen before Processing

The temperature requirements of the specimen after it is drawn must be carefully considered. For example, the result of an erythrocyte sedimentation rate will be higher if the sample was subject to higher temperatures (Bray et al. 2016). If the specimen is sent to an outside lab, the sample must not be drawn during the weekend when delivery will be delayed. Most specimens, once received by the lab, are run within a 24-h period.

Key Learning in Pediatric Blood and Urine Collection

- The size of the blood tube for collection must consider the patient's size and the minimum amount needed for processing the sample.
- Interpretation of the diagnostic laboratory test results must be age-adjusted to be correctly interpreted.
- A heel stick may be used for infants, providing you have the appropriate tubes for the collection. For children over 2 years of age, venipuncture should be used. A butterfly with a syringe is better in pediatric patients with small veins as the vein may collapse if a transfer device is used.
- Certain anticoagulants such as EDTA can cause platelet clumping, resulting in a low platelet count.

1.2 Key Concepts in the Interpretation of Lab Tests

1.2.1 Overview

Clinicians order clinical tests to either screen for a disease's presence before symptoms are present or to diagnose a disease's presence. In both cases, the clinician must understand the basic properties of diagnostic tests: sensitivity and specificity. Sensitivity (Sn) and specificity (Sp) determine a laboratory test's accuracy relative to a reference or "gold" standard (Trevethan 2017). Sn measures true positives, and Sp measures true negatives (Borysiak et al. 2016). A perfect clinical test will correctly identify all patients with the disease and all patients who do not have the disease. Unfortunately, this is rarely the case; therefore, some test results may reflect either false positives or false negatives. Therefore, clinicians must acquire a basic understanding of test properties to choose tests with acceptable test properties so that false positives and false negatives may be minimal and test results can be interpreted properly. When new clinical tests are developed (e.g., detection of COVID-19) or more

Table 1.1 Definition of terms

Term	Definition/mathematical formula
Diagnostic accuracy	A test that measures what it is supposed to measure
False negative (FN)	A negative test result in a child who has the disease
False positive (FP)	A positive test result in a disease-free child
Negative likelihood ratio (LR−)	The change in the odds of having a diagnosis for patients with a negative test $LR- = (1 - \text{sensitivity})/\text{specificity}$
Negative predictive value (NPV)	The probability that a child with a negative test result does not have the disease $NPV = TN/(TN + FN)$
Positive likelihood ratio (LR+)	The number of times more likely that a negative test comes from an individual with the disease rather than from an individual without the disease $LR+ = \text{sensitivity}/(1 - \text{specificity})$
Post-test probability	The likelihood that an event will occur following a positive or negative test result
Pretest probability	The probability that a patient has the disease before the diagnostic test is performed
Prevalence	The probability that a patient has the disease after the results of the diagnostic test
Positive predictive value (PPV)	The probability a child with a positive result does have the disease $PPV = TP/(TP + FP)$
Precision	The reproducibility of a test to give the same result if repeated on the same patient sample
Reference standard	The test is considered to be the most accurate way to test for a disease
Reliability	The repeatability or reproducibility of a laboratory test that would give you a similar result with repeat testing
Sensitivity	The probability that a child with the disease will test positive $\text{Sensitivity} = TP/TP + FN$
Specificity	The probability that a child without any disease will test negative $\text{Specificity} = TN/TN + FP$
True negative (TN)	A person without a disease who has a negative test result
True positive (TP)	A person with a disease who has a positive test result

established tests used for new purposes (e.g., ultrasound used to diagnose pediatric pneumonia), the new test's performance is compared to a reference standard. Table 1.1 provides definitions and mathematical formulas for terms that will be explained further throughout the chapter.

In evaluating whether to order a diagnostic test, there are many important considerations, including:

- How does the test you are ordering compare with other laboratory tests?
- What will the lab test do to help you care for the patient?
- Would you still order the test if the patient did not have insurance?
- Can you interpret the test?
- How will the results of the test affect your clinical decision-making? Which is the best test to eliminate the differentials and determine the diagnosis?
- Does testing improve the patient's health outcomes?
- How much does the test cost? Is the test cost-effective?
- Were the test parameters (sensitivity, specificity, accuracy, precision, and predictive values) evaluated?

1.2.2 Precision, Mean, and Standard Deviation

Precision is the reproducibility and repeatability of the test. Repeatability refers to the repeatability of the test in a single laboratory, whereas reproducibility refers to the repeatability of the test in different laboratories. It is the closeness of different independent measurements for a set of experimental tests (Borysiak, 2016).

The range of normal values for a test is decided by its 95% confidence interval or two standard deviations (SDs) from the mean. For diagnostic laboratory tests, some ranges of normal are very narrow, whereas others are much wider. When a result falls slightly outside the lower or upper limits of the 95% confidence interval, the clinician must consider whether the child's lab value may represent a value within the 99% confidence interval (three SDs from the mean).

The 99% confidence interval can easily be calculated. For example, if a child has a potassium (K) of 3.4 and the normal range is 3.5–4.9, first, calculate the mean value for K (calculated as [3.5 + 4.9]/2 = 4.2). To calculate an SD's width,

subtract the mean from the upper or lower limit of the normal range (4.9–4.2 = 0.7). Using this information, the range for three SDs from the mean would be 4.2 ± (3*0.7), representing a 99% confidence interval range between 2.7 and 5.6.

However, it would then be important to evaluate the patient for signs of hypokalemia or hyperkalemia if the patient falls out of the range of the 95% confidence interval. It is important to recognize that a K of 3.4 might be normal for that patient.

A good example of this is seen with the TSH in hypothyroidism. A TSH slightly above normal within the 99% confidence interval range may not indicate overt hypothyroidism. The TSH normally found in children with hypothyroidism is well above three SDs from the mean.

Choosing a diagnostic lab test requires thoughtful consideration of the tests' parameters and whether the diagnostic test is the best one to rule out the worst-case scenarios and confirm the most likely diagnosis.

1.2.3 The Relevance of Sensitivity and Specificity in the Diagnostic Process

The underlying reason for ordering a diagnostic test is based on knowledge of the disease's underlying pathophysiology and the test's relationship to the disease process. Most laboratory tests are ordered as part of a diagnostic process—the patient presents with a symptom that prompts the clinician to order a test. A laboratory test with poor accuracy can lead to an inaccurate diagnosis due to missing a condition where it exists (a false-negative test result) or producing a positive test result when the patient does not have a disease (a false-positive test result). Other factors in the diagnostic process, such as history, symptoms, physical examination findings, and other test results, must balance the possibility of an inaccurate test result.

Furthermore, a test's sensitivity and specificity can vary in different clinical scenarios because of changing biological variables, with age being especially important. For example, although the "mono spot" test is extremely sensitive in adults and older children, its sensitivity is less than 50% in young children (Sumaya and Ench 1985).

1.2.4 Test Accuracy

The concepts of **sensitivity** and **specificity** help describe the **validity** and **accuracy** of a laboratory or other clinical test. The higher the sensitivity and specificity, the more useful the test. The test result will never be negative if a patient has the condition (there are no false negatives) if the test is 100% sensitive. A positive test is always accurate (no false positives) if the test is 100% specific. Another way of remembering this is that specificity has a p (needs an N) and reflects the true negative rate.

Table 1.2 illustrates the concept of false positives (those without the target condition who test positive for the condition) and false negatives (those with the target condition who test negative) of a new diagnostic test compared against a reference standard.

Sensitivity is the test's ability to identify patients with the disease and is calculated as the number of true positives (TP) divided by the number of true positives plus false negatives (TP + FN). Figure 1.1 illustrates this concept. Twenty children in a sample of one thousand children have Lyme disease. The children are tested using the enzyme-linked immunosorbent assay (ELISA) test. Eighteen (true positive) of the 20 children test positive, and two children test negative (false negative).

$$\text{Sensitivity} = TP / (TP + FN) = 18 / 20 = 90\%$$

Specificity is the ability of a test to identify patients who do not have the disease and is calculated as the number of those who are disease-free and test negative (TN) divided by the number of true negatives plus false positives (TN + FP) (Baeyens et al. 2019). Of the 980 children who do not have Lyme disease. Of these, 960 children test negative (TN), and 20 children test positive (FP).

$$\text{Specificity} = TN / (TN + FP) = 960 / 980 = 97.9\% = 98\%$$

In this sample of children, while 38 children tested positive, 20 of those children did not have Lyme disease. The test had 90% sensitivity; however, there is a risk of false positives. If the ELISA test is positive for Lyme disease, a Western blot test is usually performed to confirm the diagnosis. Two-tier testing illustrates the diagnostic principle that while the result of a diagnostic test can increase the probability and level of suspicion that a person has the disease, additional testing is often required to confirm the diagnosis.

A test with high sensitivity will correctly detect patients with the disease (TP), but some people who do not have the disease will also test positive (FP). Therefore, a positive test does not mean that the clinician can be confident that the

person truly has the disease. If a test has low sensitivity, patients with the condition will be missed and are therefore not useful. When a test has high specificity, it will correctly detect most people free of that disease (TN), but some people with the disease will test negative (FN).

A test with poor specificity will result in a patient having a positive test result (FP) when they are, in fact, healthy. A test with high specificity will have a low false-positive rate. Highly specific laboratory and clinical tests are used to confirm the presence of a disease. Specificity is independent of the disease rate in a geographic area. It should be remembered that a highly specific test is unlikely to produce false-positive results.

Table 1.2 Concepts of false positives and negatives

	Reference standard	
	Target condition: positive	Target condition: negative
Tests positive with a new diagnostic test	True positive (TP)	False positive (FP)
Tests negative with a new diagnostic test	False negative (FN)	True negative (TN)
	Sensitivity = TP/TP + FN	Specificity = TN/TN + FP

Fig. 1.1 Clinical illustration of test sensitivity and specificity

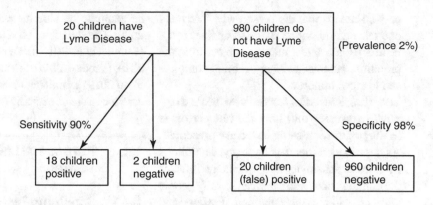

A test's sensitivity and specificity are inversely related as the sensitivity of a test increases, the specificity decreases and vice versa. A test may be better suited to either screen for a disease or diagnose the disease based on a test's sensitivity and specificity. Clinicians must always consider the purpose for which they have ordered the test: is it to screen for disease or assist in diagnosing or confirming the presence of disease? For diagnosis or confirmation of the presence of disease, the clinician must also consider the child's symptoms, risk history, results of other tests, and clinical experience to balance these risks.

1.3   Evidence-Based Practice and Diagnostic Tests

The evidence informing practice decisions accumulates and changes over time. New laboratory or other clinical tests are developed, whereas older established tests may be effectively utilized for new purposes. In both cases, diagnostic accuracy, sensitivity, and specificity of the new or repurposed test must be established. Researchers test the new test's diagnostic accuracy in high-quality cross-sectional design studies where the new test's performance compared to the current reference standard provides level 2 evidence. A meta-analysis of high quality in which test accuracy data reported in several studies where the new test has been evaluated is synthesized across studies provides level 1 evidence and a higher level of evidence than a single study (Centre for Evidence-Based Medicine 2020).

1.3.1   Appraising the Quality of a Study Evaluating Performance of a Diagnostic Test

When considering using a new test, the clinician should evaluate the study's quality that determined the new test's diagnostic accuracy. The Centre for Evidence-based Medicine on Diagnostic Accuracy (2020) suggests that clinicians appraise five key elements of diagnostic studies (Centre for Evidence-Based Medicine, https://www.cebm.net/we-content/uploads/2014/04/diagnostic-study-appraisal-worksheet.pdf). Most required information can be found in a study's methods section; test characteristics information is reported in the results section.

1. **The sample of subjects to whom the test was administered was representative of the spectrum of patients who would benefit from its use in practice.** Ideally, the new test should be administered to all (those with mild, moderate, and severe disease) representing the target disorder. The study sample should have either been randomly selected or consecutively admitted to the study in order to minimize selection bias.
2. **Both the new test and the reference standard were obtained for each subject regardless of one test result.** The reference standard should be a test as close to the truth as possible.
3. **An independent blind comparison should be made between the new test and the reference standard.** An independent blind com-

parison means that the person who interprets one test should not be aware of another test's results. When a test may be subject to interpretation, such as an X-ray, a blind comparison is more important.

4. **Test characteristics for the new test's diagnostic accuracy and how the test performs in the population being tested are presented.** As described earlier, test accuracy, determined by a test's sensitivity and specificity, informs the clinician how well a test can identify people with or without the condition. Positive and negative predictive values and positive and negative likelihood ratios inform the clinician regarding how well the test performs in the population. These values can be calculated using the test's sensitivity and specificity and will be discussed later in the chapter. Of note, predictive values are dependent on the prevalence of the condition in the population in which the study was conducted. Predictive values have less utility when community prevalence differs from the population in which the study was conducted. Likelihood ratios are not dependent on disease prevalence and are more useful in clinical practice settings.

Online evidence-based practice tools are available to simplify the calculation of test characteristics (https://www.ebm-tools.knowledgetranslation.net/calculator). The clinician can easily calculate all diagnostic test characteristics by entering information for the number of true and false positives and true and false negatives reported in an individual study.

5. **The methods for performing the test were described in sufficient detail to allow replication.**

1.3.2 Systematic Reviews and Meta-Analyses of Diagnostic Accuracy Studies

When evidence accumulates, and a sufficient number of individual studies examining a particular test have been conducted, researchers will synthesize data from these studies using systematic review meta-analytic methods to increase certainty regarding diagnostic test performance. Table 1.3 provides an example of nine meta-analyses (Brown et al. 2020; Chartrand et al. 2015; Cui et al. 2019; Holtman et al. 2016; Lean et al. 2014; Lee and Yun 2019; Pereda et al. 2015; Yoon et al. 2017; Zhao and Yuan 2019) examining diagnostic test performance across a range of pediatric conditions.

1.4 Purpose of Laboratory Testing

1.4.1 Screening Tests

An effective screening test should detect a disease. At the same time, it is asymptomatic or in a latent period to be treated early, thereby mitigating the disease process. HIV screening in adolescents is an example of a screening test that has fostered earlier identification and treatment of HIV, improving the illness course. Based on strong evidence, the US Preventive Services Task Force (USPSTF) recommends that clinicians screen all adolescents aged 15 years and older and younger adolescents at increased risk of infection for HIV (USPSTF 2019). Most patients with a positive screening test need further testing to confirm the presence of the disease. Other commonly used screening tests in pediatrics include lead tests, cholesterol screening, and newborn screening for inborn metabolism errors.

A good screening test must be highly sensitive. If a test has low sensitivity, many patients with the condition will be missed. When screening for a disease's presence before symptoms are present, the clinician does not want to miss disease detection through false negatives. The clinician would rather identify false positives because, on confirmatory testing, the person will test negative. A positive test result does not necessarily indicate a condition is present. However, when a test is highly sensitive, the clinician can have a high level of confidence that someone who tests negative will not have the disease, illustrated by the mnemonic **SnNout**. When a test has high **Sen**sitivity, a **N**egative test helps to rule **out** the disease.

For example, when performing newborn screening for inborn errors of metabolism, we would want a highly sensitive test since we want to identify all newborns who have the disease but have no symp-

Table 1.3 Systematic reviews and meta-analyses of diagnostic accuracy studies

Author	Year	Test	Reference standard	Target condition	Studies	Sensitivity (95% CI)	Specificity (95% CI)	LR+ (95% CI)	LR– (95% CI)
Brown et al.	2020	CRP	Microbiological culture	Late-onset newborn infection	22	0.98 (0.90–1.00)	0.30 (0.21–0.41)		
Chartrand et al.	2015	RADT	RT-PCR, immuno-fluorescence, viral culture	Respiratory syncytial virus	63	0.81 (0.78–0.84)	0.96 (0.95–0.98)		
Cui et al.	2019	Procalcitonin		Acute appendicitis	7	0.62 (0.57–0.66)	0.86 (0.82–0.89)	5.3 (1.8–15.8)	0.29 (0.15–0.58)
				Complicated appendicitis	4	0.89 (0.84–0.93)	0.90 (0.86–0.94)	7.7 (3.7–16.1)	0.12 (0.05–0.27)
Holtman et al.	2016	CRP	Endoscopy	IBD diagnosis in symptomatic children	9	0.63 (0.51–0.73)	0.88 (0.80–0.93)	5.1 (2.8–9.4)	0.42 (0.30–0.59)
		ESR			11	0.66 (0.58–0.73)	0.84 (0.80–0.88)	4.2 (3.3–5.3)	0.41 (0.33–0.50)
		Platelet count			8	0.55 (0.36–0.73)	0.88 (0.81–0.93)	4.7 (2.9–7.7)	0.51 (0.34–0.76)
		Hemoglobin			9	0.37 (0.24–0.52)	0.90 (0.83–0.94)	3.7 (2.3–5.9)	0.70 (0.57–0.86)
		Albumin			6	0.48 (0.31–0.66)	0.94 (0.86–0.98)	8.3 (3.7–18.7)	0.55 (0.40–0.76)
		FCal			10	0.99 (0.92–1.00)	0.65 (0.54–0.74)	2.8 (2.1–3.7)	0.01 (0.00–0.13)
Lean et al.	2014	RADT (molecular technique)	Throat culture	Group A streptococcal pharyngitis	7	0.92 (0.89–0.95)	0.99 (0.97–0.99)		
Lee, Yun.	2019	Ultrasound	X-ray	Elbow fracture	10	0.96 (0.88–0.99)	0.89 (0.82–0.94)		
Pereda et al.	2015	Ultrasound	Chest X-ray	Pneumonia	8	0.96 (0.94–0.97)	0.93 (0.90–0.96)	13.7 (6.4–36.8)	0.04 (0.03–0.12)
Yoon et al.	2017	MR enterography	Histopathologic test findings	Active inflammation with known or suspected IBD	18	0.83 (0.75–0.89)	0.93 (0.90–0.95)		
Zhao et al.	2019	FeNO	Guideline criteria	Asthma	20	0.57 (0.47–0.67)	0.61 (0.46–0.75)		

CRP C reactive protein, *MR* magnetic resonance, *IBD* inflammatory bowel disease, *RADT* rapid antigen detection test, *RSV* respiratory syncytial virus, 95% CI = 95% confidence interval toms. To assure that no newborn with the disease is missed, we understand that the test will over-identify newborns with false positives (FP). Further testing is needed to confirm an inborn error of metabolism in those with a positive test. While a test's sensitivity is critical for screening tests, it is also important that specificity is not too low; otherwise, the rate of false-positive results will be high.

In newborn screening for phenylketonuria (PKU), we accept a false-positive rate higher than we would like to avoid missing a case of PKU. Most screening tests are offered in two stages. The first testing stage is less expensive, invasive, and inaccurate, leading to false positives. The second stage of testing is more expensive and more invasive and has greater sensitivity and specificity. Follow-up testing will have high specificity and a low false-positive rate and can be used on the positive initial screening patients.

The World Health Organization (WHO) has identified other considerations for good screening tests. These are summarized in Box 1.2.

Box 1.2 WHO Screening Guidelines

1. The health problem must be important and affect a substantial number of people.
2. A recognizable asymptomatic or early mildly symptomatic disease detection can be effectively treated.
3. The health condition test must have a high level of accuracy, and the patient must accept the screening test.
4. Screening, diagnosis, and treatment must be economically balanced within the disease's societal burden (Wilson and Jungner 1968).

Screening tests should be ordered (1) if the test will detect the condition earlier than it would have been detected without screening and (2) if the early treatment will make a significant difference in the outcome. The screening test does not necessarily need to be inexpensive, but it should be cost-effective compared to society's potential symptomatic disease cost. A screening test should not be ordered if the detection of the condition does not improve health outcomes. A screening test must be highly sensitive (detecting a disease that is present). Ideally, the test should also have high specificity. However, few screening tests have both high sensitivity and specificity. Therefore, a screening test result always requires confirmation with another test to determine if a condition is truly present.

1.4.2 Diagnosis and Laboratory Tests

Clinicians frequently use laboratory and other clinical tests to help make a diagnosis. While sensitivity and specificity provide important information to evaluate a diagnostic test, it does not provide information regarding the probability of whether a child has or does not have a disease. Before testing, the clinician must consider the prevalence of the disease in the community and the child's history and physical exam findings, which have raised the clinician's suspicion that a disease may be present. Since diagnostic tests are not perfect and run the risk of both false-positive and false-negative results, the clinician must consider the probability of disease before the test is conducted (pretest probability) and how much a positive test will raise that level of certainty (post-test probability).

The prevalence of the disease in the community is the proportion of people in the community who have the condition and can be calculated as the number of cases divided by the total number of people in the population. Epidemiological studies provide estimates of disease prevalence in different populations. The clinician may not know the true prevalence of the disease in the population. However, the clinician has an index of suspicion about the probability of disease, which leads him/her to order the test. Here, this index of suspicion can be considered as an estimate of pretest probability. For example, the pretest probability that a child who went hiking with his family in a state with endemic Lyme disease has Lyme disease is higher than that of a similar child who went hiking but presents with knee swelling and a history of a tick bite. The presence of a bulls-eye lesion would further increase the pretest probability. The test result provides additional information to inform the clinician's diagnostic process (post-test probability). A positive test result will increase the probability, whereas a negative test result will decrease probability levels.

When the purpose of ordering a test is to inform the diagnosis of a condition, the test must be highly specific so that false-positive test results are minimized, and a positive test result can help to rule in the presence of a disease. If the test has low specificity, many patients who do not have the condition will have a false-positive test. When a test is highly specific, the clinician can have a high level of confidence that someone who tests positive for the condition will have the disease, illustrated by the mnemonic **SpPin**. When a test has high **Sp**ecificity, a **P**ositive test helps to rule **in** the diagnosis (Sackett et al. 2000).

The following example illustrates how a new test's diagnostic test properties would be determined in the children's population. In this example, the test performance evaluated is a COVID rapid test assessed by a saliva sample, and the reference standard is PCR antigen testing obtained by the nasopharyngeal swab. A sample of 1500 children with cough and fever are evaluated with both tests; using the reference standard, 195 children have a positive antigen test result, and 1305 children have a negative antigen test result. The prevalence of COVID in this sample determined by the reference standard is 13%. Of the 195 children with a positive antigen test result, 159 have a positive COVID rapid test result (TP), and 36 have a negative test result (FN). Of the 1305 children with a negative antigen test, 3 have a positive COVID rapid test result (FP), and 1302 have a negative test result (TN). A contingency table would be completed to calculate the sensitivity and specificity of the COVID rapid test (illustrated in Table 1.4).

Using data from the contingency table, the rapid test's sensitivity and specificity are 81.5% and 99.8%, respectively, compared to the PCR nasopharyngeal swab. While this is purely an example, a few points about diagnostic tests' utility should be made. First, while PCR antigen testing obtained by nasopharyngeal swab is used here as the reference standard, the test is imperfect, and results vary based on sampling quality (Watson et al. 2020). Based on the test performance presented here, the COVID rapid test would not be a good screening test because the number of false negatives is high. However, the test's specificity is very high, illustrating that a positive test result would help confirm the presence of COVID in a child presenting with symptoms. The clinician would need to interpret a negative test result with caution. A single negative test might not be informative for clinical decision-making, particularly if the child presented with symptoms suggestive of COVID-19. There was a history of exposure in the family or at school. The additional information obtained from positive and negative likelihood ratios will be presented later in this chapter.

1.4.3 Establishment of Test Value Cutoffs

A diagnostic test aims to be accurate as possible, but the interpretation of test results must always

Table 1.4 Contingency table illustration of test sensitivity and specificity: COVID antigen test

	COVID positive	COVID negative
Tests positive with COVID rapid test	True positive (TP) 159	False positive (FP) 3
Tests negative with COVID rapid test	False negative (FN) 36	True negative (TN) 1302
	Sensitivity = TP/TP + FN = 159/(159 + 36) = 159/195 = 81.5%	Specificity = TN/TN + FP = 1302/(1302 + 3) = 1302/1305 = 99.8%

be balanced with other test results (Borysiak et al., 2016).

A given test's normal range reflecting the 95% confidence interval will affect the test's sensitivity (Borysiak et al., 2016). The clinical cutoff for a test depends on the clinical use of the particular test. For example, suppose the test is to diagnose the presence of a deadly disease. In that case, the clinical cutoff must have a high specificity to prevent errors in diagnosing a deadly condition. In contrast, life-threatening but treatable diseases require a high sensitivity to ensure that even mild forms of the disease can be recognized and treated (Borysiak et al., 2016). If the cutoff for a disease is too low, the clinician will identify too many children who do not have the disease; if the cutoff is too high, children who have milder symptoms but would benefit from treatment will be missed. In the diagnostic process, some tests have thresholds to aid the clinician with test interpretation.

In some cases, the primary test's diagnostic accuracy can be improved if another test is added. The mono spot or heterophile antibody test for infectious mononucleosis is a good example. Although this test has good test accuracy (sensitivity 81–95%; specificity 98–100%) for people over 10 years of age, it has low sensitivity (<50%) in younger children (Marshall-Andon and Heinz 2017). In children under 4, the test's sensitivity decreases to between 10% and 50%, making it a far less accurate test (Marshall-Andon and Heinz 2017). Further, heterophile antibodies remain positive for 1 year, so a positive result may not be the reason for the current presentation (Marshall-Andon and Heinz 2017).

A test specificity can be improved when two or more tests are used. For example, when a positive heterophile antibody test for mononucleosis is augmented with a complete blood count with differential, the sensitivity increases. As the proportion of atypical lymphocytes increases, test specificity increases. A child with symptoms suggestive of infectious mononucleosis and a positive heterophile antibody test has ≥10% atypical lymphocytes, with a sensitivity of 75% and a specificity of 92%. As the atypical lymphocytes increase to ≥25% atypical lym-

phocytes, the sensitivity changes to 56% and the specificity changes to 98%. As the atypical lymphocytes count increases to ≥40%, the specificity of a test increases to 100%, while the sensitivity decreases to 25% (Ebell 2004). Note that as test specificity increases, sensitivity decreases. The two case studies below are the diagnostic testing and the symptoms of infectious mononucleosis.

1.4.4 Real-Life Examples

A 12-year-old child presents to an urgent care center with a 7-day fever history and generalized fatigue. The physical exam is positive for tonsillopharyngitis, bilateral cervical adenopathy, and an enlarged spleen 2 cm below the left costal margin. The clinician suspects infectious mononucleosis and orders a heterophil antibody test, and the test result is positive. Based on the test's sensitivity and specificity in this age group and the clinical presentation, the clinician confirms the diagnosis of infectious mononucleosis with the family.

In contrast, a 2-year-old presents a fever of 102° for 6 days and complains of a sore throat. Positive physical exam findings include cervical adenopathy and an enlarged spleen 2 cm below the left costal margin. The heterophile antibody test is negative, and a complete blood count with differential shows 12% atypical lymphocytes. To confirm a diagnosis of infectious mononucleosis, the clinician would need to do further EBV antibody testing.

Cases 1 and 2 illustrate that the interpretation of the heterophile antibody test would differ in two children with a similar presentation of symptoms but different ages. With a high degree of certainty, the clinician could tell the family of the 12-year-old that the child has infectious mononucleosis based on a positive test. However, a positive heterophile antibody test for the younger child was insufficient, and additional testing was needed because of poor test sensitivity. The proportion of atypical lymphocytes was in a range of suspicion but did not confirm the diagnosis requiring further testing.

Test sensitivity and specificity should not be misinterpreted as the probability of disease presence. While sensitivity and specificity provide important information to evaluate diagnostic test performance, it does not provide probability information about whether a child does or does not have a disease. Test results help to increase or decrease the level of diagnostic certainty. A clinician has a level of suspicion based on a child's history, symptoms and physical exam findings, and community prevalence of the disease, which prompts him/her to order a diagnostic test. This is considered a pretest probability. A positive test result will increase suspicion of the disease's presence, whereas a negative test result will decrease suspicion. This change in the level of suspicion is considered a post-test probability. The post-test probability increases or decreases based on the test's sensitivity and specificity, determining likelihood ratios.

1.5 How Will a Test Perform in a Patient Population?

A diagnostic test aims to either increase or decrease the level of certainty that a disease is present. Prevalence of disease in the community and patient history, signs, and symptoms inform the clinician's certainty level before ordering a diagnostic test. These factors constitute a pretest probability: how a positive test result will increase the certainty of a disease or a negative test will decrease the level of certainty of disease depending on the test's specific performance characteristics. This section will discuss positive and negative predictive values and positive and negative likelihood ratios and their specific utilities to the clinician.

1.5.1 Positive and Negative Predictive Values

Sensitivity and specificity focus on the probability of findings given the presence or absence of disease. Predictive values focus on the probability of disease given a positive or negative test result. A positive predictive value (PPV) is the probability that the patient has the disease if the test result is positive. A negative predictive value (NPV) is the probability that the patient does not have the disease if the test result is negative. Of note, both PPV and NPV estimations are dependent on the prevalence of the disease in the sample from which the accuracy of the test was studied.

PPV is calculated as the number of true positives. These persons have disease confirmed by the reference standard and a positive test result, divided by all persons with a positive test result (true positive + false positive). NPV is calculated as the number of true negatives, persons who do not have the disease, and a negative test result, divided by all persons with a negative test result (true negative + false negative).

To illustrate these concepts, let's estimate the PPV and NPV using data presented in Table 1.4, where a new rapid COVID test was compared to COVID antigen testing. The sample comprised 1500 children from a low-income community who were hard hit by the virus who presented to emergency rooms with COVID symptoms and tested with both the new and reference standard tests. In 159 children, both tests were positive (TP), and three children had a positive rapid test but a negative antigen test (FP). The prevalence of COVID-19 in this sample of 1500 children was 10.6%, and the PPV was 98.1%.

$$PPV = TP/(TP + FP)$$
$$PPV = 159/(159 + 3)$$
$$PPV = 159/162$$
$$PPV = 98.1\%$$

In this sample, 1302 children had a negative result for both the rapid and antigen tests (TN), and 36 children had a positive antigen test but had a negative rapid test result (FN). The NPV in this sample was 97.3%

$$NPV = TN/(TN + FN)$$
$$NPV = 1302/(1302 + 36)$$
$$NPV = 1302/1338$$
$$NPV = 97.3\%$$

In this example, both the PPV and NPV are very high. Using these estimates would suggest that the probability that the patient has the disease if the test result is positive is 98.1%. The probability that the patient does not have the disease is 97.3% if the test result is negative. However, the prevalence of COVID in the sample on which this study was based was much higher than in the community where the clinician practices. In the clinician's community, the disease prevalence was 0.5% for children. Community prevalence can often differ from the prevalence in which a new test is evaluated.

Although a test's sensitivity and specificity do not change with disease prevalence, a test's positive and negative predictive value is altered by a population's prevalence. The prevalence of a condition may also vary by age group. The following provides a few examples of age-related differences.

1.5.2 Real-Life Examples

1. While all 2-year-old children are less than 3½ feet tall, a 15-year-old adolescent who is 3½ feet tall needs to be evaluated for short stature and pituitary dysfunction.
2. Hemoglobin of 9.0 g/dl is normal for a 1-month-old infant but would need a workup for iron deficiency anemia in adolescents.
3. An elevated alkaline phosphatase level is normal in a growing child, but an elevated alkaline phosphatase level in an 18-year-old female would require further diagnostic evaluation.

The prevalence of disease may also be affected by seasonal fluctuation. For example, strep pharyngitis prevalence among children is much higher in June than in early spring. For these reasons, PPV and NPV have less diagnostic utility unless the clinician is sure that the prevalence of the disease in the study sample is similar to the local community or age group prevalence.

Key Learning about Sensitivity and Specificity

- The higher the sensitivity and specificity, the more useful the test.
- When a test is highly specific, the clinician can have a high level of confidence that someone who tests positive for the condition will have the disease, illustrated by the mnemonic **SpPin**. When a test has high **Sp**ecificity, a **P**ositive test helps to rule **in** the diagnosis.
- A test with poor specificity will result in a patient having a positive test result (FP) when he/she is, in fact, healthy. A test with high specificity will have a low false-positive rate. **SnNout**. When a test has high **Sen**sitivity, a **N**egative test helps to rule **out** the disease.
- The prevalence of a disease may be affected by seasonal variations. It is important to consider this when ordering a laboratory test.

1.5.3 Positive and Negative Likelihood Ratios

Unlike positive and negative predictive values, likelihood ratios are not dependent on either disease prevalence of the sample on which the test's sensitivity and specificity were based or community prevalence of the disease. Likelihood ratios can inform the clinician of the magnitude of change that a positive or negative test result has on post-test probability. Table 1.5 presents the formulas for calculating likelihood ratios.

Positive likelihood ratio: A positive or negative lab result must be put into the context of the possible diagnosis for which the test is performed to

Table 1.5 Formulas for estimating positive and negative likelihood ratios

Test characteristic	Formula
Positive likelihood ratio	Sensitivity/(1 − Specificity)
Negative likelihood ratio	(1 − Sensitivity)/Specificity

determine the result's accuracy (Fierz and Bossuyt 2020). A positive likelihood ratio (LR+) provides an answer to the question: "how many times more likely is it that a positive test result will occur in children with the disorder compared to those without the disorder?" (Akobeng 2006). It can be said the LR is the percentage of sick children who have the disease versus the percentage of people who are well who have a positive test result. One of the advantages of LR is that the clinician can determine the pretest probability of the child having the disease based on demographic, prevalence, and individual child considerations.

Positive likelihood ratios are calculated as sensitivity/1 − specificity). For example, Pereda et al. (2015) reported that ultrasound sensitivity and specificity to diagnose pneumonia in symptomatic children are 96% and 93%, respectively.

A test with LR+ greater than 10 means that the test is a good test to rule in the disease. A test with LR− less than 0.1 means it is a good test to rule out a disease. LR+ and LR− values of this magnitude will generate significantly large and conclusive changes from pretest to post-test probability. If the LR+ is greater than 10 or the LR− is less than 0.01, there is a good chance that the test results will be conclusive. Smaller LR values mean that the test will not improve post-test probability significantly and, therefore, will not help improve clinician certainty regarding whether a disease is present.

1.5.3.1 Fagan's Nomogram

A practical way for the clinician to utilize likelihood ratios estimated from the sensitivity and specificity of a test to improve diagnostic certainty is to plot the values using Fagan's nomogram (Caraguel and Vanderstichel 2013). Fagan's nomogram is based on Bayes' theorem, which describes the probability of an event (in this case, a diagnosis) based on prior knowledge of conditions (pretest probability and positive or negative test result) that might be related to the event. Figure 1.2 illustrates Fagan's nomogram. Pretest probability is plotted (scale on the left side of nomogram) using either community prevalence of the condition or the clinician's estimation of clinical certainty based on the child's clinical

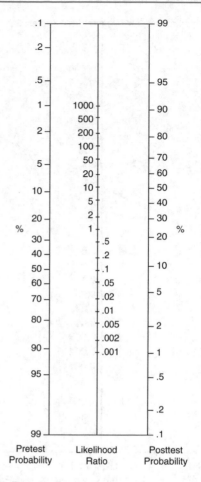

Fig. 1.2 Fagan's nomogram

presentation and physical examination finding. If the child's test result is positive, LR+ is plotted on the nomogram; if the test result is negative, LR− is plotted (middle scale of nomogram). Connecting pretest probability and likelihood ratio using a straight line will provide an estimate of post-test probability based on the test result.

In the clinical setting, the LR can interpret the results of a wide range of clinical tests (Crewe and Rowe 2011). An online calculator to plot Fagan's nomogram using test characteristics can be found at http://araw.mede.uic.edu/cgi-bin/test-calc.pl

Using the online calculator estimates the post-test probability of a positive ultrasound to diagnose pneumonia in case 3. Pretest probability was 25%, and LR+ is 13.7 and LR− is 0.04. Figure 1.3 illustrates the change from pretest

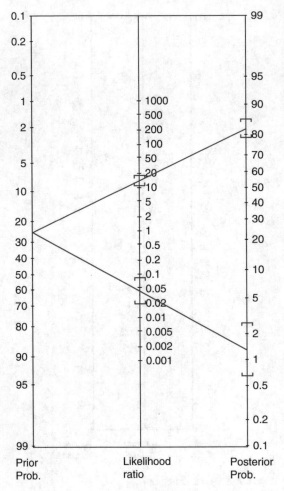

Fig. 1.3 Using Fagan's nomogram to ascertain the post-test probability

Table 1.6 Magnitude of LR effect on post-test probability (McGee S, 2002)

Positive likelihood values	Negative likelihood values
LR+ of 2 increases the post-test probability by 15%	LR− of 0.5 decreases post-test probability by 15%
LR+ of 5 increases the post-test probability by 30%	LR− of 0.2 decreases post-test probability by 30%
LR+ of 10 increases the post-test probability by 45%	LR− of 0.1 decreases post-test probability by 45%

exam. Based on the child's history and exam findings, the clinician suspects community-acquired pneumonia and estimates the pretest probability to be 25%. The ultrasound is positive. How will a positive test improve the clinician's level of certainty?

Using sensitivity and specificity, LR+ can be estimated.

$$LR+ = sensitivity/(1 - specificity)$$
$$LR+ = 0.96/(1 - 0.93)$$
$$LR+ = 0.96/0.07$$
$$LR+ = 13.7$$

Considering the same child, how will a negative ultrasound test result help the clinician make the diagnosis? The negative likelihood ratio (LR−) can be estimated using the test's sensitivity and specificity.

$$LR- = (1 - sensitivity)/specificity$$
$$LR- = (1 - 0.96)/0.93$$
$$LR- = 0.04/0.93$$
$$LR- = 0.04$$

Based on likelihood ratios, the increase or decrease in post-test probability can be estimated. The higher the LR+, the more the LR increases the post-test probability. In the example, the pre-test probability was 25%; therefore, a positive test with an LR+ of 13.7 will increase the post-test probability to 70%. Conversely, an LR− would decrease the post-test probability to 0%. Table 1.6 demonstrates how LR affects post-test probability.

probability to post-test probability using Fagan's nomogram. Post-test probability was increased to approximately 82% following a positive ultrasound result (illustrated by the blue line) and decreased to 1.5% following a negative ultrasound result (illustrated by the red line).

1.5.4 Real-Life Example

An 8-year-old child presents to the emergency room with fever and cough for the past 2 days and has diminished breath sounds on physical

1.5.5 Receiver Operating Characteristic (ROC) Curve

A receiver operating characteristic (ROC) curve represents the plot of the true positive rate against the false-positive rate within different cut points for a diagnostic test. ROC curves are derived from clinical prediction rules. The shape of ROC is calculated by knowing the LRs at various spots along the ROC curve (Fierz and Bossuyt 2020). The AUC displays the probability that a test will correctly identify a person with the disease with greater accuracy than a person without the disease. A test with higher AUC has higher likelihood ratios and is, therefore, more cost-effective and discriminatory. AUC can be categorized to describe test performance: AUC between 0.9 and 1.0 is very good; 0.8 and 0.89 is good; 0.7 and 0.79 is fair, 0.6 and 0.69 is poor. A test with AUC between 0.5 and 0.59 is not discriminatory and should not be used. The graph depicted in Fig. 1.4 illustrates three ROC curve plots. The red curve illustrates a test with good test performance (AUC 0.85); the black curve illustrates a test with fair test performance (AUC 0.70); and the orange line illustrates 0.5 AUC.

1.5.6 Real-Life Example: Case 1

The following two case studies will illustrate how to use the concepts reviewed in this section.

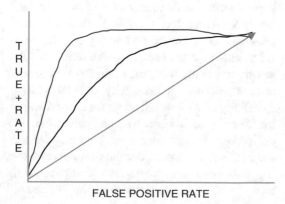

Fig. 1.4 Test performance illustrated by receiver operating characteristic curves

In early spring, a 7-year-old child presents with a sore throat, acute onset of fever (103 °F), and one episode of vomiting. You know that the incidence of strep is higher at this time of year. The family reports a recent outbreak of strep throat at their child's school. The physical exam is remarkable for erythematous, hypertrophied tonsils, and palatal petechiae.

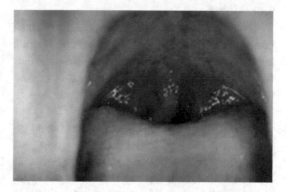

Your practice site now offers a point-of-care (POC) polymerase chain reaction (PCR) Roche cobas® Liat® Strep A test as well as the traditional rapid antigen detection test (RADT) with a confirmatory backup culture for negative tests. As a clinician, you consider the child's age, clinical history, and assessment and are sure the examiner's technique for acquiring the sample is meticulous. The patient's insurance will cover both approaches. What things should you consider?

Your pretest clinical suspicion of strep is high. Given the time of year and recent outbreaks of strep throat, the disease's prevalence is higher than your usual. You review the recent data of sensitivity and specificity. In two meta-analyses, RADT testing had a sensitivity of 86% (79–92%) and 87% (84–89%) and a specificity of 92% (88–95%) and 96% (95–97%), respectively (Stewart et al. 2014; Lean et al. 2014). If a backup culture was performed, the sensitivity was 71.8%, and the specificity was 100% (Rao et al. 2019). The POC PCR Roche cobas Liat® Strep A test had a sensitivity of 95.5% and a specificity of 99.3% (Rao et al. 2019).

Based on the child's presenting symptoms, history of a recent outbreak of strep throat at school, and time of year, you estimate the pretest probability at 40%. The RADT, because of its poorer sensitivity, requires a backup test for confirmation. The POC PCR Roche cobas Liat® Strep A test has very high sensitivity and excellent specificity. For these reasons, you will plan to apply the mnemonic of SpPin. If the POC PCR Roche cobas Liat® Strep A test is positive, how much will the test result increase post-test probability?

To answer this question, you need to calculate the LR+ and LR− using either the formulas or an online calculator such as the one found here: http://araw.mede.uic.edu/cgi-bin/testcalc.pl. The LR+ is 136 and the LR− is 0.05. A positive test result will increase post-test probability from 40% to 99%, and a negative test result will decrease post-test probability from 40% to approximately 3.5%. You can see that a backup culture is unnecessary with this test. The test has other distinct advantages since there will be fewer unnecessary antibiotic prescriptions.

While strep throat is self-limiting, a clinician treats strep throat to prevent rheumatic fever. A test with high specificity has few false positives. Therefore, there is less overprescribing with antibiotics.

1.5.7 Real-Life Example

A clinician works at an inner-city clinic where the prevalence of chlamydia among sexually active adolescent females is 11%. The clinician has some difficulty in getting adolescents back for treatment after a positive chlamydia nucleic acid amplification. Chlamydia trachomatis is the most common sexually transmitted disease globally, with possible adverse outcomes of infertility and pelvic inflammatory disease. Regular screening for chlamydia in sexually active women under the age of 25 is recommended due to the high prevalence of the disease.

A rapid point-of-care chlamydia test has a sensitivity of 82% and a specificity of 99% (Quidel 2020). You consider its use as a first-line test for your patients and then using chlamydia nucleic acid amplification test as a backup. What do you need to consider using a rapid point-of-care chlamydia test with a backup nucleic amplification test? Understanding the prevalence, sensitivity, and specificity is the first step. The prevalence of the disease is 11% in your population. The test's sensitivity is fair (82%), but the test specificity is excellent (99%). This means that there will be very few false-positive results. Using this test's reported sensitivity and specificity and a prevalence of 11%, The LR+ is 82, and the LR− is 0.18.

We know that a positive LR greater than ten and a negative LR less than 0.1 will generate significantly large and conclusive changes from pretest to post-test probability. The positive LR of 82 is significant and will increase the pretest probability of disease from 11% before conducting the test to approximately 91% and identifying adolescents who need treatment. The point-of-care result is quickly obtained, enabling early treatment and avoiding complications from untreated infections due to lack of follow-up. However, because the test has only fair sensitivity, there will be false negatives for those who have chlamydia if you use this test for screening adolescents for the presence of chlamydia.

The NAAT test has a much higher sensitivity (99%), and therefore the recommendations for a NAAT test as a first-line screening test make sense (American Academy of Pediatrics [AAP] 2018; Workowski et al. 2021). However, one must also consider the probability of follow-up for treatment. For example, if the return to follow-up were only 65%, then using a rapid point-of-care test with a sensitivity of 82% and a specificity of 99% would allow for cost-effective treatment of adolescents who had chlamydia. To decide on the right course for your population, the clinician must consider the prevalence, testing cost, treatment costs, and complications, along with test characteristics, as discussed above.

Key Learning about Likelihood Ratios

- The best way to use likelihood ratios estimated from the sensitivity and specificity of a test to improve diagnostic certainty is to plot the values using Fagan's nomogram.
- It is important to consider the pretest diagnostic probability when ordering a diagnostic laboratory test.
- The higher the LR+, the more the LR increases the post-test probability.
- A positive LR greater than 10 and a negative LR less than 0.1 will generate significantly large and conclusive changes from pretest to post-test probability.

1.6 Diagnostic Reasoning

Missed diagnosis is the most common, expensive, and harmful form than any other types of error. According to the 2015 Institute of Medicine report, it makes up to 20% of all diagnostic errors (Balogh et al. 2015). There are several types of diagnostic error types. Cognitive error is a broad category that includes confirmation bias, anchoring bias, anchoring bias, and availability bias. Confirmation bias is not considering evidence that might change your initial diagnostic impression. In contrast, anchoring bias is when the clinician fixates on a certain feature of the clinical presentation rather than considering other clinical information, which would lead to a different diagnosis. Availability bias is sticking with the first likely diagnosis rather than considering other possible causes. Instead of a pure knowledge deficit, the cognitive error tends to be more related to how information is processed when making the clinical diagnostic decision. Clinicians must recognize potential cognitive biases to avoid cognitive errors. Taken time out to think about the clinical presentation and the possible diagnoses is a way of avoiding cognitive diagnostic errors. It is estimated that 80% of

diagnoses can be made by history and another 5–10% comes after the physical exam. Diagnostic stewardship points to the need to consider pretest probability before ordering a diagnostic lab test (Morjaria and Chapin 2020).

1.6.1 Diagnostic Stewardship

The tendency to overutilize diagnostic tests has been well documented in multiple studies, with an estimate that one out of five lab tests is unnecessary (Zhi et al. 2013). The goal of diagnostic stewardship is to use the right test for the right patient at the right time to generate the right diagnosis (Morjaria and Chapin 2020). The number, type, complexity, and diversity of clinical diagnostic laboratory tests have grown enormously over the past 50 years. While newer tests have improved the clinician's ability to diagnose a wide variety of illnesses earlier, the reality of the overutilization of lab tests has increased healthcare costs. The decision to order a test should be guided by careful clinical evaluation, recognition of a clinical syndrome, and estimation of the pretest likelihood of the condition for which the test is obtained (Messacar et al. 2017). Diagnostic stewardship in a patient who likely has an infectious disease means that the clinician will use an appropriate diagnostic laboratory test to guide treatment to avoid antimicrobial resistance and optimize patient outcomes (Patel and Fang 2018). Clinicians often order common tests for patients without symptoms specific to the disease process. Positive tests may result in unnecessary therapy as the results may represent false-positive findings or result from colonization rather than true infection.

The first molecular tests for identifying infectious disease agents were first available 27 years ago, but there has been a marked increase in these tests (Graf and Pancholi 2020). Readily available molecular panels may worsen diagnostic mistakes, particularly when there is a low pretest likelihood of disease (Baird 2019). Newer and more accurate tests have led to a greater ability to diagnose, but not with absolute certainty

(Bindraban et al. 2018). Data suggest that the actual rate of inappropriate laboratory tests ranges between 23% and 67% (Lippi et al. 2015). The plethora of laboratory tests and the cost associated with those tests are significant factors in rising healthcare costs (Vegting et al. 2012). Overutilization of lab tests and the resultant false-positive and false-negative test results cause further testing and imaging that may lead to invasive procedures causing patient harm (Harb et al. 2019) and excessive medical costs (Iams et al. 2016). Diagnostic excess leads to excessive laboratory testing without much additional information (Kazmierczak 1999).

The patient's desire for laboratory tests can also lead the clinician to over-order tests; findings of a recent review demonstrated that 53% of the time, the clinician's order for a diagnostic test was influenced by patients (The ABIM Foundation 2014). Evidence-based care discourages clinician's ordering unindicated diagnostic tests. Over-testing can cause additional costs and may lead to incidental findings that lead to further testing without elucidating the diagnosis. Thus, overordering is not without risks and may lead to additional stress on guardians and children. Clinicians need to utilize shared decision-making and make sure families understand why their requested tests are not needed and must address their concerns and their values. While these kinds of conversations can be time-consuming, they can strengthen relationships between the clinician and the patient (Rolfe and Burton 2013).

The development of new and improved old diagnostic laboratory tests has challenged clinicians' ability to interpret the tests correctly (Kazmierczak 1999). Incorrectly choosing or misinterpreting diagnostic test results is another reason for diagnostic medical errors (Balogh et al. 2015). While there has been considerable focus on reducing procedure error, institutions and educational institutions have not devoted the same time and effort to reduce errors in diagnostic laboratory tests (Bindraban et al. 2018; Laposata 2018: Smith et al. 2014). Studies have shown that the time allotted for education regarding clinical diagnostic testing in medical schools is limited (Smith et al. 2014). No study has examined the amount of time allocated to clinical diagnostic testing in either nurse practitioner or physician assistant education. Clinicians are challenged as they choose between various diagnostic laboratory tests to help them make the best diagnostic and therapeutic decisions. It is estimated that 70–80% of a child's medical records is composed of laboratory data (Hallworth 2011).

Defensive medicine is another reason for overordering tests. Clinicians sometimes order tests that are not indicated to decrease the exposure to malpractice liability and make sure that they do not miss something. A recent review of the medical malpractice problem showed that 34% of physicians had been sued during the length of their careers. The rate of malpractice increases as the amount of time the clinician has been practicing (American Medical Association 2020). The most current data about nurse practitioners being named primary defendants is estimated at a 1.1% rate (American Academy of Nurse Practitioners [AANP] 2020). While it is true that clinicians need to rule out worse-case scenarios (Buppert 2018), this should be done based on the history and the assessment along with the prevalence of the disease. The practice of defensive medicine is resulting in increased healthcare spending (Kessler 2011). Estimation is that our present liability systems are about $56 billion annually, with approximately 80% of the cost related to defensive medicine (Mello et al. 2010). The perception of liability risk is a major driver of defensive medicine. Ensuring that families are happy with their care and that clinicians do not miss something is a source of increased healthcare costs.

1.6.2 Underordering Diagnostic Laboratory Tests

Clinical guidelines are constantly changing. It is critical for the clinician to track the current screening guidelines from the AAP, Centers for Disease Control (CDC), US Preventive Services Task Force (USPSTF), and specialty organizations. HIV screening in adolescents is an example of an underutilized test in primary care. An estimated 14% of Americans who have HIV do not know they are infected with the virus (CDC 2015). The 2017 HIV Surveillance Report indicated that starting at age 15, there was a significant increase in HIV diagnoses (CDC, 2017). There remain significant gaps in testing with missed opportunities for HIV testing during routine healthcare encounters (Dailey et al. 2017). Keeping up with the latest guidelines can be daunting. Still, the clinician can receive help by utilizing Choosing Wisely and PubMed and requesting email updates from MMWR, FDA, and other specialty organizations (Baird 2019).

The goal of avoiding the under- and overutilization of tests has been tried by educational plans (Kobewska et al. 2015), use of diagnostic management teams (Verna et al. 2019), use of interdisciplinary teams (Seegmiller et al. 2013), utilizing diagnostic experts (Laposata 2018), use of a clinical laboratory consult (Burke 2003), use of clinical guidelines (Iams et al. 2016), and by clinical decision support with computer-generated alerts (Jackups et al. 2017). The sustainability of these interventions over time has rarely been studied (Bindraban et al. 2018). While the intervention is reported as successful, the target for reducing the overuse of the test was not preset before the intervention. Publication bias is certainly a factor as interventions that do not show a positive effect are rarely published. Therefore, it is nearly impossible to determine what kind of intervention is the most effective in changing inappropriate test utilization (Bindraban et al. 2018).

Healthcare providers are poorly trained regarding the cost of the laboratory tests they order, and patients are not aware of the test costs until they receive the bill. Employers have developed several programs to reduce the cost of laboratory tests, including using only certain labs, passing on the test's cost to the employee by increasing the patient out-of-pocket spending, and reducing insurer spending by negotiating contracts with laboratories. One study showed that the use of reference pricing for laboratory tests reduced spending by $4.08 million over 3 years for one company (Robinson et al. 2016). Some Internet sites provide information to help clinicians see the healthcare costs of lab tests. Healthcare Bluebook is easy to use and reports cost results from five labs near your zip code (https://www.healthcarebluebook.com/ui/consumerfront). Clear health costs (https://clearhealthcosts.com) is another site to determine healthcare procedure costs near your zip code. These sites are examples of how you learn about healthcare costs before ordering tests. The American College of Radiology has developed appropriateness criteria to help clinicians make effective decisions about imaging. It should be remembered that sometimes an expensive test may be the most appropriate option to deliver high-value care when the test facilitates an accurate and fast diagnosis leading to prompt treatment.

There are several initiatives to promote the better use of lab tests. High-value care is a priority for clinicians. Provision of unnecessary services, inefficient delivery, and missed prevention opportunities lead to inefficient health care. The American College of Physicians has taken on the high-value care initiative to improve the use of clinical practice guidelines, education about high-value care by training videos and case studies, and education for patients regarding high-value care. Their website has several links to internal medicine cases that will teach you more about this concept. The Choosing Wisely campaign was also developed to avoid over- and underutilizing diagnostic tests; several national organizations have posted their guidelines. A phone application is also available. The American College of Physicians and the American Board of Internal Medicine launched the Choosing Wisely Campaign (Cassel and Guest 2012).

Key Learning about Ordering Diagnostic Laboratory Tests

- Instead of a pure knowledge deficit, the cognitive error tends to be more related to how information is processed when making the clinical diagnostic decision. Clinicians must recognize potential cognitive biases to avoid cognitive errors. Overordering and underordering laboratory tests is a reason for misdiagnosis.
- Diagnostic stewardship encourages clinicians to understand the pretest probability of the disease before ordering a test. The clinician can then order the right test for the right person at the right time.
- Several websites can help you determine the best screening and diagnostic lab tests. These include the Choosing Wisely Campaign, AAP, CDC, US Preventive Services Task Force (USPSTF), and specialty organizations.
- Cost of diagnostic laboratory tests can be determined by zip code using Healthcare Bluebook or Clear Health Costs.

Questions

Questions 1–7 apply to the following scenario: 1500 children are tested for strep tonsillitis using a rapid strep test (RST). Of these, 27 have a positive RST. A gold standard backup throat culture was also performed on all children. Of those who have a negative RST result, 1468 also have a negative throat culture. Of those with a positive RST, 20 have a positive throat culture.

1. Using these data, complete the contingency table below

2. What is the prevalence of strep tonsillitis in this population?
3. What is the sensitivity of the RST test?
4. What is the specificity of the RST test?
5. What is the positive likelihood ratio (LR+)?
6. What is the negative likelihood ratio (LR−)?
7. Using the prevalence of strep tonsillitis in this sample as the pretest probability and Fagan's nomogram, what is the post-test probability of strep tonsillitis if the RST test is positive? What is the post-test probability of strep tonsillitis if the RST test is negative?

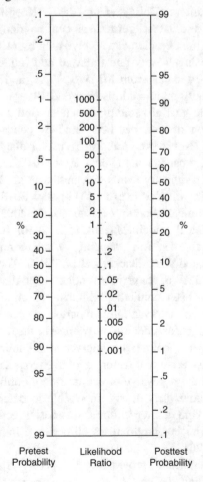

	Disease present (D+)	Disease absent (D−)	
Test positive (T+)	True positive (TP)a	False positive (FP)b	TP + FP(a + b)
Test negative (T-)	False negative (FN)c	True negative (TN)d	FN + TN(c + d)
	TP + FN(a + c)	FP + TN(b + d)	Total(a + b + c + d)

8. Procalcitonin (PCT), C-reactive protein (CRP), and white blood cell count (WBC) have all been proposed as tests to distinguish infants with bacterial infection from those without bacterial infection. All three tests were used in a group of 175 sick hospitalized infants; blood culture results (bacterial vs. non-bacterial) were the reference standard. Examine the ROC curves of the three tests.

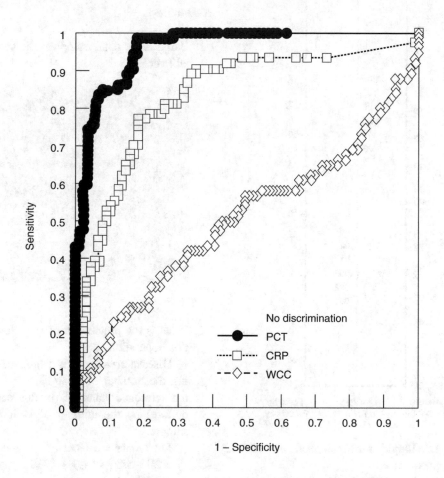

Which test had the best overall performance?

(a) PCT

(b) CRP

(c) WBC

9. The prevalence of a disease in your population is 10%. A patient presents to the clinic with symptoms suggestive of the disease, thereby raising your suspicion of disease to 25%. The lab test has an LR+ of 10 and an LR− of 0.5. The test result is positive. Using the nomogram below, what is the post-test probability that the disease is present, given that the patient has a positive test?

(a) 45%

(b) 60%

(c) 75%

(d) 90%

10. Which of the following statements most accurately describes likelihood ratios?

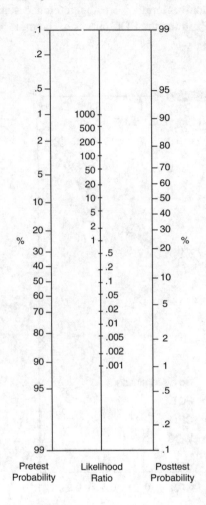

Pretest Probability — Likelihood Ratio — Posttest Probability

(a) Likelihood ratios depend on disease prevalence.
(b) A positive likelihood ratio greater than 3 means the test is useful.
(c) Likelihood ratios help clinicians decide how certain they can be about the presence of disease after conducting a diagnostic test.
(d) A negative likelihood ratio greater than 1 means the test is useful.

11. Which of the following statements best describes the utility of a receiver operator curve (ROC)?
    (a) The closer the curve comes to the 45-degree diagonal, the more accurate the test is.

(b) The area under the curve is a measure of overall test accuracy.
(c) An area under the curve (AUC) 0.77 can be interpreted as excellent test performance.

Rationale

1. Using these data, complete the contingency table below

		Target disorder (strep tonsillitis) by throat culture		
		Present	Absent	
Index test result	Positive RST	True positive (a) 20	False positive (b) 7	27
	Negative RST	False negative (c) 5	True negative (d) 1468	1473
		25 (a + c)	1475 (b + d)	1500

2. What is the prevalence of strep tonsillitis in this population?

Disease prevalence is calculated by dividing the number of strep cases validated by the reference standard (in this case, throat culture) by the number of children in the sample.

Prevalence = a + c/a + b + c + d
= 20 + 5/20 + 5+ 7 + 1468
= 25/1500
= 0.0166
= 1.7%

3. What is the sensitivity of the RST test?

Sensitivity reflects the number of true positives divided by the number of people who have the disease validated by the reference standard. The sensitivity of the RST test in this sample is 80%.

Sensitivity = a/a + b.
= 20/25
= 0.80
= 80%

4. What is the specificity of the RST test?

Specificity reflects the number of true negatives divided by the number of people without the disease validated by the reference standard. The specificity of the RST test in this sample is 99.5%.

Specificity = d/c + d.

= 1468/1475

= 0.9952

= 99.5%

5. What is the positive likelihood ratio (LR+)?

The positive likelihood ratio (LR+) reflects test sensitivity divided by 1-specificity. The LR+ of this test is 160.

LR+ = sensitivity/(1 − specificity)

= 0.80/(1-0.995)

= 0.80/0.005

= 160

6. What is the negative Likelihood ratio (LR−)?

The negative likelihood ratio (LR−) reflects 1-sensitivity/specificity. The LR− of this test is 0.20.

LR− = 1-sensitivity/specificity

= (1-0.80)/0.995

= 0.20/0.995

= 0.20

7. Using the prevalence of strep tonsillitis in this sample as the pretest probability and Fagan's nomogram, what is the post-test probability of strep tonsillitis if the RST test is positive? What is the post-test probability of strep tonsillitis if the RST test is negative?

Using Fagan's nomogram to determine the post-test probability of strep tonsillitis when the RST test is positive, plot disease prevalence 1.7% as prior or pretest probability, and the LR+ 160. The post-test probability has increased from 1.7% to approximately 73%.

Using Fagan's nomogram, determine post-test probability of strep tonsillitis if the RST test is negative, plot disease prevalence 1.7% as prior or pretest probability, and the LR− 0.20. The post-test probability has decreased from 1.7% to approximately 0.4%.

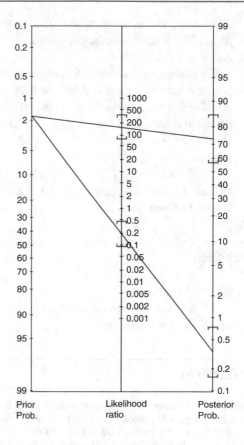

Procalcitonin (PCT), C-reactive protein (CRP), and white blood cell count (WBC) have all been proposed as tests to distinguish infants with bacterial infection from those without bacterial infection. All three tests were used in a group of 175 sick hospitalized infants; blood culture results (bacterial vs. non-bacterial) were the reference standard.

8. Answer: a

The ROC is a plot of a test's sensitivity against 1-specificity and illustrates overall test performance. A curve that hugs the outer edges of the graph represents a test with high sensitivity and specificity. Of the three ROC curves presented, the PCT had the best overall test performance.

9. Answer: c

The blue line in the figure below illustrates the estimation of the post-test probability using Fagan's nomogram. The pretest probability is 25%, and the LR+ is 10.

10. Answer: c

Likelihood ratios enable the estimation of post-test probability based on positive or negative test results. For the best clinical utility, LR+ should be 10 or higher, and LR− should be 0.1 or lower.

11. Answer: b

The ROC is a plot of a test's sensitivity against 1-specificity and illustrates a test's overall performance.

Websites

https://arupconsult.com/
https://ebm-tools.knowledgetranslation.net/
https://labtestsonline.org/

References

Akobeng A. Understanding diagnostic tests 2; likelihood ratios, pre-post-test probabilities and their use in clinical practice. Acta Paediatr. 2006;96(4):487–91.

American Academy of Nurse Practitioners. NP fact sheet. Accessed on Aug 1, 2020., https://www.aanp.org/about/all-about-nps/np-fact-sheet

American Academy of Pediatrics. Committee on Infectious Diseases. Red Book: Report of the Committee on Infectious Diseases. 31st ed. Elk Grove Village, IL: American Academy of Pediatrics; 2018.

American Medical Association. Medical Liability Reform NOW! The facts you need to know to address the broken medical liability system. 2020; Accessed Aug 1, 2020, from https://www.ama-assn.org/system/files/2020-05/mlr-now.pdf

Baeyens JP, Serrien B, Goossens M, Clijsen R. Questioning the "SPIN and SNOUT" rule in clinical testing. Arch Physiother. 2019; Mar 7;9:4 Retrieved on November 30, 2020, from https://www.ncbi.nlm.nih.gov/pmc/articles/PMC6407254/

Baird G. The choosing wisely initiative and laboratory test stewardship. Diagnosi. 2019;6(1):15–23.

Balogh EP, Miller BT, Ball JR, editors. Improving Diagnosis in Health Care. Committee on Diagnostic Error in Health Care, Board on Health Care Services, Institute of Medicine, The National Academies of Sciences, Engineering, and Medicine. Washington, DC: National Academies Press; 2015. PMID: 26803862

Bindraban RS, Ten Berg MJ, Naaklgeboren CA, Kramer MHH, Vansolinge WW, Nanayakkara PWB. Reducing test utilization in a hospital setting: a narrative review. Ann Lab Med. 2018;38:402–12.

Blankenstein O, Pedersen BT, Schlump M, Andreasen AH, Júlíusson PB. Management and interpretation of heterogeneous observational data: using insulin-like growth factor-1 data from the NordiNet International Outcome study. Growth Hormon IGF Res. 2015;25:41–6.

Borysiak MD, Thompson MJ, Posner JD. Translating diagnostic assays from the laboratory to the clinic: analytical and clinical metrics for device development and evaluation. Lab Chip. 2016;16(8):1293–313.

Boyd C, Wood K, Whitaker D, Ashorobi O, Harvey L, Oster R, et al. Accuracy in 24-hour urine collection at a tertiary center. Rev Urol. 2018;20(3):119–24.

Bray C, Bell LN, Liang H, Haykal R, Kalksow F, Mazza JJ, Yale SH. Erythrocyte sedimentation rate and C-reactive protein measures and their relevance in clinical medicine. WMJ. 2016;115(6):317–21.

Brown JVE, Meader N, Wright K, Cleminson J, McGuire W. Assessment of C-reactive protein diagnostic test accuracy for late-onset infection in newborn infants: a systematic review and meta-analysis. JAMA Pediatr. 2020;174(3):260–8.

Buppert C. Nurse practitioner's business practice and legal guide. 6th ed. Burlington, MA: Jones and Barlett; 2018.

Burke MD. Clinical laboratory consultation: appropriateness to laboratory medicine. Clin Chim Acta. 2003;333:125–9.

Caraguel CGB, Vanderstichel R. The two-step Fagan's nomogram: ad hoc interpretation of a diagnostic test result without calculation. Evid Based Med. 2013;18(4):125–8.

Cassel CK, Guest JA. Choosing wisely: helping physicians and patients make smart decisions about their care. JAMA. 2012;307:1801–2.

Centers for Disease Control and Prevention. HIV Surveillance report. 2015. https://www.cdc.gov/hiv/pdf/library/reports/surveillance/cdc-hiv-surveillance-report-2015-vol-27.pdf

Centers for Disease Control and Prevention (CDC). Diagnoses of HIV Infection in the United States and Dependent Areas, 2017. CDC website. https://www.cdc.gov/hiv/pdf/library/reports/surveillance/cdc-hiv-surveillance-report-2017-vol-29.pdf. Published November 2018. Accessed Aug 1, 2020.

Centre for Evidence-Based Medicine. OCEBM levels of evidence. https://cebm.ox.ac.uk/resources/levels-of-evidence/ocebm-levels-of-evidence. Accessed November 3, 2020.

Centre for Evidence-Based Medicine, Diagnostic Accuracy Studies. https://www.cebm.net/wecontent/uploads/2014/04/diagnostic-study-appraisal-worksheet.pdf. Accessed November 3, 2020.

Chartrand C, Tremblay N, Renaud C, Papenburg J. Diagnostic accuracy of rapid antigen detection test for respiratory syncytial virus infection: systematic review and meta-analysis. J Clin Microbiol. 2015;53(12):3738–49.

Crewe S, Rowe PC. Likelihood ratio in diagnosis. Pediatr Rev. 2011;22(7):296–9.

Cui W, Liu H, Ni H, Qin X, Zhu L. Diagnostic accuracy of procalcitonin for overall and complicated acute appendicitis in children: a meta-analysis. Ital J Pediatr. 2019;45:78.

Dailey AF, Hoots BE, Hall HI, Song R, Hayes D, Fulton P, et al. Vital signs: human immunodeficiency virus testing and diagnosis delays—United States. MMWR Morb Mortal Wkly Rep. 2017;66:1300–6.

Ebell MH. Epstein-Barr virus infectious mononucleosis. Am Fam Physician. 2004;70(7):1279–87.

Fang C, Chien Y, Yang L, Lu W, Lin M. EDTA-dependent pseudothrombocytopenia. Formosan J Surg. 2015;48(3):107–9.

Fierz W, Bossuyt X. Likelihood ratios as a value proposition for diagnostic laboratory tests. Am Ass Clin Chem. 2020:1–9.

Gaglani A, Gross T. Pediatric pain management. Emerg Med Clin North Am. 2018;36(2):323–34.

Graf EH, Pancholi P. Appropriate use of future directions of molecular diagnostic testing. Curr Infect Dis Rep. 2020;22:5.

Hallworth MJ. The "70% claim". Ann Clin Biochem. 2011;48:487–8.

Harb R, Hajdasz D, Landry M, Sussman LS. Improving laboratory test utilization at the multihospital Yale-New Haven Health System. BMJ Qual. 2019;8(3):e0000689.

Holtman GA, Lisman-van Leeuwen Y, Reitsma JB, Berger MY. Noninvasive test for inflammatory bowel disease: a meta-analysis. Pediatrics. 2016;137(1):e20152026.

Iams W, Heck J, Kapp M, Leverenz D, Velia M, Szentirmai E, et al. A multidisciplinary house staff lead initiative to safely reduce daily laboratory testing. Acad Med. 2016;91(6):813–20.

Jackson E. Urinary tract infections in children: knowledge updates and a salute to the future. Pediatr Rev. 2015;36(4):153–66.

Jackups R, Szymnaski JJ, Persaud SP. Clinical decision support for hematology laboratory test utilization. Int J Lab Hematol. 2017; Retrieved on November 30, 2020, https://onlinelibrary.wiley.com/doi/full/10.1111/ijlh.12679

Kaminska J, Dymicka-Perkarska V, Tomaszewska J, Matowicka-Karna J, Koper-Lenkiewicz O. Diagnostic utility of protein to creatinine ratio (P/C ratio) in spot urine sample within routine clinical practice. Crit Rev Clin Lab Sci. 2020;57(5):345–64.

Kazmierczak S. Statistical techniques for evaluating the diagnostic utility of laboratory tests. Clin Chem Lab Med. 1999;37(11-12):1001–9.

Kessler DP. Evaluating the medical malpractice system and options for reform. J Econ Perspect. 2011;25:93–110. PMID: 21595327

Kobewska DM, Ronksley PE, Mckay JA, Forster AJ, Van Walraven C. Influence of educational, audit and feedback, system-based and incentive and penalty interventions to reduce laboratory test utilization: a systematic review. Clin Chem Lab Med. 2015;53:157–83.

Laposata M. Obtaining a correct diagnosis rapidly in the United States in association with many barriers not present in other countries. Am J Clin Pathol. 2018;149:458–60.

Lean WL, Arnup S, Danchin M, Steer AC. Rapid diagnostic tests for group A streptococcal pharyngitis: a meta-analysis. Pediatrics. 2014;134(4):771–81.

Lee SH, Yun SJ. Diagnostic performance of ultrasonography for detection of pediatric elbow fracture: a meta-analysis. Ann Emerg Med. 2019;74(4):493–502.

Lippi G, Brambilla M, Bonelli P, Aloe R, Balestrino A, Nardelli A, et al. Effectiveness of a computerized alert system based on re-testing intervals for limiting the inappropriateness of laboratory test requests. Clin Biochem. 2015;48:1174–6.

Marshall-Andon T, Heinz P. How to use … the Monospot and other heterophile antibody tests. Archives of Disease in Childhood – Educaiton and Practice. 2017; 102:188–93.

McGee S. Simpifying likelihood ratios. J Gen Intern Med. 2002;17:647–50.

Mello MM, Chandra A, Gawande AA, Studdert DM. National costs of the medical liability system. Health Aff (Millwood). 2010;29:1569–77.

Messacar K, Parker SK, Todd JK, Dominguez SR. Implementation of rapid molecular infectious disease diagnostics: the role of diagnostic and antimicrobial stewardship. J Clin Microbiol. 2017;55(3):715–23.

Morjaria S, Chapin KP. Who to test, when and for what. J Mol Diagn. 2020;22:9.

Nagler M, Keller P, Siegrist D, Alberio L. A case of EDTA-dependent pseudothrombocytopenia: simple recognition of an underdiagnosed and misleading phenomenon. BMC Clin Pathol. 2014;14:article 19. Retrieved on August 2, 2020, https://bmcclinpathol.biomedcentral.com/articles/10.1186/1472-6890-14-19

Patel R, Fang FC. Diagnostic stewardship: opportunity for a laboratory-infectious diseases partnership. Clin Infect Dis. 2018;67(5):799–801.

Pereda MA, Chavez MA, Hooper-Miele CC, Gilman RH, Steinhoff MC, Ellington LE, et al. Lung ultrasound for the diagnosis of pneumonia in children: a meta-analysis. Pediatrics. 2015;135(4):714–22.

Quidel. QueVue Chlamydia Test. Retrieved August 20, 2020., https://www.quidel.com/sites/default/files/product/documents/EF0562610EN00_%2808_19%29_QuickVue_Chlamydia_Pkg_Insert.pdf

Rao A, Berg B, Quezada T, Fader R, Walker K, Tang S, et al. Diagnosis and antibiotic treatment of group a streptococcal pharyngitis in children in a primary care setting: impact of point-of-care polymerase chain reaction. BMC Pediatr. 2019;19:24. Retrieved on August 2, 202. https://doi.org/10.1186/s12887-019-1393-y.

Ridefelt P, Gustafsson J, Aldrimer M, Hellberg D. Alkaline phosphatase in healthy children reference intervals and prevalence of elevated levels. Horm Res Paediatr. 2014;82:399–404.

Robinson JC, Whaley C, Brown TT. Association of reference pricing for diagnostic laboratory testing with changes in patient choices, prices and total spending for diagnostic tests. JAMA Intern Med. 2016;176(9):1353–9.

Rolfe A, Burton C. Reassurance after diagnostic testing with a low pretest probability of serious disease: systematic review and meta-analysis. JAMA Intern Med. 2013;173:407–16.

Sackett D, Strauss S, Richardson WS, Rosenberg W, Haynes RB. Evidence-based medicine: how to practice and teach EBM. Edinburgh: Churchill Livingstone; 2000.

Seegmiller AC, Kim AS, Mosse CA, Levy MA, Thompson MA, Jagasia MH, et al. Optimizing personalized bone marrow testing using an evidence-based, interdisciplinary team approach. Am J Clin Pathol. 2013;140:643–50.

Segel GB, Halterman J. Neutropenia in pediatric practice. Pediatr Rev. 2008;29:12–25.

Smith B, Kamoun M, Hickner J. Laboratory Medicine Education at U.S. Medical Schools: a 2014 Status Report. Acad Med. 2014;91(1):107–12.

Stewart EH, Davis B, Clemans-Taylor BL, Littenberg B, Estrada CA, Centor RM. Rapid antigen group a streptococcus test to diagnose pharyngitis: a systematic review and meta-analysis. PLoS One. 2014;9(11):e111727.

Sumaya CV, Ench Y. Epstein-Barr virus infectious mononucleosis in children: heterophile antibody and viral-specific responses. Pediatrics. 1985;75(6):1011–9.

Tan G, Stalling M, Dennis G, Nunez M, Kahwash SB. Pseudothrombocytopenia due to platelet clumping: a case report and brief review of the literature. Case Rep Hematol. 2016;3036476. Retrieved on August 2, 2020, https://www.hindawi.com/journals/crihem/2016/3036476/

The ABIM Foundation. Unnecessary tests and procedures in the health care system: what physicians say about the problem, the causes and the solutions. Results from a national survey of physicians. May 1, 2014. Accessed on July 30, 2020, at https://www.choosingwisely.org/wp-content/uploads/2015/04/Final-Choosing-Wisely-Survey-Report.pdf.

Trevethan R. Sensitivity, specificity and predictive values: foundations pliabilities, and pitfalls in research and practice. Front Public Health. 2017;5:307–13.

US Preventive Services Task Force [USPSTF]. Screening for HIV infection: US Preventive Services Task Force recommendation statement. JAMA 2019; Retrieved on November 30, 2020, from https://jamanetwork.com/journals/jama/fullarticle/2735345

Vegting L, Beneden M, Kramer H, Piet A, Prabath K, Nanayakkara WB. How to save costs by reducing unnecessary testing: lean thinking in clinical practice. Eur J Intern Med. 2012;23(1):70–5.

Verna R, Velazquez A, Laposata M. Reducing diagnostic errors worldwide through diagnostic management teams. Ann Lab Med. 2019;39:121–4.

Watson J, Whiting PF, Brush JE. Interpreting a COVID-19 test result. BMJ. 2020;369:m1808. Retrieved November 30, 2020 from https://www.bmj.com/content/369/bmj.m1808

Wilson JMG, Jungner G. Principles and practices of screening for disease. Geneva: World Health Organization; 1968. Report No.: Public Health Papers No. 34

Workowski KA, Bachmann LH, Chan PA, Johnston CM, Muzny CA, Park I, et al. Sexually transmitted infections treatment guidelines, 2021. MMWR Recomm Rep. 2021;70(4):1–187.

Yoon HM, Suh CH, Kim JR, Lee JS, Jung AY, Cho YA. Diagnostic performance of magnetic resonance enterography for detection of active inflammation in children and adolescents with inflammatory bowel disease: a systematic review and meta-analysis. JAMA Pediatr. 2017;171(12):1208–16.

Yuksel S, Yusel G, Oncel S, Divanli E. Osteomyelitis of the calcaneus in the newborn: an ongoing complication of the Guthrie test. Eur J Pediatr. 2007;166(1):503–4.

Zhao C, Yuan B. Evaluation of the accuracy of FeNO in pediatric asthma diagnosis: a meta-analysis. Int J Clin Exp Med. 2019;12(5):4517–27.

Zhi M, Ding EL, Theisen-Toupal J, Whelan J, Arnaout R. The landscape of inappropriate laboratory testing: a 15-year meta-analysis. PLoS One. 2013;8:e78962.

Laboratory Screening and Diagnostic Testing in Antepartum Care

Adena Bargad and Hannah VogtSchaller

Learning Objectives

After completing the chapter, the learner should be able to:

1. Describe qualitative versus quantitative pregnancy tests and interpret them.
2. List the routine lab tests for an initial prenatal visit.
3. Discuss testing for sexually transmitted infections in pregnant adolescents.
4. Discuss routine late pregnancy screening tests for gestational diabetes and Group Beta Strep.
5. Explain the difference between screening and diagnostic testing for aneuploidies and the different associated screening protocols and testing procedures available.
6. Understand the use of cfDNA to screen for chromosomal abnormalities and to identify fetal blood and Rh type.
7. Discuss carrier screening for genetic conditions.
8. Identify the diagnostic criteria for preeclampsia.
9. Identify modes of fetal surveillance to evaluate the health of the fetus throughout pregnancy.
10. Recognize issues related to confidentiality, pregnancy options counseling, and social determinants of health in caring for pregnant adolescents.

2.1 Introduction

The developmental and psychosocial demands of adolescence make teens and young adults particularly vulnerable to sexual and reproductive health risks. Despite major declines in recent years, primarily attributable to the increased availability and use of highly effective contraceptives, the birth rate among adolescents aged 15–19 in the USA remains considerably higher than the international average in high-income countries (Lindberg et al. 2018; World Bank 2018a; World Bank 2018b). Girls aged 15–19 have the highest rates of both unintended pregnancy (mistimed or unwanted pregnancy) and rapid repeat pregnancy (within less than 2 years) of any age group of women in the USA (Guttmacher Institute 2019). Adolescent pregnancy is associated with both maternal and neonatal risks, including but not limited to increased risk for anemia and infections, preterm labor and birth, and neonatal low birth weight and respiratory distress syndrome (Jeha et al. 2015). While these risks have been variously attributed to both

A. Bargad (✉)
Columbia University School of Nursing,
New York, NY, USA
e-mail: ab3120@columbia.edu

H. VogtSchaller
Denver Health, Denver, CO, USA

© The Author(s), under exclusive license to Springer Nature Switzerland AG 2022
R. M. John (ed.), *Pediatric Diagnostic Labs for Primary Care: An Evidence-based Approach*,
https://doi.org/10.1007/978-3-030-90642-9_2

physiologic and social factors, there is consensus that without adequate prenatal care and socioeconomic and emotional support, teen parents and their children experience a wide range of long-term educational, socioeconomic, and developmental disadvantages (Leftwich and Alves 2017).

2.2 Health Disparities

Importantly, these disadvantages are disproportionately experienced by poor adolescent mothers of color and their children. Those in the child welfare system are at particularly high risk for unintended pregnancy and its potential adverse sequelae (Fasula et al. 2019; Penman-Aguilar et al. 2013). Indeed, disadvantaged social contexts have been consistently associated with teen pregnancy and birth. Significant racial and ethnic, geographic, and socioeconomic disparities in teen pregnancy, teen birth, and maternal and neonatal adverse consequences persist. However, there is consensus that adolescent pregnancy prevention alone cannot ameliorate the myriad social determinants of health that underlie perinatal health disparities or the associated intergenerational social and economic disadvantages experienced disproportionately by teen parents and their children (Fuller et al. 2018). Segregated neighborhoods and schools, living in food deserts, and disproportionate exposure to environmental toxins are just a few societal contributors to perinatal health disparities for pregnant adolescents and adults in marginalized communities (Centers for Disease Control and Prevention 2020a, b, c, d, e, f).

Further, there is considerable evidence for a biopsychosocial model of the impact of racism on health. The chronic stress of actual or even perceived racism has detrimental effects on health in general and adverse birth outcomes in particular (Black et al. 2015; Braveman et al. 2017; Lee et al. 2018). All these social determinants play an important role in the significantly higher infant mortality rates among Black pregnant teens aged 15–19 relative to their White and Latinx counterparts from largely preventable causes, including preterm labor and birth, low birth weight, congenital anomalies, unintentional injuries, and maternal complications of pregnancy (Black et al. 2015).

While most states allow minors to receive confidential prenatal, labor/delivery, and postpartum care, pediatric providers should be familiar with minors' rights to access and consent to prenatal care and practice under state laws. The Guttmacher Institute maintains updated resources regarding the laws that govern a minor's ability to access prenatal care (Guttmacher Institute 2021). The Society for Adolescent Health and Medicine (SAHM), the American Academy of Pediatrics (AAP), and the American College of Obstetrics and Gynecology (ACOG) jointly provide detailed guidance regarding confidentiality issues as they pertain to insurance and billing for adolescent health-care providers (SAHM, AAP, and ACOG 2016). It should be noted that pregnancy among preteens or in early adolescence is rare and should always raise suspicion for sexual abuse or nonconsensual sex. Providers must also be aware of mandated child abuse reporting laws in their states.

Pregnant adolescents often present initially with generalized abdominal, genitourinary, and/or menstrual complaints and may deny sexual activity. Therefore, pediatric health-care providers should have a low threshold for considering pregnancy as a differential diagnosis in adolescent females with such complaints. Pediatric providers should be prepared to provide pregnancy testing, patient-centered pregnancy decision-making support, and basic pregnancy resolution options counseling, including pregnancy continuation, abortion, and adoption plans. Adolescents should always be asked how they would feel about a positive pregnancy test before a test is performed so that the provider can be prepared with appropriate support and interventions. Finally, the teen's feelings around whether and how they might share the information with parents, guardians or partners should also be explored.

When an adolescent decides to continue a pregnancy, professional society guidelines, individual risk assessment, and individual needs will determine the schedule of prenatal visits and laboratory testing. At a minimum, the AAP's Guidelines for Perinatal Care (Kilpatrick et al.

2017), written jointly by the AAP's Committee on the Fetus and Newborn and ACOG's Committee on Obstetric Practice, recommend an initial visit in the first trimester, monthly visits until 28 weeks, visits every 2–3 weeks up to 36 weeks gestation, and then weekly visits until delivery. However, both professional organizations emphasize that clinical judgment should tailor the schedule of visits to the individual pregnant patient's needs consistent with achieving prenatal care's fundamental goals. These goals include early and accurate estimation of gestational age, assessing maternal and fetal risk factors and ongoing assessment of maternal-fetal well-being, providing timely patient education, offering reassurance and referrals as needed, and completing routine laboratory screening and testing. Thoroughly executing these prenatal care elements helps prevent preterm birth (delivery before 37 weeks), a leading cause of neonatal death and long-term disability (CDC 2020a). In addition, new recommendations for preventive postpartum health including much earlier post partum visits and assessments can reduce maternal and neonatal morbidity and mortality and encourage long-term health and well-being for both mother and child (ACOG 2018e, reaffirmed 2021).

2.3 Laboratory Tests and Pregnancy

Pregnancy can be confirmed by urine or serum pregnancy testing or by ultrasound. Both urine and serum pregnancy tests detect human chorionic gonadotropin (HCG), the "pregnancy hormone." HCG is initially released by the fertilized egg and later by the placenta. Still, it is not detectable in urine or blood until after implantation of the fertilized egg in the uterine lining.

2.3.1 Understanding Pregnancy Diagnostic Testing

Urine pregnancy tests are usually positive by 14 days after fertilization and are most reliable after

a missed menses. The accuracy of over-the-counter and point-of-care urine tests varies. While false positives are rare, false negatives are common, especially in the first few weeks after conception (Cole 2012). Serum pregnancy tests can be reliably positive 7–10 days after fertilization. More information about point-of-care pregnancy tests and their pitfalls can be found in Chap. 5, Section 5.8.2.

2.3.1.1 Urine Pregnancy Test

A urine pregnancy test is a "qualitative" test, meaning that results indicate only positive or negative with no specified quantification of HCG level. High sensitivity urine pregnancy tests (HSPT) read positive when the serum HCG level reaches 25 mIU/mL.

2.3.1.2 Serum Pregnancy Test

Serum tests can be either qualitative or quantitative, the quantitative tests providing a numeric level in mIUs/mL of HCG in the bloodstream. Serum HCG levels rise in early pregnancy at a predictable rate. Serial levels can be used to assess whether early pregnancies are developing normally or abnormally, as in ectopic pregnancy or an early pregnancy loss (miscarriage). Table 2.1 shows expected serum HCG levels associated with particular conditions and at various points in pregnancy.

Table 2.1 Serum HCG levels associated with conditions and points in pregnancy

Condition/gestational age	HCG level in serum (mIU/mL)
Non-pregnant	<5
Equivocal (requires retesting)	6–25
9–12 weeks gestational age	25,000–300,000 (peak)
Intrauterine gestational sac visible on ultrasound	1500–3000 (practice site protocols vary)
4-12 weeks post-delivery or abortion	<5
Viable normal pregnancy	Serial levels typically double over 72 hours
Ectopic pregnancy or early pregnancy loss	Serial levels plateau or decrease over 72 hours

Sources: ACOG 2018a; Larsen et al. 2013; American Pregnancy Association 2020

2.4 Diagnostic Testing to Confirm Gestational Age

Early and accurate gestational age determination is of primary importance in prenatal care and should be documented clearly in the medical record. Assessments of fetal growth and well-being, timing and interpretation of laboratory tests, and decision-making about interventions to prevent pre- and post-term births depend entirely on the accuracy of early pregnancy dating and the assigned estimated delivery date (EDD). Based on considerable evidence, ACOG, the American Institute of Ultrasound in Medicine, and the Society for Maternal-Fetal Medicine endorse ultrasound in the first trimester up to and including 13 weeks 6 days (13 6/7) estimated gestational age (EGA) as the most accurate method to determine or confirm gestational age (ACOG 2017a). Therefore, redating a pregnancy based on discrepancies between the EDD as determined by the last menstrual period (LMP) and the EDD established by ultrasound should rarely be done. Table 2.2 shows the recommended parameters for redating pregnancy when such discrepancies exist.

Providers of early pregnancy care should be able to identify the physical landmarks of early pregnancy in ultrasound images. Figure 2.1 illustrates the earliest physical landmarks of pregnancy visible on ultrasound. These landmarks include the gestational sac, the fluid-filled cavity or chorionic cavity that is the first

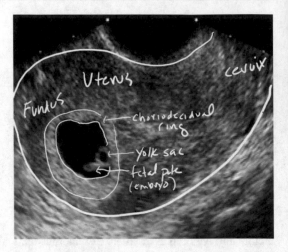

Fig. 2.1 Ultrasound of intrauterine pregnancy. Photo courtesy of R. Bargad

sign of pregnancy (visible at approximately 3–5 weeks), the yolk sac (a membranous sac that serves several nutritive purposes and is only visible with an intrauterine pregnancy (visible at approximately 5.5 weeks), and the fetal pole or embryo (visible at approximately 6 weeks). The pregnancy pictured in Fig. 2.1 meets the visual criteria for a normal, intrauterine pregnancy at approximately 6 weeks EGA with a gestational sac that is located at the fundus, elliptical in shape, and eccentrically implanted on the endometrium. The image also demonstrates the double decidual ring sign or choriodecidual reaction. The hyperechoic (white) concentric rings surrounding the anechoic (black) gestational sac where the decidua of the uterus and the decidua of the gestational sac intersect. Note that embryonic cardiac motion is visible on ultrasound at 5.5–6 weeks.

2.5 Initial Visit

The clinician working in primary care may be the first person to identify a pregnant adolescent. Initial visits with the obstetrical clinician can be delayed due to overwhelming demand. The primary care clinician may order initial labs, start prenatal vitamins, and order the first obstetrical ultrasound, depending on the resources.

Table 2.2 Guidelines for redating gestational age (EGA) and estimated date of delivery (EDD)

Gestational age range in weeks based on last menstrual period (LMP)	Redate if the discrepancy between ultrasound dating and LMP is as follows
First trimester	
≤8 6/7	>5 days
9 0/7 to 13 6/7	>7 days
14 0/7 to 15 6/7	>7 days
16 0/7 to 21 6/7	>10 days
22 0/7 to 27 6/7	>14 days
28 0/7 and beyond	>21 days

Adapted from ACOG 2017a

2.5.1 Routine Prenatal Labs

A routine laboratory test panel is performed for all pregnant patients at their initial prenatal visit. The need for supplemental testing is based on individual risk factors or patient preferences. ACOG's Obstetric Patient Record Forms, including an Antepartum Record, Obstetric Medical History Form, and Postpartum Care Plan Form, detail the recommended form and content for documentation of laboratory and diagnostic tests in antepartum and postpartum care and are available here: https://www.acog.org/clinical-information/obstetric-patient-record-forms.

2.5.1.1 ABO and Rh Blood Typing

A pregnant woman's blood type is designated using the standard ABO blood typing system, which includes whether her blood is positive or negative for Rh (Rhesus) factors or antigens. Rh antigens are a set of proteins on the red cell surface that play a role in cell membrane integrity. While there are more than 50 known Rh antigen types, five account for the most significant clinical issues (identified as D, C, c, E, and e antigens). The presence or absence of the RhD antigen on red blood cells determines whether a person is Rh-positive (antigen present) or Rh-negative (antigen absent). RhD antigen positivity or negativity is inherited, and the Rh-positive gene is dominant, resulting in approximately 85% of the US population being Rh-positive (Garratty et al. 2004). Importantly, suppose an Rh-negative person conceives a baby with an Rh-positive person. In that case, the fetus could have Rh-positive blood, a dynamic referred to as maternal-fetal Rh incompatibility, which can have dire consequences for the fetus. If paternity is certain, the father of the baby of an Rh-negative pregnant woman can be tested, and, if the father of the baby is also negative, the fetus is not at risk.

With maternal-fetal Rh incompatibility, an Rh-negative mother can develop antibodies to the fetal Rh-positive blood when any fetal blood enters the maternal circulation. This fetomaternal blood exchange occurs primarily at the time of delivery. It can also occur during antenatal procedures such as amniocentesis or chorionic villus sampling, with conditions such as placenta previa, placental abruption, or with abdominal trauma, pregnancy loss, or abortion. The resultant maternal production of antibodies to the fetal blood is an immunologic response referred to variously as maternal Rh sensitization, isoimmunization, or alloimmunization. When these antibodies cross the placenta, they can destroy an Rh-positive fetus's red blood cells. In severe cases, maternal RhD alloimmunization results in hemolytic disease of the newborn (HDN) marked by congenital neurologic consequences for the infant (kernicterus) or even neonatal death (*hydrops fetalis*).

The fetus in the first pregnancy with maternal-fetal Rh incompatibility is generally unaffected given that the primary risk of exposure to fetal blood is during delivery. Still, the risk for maternal anti-RhD antibody production increases with each subsequent pregnancy. An injection of anti-D immune globulin such as Rhogam protects maternal alloimmunization by preventing the maternal antibody immune response to Rh-positive fetal red blood cells and effectively preventing HDN. This medication is routinely given to Rh-negative women at 28 weeks of pregnancy, within 3 days postpartum when the neonate is determined to be Rh D-positive and/or during pregnancy at the time of any procedure or event that is high risk for the intermixing of fetal and maternal blood (ACOG 2017b).

2.5.1.2 Antibody Screen

It is standard of care in the USA to routinely screen all pregnant people, regardless of blood type, for the presence of any red blood cell antibodies in the maternal circulation with an antibody screen or indirect Coombs test. Red blood cells are incubated with maternal plasma, mixed with Coombs serum, and examined for agglutination, the visible expression of the aggregation of antibodies. In maternal-fetal Rh incompatibility, if the red cells are coated with maternal anti-D antibodies, the indirect Coombs test is considered positive. Note that a direct Coombs test is performed directly on red blood cells, not plasma, as when a hemolytic disease of the newborn is suspected.

An indirect Coombs titer can then be calculated to determine the approach to management. An antibody titer reflects the concentration of antibodies in solution over serial dilutions. In the case of prenatal antibody testing, a positive indirect Coombs titer higher than 1:4 should be considered indicative of alloimmunization. Titers 1:8 or lower can be managed by serial monitoring of maternal antibody titers, but titers 1:16 or higher require fetal monitoring and assessment by ultrasonography or serial amniocentesis (Cacciatore et al. 2009). While other tests exist for maternal antibody screening, including gel microcolumn assay and automated enzymatic methods, they are not recommended for routine use. Ultimately, accurate quantitation of fetal red blood cells in the maternal circulation is necessary to determine adequate immunoglobulin (Rhogam) dosage. Several tests are used for this purpose, including the qualitative Rosette test, the quantitative Kleihauer-Betke test (acid elution assay), and flow cytometry. The flow cytometry method is preferred and processes maternal blood through an instrument at high speed, separating and counting fetal blood cells resulting in a computerized, digital readout of the degree of maternal alloimmunization (Farias et al. 2016).

Less common causes of HDN include antibodies directed against antigens of the Kell blood group (e.g., anti-K and anti-k), Kidd blood group (e.g., anti-Jka and anti-Jkb), Duffy blood group (e.g., anti-Fya), and MNS and s blood group antibodies. ABO maternal-fetal incompatibilities can also occur among type O women carrying a fetus with a different blood type. HDN due to ABO incompatibility is usually less severe than Rh incompatibility. In contrast to the Rh antigens, the ABO blood group antigens are expressed by various fetal tissues, reducing the binding of target antigens on the fetal RBCs alone (Dean 2005). As a result, ABO maternal-fetal incompatibility generally results in mild jaundice and has not been found to increase in severity with subsequent pregnancies (Blackburn 2017). Any positive antibody screen/direct Coombs requires further testing to determine the specific type of maternal-fetal incompatibility, the degree of maternal alloimmunization, and subsequent neonatal risk for HDN and related consequences.

2.5.1.3 Noninvasive Prenatal Testing for Fetal Blood and Rh Type

Importantly, advances in noninvasive prenatal testing (NIPT) that allow for the detection of cell-free fetal DNA (cfDNA) in the maternal serum have made prenatal fetal blood typing, including Rh typing, reliable as early as the tenth week of pregnancy via a single maternal blood sample (see more on NIPT below). Some countries have already replaced routine Rh-D immunoglobulin prophylaxis of all Rh-negative women with targeted Rh-D immunoglobulin prophylaxis only for Rh-D negative women whose fetus's blood type is determined at 24–27 weeks (or earlier) via NIPT to be Rh-positive. Some of the benefits of targeted prophylaxis include eliminating or greatly reducing the need for postpartum cord blood or neonatal heel-stick blood sampling, increasing the worldwide availability of Rh-D immunoglobulin, and reducing overall costs associated with obstetric and neonatal care. However, in most countries, including the USA, the current protocol remains to routinely administer anti-D immune globulin to non-sensitized, RhD-negative pregnant women in the 28th week of gestation and again postpartum, unless the fetal cord blood is phenotyped and the neonate is also Rh-negative (Runkel et al. 2020).

2.5.1.4 Complete Blood Count

A complete blood count (CBC), including hemoglobin and hematocrit, is performed at the initial prenatal visit and is repeated at 24–28 weeks to screen for anemia. One of the normal hematological changes of pregnancy is the "dilutional" anemia created by a greater increase in plasma volume (45%) relative to the increase in red cell mass (25%). This disproportionate dynamic results in the physiologic decrease of the red cell count, hemoglobin, and hematocrit levels, requiring trimester-specific standards for diagnosing anemia in pregnancy. Table 2.3 indicates the trimester-specific criteria for anemia in preg-

Table 2.3 Diagnosis of anemia in pregnancy

First trimester	Hgb < 11.0 g/dL	Hct < 33%
Second trimester	Hgb <10.5 g/dL	Hct < 32%
Third trimester	Hgb < 11.0 g/dL	Hct 33%

Adapted from ACOG 2017c, 2021

nancy. A review of the evaluation of the pediatric patient with anemia can be found in Sect. 8.6.

Iron deficiency anemia, a microcytic anemia, is by far the most common cause of anemia in pregnancy and has been associated with a wide range of adverse maternal and neonatal outcomes, including increased risk for cesarean birth, postpartum hemorrhage, preterm birth, low birth weight, deficits in early neonatal behavioral and cognitive indices, and increased perinatal mortality (Dilla et al. 2013; Rahman et al. 2016; Menon et al. 2016). Formulations contain 30 mg of recommended daily iron intake in pregnancy. ACOG and the CDC recommend routine low dose iron supplementation starting in the first trimester (ACOG 2021). Experts recommend additional supplementation as needed for anemia in pregnancy with a follow-up CBC and serum ferritin 3–4 weeks after therapy is initiated to evaluate the adequacy of the response. ACOG recommends that women with hematocrit <30% near term have an active type and cross-match at delivery for potential blood transfusion (ACOG 2017d).

2.5.1.5 Platelet Count

Platelet counts in uncomplicated pregnancies gradually decrease at approximately the same rate throughout pregnancy. This physiologic, gestational thrombocytopenia results from expanded intravascular volume and increased aggregation of platelets in the spleen and the placenta resulting in lower peripheral platelet levels (Reese et al. 2019). Therefore, decreased platelet counts between 100,000 and 150,000/µL in pregnancy are considered normal. However, platelet counts below 100,000/µL usually result from underlying medical conditions, including immune thrombocytopenia, preeclampsia, or HELLP (hemolysis, elevated liver enzymes, and low platelet count) syndrome. When the platelet count falls below 150,000/µL, evaluation and continued monitoring are warranted, and in patients with preeclampsia or HELLP syndrome, low platelet levels may require induction of labor (Reese et al. 2018).

2.5.1.6 Hemoglobin Electrophoresis

Blood contains different types of hemoglobin, the oxygen-carrying substance in red blood cells.

Normal adult hemoglobin contains 95–98% hemoglobin A (two alpha-chains and two beta-chains), 2–3% hemoglobin A2, and 1–2% fetal hemoglobin. Hemoglobin electrophoresis is a laboratory test whereby an electrical current is passed through the hemoglobin in a blood sample, causing the different hemoglobin types to separate into different bands. The blood sample is then compared to a healthy sample to determine which types of hemoglobin are present and in what proportion.

In the USA, all newborns are screened with hemoglobin electrophoresis as part of routine newborn screening. In pregnant patients, screening for hemoglobinopathies with a hemoglobin electrophoresis test is sometimes reserved for populations known to be at increased risk for thalassemia (patients from some regions of Africa, the Caribbean, the Mediterranean, the Middle East, South America, Southeast Asia, or the Western Pacific) or SCD (African-American, South American, Caribbean) or patients with any abnormal red cell indices (ACOG 2017b). However, given changing migration patterns, interethnic coupling, and the ethnic diversity of large urban areas, most obstetric providers routinely order hemoglobin electrophoresis for their obstetric patients to rule out potential hemoglobinopathies. More information about hemoglobin electrophoresis can be found in Chap. 8, Sects. 8.8.2, 8.8.6.1, and 8.11, and Table 2.4 reviews the differential lab findings for selected hematological conditions in pregnancy.

2.5.1.7 Urine Culture/Screen

Hormonal and anatomic changes in pregnancy provoke renal adaptations that result in increased urinary stasis and decreased resistance to bacteria. The result is an increased risk for urinary tract infection that can more rapidly progress to pyelonephritis. Both are associated with adverse maternal and fetal outcomes, including preeclampsia, preterm birth, and low birth weight (Matuszkiewicz-Rowinska et al. 2015; Yan et al. 2018). Therefore, professional guidelines recommend that all pregnant patients be screened via a urine culture and sensitivity at the initial prenatal visit. Unlike in non-pregnant patients, asymptomatic bacteriuria (ASB) in pregnant patients that meets colony-forming

Table 2.4 Differential laboratory findings for hematologic conditions in pregnancy

Condition	MCV (fL)	MCH (pg/cell)	Ferritin (mg/dL)	Hgb electrophoresis	Management
IDA	NML or <80 Microcytic	Nml or <27	<12	Nml Hgb A	Supplement
Thalassemia	<80 Microcytic	<25	NML	Alpha: Hgb Bart's or Hgb H Beta: Reduced or absent HgbA; elevated HgbA2; increased Hgb F	Test FOB Genetics Amniocentesis Refer to MFM
Sickle cell	NML or decreased	NML or Decreased	NML	Decreased or absent Hgb A Hgb S or C	Test FOB Genetic amniocentesis Refer to MFM
Folate deficiency	>100 Macrocytic		NML	Nml Hgb A	Supplement
B12 deficiency	>100 Macrocytic		NML	Nml Hgb A	Supplement

Adapted from ACOG 2017d; Lazar et al. 2019

Table 2.5 Laboratory testing for urinary tract infection in pregnancy

Test	Population/timing	Characteristics	Pertinent results
Urine culture and sensitivity	All pregnant women at the initial visit Women with UTI symptoms q trimester: DM, sickle cell trait q month: Treated for asymptomatic bacteriuria (ASB) current pregnancy or recurrent UTIs	Identifies asymptomatic bacteriuria Identifies and quantifies specific organisms and antibiotic sensitivities	ASB: ≥100,000 cfu/mL Symptomatic: Any CFL Any amount of GBS in clean-catch midstream urine specimen requires intrapartum prophylaxis
Urinalysis (microscopic analysis)	Women with symptoms	Faster processing than culture	Nitrites, WBC/leukocyte esterase, WBC casts, RBCs/heme, bacteria
Urine dip (reagent strip)	Women with symptoms Routine q prenatal care visit	Fastest, screening only, inexpensive, lowest sensitivity and specificity	Nitrites, WBC/leukocyte esterase, RBCs/heme

Adapted from Aurthur and Walsh 2019

unit (CFU) count criteria is treated in pregnancy to prevent maternal and fetal morbidity and mortality. A test of cure is recommended after completing the recommended antibiotic course (Kilpatrick et al. 2017). *E. coli* is the most common pathogen identified in symptomatic and asymptomatic urinary tract infections originating from the periurethral; however, several other pathogens can cause UTIs in pregnancy, including *Klebsiella pneumoniae*, *Proteus mirabilis*, *Enterobacter* species, *Staphylococcus saprophyticus*, and *Proteus* species. Groups B streptococcus is an important pathogen in pregnancy that can result in invasive GBS disease and sepsis in the newborn (discussed separately below).

Note that evidence regarding an association between the use of the most common antibiotics for UTIs, nitrofurantoin and sulfonamides, and congenital disabilities has been mixed. ACOG guidelines recommend these agents for first-line use in the second and third trimesters but in the first trimester only when no alternative antibiotics are available (ACOG 2017e). Table 2.5 reviews the different laboratory testing for urinary tract infection options, interpretations, and recommendations for pregnant patients. Note that negative nitrites do not rule out infection, RBCs and WBCs can reflect vaginal discharge, WBC casts are common in pyelonephritis, and leukocyte esterase increases the likelihood of the presence of infection (Aurthur and Walsh 2019).

2.5.1.8 Urine Dipstick

The utility of routine urine dipstick/reagent strip testing at every prenatal visit to detect proteinuria as a diagnostic criterion for preeclampsia has been debated for years. Preeclampsia is a pregnancy complication characterized by high blood pressure and signs of kidney and liver organ damage. Based on studies indicating minimal predictive utility in low-risk, asymptomatic patients, the US Preventive Services Task Force (USPSTF) recommends against screening for preeclampsia with point-of-care urine dipsticks in asymptomatic patients. Both the USPSTF and ACOG recommend that the best laboratory studies to confirm a diagnosis of preeclampsia are a 24-hour urine collection or protein to creatinine ratio (P-C ratio) in a single voided urine. A ratio > 0.3 mg/dL has been shown to meet or exceed 300 mg protein in a 24 hr. urine collection and is diagnostic for preeclampsia. Also, both the USPSTF and ACOG agree that proteinuria is often but not always present in the setting of preeclampsia, and guidelines indicate that the diagnosis of preeclampsia can be made without proteinuria when other clinical signs are present. In contrast, given the well-established accuracy and predictive validity for preeclampsia of blood pressure readings, the USPSTF and ACOG have concluded substantial benefits for routine blood pressure screenings at every prenatal visit (US Preventive Services Task Force, Bibbins-Domingo, Grossman, Curry, Barry, and Davidson 2017; ACOG 2020a). Box 2.1 outlines the diagnostic criteria for preeclampsia.

Box 2.1 Diagnostic Criteria for Preeclampsia

Elevated blood pressure:

- If a pregnant woman who is more than 20 weeks of gestation and who had previously normal blood pressure has a BP >140 mm Hg/ 90 mm Hg done on two occasions at least 4 hours apart.
- If the BP >160 mm Hg/110 mm Hg on two separate occasions within a short interval (minutes).

Proteinuria:

- >300 mg per 24-hour urine collection
- Protein/creatinine ratio 0. > 3 mg/dL.
- Urine dipstick reading of >2+ (used only if other quantitative methods not available).

In the absence of proteinuria, new-onset hypertension with the new onset of any of the following:

- Thrombocytopenia with a platelet count less than 100×10^9/L.
- Renal insufficiency: creatinine concentrations >1.1 mg/dL or doubling of the serum creatinine concentration from a previous result.
- Impaired liver function: elevated blood concentrations of liver transaminases to twice normal concentration.
- Pulmonary edema.
- New-onset headache unresponsive to medication and not accounted for by alternative diagnoses or visual symptoms.

Adapted from American College of Obstetrics and Gynecologists 2013

2.5.2 Real-World Example

A 15 year old presents for a sick visit reporting daily nausea and vomiting and fatigue for a few weeks. A urine pregnancy test is positive and, on exam, the uterine fundus is at the symphysis, consistent with approximately 12 weeks EGA. The patient reports consensual sex with a same age partner. She is vague and mildly upset in response to being asked how she feels about the positive pregnancy test. Patient education is provided on all pregnancy resolution options: continuation, termination, and adoption and resources for each are given. The patient's social supports are assessed, and she is encouraged to discuss the situation with a trusted adult. Given the patient's indecision, an ultrasound to confirm pregnancy dating is ordered for the next day, routine prenatal labs are drawn, prenatal vitamins are provided and a follow up appointment is scheduled for 1 week while the patient is encouraged to make a decision regarding the pregnancy as soon as possible.

Key Learning About Diagnosing Pregnancy, Rh Incompatibility, and Routine Urine Dipstick Testing in Prenatal Care

- Urine pregnancy tests are reliably positive 14 days after fertilization.
- Serum pregnancy tests can be reliably positive 7–10 days after fertilization.
- First trimester ultrasound is the most reliable method for dating a pregnancy.
- ABO and Rh factor blood typing and antibody screening are routine in pregnancy.
- The fetus in the first pregnancy with maternal-fetal Rh incompatibility is generally unaffected but the risk for maternal anti-RhD antibody production increases with each subsequent pregnancy. An injection of anti-D immune globulin such as Rhogam prevents maternal alloimmunization and HDN.
- Urine culture and sensitivity is routine at the initial visit.
- Urine dipstick for protein has low predictive validity for preeclampsia in low-risk, asymptomatic pregnant patients, but routine blood pressure screening at every prenatal visit is recommended.

2.6   Sexually Transmitted Infections

Sexually transmitted infections (STIs) during pregnancy have been associated with preterm labor and birth, neonatal congenital infections and anomalies, and neonatal death. Female anatomy increases the risk of acquiring STIs as the thin vaginal epithelium and moist vaginal environment allow bacteria to penetrate and grow easily. Cervical ectropion, the exposure of endocervical cells on the face of the cervix common during adolescence, can also favor acquiring both viruses and bacteria. Importantly, recent estimates indicate youth ages 15–24 account for nearly half of all newly acquired STIs annually (CDC 2021a).

2.6.1   Testing for Sexually Transmitted Infections

Some infections are transmitted in utero, while others are transmitted only during labor and delivery or breastfeeding. As of 2020, all states have laws that explicitly allow minors to give informed consent to receive STD diagnosis and treatment services (CDC 2021b). Pediatric providers should be prepared to emphasize confidentiality, which has been shown to increase STI testing and treatment among teens (Leichliter et al. 2017). CDC guidelines recommend that all pregnant people under 25 be routinely screened for the STIs discussed below when they present for prenatal care (CDC 2019a). To prevent congenital syphilis, pregnant adolescents who are at high risk should be screened at 28 weeks and delivery (Workowski et al. 2021).

2.6.1.1 Gonorrhea and Chlamydia

Gonorrhea and chlamydia can cause neonatal conjunctivitis and pneumonia when transmitted during labor and delivery. Nucleic acid amplification testing (NAAT) via clinician- or patient-collected (equivalent sensitivity and specificity) vaginal swab is the preferred testing method; however, cervical and urine samples can also be used (Rönn et al. 2019; CDC 2014). Pharyngeal or rectal swabs should be collected for patients reporting oral and/or anal sexual behaviors. In pregnancy, a test of cure for chlamydia should be performed 4 weeks after treatment and again 3 months after treatment (Workowski et al. 2021). Pregnant adolescent patients should be re-screened in the third trimester regardless of STI history in the current pregnancy.

Pregnant women aged <25 years are at increased risk for gonorrhea, and the risk increases when there are other STIs or have multiple partners or the partner has an STI. Therefore, they should be screened for gonorrhea during the first prenatal visit and, if the risk continues, should be screened again in the third trimester (Workowski et al. 2021). Additional information about point-of-care tests for STIs is found in Chap. 4, Section 4.9.

2.6.1.2 Syphilis

Syphilis easily crosses the placenta, potentially causing long-term adverse effects on any fetal organ system, and 40% of newborn (congenital) syphilis cases result in miscarriage, stillbirth, or neonatal death (CDC 2020b). Increasing rates of congenital syphilis are largely due to gaps in testing and treatment during prenatal care (Kimball et al. 2020). Providers are responsible for knowing area prevalence rates, available via CDC or local health department surveillance reports. The CDC recommends retesting in the third trimester and before delivery for high-risk patients. Some states require syphilis testing at delivery, with penalties imposed on providers who fail to do so (CDC 2020c).

Screening is via one of the following tests: non-treponemal tests (rapid plasma reagin (RPR), venereal disease research laboratory (VDRL), toluidine red unheated serum test (TRUST)) or treponemal tests (fluorescent treponemal antibody absorption (FTA-ABS), microhemagglutination test for antibodies to *T. pallidum* (MHA-TP), *T. pallidum* particle agglutination assay (TPPA), *T. pallidum* enzyme immunoassay (TP-EIA), chemiluminescence immunoassay (CIA), Syphilis Health Check (point of care, rapid test)). Confirmatory testing depends on institutional serologic testing algorithms and availability. More information about syphilis can be found in Chap. 6, Section 6.4.1.

2.6.1.3 HIV

HIV can be transmitted anytime during pregnancy, labor, and delivery or during breastfeeding; however, maternal and neonatal antiviral treatment has been shown to reduce prenatal transmission risk by 99% (CDC 2006). The CDC, ACOG, and AAP all endorse universal screening for all pregnant patients as early as possible using an opt-out approach, legal in all US states and territories, whereby patients are informed that

HIV testing is part of the routine prenatal lab panel unless they specifically decline it (ACOG 2018b). Documentation is required if a pregnant patient declines HIV testing. When the patient's HIV status is unknown at the time of delivery, CDC guidelines state newborn testing should be performed as soon as possible so that antiretroviral prophylaxis can be offered to HIV-exposed infants. Women should be informed that a positive HIV test in the infant confirms that the mother is also infected with HIV and that neonatal antiretroviral prophylaxis benefits are maximized when initiated ≤12 h after birth (ACOG 2018b). Perinatal HIV testing laws vary among states as to whether they require testing in the third trimester, at labor and delivery if prenatal HIV testing/status is not documented, or of the newborn, with or without maternal consent, when the mother's HIV status is unknown (Salvant-Valentine and Poulin 2018). Testing is via nucleic acid test (NAT); antigen/antibody combination assay tests capable of detecting HIV-1 antibodies, HIV-2 antibodies, and HIV-1 p24 antigen; or antibody-only tests (rapid tests) with reactive antigen/antibody combination immunoassays tested further with an HIV-1/HIV-2 antibody differentiation assay (supplemental testing) and confirmatory testing based on institutional testing algorithms (Branson et al. 2014). More information about HIV can be found in Chap. 6, Sects. 6.3.5 and 6.4.6 and in Chap. 4, Sect. 4.9.2.

2.6.1.4 Hepatitis B Virus

Hepatitis B virus does not cross the placenta, so most infections occur during labor and delivery or postpartum with infant exposure to maternal blood or secretions (Dionne-Odom et al. 2016). All pregnant women are screened for HBV, regardless of prior testing or vaccination status, by testing for the hepatitis B surface antigen (HBsAg) (Workowski et al. 2021). Reactive HBsAg tests can indicate either acute infection or chronic carrier status, and further antigen and antibody testing are required to determine maternal status accurately. The risk of perinatal transmission is greatest if acquired in the third trimester and if further testing indicates they are HBeAg positive, indicative of acute or chronic infection with active viral replication and infectivity.

The HBV vaccine series and a single HBIG dose prevent chronic HBV in most exposed infants. Pregnant patients should be re-screened in the third trimester for any first trimester positive results if they remain in a high-risk group for reinfection or if they engage in high-risk behaviors including using non-medical drugs, exchanging sex for money or drugs, or living in high infection prevalence areas, are symptomatic, or have partners in any of those risk groups (Kilpatrick et al. 2017). More information about hepatitis B can be found in Chap. 6, Sect. 6.5.2.

2.6.1.5 Trichomonas, Bacterial Vaginosis, and HSV

The CDC currently recommends against routine screening of asymptomatic pregnant patients for bacterial vaginosis, trichomonas, and herpes simplex virus (HSV) (CDC 2019a). More information about HSV can be found in Chap. 6, Section 6.3.4, and information about trichomonas and other sexually transmitted infections can be found in Chap. 4, Sects. 4.9 and 4.9.1.

2.7 Other Infectious Diseases: TORCH Infections

The TORCH acronym was originally intended to aid in the diagnosis of neonatal congenital infections by grouping those marked by rashes or skin lesions and included toxoplasmosis (T), other agents (O, syphilis), rubella (R, German measles), cytomegalovirus (C), and herpes simplex virus (H). Of these original TORCH infections, ACOG recommends routine screening only for syphilis (discussed above) and rubella. Chapters 3 and 6 have more details about these infections.

2.7.1 Rubella

While rubella has been essentially eliminated in the US population since 2004, periodic outbreaks occur, and infection, particularly in the first half of pregnancy, can result in congenital rubella syndrome (CRS). CRS encompasses a range of sequelae from spontaneous abortion to cardiac, visual, and auditory congenital anomalies. Women who are not immune can be offered vaccination postpartum.

2.7.1.1 Rubella IgG

Rubella immunity is assessed routinely during the initial prenatal lab panel via serologic enzyme immunoassay testing for rubella IgG only (CDC 2020d). Specific reference ranges vary by the laboratory; however, results are always reported as negative, equivocal, or positive. A positive result indicates the presence of IgG and immunity. Negative or equivocal results can be followed up with further laboratory testing with enzyme immunoassays for IgM antibodies; however, the CDC warns against false-positive IgM results and recommends IgG and IgM retesting 5–10 days after an initial positive IgM result (CDC 2020c). IgG avidity testing, an indication of the acuity of rubella infection, can help to distinguish acute infection (IgM positive, low avidity, rising IgM) versus a false positive or re-infection (IgG and IgM positive, high avidity) (CDC 2020d).

2.7.2 HSV

HSV screening is not routinely recommended and can be considered for pregnant patients who engage in high-risk behaviors or are in a high-risk group or if their sexual partner is HSV positive, as HSV testing can be useful for discordant partners in guiding sexual behavior, particularly in the third trimester when a new infection would pose the greatest risk to the fetus (CDC 2020e). HSV testing is discussed in Chap. 6, Sect. 6.3.4.

2.7.3 Hepatitis C

The 2020 CDC updated guidelines state that all pregnant patients should be screened for hepatitis C virus (HCV) unless geographic prevalence rates are <0.1% (Schillie et al. 2020). Note that the 2020 USPSTF guidelines state that all pregnant *adults* should be screened for HCV and that, given the increasing prevalence of hepatitis C virus (HCV) in women aged 15–44 and in infants born to HCV-infected mothers, clinicians "may want to consider" screening pregnant persons younger than 18 years old (Chou et al. 2020). More information about hepatitis C can be found in Chap. 6, Sect. 6.5.3.

Numerous other infectious agents can cause congenital infections and should be considered in the complex differential diagnosis of neonatal congenital infections. These agents include parvovirus B19, enterovirus, varicella, Group Beta Strep (GBS, discussed separately below), hepatitis A, and emerging infections like Ebola and Zika viruses. Laboratory testing for infectious diseases involves pathogen-specific serological testing for IgG and IgM and the appropriate interpretation for acuity and perinatal transmissibility. It should be noted that some states have instituted routine infant screening for toxoplasmosis and targeted screening for cytomegalovirus in newborns with hearing deficits. However, there is a consensus that universal screening for TORCH infections is neither cost-effective nor a productive diagnostic approach and that newborns should be tested with the appropriate diagnostic samples (e.g., amniotic fluid, serum, blood, urine, nasopharyngeal or conjunctival swab) for specific pathogens based on specific symptoms and the entire clinical picture including a maternal history of exposures (de Jong et al. 2013). Section 3.4 of Chap. 3 reviews common infections in the newborn.

2.7.4 Cervical Cancer and Human Papilloma Virus Screening

Guidelines for frequency of cervical cancer screening via pap smear or human papilloma virus (HPV) testing do not change for pregnant patients. Pediatric providers should generally not have cause to perform cervical cancer or HPV screening as all professional organizations' guidelines indicate that such screening should not be initiated until age 21. The most recent American Cancer Society Guidelines (ACS 2020) recommend that this screening not be initiated until age 25 and that the preferred screening method is primary HPV testing (as opposed to a pap smear) via cervical swab (Fontham et al. 2020).

2.7.5 Screening for Tuberculosis

While the overall incidence of tuberculosis (TB) among adolescents in the USA is low, the incidence is disproportionately higher among adolescents of all non-White racial or ethnic groups, adolescents living in US-affiliated islands, or adolescents whose parents are from tuberculosis-endemic countries (Cowger et al. 2019). Congenital neonatal TB infection is rare but is associated with considerable morbidity and mortality. The majority of neonatal infections are acquired postpartum via exposure to maternal aerosolized contagious respiratory secretions. Untreated TB poses greater potential risks to the developing fetus and the newborn than maternal treatment with standard medication regimens, and, while TB medications cross the placenta and are found in breast milk, they are not teratogenic (Malhamé et al. 2016; Gould and Aronoff 2016). Importantly, the symptoms of tuberculosis are nonspecific and can mimic normal physiologic changes in pregnancy that result in increased respiratory rate, poor appetite, and fatigue. Still, symptoms compatible with a diagnosis of TB should always be evaluated, but the AAP/ACOG Guidelines for Perinatal Care (Kilpatrick et al. 2017) do not recommend routine TB screening for low-risk women. They do, however, recommend TB screening for pregnant patients with the following high-risk factors:

- Known HIV infection.
- Close contact with individuals known or suspected to have TB.
- Medical risk factors are known to increase the risk of disease if infected (such as diabetes, lupus, cancer, alcoholism, and drug addiction).
- Birth in or emigration from high-prevalent countries.
- Being medically underserved.
- Homelessness, living or working in long-term care facilities, such as correctional institutions, mental health institutions, and nursing homes (Kilpatrick et al. 2017).

There are two types of tests available to screen pregnant patients for TB infection, the tuberculin skin test (TST or Mantoux test) and a blood test, an interferon-gamma release assay (IGRA). These are discussed in detail in Chap. 6, Section 6.4.2.

2.7.6 Real-Life Example

A 15 year-old patient presents for an initial prenatal visit at 12 weeks EGA. She has no complaints. Routine prenatal labs were done including routine screening for GC, CT, HIV, and Hep C. Results were positive for GC and CT which were treated per CDC protocol and expedited partner therapy was provided. Patient education on condom use for STI prevention and STI rescreening every trimester was discussed.

Key Learning about Sexual Transmitted Infections

- The CDC, ACOG, and AAP all endorse universal screening for HIV for all pregnant patients as early as possible using an opt-out approach.
- For GC and CT, NAAT testing via clinician- or patient-collected (equivalent sensitivity and specificity) vaginal swab is the preferred testing method; however, cervical and urine samples can also be used.
- HSV screening is not routinely recommended.
- Syphilis easily crosses the placenta, potentially causing long-term adverse effects on any fetal organ system, and 40% of newborn (congenital) syphilis cases result in miscarriage, stillbirth, or neonatal death.
- Pregnant patients should be re-screened in the third trimester for any first-trimester positive results if they remain in a high-risk group for reinfection or if they engage in high-risk behaviors.
- The 2020 CDC updated guidelines state that all pregnant patients should be screened for hepatitis C virus (HCV) unless geographic prevalence rates are <0.1%.

2.8 Blood Lead Level Screening

Blood lead levels increase during pregnancy due to physiologic changes in calcium metabolism in the bone that facilitate the bioavailability of lead in the bloodstream. Maternal lead levels correlate with neonatal cord blood levels confirming that lead crosses the placenta, and prenatal lead exposure at a wide range of levels has been associated with several adverse perinatal outcomes, including spontaneous abortion, gestational hypertension, low birth weight, and impaired neurodevelopment. At present, ACOG (2019), in line with the CDC, does not recommend routine lead screening for all pregnant patients in favor of a risk-based approach which calls for state and local health departments to provide clinicians with guidelines to inform population-specific screening guidelines.

Recent public health crises in Flint, Michigan, and East Chicago, Indiana, have brought to light that children in many communities in the USA, particularly in poor communities of color, are at high risk for lead exposure (Sacks and Balding 2018). Thousands of municipalities across the country have been identified as high-risk lead exposure areas, particularly in urban and industrial parts of the country, and these high-risk areas closely correlate with elevated blood levels in children (Frostenson and Kliff 2016; Marshall et al. 2020). Pregnant women have exposures similar to young children, providing a rationale for universal risk assessment of pregnant women based on questionnaires already in use to identify children at risk which have been shown to have acceptable sensitivity and specificity for identifying pregnant women with elevated lead levels (Gardella 2001). Risk factors for lead poisoning are found in Chap. 4, Sect. 4.4.

Table 2.6 outlines blood level parameters and associated recommended follow-up testing in pregnancy.

2.9 Late Pregnancy Laboratory Screening and Testing

Testing in the last trimester includes testing for gestational diabetes, for Group B Strep (GBS), and potentially for rupture of membranes. These

Table 2.6 Recommended blood lead level follow-up during pregnancy

Venous blood lead level	<5 mcg/dL	5–14 mcg/dL	15–24 mcg/dL	25–44 mcg/dL	≥45 mcg/dL
Recommended follow-up testing	None needed	Within 1 month and at delivery (maternal)	Within 1 month, then q 2–3 months and at delivery (maternal or cord blood)	Within 1–4 weeks, then q months and at delivery (maternal or cord blood)	Within 24 hrs.; interval frequency depends on trending levels; at delivery (maternal or cord blood) Note: Specialist referral required and recommended against breastfeeding

Adapted from ACOG (2019)

tests are included here for pediatric providers of obstetrical care in primary care settings for adolescents who might not get regular, specialty obstetric care.

2.9.1 Gestational Diabetes Mellitus Screening (24–28 Weeks)

The normal hormonal and metabolic changes of pregnancy promote insulin resistance in the late second and third trimesters of pregnancy, providing the fetus with a consistent and adequate supply of nutrients. Most pregnant people maintain euglycemia despite this physiologic insulin resistance; however, those who cannot produce enough extra insulin necessary to maintain euglycemia are at risk for developing gestational diabetes mellitus (GDM). The American Diabetes Association (ADA) defines GDM as diabetes diagnosed in the second or third trimester of pregnancy which was not overt diabetes before the pregnancy (ADA 2020). GDM complicates up to 16% of pregnancies in the USA (Correa et al. 2015). The resultant alterations in fetal glucose and lipid metabolism commonly provoke excessive fetal growth or macrosomia. Macrosomia underlies many of the adverse outcomes associated with GDM, including preterm labor and birth, the need for cesarean birth, and neonatal birth injuries (ACOG 2018c). While for most people euglycemia returns almost immediately after delivery, GDM increases the risk for developing type 2 diabetes mellitus later in life and is also an independent risk factor for child-

hood overweight and obesity and metabolic syndrome in the offspring (Garcia-Vargas et al. 2012; Vounzoulaki et al. 2020; Wang et al. 2018). While the risk of GDM increases with maternal age, several other risk factors, including overweight/obesity, having a first-degree relative with diabetes, or being a member of higher risk racial or ethnic groups, increase GDM risk among pregnant adolescents to the same degree as pregnant adults.

There is currently little to no consensus among the different national and international professional organizations regarding screening guidelines or diagnostic criteria for GDM. The main issues that drive guideline variations include whether or not to screen asymptomatic pregnant people before 24 weeks EGA, what screening regimen to use, and what glucose levels are diagnostic for GDM. The lack of consensus results from evaluations of the available evidence that differentially weigh the benefits and harms of screening asymptomatic women early in pregnancy and the lack of an evidence-based cutoff threshold for the maternal glucose level at which adverse perinatal outcomes occur. Essentially, the strategies vary in their risk for over- or under-diagnoses (sensitivity and specificity), and there are data to support various strategies and diagnostic criteria. Further research is needed to resolve the ongoing debates regarding the screening, diagnosis, and treatment of GDM (Bilous et al. 2021).

The majority of US obstetric care providers adhere to the ADA (2020) and ACOG (2018c) guidelines which call for universal screening at

24–28 weeks. Both professional organizations also agree that early screening at the initial prenatal visit should be considered for high-risk patients who are overweight or obese (BMI $\geq$ 25 kg/m^2 or $\geq$ 23 kg/m^2 in Asian Americans) and have one or more of the following additional risk factors for diabetes:

- History of GDM or birth of an infant weighing $\geq$4000 g in a previous pregnancy or adolescent's mother with a history of DM or GDM during the adolescent's gestation.
- First- or second-degree relative with diabetes.
- Sedentary lifestyle.
- Hgb A1C $\geq$5.7% (39 mmol/mol); impaired glucose tolerance or impaired fasting glucose on any previous testing.
- High-risk race/ethnicity (African American, Latino, Native American, Asian American, Pacific Islander).
- History of cardiovascular disease, elevated HDL or triglycerides, hypertension ($\geq$140/90 mmHg), or hypertension therapy.
- Other clinical conditions associated with insulin resistance (severe obesity, hyperandrogenic disorder).

If an early (first trimester) screening test is negative, laboratory screening is repeated at 24–28 weeks gestation. If an early screening test is positive, but follow-up diagnostic testing is negative, only the diagnostic testing must be repeated at 24–28 weeks gestation.

Two screening and diagnostic methods are endorsed by the ADA, a two-step and a one-step method. The two-step method, also endorsed by ACOG and the National Institutes of Health (NIH), currently remains the most common protocol utilized in the USA.

2.9.1.1 Screening for Gestational Diabetes: The One-Step Method

The one-step method was advanced by the International Association of Diabetes and Pregnancy Study Group (IADPSG) based on results of a large-scale, prospective study of GDM called the Hyperglycemia and Adverse Pregnancy Outcomes (HAPO; HAPO Hyperglycemia and Adverse Perinatal Outcomes Study Cooperative Research Group et al. 2008) study. In addition to the ADA supporting the one-step protocol as an option, it is endorsed by several international professional organizations including the International Federation of Gynecology and Obstetrics, the Australasian Diabetes in Pregnancy Society, and the WHO as well as the Endocrine Society in the USA.

Step 1 is the 1-h glucose challenge test (OGCT), whereby the patient (non-fasting) drinks a concentrated glucose solution (50 g of sugar dissolved in 8 oz. of water) and has plasma glucose levels assessed after 1 h. In using a single step, the protocol acts simultaneously as a screening and diagnostic test. A fasting plasma glucose level is drawn, and a 75-gram oral glucose load is administered, after which 1- and 2-h plasma glucose levels are assessed. Only one abnormal value is required for the diagnosis of GDM. The specific plasma glucose cutoff level for a positive screen is 130, 135, or 140 mg/dL. The cutoff is generally based on community prevalence rates of GDM, and ACOG favors a cutoff of $\geq$135 mg/dL. Levels above the cutoff threshold prompt the second step, with the exception that a plasma glucose level $\geq$ 200 mg/dL at the first step is considered diagnostic for GDM.

2.9.1.2 Screening for Gestational Diabetes: The Two-Step Method

Step 2 is a 3-h glucose tolerance test (OGTT) whereby the patient's blood (plasma or serum) glucose level is assessed after an overnight fast (no caloric intake for at least 8 h). The patient drinks a concentrated glucose solution (100 g of sugar dissolved in 8 oz. of water), and blood glucose levels are assessed at 1, 2, and 3 h post-glucose solution administration. There are different criteria for cutoff levels for abnormal results, one proposed by the National Diabetes Data Group (NDDG 1979) and the other by Carpenter and Coustan (1982). Again, one is not recommended over the other, but providers and institutions are encouraged to adopt and adhere to a single standardization protocol. While the standard practice has long required two abnormal levels out of the four assessed to diagnose GDM, ACOG endorses the use of either one or two abnormal values based on a growing body of evidence that even one abnormal value is associated with adverse perinatal outcomes (Cheng et al. 2009; ACOG 2018c).

Table 2.7 indicates the diagnostic cutoff criteria for GDM. Glucose levels greater than or equal to the thresholds meet the criteria for the diagnosis of GDM. One or two abnormal levels may be used to diagnose the two-step protocols depending on patient population and practice protocols; just one abnormal level is needed in the one-step protocol.

2.9.1.3 Other Laboratory Tests Used, but Not Recommended for Gestational Diabetes

A urine dipstick positive for glycosuria with a normal blood glucose level is common in pregnant women. Pregnancy is associated with reductions in reabsorption of glucose, resulting in higher rates of urinary excretion. Therefore, glycosuria has both poor positive and negative predictive validity for GDM. Similarly, the sensitivity of hemoglobin A1C, a measure of average blood sugar levels over the previous 2–3 months, can be affected by race/ethnicity, hemoglobinopathies, HIV, and pregnancy itself (second trimester). All of these factors alter the relationship of A1C to plasma blood sugar levels.

For this reason, A1C is not the preferred screening or diagnostic test for GDM, especially after the second trimester. However, the ADA (2020) uses standard diagnostic criteria for overt diabetes in high-risk pregnant patients screened in the first trimester. The ADA Standard Criteria for the Diagnosis of Diabetes is found in Chap. 4, Table 4.9. These criteria can be used for high-risk pregnant patients screened in the first trimester, and the ADA guidelines further specify that "in the absence of unequivocal hyperglycemia, diagnosis requires two abnormal test results from the same sample or in two separate test samples" (ADA 2020, p. S16).

There is consensus in the scientific and medical communities that interventions improve glycemic control and perinatal outcomes (Hartling et al. 2013). Nutrition and exercise therapy is the cornerstone of treatment for GDM (class A1GDM), with the addition of insulin therapy

when daily self-monitoring indicates that the goal of glycemic control is not being met by nutritional and exercise-based interventions (class A2GDM). Patient self-glucose monitoring includes four daily capillary blood glucose levels, and based on expert opinion, the following are the abnormal level thresholds: fasting, ≥95 md/dL; 1-hour postprandial, ≥ 140 mg/dL; 2-hour postprandial, ≥120 mg/dL; and 2 a.m.–6 a.m., ≤60 mg/dL) (ACOG 2018d). Management also involves the increased frequency of prenatal visits, additional maternal and fetal monitoring, and possibly planned induction of labor or C-section. Multiple barriers exist to pregnant adolescents modifying their diet and exercise and carefully monitoring their glucose levels. A team approach utilizing social workers, dieticians, and diabetes educators is necessary to ensure optimal outcomes.

Finally, a systematic review of the literature found that patients with GDM have nearly ten times the risk of developing type 2 diabetes mellitus (T2DM) later in life than people who do not have GDM. The authors further concluded that GDM could essentially be a reliable predictor of later development of T2DM (Vounzoulaki et al. 2020). It follows that postpartum follow-up is key to identifying T2DM in the GDM population; however, numerous studies have indicated that adherence to postpartum screening guidelines

Table 2.7 Diagnostic cutoff criteria for GDM

Two-step Carpenter and Coustan (1982) (plasma or serum level)	Two-step National Diabetes Data Group (1979) (plasma level)	One-step International Association of Diabetes and Pregnancy Study Groups Consensus Panel et al. (2010) (plasma level)
Fasting: 95 mg/dL 1 hour: 180 mg/dL 2 hours: 155 mg/dL 3 hours: 140 mg/dL	Fasting: 105 mg/dL 1 hour: 190 mg/dL 2 hours: 165 mg/dL 3 hours: 145 mg/dL	Fasting: 92 mg/dL 1 hour: 180 mg/dL 2 hours: 153 mg/dL

Adapted from Carpenter and Coustan 1982; National Diabetes Data Group 1979; International Association of Diabetes and Pregnancy Study Groups Consensus Panel et al. 2010 is poorly followed by both patients and providers (Seidu and Khunti 2012). Some studies (Hale et al. 2012; Hunt et al. 2010) estimate that more than half of GDM patients do not receive the follow-up screenings recommended by the ADA (2020), which include the following:

- Four to twelve weeks postpartum screening with a 75-g oral glucose tolerance test and clinically appropriate non-pregnancy diagnostic criteria.
- Lifelong screening for the development of diabetes or prediabetes at least every 3 years (fasting blood glucose, random plasma glucose, or A1C).
- Prediabetic patients with a history of GDM should receive intensive lifestyle interventions and/or metformin to prevent diabetes.

The same barriers that can prevent adolescents from adequately managing GDM could prevent adequate follow-up postpartum screening. One study suggests that a normal postpartum day two screening OGTT before hospital discharge after delivery appears to exclude type 2 diabetes at the 4–12-week screening test and may be useful given the challenges of follow-up after discharge (Carter et al. 2018). Finally, the ADA recommends that once females with diabetes reach puberty, preconception counseling should be a routine part of their health care (ADA 2020).

2.9.1.4 Group B Streptococcal Screening (36–38 Weeks)

For some people, Group B Streptococcal (GBS), a gram-positive bacterium, is a natural part of the gastrointestinal and vaginal microbiome. Colonization in the vagina and rectum occurs in 10–30% of pregnant women and may be transient or continuous colonization. GBS infection is the most frequent neonatal infection. Without adequate treatment in labor, it has a 50% chance of vertical transmission, with 1–2% of those cases developing into GBS early-onset disease in the newborn. GBS early-onset disease is defined as symptom development, most frequently sepsis and pneumonia, during the first 7 days of life. GBS screening during the prenatal period is vital to ensure delivery providers can adequately treat during labor to prevent vertical transmission (ACOG 2020b).

Universal screening for GBS is recommended for every pregnant person regardless of the planned mode of delivery. Screening is performed during the third trimester, between 36 0/7 and 37 6/7 weeks gestation. The sample is collected by swabbing the introitus of the vagina first and then, with the same swab, the rectum through the anal sphincter (ACOG 2020b). The swab should be moved from side to side or rotated at the collection site, allowing several seconds to absorb organisms. Cervical, perianal, perirectal, or perineal specimens are unacceptable, and a speculum should not be used for culture collection. The swab is placed in a tube with a transport medium, and the lab order is for Group B *Streptococcus* colonization detection culture with reflex to susceptibilities. Importantly, if any prenatal urine culture is positive for GBS bacteremia at any point in a pregnancy, treatment is required both at the time of detection and during labor. In that case, the 36–38-week GBS screening can be omitted. Because GBS can be a transient infection, it is reassessed in each pregnancy to determine if treatment is indicated. GBS status should be documented in the patient's prenatal chart so that delivery providers know the need for treatment upon admission to the hospital. Finally, screening during subsequent pregnancy can be entirely omitted for patients with a history of an infant diagnosed with GBS early-onset disease since these patients should automatically be treated during labor in subsequent pregnancies (ACOG 2020b).

2.9.2 Testing for Rupture of Membranes

Some studies have shown that the incidence of prelabor rupture of membranes (PROM) and preterm PROM is higher in adolescent pregnancies (Marković et al. 2020; Bostancı Ergen et al. 2017), so all providers who care for adolescents may need to diagnose PROM. PROM refers to the rupture of the amniotic sac before the onset of labor contractions and, when labor doesn't begin within 24 h after the rupture, can pose a risk for infection.

Preterm PROM is a rupture of membranes that occurs before 37 weeks, and it poses all the consequent risks of prematurity. Fluid samples can be evaluated for nitrazine strip/pH testing (amniotic fluid pH is ≥ 7 compared to vaginal pH = 3.8–4.5), microscopic observation of ferning (the characteristic unique crystallization pattern of amniotic fluid when it dries), evaluation for the presence of fetal fibronectin (a protein at the interface of the amniotic sac and the uterine lining), or commercially available tests for the presence of other amniotic proteins (ACOG 2020c).

2.9.2.1 Nitrazine Strip/pH Testing

The diagnosis of PROM and preterm PROM is based on history, physical examination, and positive point-of-care testing. Digital exams are avoided to reduce the risk of infection. A sterile speculum exam allows observation of fluid at the cervical os and pooling of fluid in the vagina. ROM is typically diagnosed based on history and exam, but no single observation or test confirms ROM. For example, observation of pooling of fluid in the posterior fornix of the vagina via a sterile speculum exam alone is not diagnostic for rupture of membranes without confirmation via ferning or nitrazine testing (Hunter 2015).

2.9.2.2 Point of Care Fetal Fibronectin Tests/Amniotic Proteins

The sensitivity of point-of-care fetal fibronectin tests and the specificity of point-of-care tests for amniotic proteins have been called into question. Neither is to be used independently of other assessments to diagnose ROM (ACOG 2020c). Both term PROM and preterm PROM will necessitate patients to have further workup and monitoring at a hospital with labor and delivery capacity and possibly a NICU.

2.9.3 Real-Life Example

A 17 year old, BMI 44, presents to the ED reporting abdominal pain and states "I feel like I'm peeing on myself." Her history included irregular menses since menarche including long stretches of up to several months of amenorrhea. She could not recall her LMP. Physical exam and ultrasound were consistent with pregnancy of 40 weeks EGA, nitrazine strip testing was positive for amniotic fluid, and the cervix was fully dilated indicating active labor. Within 30 min of her arrival at the ED, she delivered a healthy infant. The adolescent reported she was unaware she was pregnant because she associated her symptoms over the past 10 months with GI upset which was common for her. In addition, she was used to many months of amenorrhea, related to obesity which can result in anovulatory cycles.

Key Learning about Third-Trimester Screening

- Testing in the last trimester includes testing for gestational diabetes, for Group B Strep (GBS), and potentially for rupture of membranes.
- GBS infection is the most frequent neonatal infection, and GBS screening should be done at 36–38 weeks of gestation.
- PROM refers to the rupture of the amniotic sac before the onset of labor contractions and, when labor doesn't begin within 24 h after the rupture, can pose a risk for infection.
- Fluid samples from the mother can be evaluated for nitrazine strip/pH testing, microscopic observation of ferning, evaluation for the presence of fetal fibronectin, or commercially available tests for the presence of other amniotic proteins.

2.10 Fetal Surveillance

2.10.1 Methods of Fetal Surveillance

In addition to augmented laboratory testing, many obstetric conditions may warrant increased fetal surveillance during pregnancy. Some obstetric care providers with experience, training, and demonstrated competence may engage in interprofessional collaborative care for patients with pre-existing conditions or gestational conditions requiring additional fetal surveillance. There are guidelines for increased fetal surveillance for intrauterine growth restriction, gestational diabetes, or hypertensive disorders. Some of the basic clinical tools for additional fetal surveillance are discussed briefly below. In general, fetal surveillance methods include monitoring fetal heart rate, fetal movement, amniotic fluid levels, or umbilical artery blood flow. These methods help identify the risk for fetal hypoxia and/or whether the fetus is neurologically intact. Note that, minimally, consultation, but likely referral to obstetric or maternal-fetal medicine specialists, would be required when additional fetal surveillance is necessary.

2.10.1.1 The Nonstress Test (NST)

The nonstress test (NST) records a fetal heart rate tracing from an external ultrasonographic monitor on the maternal abdomen for at least 20 minutes. Normal fetal heart rate is between 110 and 160 bpm. The NST assesses the baseline fetal heart rate (sustained fetal heart rate for 2 min out of 10) and accelerations and decelerations from the baseline. Acceleration is defined as an increase above the baseline by at least 15 bpm for at least 15 seconds, or for a fetus ≤32 6/7 weeks gestation or less, at least 10 bpm for at least 10 s (ACOG 2014, reaffirmed 2020; Glantz and Bertoia 2011). A normal, reactive NST has two heart rate accelerations from baseline within 20 minutes, which is reassuring of fetal well-being because accelerations reflect an appropriate increase in heart rate in response to fetal movement, suggesting that the fetus is neurologically intact and not acidotic. An abnormal, nonreactive NST with no accelerations after 40 mins with or without vibroacoustic stimulation, such as clapping near the maternal abdomen or using a device such as an artificial larynx (Hasanpour et al. 2013), warrants further testing as a biophysical profile (discussed below). NSTs are used to monitor fetal well-being weekly or twice weekly for many conditions in pregnancy and for post-term pregnancies or to evaluate a maternal report of decreased fetal movement, and standards for the evaluation of fetal heart rate tracings were established by the National Institute of Child Health and Human Development Workshop Report on Electronic Fetal Monitoring (Macones et al. 2008).

2.10.1.2 The Contraction Stress Test (CST)

The contraction stress test (CST) assesses fetal heart rate in response to maternal contractions induced by intravenous Pitocin or patient self-stimulation of the nipples if they are not occurring naturally at the time of the test (ACOG 2014, reaffirmed 2020). The CST is used far less frequently than the NST. Since the CST can induce labor, it is contraindicated when labor and delivery would be contraindicated (e.g., preterm gestation, placenta previa, maternal history of uterine surgery). For this reason, the majority of professional organizations recommend the use of NSTs versus CSTs for antenatal fetal surveillance (Johnson et al. 2018). The fetal heart rate is traced and observed for the presence or absence of late decelerations. Late deceleration is a gradual decline of the fetal heart rate over at least 30 s from start to nadir that occurs after the contraction peak. This late deceleration pattern indicates poor fetal recovery from the stressor of the contraction. If late decelerations follow ≥50% of contractions, the test is considered positive/abnormal.

2.10.1.3 Amniotic Fluid Index (AFI) and Maximum Vertical Pocket (MVP)

Amniotic fluid index (AFI) and maximum vertical pocket (MVP) measure the level of amniotic fluid volume via abdominal ultrasound. Amniotic fluid volume is considered a fetal vital sign as it reflects the function of several fetal organ systems. AFI measures the anteroposterior diameters in centimeters of the deepest, unobstructed pocket of amniotic fluid in four quadrants of the uterus and adds them together. An 8–18 cm AFI score is normal, while measurements under 8 cm and over 24 cm require further assessment. The MVP is the deepest unobstructed vertical pocket in any quadrant of the uterus, and ≥2 cm is considered within normal limits.

2.10.1.4 Biophysical Profile (BPP)

A biophysical profile (BPP) combines five different elements, including the NST and AFI assessments, to produce a score out of 10 possible points

(2 if the element is present, 0 if not present). BPP scores of 8–10 are normal, 5–7 are equivocal/abnormal, 4 or less is abnormal and indicates fetal distress requiring emergency delivery. It can be used for routine or scheduled surveillance for high-risk maternal and fetal conditions, a further assessment of a non-reactive NST, or further assessment of an abnormal AFI. The five elements include (ACOG 2014, reaffirmed 2020):

1. Nonstress test – 2 points for a reactive test.
2. Fetal breathing movements – 2 points for one or more episodes of rhythmic fetal breathing within a 30-minute timeframe.
3. Fetal movement – 2 points for three or more body or limb movements within a 30-minute timeframe.
4. Fetal tone – 2 points for one or more fetal extensions and return to flexion within a 30-minute timeframe.
5. Amniotic fluid volume – 2 points for a single vertical pocket of greater than 2 cm.

2.10.1.5 Umbilical Artery Doppler Velocimetry

Doppler velocimetry is an ultrasound technique used to assess circulation in many clinical conditions. Flow velocity in the umbilical artery of growth-restricted fetuses differs from normally developing fetuses, and abnormal velocity waveforms are associated with neonatal morbidity and mortality. Umbilical artery Doppler waveforms can also differentiate pathological growth restriction from a small but healthy developing fetus. Its use is associated with significantly reduced stillbirth rates in the setting of fetal growth restriction. (ACOG 2014, 2021).

2.10.1.6 Maternal-Fetal Movement Assessment

Maternal perception of decreased fetal activity has long been associated with an increased risk of stillbirth (Sadovsky and Yaffe 1973; Leader et al. 1981). Heazell et al. (2018) found that women who experienced a stillbirth reported less overall monitoring of fetal activity. They reported that providers did not instruct them to monitor fetal activity. Also, they reported a significantly decreased or a marked increase in the usual fetal movement patterns in the 2 weeks before fetal demise. While no single method of fetal movement counting is superior to another, one common method considers ten movements in 2 h to be reassuring. The mean time to a count of 10 is approximately 21 min (Moore and Piacquadio 1989). More importantly, all pregnant patients should be educated that fetal movement is an important indicator of fetal well-being. Any significant change in fetal movement patterns should be reported to a provider.

2.10.2 Real-Life Example

A 17 year old at 38 weeks EGA followed her providers instructions and called to report decreased fetal movement for the past 12 hours. The provider sent the teen to Labor and Delivery where the NST was nonreactive and BPP score was 5. The infant was delivered via emergency c-section, was determined to be low birth weight, spent 3 days in the NICU and was discharged to home doing well.

Key Learning about Fetal Surveillance

- A nonstress test (NST) records a fetal heart rate tracing from an external ultrasonographic monitor on the maternal abdomen for at least 20 min.
- A biophysical profile includes a nonstress test, fetal breathing movements, fetal body/limb movement, fetal tone, and amniotic fluid volume. Each element is scored 0–2 points and a score of 8–10 is reassuring.
- A contraction stress test (CST) assesses fetal heart rate in response to maternal contractions induced by intravenous Pitocin or patient self-stimulation of the nipples if they are not occurring naturally at the time of the test.
- Education about fetal movement is important as decreased fetal activity is associated with stillbirth. Ten movements in 2 h are considered within normal ranges.

2.11 Genetic Screening and Testing

The number and complexity of prenatal genetic screening and diagnostic tests have grown exponentially in recent years with technological advances in genetics and genomics. Currently available options allow for noninvasive, highly sensitive, and specific prenatal screening for and diagnosis of hundreds of genetic conditions. Prenatal diagnosis of fetal genetic conditions and congenital anomalies can help pregnant patients and their families prepare to care for an infant with special needs or inform the decision on whether to continue or terminate a pregnancy. Prenatal genetic screening and testing results must be communicated to consider further diagnostic testing and all management options.

Given the evolving complexity of the genetic screening and testing landscape, patient-centered counseling and shared decision-making that foster patient autonomy and informed consent are of utmost importance. All providers who offer prenatal genetic testing must understand the risks, benefits, and limitations of available screening and testing options and be prepared to utilize genetics professionals to interpret genetic testing results (ACOG 2018d; Knutzen and Stoll 2019). Health-care providers who do not have the necessary knowledge of genetics to counsel patients appropriately should refer to a genetic counselor or maternal-fetal medicine specialist. Numerous resources exist to inform providers which screening or diagnostic tests should be offered based on availability, insurance coverage, and timing of a patient's entry into prenatal care. Table 2.8 shows a selection of genetics-related resources.

2.11.1 Prenatal Screening Versus Diagnostic Testing

Patients and providers need to be clear about the difference between screening and diagnostic testing. Screening tests assess whether a pregnant patient is at increased risk for having an affected fetus, while diagnostic tests definitively diagnose whether a condition is present in the fetus of a patient identified to be at elevated risk. The only diagnostic tests for genetic disorders in prenatal care are chorionic villus sampling (CVS) or amniocentesis, and ultrasound alone can diagnose certain structural anomalies, including heart defects or open neural tube defects (ONTDs) like spina bifida. The remaining tests, including first- and second-trimester integrated or sequential screening for aneuploidy, carrier testing for genetic conditions, or cell-free DNA testing, are all considered screening tests that only estimate the chances that a fetus will have a condition. These tests also vary in their sensitivity, the degree to which the test correctly identifies a fetus with a condition, and specificity, the degree to which the test correctly identifies a fetus without a condition. Therefore, follow-up diagnostic testing is always necessary to confirm any screening test result. It is important to note that ACOG recommends offering all screening and diagnostic options to all pregnant patients regardless of age or risk profile, with appropriate and thorough counseling regarding the risks, benefits, and limitations of any approach and the opportunity to accept or decline any or all such testing (ACOG 2020d).

Once the patient has been counseled on the testing options (screening or diagnostic testing or

Table 2.8 Genetics counseling resources

Organization/resource	URL
National Society of Genetic Counselors NIPT cFDNA Screening Predictive Value Calculator	https://www.perinatalquality.org/Vendors/NSGC/NIPT/
National Society of Genetic Counselors Finding a genetic counselor	https://findageneticcounselor.nsgc.org/
Genetic Support Foundation/Washington State Department of Health Video Series	https://geneticsupportfoundation.org/
ACOG Cell-Free DNA Infographic	https://www.acog.org/womens-health/infographics/cell-free-dna-prenatal-screening-test

Table developed by authors

neither), if they choose screening testing, they must be counseled on the screening test options available to them for their gestational age. There are several screening protocols; however, only one should be used at a time. Further, only one protocol may be appropriate to offer given the EGA, community or institutional standards of practice, or insurance coverage issues. Patients should be counseled that a negative or normal screening test result does not rule out all risk, and each testing protocol has the potential for false-negative results. The tests include ultrasound and maternal blood tests that assess protein biomarker levels or analytes produced by the placenta, which can be found in the maternal circulation and correlate with different aneuploidies and NTDs. In general, regarding ultrasound and analytes, the greater the number of individual pieces of information that contribute to the screening test picture, the more sensitive and specific it becomes, providing a more accurate estimate of the presence of an anomaly in an affected fetus and decreasing the likelihood of falsely identifying increased risk when none exists.

2.11.1.1 Carrier Screening for Genetic Conditions

Mutations can cause a genetic disorder in one gene (e.g., cystic fibrosis, thalassemia, or sickle cell disease), a combination of gene mutations and environmental factors (e.g., many cancers, type 2 diabetes, obesity), or damage to the structure or number of chromosomes (e.g., Trisomy 21 or Down syndrome). Carrier screening for genetic conditions identifies autosomal recessive disorders that can be inherited throughout generations of a family without anyone's knowledge. While carrier screening is ideally performed before pregnancy as part of preconception care, most carrier screening is performed at an initial prenatal visit.

Some genetic conditions have higher prevalence rates within specific populations, and targeted screening, limited to those high-risk populations, is one screening option. However, given that the USA is a multiracial and multiethnic country, ACOG (2017f) recommends offering expanded or panethnic carrier screening to all pregnant patients regardless of ancestry. While expanded carrier screening panels can include hundreds of genetic disorders, ACOG recommends that, at a minimum, an expanded carrier screening panel should routinely include screening for cystic fibrosis, spinal muscular atrophy, thalassemia, and hemoglobinopathies (ACOG 2017f).

Any positive genetic screening result should prompt screening of the reproductive partner because, if both parents are carriers of the same genetic condition, their offspring have a 25% chance of having the condition, a 50% chance of being a carrier, and a 25% chance of not having or being a carrier of the condition. If both parents have positive carrier screening tests for the same condition, diagnostic testing (CVS or amniocentesis) appropriate to fetal EGA can be offered. Table 2.9 reviews the increased carrier frequency of particular genetic conditions by ancestry, reliable resources for condition information, screening recommendations, and associated genetic mutation and condition characteristics.

2.11.2 First-Trimester Screening

First-trimester screening includes ultrasound measurement of the nuchal fold, or nuchal translucency, and two analytes, pregnancy-associated plasma protein-A (PAPP-A) and human chorionic gonadotropin (HCG). The nuchal fold is a fluid-filled space on the dorsum of the fetal neck. A measurement ≥ 3.0 mm is considered enlarged, and the degree of enlargement correlates with the degree of increased risk. The ultrasound portion is independently associated with an increased risk of fetal aneuploidies and other structural abnormalities. Elevated or decreased analyte levels are differentially associated with different fetal anomalies. For example, elevated HCG is associated with an increased risk for Trisomy 21 (Down syndrome).

2.11.2.1 Cell-Free DNA (cfDNA)

cfDNA is a screening test using a maternal blood sample that can be performed beginning at 9 weeks of gestation. To date, while ACOG and

Table 2.9 Increased carrier frequency by ancestry/population

Condition and resource	High-risk ancestry	Carrier frequency	Genetic mutation and condition characteristics
Cystic fibrosis https://www.cff.org/ What-is-CF/ About-Cystic-Fibrosis/	Caucasian Ashkenazi Jewish	1/29 1/29	Mutation in the CFTR gene: Result in a buildup of thick mucus in the lungs and GI tract; average life span of 30–40 years
Tay-Sachs disease http://www.curetay-sachs.org/	Ashkenazi Jewish French Canadian Cajun (LA)	1/30 1/15–1/30 1/27	Mutation in the hexosaminidase subunit alpha (HEXA) gene results in fatty deposits in the brain; average life span of 3–5 years
Canavan disease https://www.ninds.nih.gov/ disorders/All-disorders/ canavan-disease-information-page	Ashkenazi Jewish	1/40–58	Mutations in the ASPA gene results in the accumulation of NAA in brain tissue, resulting in damage to white matter; life span up to 10 years
Familial dystonia https://rarediseases.org/ rare-diseases/dystonia/	Ashkenazi Jewish	1/27	Mutations in several genes result in involuntary muscle contractions, twisting of specific body parts, tremors, and other uncontrolled movements; average life span of 30 years
Spinal muscular dystrophy https://smafoundation.org/	Caucasian Asian Ashkenazi Jewish	1/47 1/59 1/67	Mutation in the SMN1 gene on chromosome 5 causes failure to produce the survival motor neuron (SMN) protein; results in motor neuron loss in the spinal cord and lower brainstem, muscle weakness, and atrophy; average life span of 2 years
Fragile X syndrome https://fragilex.org/	Females Males	1/151 1/458	Mutation in the FMR1 gene decreases the production of the protein FMRP needed for brain development; results in characteristic physical features and developmental and intellectual delays; normal life span

Adapted from Jordan 2019. Additional sources: websites of national organizations as indicated

the Society for Maternal-Fetal Medicine recommend all screening and diagnostic options available be offered to all pregnant women regardless of age or risk, current guidelines recommend the use of cfDNA only in high-risk populations as its sensitivity and specificity depend on the patient's background risk level and several other factors, making false positives common in low-risk populations (ACOG 2020d). Because maternal blood has maternal and fetal cfDNA, which is more accurately placental DNA, the test's accuracy relies on the fetal fraction of total cf. DNA in the maternal bloodstream. Notably, cfDNA is used to diagnose fetal sex and blood type (with 96.6% sensitivity and 98.9% specificity), but, while it is the most sensitive and specific screening test for the common aneuploidies, it is not currently considered diagnostic for chromosomal conditions because the placental karyotype and fetal karyotype can differ somewhat molecularly (Brison et al. 2018; Pertile et al. 2017; Wright et al. 2012). Note that new protocols, particularly for contingent screening, that utilize cfDNA following first- and/or second-trimester screening results have shown high levels of sensitivity and specificity relative to CVS and amniocentesis and are increasingly being investigated and introduced (Galeva et al. 2019).

It is important to note that, at the time of the publication of this text, a paradigm shift in the field of antepartum screening for fetal genetic and chromosomal disorders is on the horizon. The usefulness of NT assessment and the various screening paradigm options indicated in Table 2.10 are under investigation given the ease and rapidly increasing availability and affordability of cfDNA testing and its robust sensitivity and specificity for detecting both common and rare chromosomal abnormalities (Huang et al. 2018; Kane et al. 2021). cfDNA testing is also potentially poised to largely replace invasive CVS and amniocentesis procedures (discussed below). Prenatal care providers should remain vigilant for professional society guideline updates from

Table 2.10 Current prenatal screening and diagnostic testing options

Gestational age for timing of test	Tests and analytes	Detection rates Trisomy 21[a] (test sensitivity)
	Screening tests	
First trimester 10–14 weeks	Ultrasound: Nuchal translucency (NT) Papp-A and hCG	NT alone: 60–70% Analytes alone: 67% Combined: 85%
Second trimester 15–18 weeks	Routine ultrasound: Anatomy scan Triple screen Quad screen	Ultrasound alone: 73% 3 analytes alone: 60–70% 4 analytes alone: 75–80% Combined: 83%
Integrated screening	Combines: First-trimester NT, Papp-A, and hCG With second-trimester quad screen and anatomy scan Final results: Only after second-trimester testing	85–96%
Sequential Stepwise Contingent	First-trimester NT, Papp-A, hCG If positive, no second-trimester screening tests (proceed to diagnostic testing) If negative: Proceed to second-trimester screening First-trimester NT, Papp-A, and hCG Next tests "contingent" on first-trimester level of risk: High: Diagnostic testing Moderate: second-trimester screening Low risk: No further testing	93–95%
NIPT 9+ weeks	Cell-free DNA (cfDNA) Massive and targeted DNA sequencing	99–100 (false-positive rate: <0.2)
	Diagnostic tests	
Amniocentesis 15+ weeks (typically 15–20)	Amniotic fluid Karyotyping, CMA, or direct DNA sequencing	99.5 (false-positive rate: < 0.04%)
CVS 10–14 weeks	Placental chorionic villi Karyotyping, CMA, or direct DNA sequencing	98% (false-positive rate: <0.04%)

Adapted from Bunt and Bunt 2014; Latendresse and Deneris 2015; ACOG 2016, reaffirmed 2020; Malone et al. (2005); Alldred et al. 2012; Simpson 2013; Latendresse 2015
[a]False-positive rate: 4–5% unless otherwise indicated

the American College of Obstetrics and Gynecology and the Society for Maternal-Fetal Medicine regarding recommended modes and protocols for antepartum screening for fetal aneuploidies and other conditions.

2.11.2.2 Diagnostic Testing Options: Chorionic Villus Sampling and Amniocentesis

During chorionic villus sampling, performed between 10 and 13 weeks gestation, the provider removes a small sample of the placenta's chorionic villi using an ultrasound-guided needle via a transabdominal or transcervical approach to obtain fetal DNA directly. During **amniocentesis,** performed between 15 and 22 weeks gestation, ultrasound visualization guides the insertion of a needle through the abdominal wall and into the uterus to obtain a sample of the amniotic fluid. An advantage of amniocentesis over CVS is that amniotic fluid can also be tested for alpha-fetoprotein to diagnose open neural tube defects (Knutzen and Stoll 2019). Both procedures can be done with a local anesthetic. Most women describe only mild cramping pain with these procedures and can return to non-strenuous activities the same day. A recent systematic review of the literature and updated meta-analysis concluded that CVS and amniocentesis do not significantly increase the risk of miscarriage over the background risk that prompted the testing. The safety profile is the same for both procedures (Salomon et al. 2019).

The samples obtained from CVS and amniocentesis can be examined using several processes, including molecular DNA testing, karyotyping, fluorescent in situ hybridization (FISH), or chromosomal microarray analysis (CMA). Each method of analysis differs in the conditions it is most useful for detecting. Molecular DNA detects genetic mutations. Karyotyping is a laboratory technique whereby an image of stained chromosomes highlights abnormal chromosome numbers or structures. FISH also allows for visualization of chromosomes but can detect minute parts of chromosomal microdeletions or duplications that karyotyping cannot detect. CMA screens the whole genome for copy number variants (ACOG 2016, reaffirmed 2020).

2.11.3 Second-Trimester Screening

Second-trimester screening for fetal anomalies includes a routine ultrasound anatomy scan at 18–23 weeks for all pregnant women regardless of risk factors or screening protocol choice. This ultrasound provides a complete survey of the fetal anatomy and biometry and assesses the amniotic fluid level and the placental location. In the context of aneuploidies, this ultrasound can detect soft markers of the physical abnormalities the aneuploidy would produce. If these soft markers are identified on ultrasound, a review of prior testing and future testing options would be discussed (Latendresse and Deneris 2015; Rose et al. 2020).

2.11.3.1 Triple and Quadruple Screen

In addition to the anatomy scan ultrasound, second-trimester screening can include a triple screen for the analytes alpha-fetoprotein (AFP), human chorionic gonadotropin (hCG), and unconjugated estriol (uE3), a quadruple (quad) screen which includes the three triple screen analytes plus dimeric inhibin A (DIA) or a Penta screen which includes all four quad-screen analytes plus hyperglycosylated human chorionic gonadotropin (h-hCG). Integrated sequential or contingent testing protocols combine first- and second-trimester screening results in different ways.

Analyte levels are reported as an MoM or multiple of the median, indicating how far the test result deviates from the median (middle) value of a large set of results obtained from unaffected pregnancies. An MoM ≥ 2.0 or 2.5 (lab dependent) is considered abnormal, and, to reiterate, abnormal screening test results reflect increased risk but always require follow-up for definitive diagnosis. Most importantly, because normal ranges for the analytes are specific to EGA, maternal age, race/ethnicity, and BMI, the accuracy of these patient demographics on laboratory testing orders is of utmost importance for the accuracy of risk level assessment and should be confirmed when any screening test indicates elevated risk. Table 2.10 reviews test timing, analytes, and, for example, detection and false-positive rates for the different screening and diagnostic tests for Trisomy 21 (Down syndrome).

2.11.3.2 Aneuploidy

While chromosomal abnormalities are significantly more common with advanced maternal age, particularly after age 35, they can occur in any pregnancy (Mikwar et al. 2020). Aneuploidies are an abnormal number of chromosomes in a cell, while microdeletions refer to whole missing chromosomes, and copy number variants are duplications of small parts of chromosomes (Rose et al. 2020). The trisomy aneuploidies, Down syndrome (Trisomy 21), Patau syndrome (Trisomy 13), and Edwards syndrome (Trisomy 18), result from a third chromosome, instead of the normal two, on the identified chromosome number for a total of 47 chromosomes in each cell, instead of the normal total of 46 (22 from the mother, 22 from the father, and 1 sex chromosome from each parent). Klinefelter syndrome, the most common sex chromosome-related disorder, results in males having an extra X sex chromosome (XXY). It should be made clear to patients that the results of either screening or diagnostic testing for aneuploidies will not lead to treatment options but can inform decision-making during pregnancy and after delivery (Latendresse and Deneris 2015). The complexity of screening tests for aneuploidies requires thorough pretest and posttest counseling and referral to genetic counseling for patients with risk factors and accurate interpretation of positive screening results (ACOG 2020d; Latendresse and Deneris 2015).

2.11.4 Neural Tube Defects

Neural tube defects (NTDs) result from the failure of the closure of the neural tube during embryological development, either at the cranial end (anencephaly) or the caudal end (myelomeningocele or spina bifida). NTDs have a genetic component such that maternal or paternal personal history of an NTD or having a prior child with an NTD increases the risk or having an affected pregnancy (March of Dimes 2022). However, the genetics are not well understood and specific genetic tests for NTD have yet to be developed (Dupépé et al. 2017). It is well established, however, that the risk for NTDs increases with certain maternal characteristics, such as, diabetes or obesity, and can also occur as a result of teratogenic exposures from medications, such as opioids or some anti-seizure medications, and some environmental exposures, such as high body temperature. The risk for NTDs is highest when exposures occur when the neural tube forms in the first month of pregnancy (Copp et al 2017; Egbe 2015; March of Dimes 2022; Rasmussen et al. 2008). The severity of clinical manifestations ranges for the different NTDs from mild to fatal. The diagnosis of an NTD requires specialized, interprofessional, collaborative care among maternal-fetal medicine, neonatology, pediatric neurosurgery, and genetics (ACOG 2017g; ACOG 2020d; Latendresse and Deneris 2015). Because numerous, large-scale, randomized clinical trials (Medical Research Council 1991) found adequate folic acid intake to be directly associated with decreases in the occurrence NTDs, the CDC and USPSTF have recently recommended that all reproductive-age women have a daily folic acid intake of 400mcg for the prevention of NTDs which can occur even before a person knows they are pregnant (CDC 2019b). Up to 95% of neural tube defects can be detected by the routine second-trimester anatomy scan ultrasound alone.

2.11.5 Real-Life Example

An 18 year old who has a younger sister with Cystic Fibrosis states she is currently trying for a pregnancy with her male partner who has a child with an NTD. Preconception genetic testing is recommended for both she adn her partner, and a referral to a genetic counselor is made. Folic acid 400mcg daily is recommended to be started the same day with the explanation that it can help to prevent NTDs when taken in the first 4 weeks of pregnancy, before she may even know she is pregnant.

> **Key Learning about Screening for Genetic and Chromosomal Abnormalities**
> - Carrier screening for heritable conditions is ideally done preconception so that explanations of genetic risk can be offered before pregnancy.
> - Second-trimester screening for aneuploidies and NTDs can include a triple screen for the analytes alpha-fetoprotein (AFP), human chorionic gonadotropin (hCG), and unconjugated estriol (uE3), a quadruple (quad) screen which includes the three triple screen analytes plus dimeric inhibin A (DIA) or a Penta screen which includes all four quad-screen analytes plus hyperglycosylated human chorionic gonadotropin.
> - cfDNA is a screening test using a maternal blood sample that can be performed beginning at 9 weeks of gestation. The test has a high degree of sensitivity and specificity for fetal sex, Rh type, and aneuploidies and is increasingly becoming a routine prenatal lab test that may replace cumbersome screening protocols for analytes.
> - Neural tube defects have a genetic component that is not well understood, however daily folic acid intake of 400mcg in the first weeks of pregnancy can aid in the prevention of NTDs, the vast majority of which are detected on routine, 2nd trimester anatomy scan.

2.12 Summary and Conclusions

Advanced practice pediatric providers with experience, training, and demonstrated competence could engage in preconception, prenatal, and postpartum collaborative care and provide appropriate referrals to obstetricians and maternal-fetal medicine specialists as needed. In caring for pregnant adolescents, pediatric providers are tasked with ordering and interpreting the necessary laboratory tests to maximize maternal and fetal well-being. Understanding pregnancy testing and interpretation and preparing to provide pregnancy decision-making counseling; conducting, ordering, and interpreting early ultrasounds for gestational age dating; and ordering the routine prenatal lab panel all serve to identify those pregnant teens potentially at risk for poor perinatal outcomes. Early screening for genetic conditions and chromosomal anomalies is part of routine antepartum care. All screening and testing options are offered to all pregnant patients, regardless of age or risk factors, but commensurate with EGA, test availability, and institutional protocols. The increasingly complex field of genetic testing requires patient-centered pre- and post-test counseling that explains the benefits and limitations of the complex array of screening and testing options and utilizes genetic professionals' expertise. Testing results can inform patient decision-making regarding pregnancy continuation or the need for increased fetal surveillance via the various modes of fetal surveillance available.

In addition to quality antepartum care, comprehensive preconception health education and adherence to postpartum care and screening recommendations could substantially decrease young parents and their children's health burdens. Addressing social determinants of health and providing health interventions that are culturally consonant with the communities they are intended to serve can help target persistent health disparities that disproportionately impact the most vulnerable adolescents (King-Bowes et al. 2018). Recent paradigm shifts in the delivery of postpartum care propose more individualized, ongoing postpartum care with earlier postpartum contact (all women within 3 weeks) and medical evaluation (BP check 3–10 days postpartum), recognizing that preventive postpartum health care can encourage long-term health and well-being for both mother and child (ACOG 2018e, reaffirmed 2021).

Also, it is clear that digital technologies, from the internet to mobile phones to gaming, all increasingly influence adolescents' lives. Numerous digital technological interventions show promise for improving adolescents' sexual and reproductive health behaviors, including antepartum health behaviors and perinatal outcomes (Immanuel and Simmons 2021; Mesnick et al. 2013). Finally, pediatric providers can rely on regularly updated antepartum laboratory testing guidelines provided by obstetric care professional organizations such as the American College of Obstetrics and Gynecology, Society for Maternal-Fetal Medicine, CDC, and USPSTF. By adhering to evidence-based guidelines, following state laws regarding minors' rights to access and consent to prenatal care, pediatric providers can ensure they can tailor obstetric care to the unique needs of the adolescents they serve. By helping to ensure adolescents have healthy pregnancies, pediatric providers of adolescent pregnancy care can play a role in reducing adverse perinatal outcomes and positively influence the lifelong health trajectories for adolescent parents and their children.

Questions

1. Which of the following is/are true regarding pregnancy testing?
   (a) Urine pregnancy tests are reliably positive 14 days after fertilization, but most reliable after a missed menses.
   (b) False-positive urine pregnancy tests are rare, but false negatives are common, especially in the first few weeks after conception.
   (c) Serial quantitative HCG tests can identify normally or abnormally developing pregnancies because HCG levels rise at a predictable rate in early pregnancy.
   (d) All the above.

2. Which of the following is/are true regarding determining the estimated gestational age (EGA) of a pregnancy?
   (a) Last menstrual period (LMP) is always the most accurate method to date a pregnancy.
   (b) ACOG endorses first-trimester ultrasound as the most accurate method to determine or confirm EGA.
   (c) Discrepancies between the EGA established by LMP and first-trimester ultrasound should always favor the LMP dating.
   (d) Structural landmarks like the gestational sac, yolk sac, and fetal pole aren't visible on ultrasound before 6 weeks EGA.

3. What is included in a routine prenatal lab panel?
   (a) CBC, blood type and RH, hemoglobin electrophoresis, urine culture and sensitivity, and select STIs.
   (b) CBC, blood type and RH, lead levels, urine culture and sensitivity, and select STIs.
   (c) CBC, blood type and RH, cfDNA, urine culture and sensitivity, and select STIs.
   (d) CBC, blood type and RH, antibody screen, hepatitis C virus, HBsAg, rubella immunity, urine culture and sensitivity, and select STIs.

4. Which of the following STIs are included in a routine lab panel in prenatal care for an adolescent?
   (a) Gonorrhea, chlamydia, HIV, and syphilis.
   (b) Gonorrhea, chlamydia, herpes simplex virus (HSV), and syphilis.
   (c) Gonorrhea, chlamydia, trichomonas, and bacterial vaginosis.
   (d) Gonorrhea, chlamydia, HIV, and human papilloma virus (HPV).

5. Which screening test is most appropriately performed at 24–28 weeks EGA?
   (a) Group Beta Strep (GBS).
   (b) Oral glucose challenge test (OGCT).
   (c) Human chorionic gonadotropin (HCG).
   (d) Syphilis.

6. Which of the following would indicate a pregnant teen's needing an early screen for gestational diabetes?

   (a) Glycosuria on urine dipstick.
   (b) First- or second-degree relative with diabetes.
   (c) BMI>30 (answer and rationale do not need to be changed).
   (d) B and C.

7. An adolescent patient with an uncomplicated pregnancy has walked into your clinic today at 36 weeks EGA with no complaints but asking for a prenatal checkup. She states she missed several OB appointments due to a lack of transportation. Which screening test should you perform?
   (a) Group Beta Strep (GBS).
   (b) Glucose challenge test (GCT).
   (c) Human chorionic gonadotropin (HCG).
   (d) cfDNA.

8. A pregnant adolescent patient is 11 weeks EGA. You are explaining her options for testing for chromosomal abnormalities (aneuploidies) appropriate for her EGA. Which of the following options will you discuss?
   (a) Screening with ultrasound for nuchal translucency (NT) and blood test for two analytes, Papp-A and hCG; screening via noninvasive prenatal testing (NIPT) for cell-free DNA (cfDNA), or diagnostic testing via amniocentesis.
   (b) Screening with ultrasound for nuchal translucency (NT) and a for two analytes, Papp-A and hCG, screening via NIPT for cfDNA, or diagnostic testing via chorionic villus sampling (CVS).
   (c) Screening with an ultrasound for nuchal translucency (NT) and a "quad screen" blood test for four analytes, NIPT for cfDNA, or diagnostic testing via amniocentesis.
   (d) Screening with an ultrasound for nuchal translucency (NT) and a "Penta screen" blood test for five analytes, NIPT for cfDNA, or expanded carrier screening.

9. cfDNA testing relies on the fetal (placental) fraction of total cf. DNA in the maternal bloodstream and:
   (a) Can reliably determine fetal sex and blood and Rh type after the ninth week of gestation.

(b) Is the most sensitive and specific screening test for common aneuploidies.

(c) Is rapidly replacing other cumbersome screening protocols due to its ease, rapidly increasing availability and sensitivity and specificity for detecting both common and rare chromosomal abnormalities.

(d) All the above.

10. When can the diagnosis of preeclampsia be made after 20 weeks EGA without proteinuria when other clinical signs are present?

(a) BP >130 mm Hg/90 mm Hg on two occasions, 4 h apart or BP >150 mm Hg/110 mm Hg on two separate occasions within a short interval (minutes).

(b) BP >140 mm Hg/90 mm Hg on two occasions, 4 h apart or BP >160 mm Hg/110 mm Hg on two separate occasions within a short interval (minutes).

(c) BP >130 mm Hg/100 mm Hg on two occasions, 4 h apart or BP >150 mm Hg/110 mm Hg on two separate occasions within a short interval (minutes).

(d) BP >140 mm Hg/100 mm Hg on two occasions, 4 h apart or BP >130 mm Hg/110 mm Hg on two separate occasions within a short interval (minutes).

11. Which of the following is an example of targeted screening for genetic mutations?

(a) Offering all patients screening for cystic fibrosis, spinal muscular atrophy, thalassemia, and hemoglobinopathies as ACOG recommends.

(b) Offering Tay-Sachs disease screening only to patients of Ashkenazi Jewish and French Canadian descent.

(c) Offering screening for genetic disorders as part of preconception care.

(d) Offering a reproductive partner genetic screening following a positive genetic screening result for the pregnant patient.

12. Which of the following is true regarding fetal surveillance to ensure fetal well-being?

(a) The use of umbilical artery Doppler velocimetry has not been associated with significantly reduced stillbirth rates in fetal growth restriction and hypertensive disorders of pregnancy.

(b) The contraction stress test (CST) is used more often than a non-stress test (NST) because it is associated with less risk of inducing labor.

(c) All pregnant patients should be educated that fetal movement is an important indicator of fetal well-being.

(d) A biophysical profile (BPP) combines several methods of fetal surveillance, including the NST, CST, and umbilical Doppler velocimetry.

Rationale

1. Answer: d

HCG is not detectable in urine or blood until after implantation of the fertilized egg in the uterine lining. As a result, urine pregnancy tests can be positive as soon as 7–10 days after fertilization, are more reliable 14 days after fertilization (not 7 days after implantation), and are most reliable after a missed menses. False negatives are common if done before implantation. Serum HCG levels rise predictably in early pregnancy such that levels double every 2–3 days in normally developing pregnancies and plateau or decrease in ectopic or early pregnancy loss.

2. Answer: b

Early and accurate gestational age determination is of primary importance in prenatal care and ACOG, endorses ultrasound in the first trimester up to and including 13 weeks 6 days (13 6/7). Estimated gestational age (EGA) is the most accurate method to determine or confirm gestational age. Redating a pregnancy based on discrepancies between the EDD as determined by the last menstrual period (LMP) and the EDD established by ultrasound should rarely be done. Whether LMP or ultrasound dating is used depends on the degree of discrepancy. The gestational sac and yolk sac are visible on ultrasound as early as 3–5 weeks and the fetal pole by 6 weeks.

3. Answer: d

Hemoglobin electrophoresis and lead levels are not considered routine in an initial lab panel and instead rely on a risk-based approach that may target at-risk populations (hemoglobin electrophoresis) and comply with local health departments' guidelines population-specific screening guidelines (lead screening) or institutional protocols. While cfDNA will eventually become a routine lab test, it can only be done after 10 weeks EGA. The 2020 CDC updated guidelines state that all pregnant patients should be screened for hepatitis C virus (HCV) unless geographic prevalence rates are <0.1%.

4. Answer: a

CDC guidelines recommend that all pregnant people less than 25 years old be routinely screened for gonorrhea, chlamydia, HIV, and syphilis. Rates of chlamydia are consistently highest among females aged 15–24, and rates of gonorrhea are highest among males aged 15–24 years. The CDC, ACOG, and AAP all endorse universal screening for HIV for all pregnant patients as early as possible using an opt-out approach, legal in all US states and territories, whereby patients are informed that HIV testing is part of the routine prenatal lab panel unless they specifically decline it. Increasing rates of congenital syphilis are largely due to gaps in testing, and routine screening as part of an initial prenatal lab panel is recommended. Herpes simplex virus, trichomonas, and bacterial vaginosis would only be tested if a pregnant patient's partner was positive and/or the patient was symptomatic. Adolescents should never be tested for HPV.

5. Answer: b

The majority of US obstetric care providers adhere to the ADA (2020) and ACOG (2018c) guidelines which call for universal screening for gestational diabetes at 24–28 weeks. Screening for GDM occurs from 24 to 28 weeks EGA because insulin resistance increases naturally during the second trimester of pregnancy. For women who

cannot produce enough insulin to adapt to this resistance, glucose levels will rise commensurately, so testing at 24–28 weeks will maximize identifying patients with GDM. HCG is the basis for pregnancy testing, syphilis is screened for early in pregnancy and again in the third trimester for high-risk patients, and GBS screening is performed at 36–37 weeks EGA, near term, to determine if treatment during labor is required.

6. Answer: d

While the risk of GDM increases with maternal age, several other risk factors, including overweight/obesity, having a first-degree relative with diabetes, or being a member of higher-risk racial or ethnic groups, increase GDM risk among pregnant adolescents to the same degree as pregnant adults. A urine dipstick positive for glycosuria with a normal blood glucose level is common in pregnant women. Pregnancy normally results in increased reabsorption of glucose and higher urinary excretion rates. Therefore, glycosuria has both poor positive and negative predictive validity for GDM.

7. Answer: a

GBS screening is performed at 36–37 weeks EGA, near term, to determine if treatment during labor is required. Screening for GDM occurs from 24 to 28 weeks EGA because insulin resistance increases naturally during the second trimester of pregnancy, so screening at that time will maximize identifying patients who are unable to increase insulin production resulting in GDM. HCG is the basis for pregnancy testing, and cfDNA tests for chromosomal abnormalities are currently offered primarily to high-risk patients.

8. Answer: b

At 11 weeks EGA, a first-trimester screening protocol is appropriate based on the detectable levels of specific analytes at that time and the ability to visualize the nuchal fold. cfDNA can be offered any time from 9 weeks EGA. It requires fetal/placental DNA to reach a certain level in the maternal circulation to achieve a high degree of sensitivity and specificity. CVS can be offered as early as 10 weeks, but amniocentesis is offered after 15 weeks EGA to decrease the risk of miscarriage. Quad and Penta screens are offered as part of second-trimester screening as the analytes tested need time to reach testable levels in the maternal circulation. Expanded carrier screening refers to offering a range of genetic tests to people regardless of ancestry or risk.

9. Answer: d

Advances in noninvasive prenatal testing (NIPT) that allow for detecting cell-free fetal DNA (cfDNA) in the maternal serum have identified fetal sex and blood and Rh type reliable as early as the ninth week of pregnancy via a single maternal blood sample. Some countries have already replaced routine Rh-D immunoglobulin prophylaxis of all Rh-negative women with targeted Rh-D immunoglobulin prophylaxis only for Rh-D negative women whose fetus's blood type is determined at 24–27 weeks (or earlier) via NIPT to be Rh-positive. While it is the most sensitive and specific screening test for the common aneuploidies, it is not currently considered diagnostic for chromosomal conditions because the cfDNA reflects the placental karyotype, which can differ somewhat from fetal karyotype molecularly. New protocols, particularly for contingent screening, that utilize cfDNA following first and/or second-trimester aneuploidy screening results have shown high sensitivity and specificity relative to CVS and amniocentesis.

10. Answer: b

Both the USPSTF and ACOG agree that proteinuria is often but not always present in the setting of preeclampsia, and guidelines indicate that the diagnosis of preeclampsia can be made without proteinuria when other clinical signs are present. In contrast, given the well-established accuracy and predictive validity for preeclampsia of blood pressure readings, the USPSTF and ACOG have concluded substantial benefit for routine blood pressure screenings at every visit, and the specific criteria for preeclampsia are stated in option b: BP >140 mm Hg/ 90 mm Hg on two occasions, 4 h apart or BP >160 mm Hg/110 mm Hg on two separate occasions within a short interval (minutes).

11. Answer: b

Some genetic conditions have higher prevalence rates within specific populations. Targeted screening refers to limiting screening for those conditions to those high-risk populations, such as offering Tay-Sachs disease screening only to patients of Ashkenazi Jewish and French Canadian descent. The USA is a multiracial and multiethnic country, so ACOG recommends offering expanded or panethnic carrier screening to pregnant patients regardless of ancestry. Screening for genetic disorders is ideally performed as part of preconception care but can be either targeted or expanded screening. Following a pregnant patient's positive screening result for being a carrier of a gene for a genetic disorder, the patient's reproductive partner should always be tested to determine whether the fetus is at risk for expressing the condition.

12. Answer: c

Maternal perception of decreased fetal activity has long been associated with an increased risk of stillbirth. All pregnant patients should be educated that fetal movement is an important indicator of fetal well-being. Any significant change in fetal movement patterns should be reported to a provider. Abnormal velocity waveforms detected by umbilical artery Doppler velocimetry are associated with neonatal morbidity and mortality. Its use is associated with significantly reduced stillbirth rates in fetal growth restriction and hypertensive disorders of pregnancy. The CST is used far less than the NST because it poses a risk for inducing labor since it induces contractions. A biophysical profile (BPP) combines five different elements: the NST, the AFI, fetal breathing movements, fetal body/limb movements, and fetal tone (extension and flexion).

References

Alldred SK, Deeks JJ, Guo B, Neilson JP, Alfirevic Z. Second trimester serum tests for Down's syndrome screening. Cochrane Database Syst Rev. 2012;6:CD009925.

American Cancer Society (2020). Guidelines for the prevention and early detection of cervical cancer. https://www.cancer.org/cancer/cervical-cancer/detection-diagnosis-staging/cervical-cancer-screening-guidelines.html. Accessed 4 Feb 2021.

American College of Obstetricians and Gynecologists. ACOG practice bulletin no. 145: antepartum fetal surveillance. Obstet Gynecol. 2014. reaffirmed 2020;124:182–92.

American College of Obstetricians and Gynecologists. Anemia in pregnancy. ACOG Practice Bulletin No. 233. Obstet Gynecol. 2021;138:e55–64.

American College of Obstetricians and Gynecologists. Antepartum fetal surveillance. Practice Bulletin No. 229. Obstet Gynecol. 2021;137:e116–27.

American College of Obstetricians and Gynecologists. Methods for estimating the due date: ACOG Committee Opinion Number 700. Obstet Gynecol. 2017a;129:150–4.

American College of Obstetricians and Gynecologists. Prevention of Rh D Alloimmunization. ACOG Practice Bulletin, Number 181. Obstet Gynecol. 2017b;130:e57–70.

American College of Obstetricians and Gynecologists. Anemia in pregnancy. ACOG Practice Bulletin No. 95. Obstet Gynecol. 2017c;112:201–7.

American College of Obstetricians and Gynecologists. Postpartum hemorrhage. ACOG Practice Bulletin No. 183. Obstet Gynecol. 2017d;130:e168–86.

American College of Obstetricians and Gynecologists. Sulfonamides, nitrofurantoin, and risk of birth defects. ACOG Committee Opinion No. 717. Obstet Gynecol. 2017e;130:e150–2.

American College of Obstetricians and Gynecologists. Carrier screening for genetic disorders, ACOG Committee Opinion #691. Obstet Gynecol. 2017f;129:41–55.

American College of Obstetricians and Gynecologists. Neural tube defects. Practice Bulletin No. 187. Obstet Gynecol. 2017g;130:e279–90.

American College of Obstetricians and Gynecologists. Tubal ectopic pregnancy. ACOG Practice Bulletin No. 193. Obstet Gynecol. 2018a;131:e91–103.

American College of Obstetricians and Gynecologists. Prenatal and perinatal human immunodeficiency virus testing. ACOG Committee opinion no. 752. Obstet Gynecol. 2018b;132:e138–42.

American College of Obstetricians and Gynecologists. Gestational diabetes mellitus. ACOG practice bulletin no. 190. Obstet Gynecol. 2018c;131:e49–64.

American College of Obstetricians and Gynecologists. Optimizing postpartum care. ACOG Committee Opinion No. 736. Obstet Gynecol. 2018d., reaffirmed 2021;131:e140–50.

American College of Obstetricians and Gynecologists. Modern genetics in obstetrics and gynecology. ACOG Technology Assessment in Obstetrics and Gynecology No. 14. Obstet Gynecol. 2018e;132:e143–68.

American College of Obstetricians and Gynecologists. Committee Opinion No. 533 Lead screening during pregnancy and lactation. Obstet Gynecol. 2019;120:416–20.

American College of Obstetricians and Gynecologists. Gestational hypertension and preeclampsia. ACOG Practice Bulletin No. 222. Obstet Gynecol. 2020a;135:e237–60.

American College of Obstetricians and Gynecologists. Prevention of group B streptococcal early-onset disease in Newborns: ACOG Committee opinion, number 797. Obstet Gynecol. 2020b;135:e51–72.

American College of Obstetricians and Gynecologists. ACOGPrelabor rupture of membranes. ACOG practice bulletin, number 217. Obstet Gynecol. 2020c;135:e80–97.

American College of Obstetricians and Gynecologists. Committee on Practice Bulletins—Obstetrics, Committee on Genetics, Society for Maternal-Fetal Medicine. Screening for Fetal chromosomal abnormalities: ACOG practice bulletin, number 226. Obstet Gynecol. 2020d;136:e48–69.

American College of Obstetricians and Gynecologists. Committee opinion no. 682 summary: microarrays and next-generation sequencing technology: the use of advanced genetic diagnostic tools in obstetrics and Gynecology. Obstet Gynecol. 2016., reaffirmed 2020;128:1462–3.

American College of Obstetrics and Gynecologists. Hypertension in pregnancyReport of the American College of Obstetricians and Gynecologists' Task Force on Hypertension in Pregnancy. Obstet Gynecol. 2013;122:1122–31.

American Diabetes Association. Classification and diagnosis of diabetes: standards of medical Care in Diabetes. Diabetes Care. 2020;43:S14–31.

American Pregnancy Association. What is HCG? Retrieved January 1, 2021, 2020. https://american-pregnancy.org/getting-pregnant/hcg-levels-71048/.

Aurthur R, Walsh NP. Urinary tract disorders. In: Jordan RG, Farley CL, Grace KT, editors. Prenatal and postnatal care: a woman-centered approach. Hoboken, New Jersey: John Wiley & Sons, Inc.; 2019. p. 673–80.

Bilous RW, Jacklin PB, Maresh MJ, Sacks DA. Resolving the gestational diabetes diagnosis conundrum: the need for a randomized controlled trial of treatment. Diabetes Care. 2021;44:858–64.

Black LL, Johnson R, VanHoose L. The relationship between perceived racism/discrimination and health among Black American women: a review of the literature from 2003 to 2013. J Racial Ethn Health Disparities. 2015;2:11–20.

Blackburn S. Maternal, fetal, & neonatal physiology: a clinical perspective. 5th ed. Amsterdam: Elsevier; 2017.

Bostancı Ergen E, Abide Yayla C, Sanverdi I, Ozkaya E, Kilicci C, Kabaca KC. Maternal-fetal outcome associated with adolescent pregnancy in a tertiary referral center: a cross-sectional study. Ginekol Pol. 2017;88:674–67.

Branson B, Owen S, Bennett B, Wesolowski L, Werner B, Wroblewski K, and Pentella M. Laboratory testing for the diagnosis of HIV infection: Updated recommendations for Centers for Disease Control and Prevention 2014. Retrieved on April 22, 2021, https://www.medbox.org/document/laboratory-testing-for-the-diagnosis-of-hiv-infection-updated-recommendations#GO.

Braveman P, Heck K, Egerter S, Dominguez TP, Rinki C, Marchi KS, Curtis M. Worry about racial discrimination: a missing piece of the puzzle of Black-White disparities in preterm birth? PLoS One. 2017;12:e0186151.

Brison N, Neofytou M, Dehaspe L, Bayindir B, Van Den Bogaert K, Dardour L, et al. Predicting fetoplacental chromosomal mosaicism during non-invasive prenatal testing. Prenat Diagn. 2018;38(4):258–66.

Bunt CW, Bunt SK. Role of the family physician in the care of children with down syndrome. Am Fam Physician. 2014;90(12):851–8.

Cacciatore A, Rapiti S, Carrara S, Cavaliere A, Santina E, Dinatale A, et al. Obstetric management in Rh alloimmunized pregnancy. J Prenat Med. 2009;3:25–7.

Carpenter MW, Coustan DR. Criteria for screening tests for gestational diabetes. Am J Obstet Gynecol. 1982;144:768–73.

Carter EB, Martin S, Temming LA, Colditz GA, Macones GA, Tuuli MG. Early versus 6–12-week postpartum glucose tolerance testing for women with gestational diabetes. J Perinatol. 2018;38:118–21.

Centers for Disease Control and Prevention. Achievements in public health: reduction in perinatal transmission of HIV infection—United States, 1985–2005. Morb Mortal Wkly Rep. 2006;52:592–7. Retrieved on January 14, 2021, from https://www.cdc.gov/mmwr/preview/mmwrhtml/mm5521a3.htm

Centers for Disease Control and Prevention. Recommendations for the laboratory-based detection of chlamydia trachomatis Neisseria gonorrhea-2014. Morb Mortal Wkly Rep. 2014;63:1–19. Retrieved on January 14, 2021, from https://www.cdc.gov/mmwr/preview/mmwrhtml/rr6302a1.htm

Centers for Disease Control and Prevention. STD screening recommendations 2019a. Retrieved January 15, 2021, https://www.cdc.gov/std/tg2015/screening-recommendations-wide.htm

Centers for Disease Control and Prevention. Recommendations: Women & Folic Acid. 2019b. Retrieved on March 11, 2021, https://www.cdc.gov/ncbddd/folicacid/recommendations.html

Centers for Disease Control and Prevention. Preterm birth, 2020a. Retrieved April 10, 2021, from https://www.cdc.gov/reproductivehealth/maternalinfanthealth/pretermbirth.htm

Centers for Disease Control and Prevention. Pregnancy and HIV, viral hepatitis, STI and TB prevention: Syphilis.

2020b Retrieved February 1, 2021, https://www.cdc.gov/nchhstp/pregnancy/effects/syphilis.html

Centers for Disease Control and Prevention. Prenatal syphilis screening laws. 2020c. Retrieved January 28, 2021. https://www.cdc.gov/std/treatment/syphilis-screenings-2018.htm

Centers for Disease Control and Prevention. 2020d Rubella. Retrieved January 28, 2021, https://www.cdc.gov/rubella/lab/serology.html

Centers for Disease Control and Prevention. Genital Herpes Screening. 2020e. Retrieved February 4, 2021. https://www.cdc.gov/std/herpes/screening.htm

Centers for Disease Control and Prevention. Social determinants and eliminating disparities in teen pregnancy. 2020f. Retrieved February 28, 2021, from https://www.cdc.gov/teenpregnancy/about/social-determinants-disparities-teen-pregnancy.htm

Centers for Disease Control and Prevention. Adolescents and young adults 2021a. Retrieved February 1, 2021, from https://www.cdc.gov/std/life-stages-populations/adolescents-youngadults.htm

Centers for Disease Control and Prevention. Minors' consent laws. 2021b. Retrieved February 1, 2021, from https://www.cdc.gov/hiv/policies/law/states/minors.html

Cheng YW, Block-Kurbisch I, Caughey AB. Carpenter-Coustan criteria compared with the national diabetes data group thresholds for gestational diabetes mellitus. Obstet Gynecol. 2009;114:326–32.

Chou R, Dana T, Fu R, et al. Screening for Hepatitis C Virus Infection in Adolescents and Adults: A Systematic Review Update for the U.S. Preventive Services Task Force. Evidence Synthesis No. 188. Agency for Healthcare Research and Quality; 2020. AHRQ Publication No. 19-05256-EF-1.

Cole LA. The hCG assay or pregnancy test. Clin Chem Lab Med. 2012;50:617–30.

Copp AJ, Stanier P, Greene NDE. Genetic Basis of Neural Tube Defects. In: Di Rocco C, Pang D, Rutka JT (eds) Textbook of Pediatric Neurosurgery. Springer International Publishing, Cham. 2017;1–28.

Correa A, Bardenheier B, Elixhauser A, Geiss LS, Gregg E. Trends in prevalence of diabetes among delivery hospitalizations, United States, 1993-2009. Matern Child Health J. 2015;19:635–42.

Cowger TL, Wortham JM, Burton DC. Epidemiology of tuberculosis among children and adolescents in the USA, 2007-17: an analysis of national surveillance data. Lancet Public Health. 2019;4:e506–16.

de Jong EP, Vossen ACTM, Walther FJ, Lopriore E. How to use... Neonatal TORCH testing. Arch Dis Child Educ Pract Ed. 2013;98:93–8.

Dean L. Blood groups and red cell antigens. National Center for Biotechnology Information: (US). 2005. Retrieved February 2, 2021, from https://www.ncbi.nlm.nih.gov/books/NBK2275/?report=reader

Dilla AJ, Waters JH, Yazer MH. Clinical validation of risk stratification criteria for peripartum hemorrhage. Obstet Gynecol. 2013;122:120–6.

Dionne-Odom J, Tita ATN, Silverman NS. Society for maternal-fetal medicine #38: hepatitis B in pregnancy screening, treatment, and prevention of vertical trans-mission. Am J Obstet Gynecol. 2016;214:6–14.

Dupépé EB, Patel DM, Rocque BG, Hopson B, Arynchyna AA, Bishop ER, Blount JP. Surveillance survey of family history in children with neural tube defects. J Neurosurg Pediatr. 2017;19:690–5.

Egbe AC. Birth defects in the newborn population: race and ethnicity. Pediatr Neonatol. 2015;56:183–8.

Farias MG, Dal Bó S, de Castro SM, da Silva AR, Bonazzoni J, Scotti L, Costa SH. Flow cytometry in detection of Fetal red blood cells and maternal F cells to identify Fetomaternal Hemorrhage. Fetal Pediatr Pathol. 2016;35:385–91.

Fasula AM, Chia V, Murray CC, Brittain A, Tevendale H, Koumans EH. Socioecological risk factors associated with teen pregnancy or birth for young men: a scoping review. J Adolesc. 2019;74:130–45.

Fontham ETH, Wolf AMD, Church TR, et al. Cervical cancer screening for individuals at average risk: 2020 guideline update from the American Cancer Society. CA Cancer J Clin. 2020;70:321–46.

Frostenson S, Kliff S. The risk of lead poisoning isn't just in Flint. 2016. Retrieved on March 1, 2021, from https://www.vox.com/a/lead-exposure-risk-map

Fuller TR, White CP, Chu J, Dean D, Clemmons N, Chaparro C, et al. Social determinants and teen preg-nancy prevention: exploring the role of nontraditional partnerships. Health Promot Pract. 2018;19:23–30.

Galeva S, Konstantinidou L, Gil MM, Akolekar R, Nicolaides KH. Routine first-trimester screening for fetal trisomies in twin pregnancy: cell-free DNA test contingent on results from combined test. Ultrasound Obstet Gynecol. 2019;53:208–13.

Garcia-Vargas L, Addison SS, Nistala R, Kurukulasuriya D, Sowers JR. Gestational diabetes and the offspring: implications in the development of the cardiorenal metabolic syndrome in offspring. Cardiorenal Med. 2012;2:134–42.

Gardella C. Lead exposure in pregnancy: a review of the literature and argument for routine prenatal screening. Obstet Gynecol Surv. 2001;56:231–8.

Garratty G, Glynn SA, McEntire R. Retrovirus epidemiol-ogy donor study. ABO and Rh(D) phenotype frequen-cies of different racial/ethnic groups in the United States. Transfusion. 2004;44(5):703–6.

Glantz JC, Bertoia N. Preterm nonstress testing: 10-beat compared with 15-beat criteria. Obstet Gynecol. 2011;118:87–93.

Gould JM, Aronoff SC. Tuberculosis and pregnancy-maternal, fetal, and neonatal considerations. Microbiol Spectr. 2016;4:6.

Guttmacher Institute. Fact sheet: Unintended pregnancy in the US. 2019. Retrieved November 20, 2020, from https://www.guttmacher.org/sites/default/files/fact-sheet/fb-unintended-pregnancy-us.pdf

Guttmacher Institute. Minors' access to prena-tal care. 2021. Retrieved April 5, 2020, from https://www.guttmacher.org/state-policy/explore/minors-access-prenatal-care

Hale NL, Probst JC, Liu J, Martin AB, Bennett KJ, Glover S. Postpartum screening for diabetes among Medicaid-eligible South Carolina women with gestational diabe-tes. Womens Health Issues. 2012;22:e163–9.

HAPO Hyperglycemia and Adverse Perinatal Outcomes Study Cooperative Research Group, Metzger BE, Lowe LP, et al. Hyperglycemia and adverse pregnancy outcomes. N Engl J Med. 2008;358:1991–2002.

Hartling L, Dryden DM, Guthrie A, Muise M, Vandermeer B, Donovan L. Benefits and harms of treating ges-tational diabetes mellitus: a systematic review and meta-analysis for the U.S. Preventive Services Task Force and the National Institutes of Health Office of Medical Applications of Research. Ann Intern Med. 2013;159:123–9.

Hasanpour S, Raouf S, Shamsalizadeh N, Bani S, Ghojazadeh M, Sheikhan F. Evaluation of the effects of acoustic stimulation and feeding mother stimulation on non-reactive non-stress test: a randomized clinical trial. Arch Gynecol Obstet. 2013;287:1105–10.

Heazell AEP, Budd J, Li M, Cronin R, Bradford B, McCowan LME, et al. Alterations in maternally per-ceived fetal movement and their association with late stillbirth: findings from the Midland and north of England stillbirth case-control study. BMJ Open. 2018;8(7):e020031.

Huang L-Y, Pan M, Han J, Zhen L, Yang X, Li D-Z. What would be missed in the first trimester if nuchal trans-lucency measurement is replaced by cell-free DNA foetal aneuploidy screening? J Obstet Gynaecol. 2018;38:498–501.

Hunt KJ, Logan SL, Conway DL, Korte JE. Postpartum screening following GDM: how well are we doing? Curr Diab Rep. 2010;10:235–41.

Hunter LA. Complications during labor and birth. In: King TL, Brucker MC, Kriebs JM, Fahey JO, Gregor CL, Varney H, editors. Varney's midwifery. 5th ed. Massachusett: Jones and Bartlett Publisher; 2015. p. 971–1019.

Immanuel J, Simmons D. Apps and the woman with gestational diabetes mellitus. Diabetes Care. 2021;44:313–5.

International Association of Diabetes and Pregnancy Study Groups Consensus Panel, Metzger BE, Gabbe SG, et al. International association of diabetes and pregnancy study groups recommendations on the diagnosis and classification of hyperglycemia in preg-nancy. Diabetes Care. 2010;33:676–82.

Jeha D, Usta I, Ghulmiyyah L, Nassar A. A review of the risks and consequences of adolescent preg-nancy. J Neonatal Perinatal Med. 2015; https://doi.org/10.3233/NPM-15814038.

Johnson GJ, Clark SL, Turrentine MA. Antepartum test-ing for the prevention of stillbirth: where do we go from here? Obstet Gynecol. 2018;132:1407–11.

Jordan RG. Genetic counseling, screening, and diagnosis. In: Jordan RG, Farley CL, Grace KT, editors. Prenatal and postnatal care: a woman-centered approach. John Wiley & Sons, Inc; 2019. p. 181–94.

Kane D, D'Alton ME, Malone FD. Rare chromosomal abnormalities: can they be identified using conventional first trimester combined screening methods? Eur J Obstet Gynecol Reprod Biol X. 2021;10:100123.

Kilpatrick SJ, et al. Guidelines for perinatal care. 8th ed. Elk Grove Village, Illinois: American Academy of Pediatrics; 2017.

Kimball A, Torrone E, Miele K, Bachmann L, Thorpe P, Weinstock H, Bowen V. Missed opportunities for prevention of congenital syphilis—United States, 2018. MMWR Morb Mortal Wkly Rep. 2020;69:661–5.

King-Bowes K, Burrus BB, Axelson S, Garrido M, Kimbriel A, Abramson L, et al. Reducing disparities in adolescent pregnancy among US tribal youths. Am J Public Health. 2018;108:S23–4.

Knutzen D, Stoll K. Beyond the brochure: innovations in clinical counseling practices for prenatal genetic testing options. J Perinat Neonatal Nurs. 2019;33:12–25.

Larsen J, Buchanan P, Johnson S, Godbert S, Zinaman M. Human chorionic gonadotropin as a measure of pregnancy duration. Int J Gynaecol Obstet. 2013;123:189–95.

Latendresse G. Genetics. In: King TL, Brucker MC, Kriebs JM, Fahey JO, Gregor CL, Varney H, editors. Varney's midwifery. 5th ed. Massachusetts: Jones and Bartlett; 2015. p. 629–56.

Latendresse G, Deneris A. An update on current prenatal testing options: first trimester and noninvasive prenatal testing. J Midwifery Womens Health. 2015;60:24–36.

Lazar J, Grace KT, Jordan RG. Hematologic and thromboembolic disorders. In: Jordan RG, Farley CL, Grace KT, editors. Prenatal and postnatal care: a woman-centered approach (pp. 651–664). Hoboken, New Jersey: John Wiley & Sons, Inc; 2019. p. 651–554.

Leader LR, Baillie P, Van Schalkwyk DJ. Fetal movements and fetal outcome: a prospective study. Obstet Gynecol. 1981;57:431–6.

Lee DB, Peckins MK, Heinze JE, Miller AL, Assari S, Zimmerman MA. Psychological pathways from racial discrimination to cortisol in African American males and females. J Behav Med. 2018;41:208–20.

Leftwich HK, Alves MV. Adolescent Pregnancy. Pediatr Clin N Am. 2017;64:381–8.

Leichliter JS, Copen C, Dittus PJ. Confidentiality issues and use of sexually transmitted disease services among sexually experienced persons aged 15-25 years—United States, 2013-2015. MMWR Morb Mortal Wkly Rep. 2017;66:237–41.

Lindberg LD, Santelli JS, Desai S. Changing patterns of contraceptive use and the decline in rates of pregnancy and birth among U.S. adolescents, 2007–2014. J Adolesc Health. 2018;63:253–6.

Macones GA, Hankins GDV, Spong CY, Hauth J, Moore T. The 2008 National Institute of Child Health and Human Development workshop report on electronic Fetal monitoring. Obstet Gynecol. 2008;112:661–6.

Malhamé I, Cormier M, Sugarman J, Schwartzman K. Latent tuberculosis in pregnancy: a systematic review. PLoS One. 2016;11:e0154825.

Malone FD, Canick JA, Ball RH. First-trimester or second-trimester screening, or both, for Down's syndrome. N Engl J Med. 2005;353:2001–11.

March of Dimes. Neural tube defects. 2022. https://www.marchofdimes.org/complications/neural-tube-defects.aspx. Accessed 27 Jan 2022.

Marković S, Bogdanović G, Cerovac A. Premature and preterm premature rupture of membranes in adolescent compared to adult pregnancy. Med Glas. 2020;17:136–40.

Marshall AT, Betts S, Kan EC, McConnell R, Lanphear BP, Sowell ER. Association of lead-exposure risk and family income with childhood brain outcomes. Nat Med. 2020;26:91–7.

Matuszkiewicz-Rowinska J, Malyszko J, Wieliczko M. State of the art paper: urinary tract infections in pregnancy: old and new unresolved diagnostic and therapeutic problems. Arch Med Sci; Poznan. 2015;11:67–77.

Medical Research Council. (MRC) Vitamin Research GroupPrevention of neural tube defects: results of the Medical Research Council vitamin study. Lancet. 1991;338:131–7.

Menon KC, Ferguson EL, Thomson CD, Gray AR, Zodpey S, Saraf A, et al. Effects of anemia at different stages of gestation on infant outcomes. Nutrition. 2016;32:61–5.

Mesnick KR, Liddon N, Kapsimalis C, Habel M, David-Ferdon C, Brown K, et al. Adolescents, technology and reducing risk for HIV, STDs and pregnancy. Atlanta, GA: Centers for Disease Control and Prevention; 2013. Retrieved on March 1, 2021, from https://www.cdc.gov/std/life-stages-populations/adolescents-tech.htm

Mikwar M, MacFarlane AJ, Marchetti F. Mechanisms of oocyte aneuploidy associated with advanced maternal age. Mutat Res. 2020;785:108320.

Moore TR, Piacquadio K. A prospective evaluation of fetal movement screening to reduce the incidence of antepartum fetal death. Am J Obstet Gynecol. 1989;160:1075–80.

National Diabetes Data Group. Classification and diagnosis of diabetes mellitus and other categories of glucose intolerance. Diabetes. 1979;28:1039–57.

Penman-Aguilar A, Carter M, Snead MC, Kourtis AP. Socioeconomic disadvantage as a social determinant of teen childbearing in the U.S. Public Health Rep. 2013;128(Suppl 1):5–22.

Pertile MD, Halks-Miller M, Flowers N, Barbacioru C, Kinnings SL, Vavrek D, et al. Rare autosomal trisomies, revealed by maternal plasma DNA sequencing, suggest increased risk of feto-placental disease. Sci Transl Med. 2017;9(405):eaan1240.

Rahman MM, Abe SK, Rahman MS, Kanda M, Narita S, Bilano V, et al. Maternal anemia and risk of adverse birth and health outcomes in low- and middle-income countries: systematic review and meta-analysis. Am J Clin Nutr. 2016;103:495–504.

Rasmussen SA, Chu SY, Kim SY, Schmid CH, Lau J. Maternal obesity and risk of neural tube defects: a meta-analysis. Am J Obstet Gynecol. 2008;198:611–9.

Reese JA, Peck JD, Deschamps DR, McIntosh JJ, Knudtson EJ, Terrell DR, et al. Platelet counts during pregnancy. N Engl J Med. 2018;379:32–43.

Reese JA, Peck JD, Yu Z, Scordino TA, Deschamps DR, McIntosh JJ, Terrell DR, et al. Platelet sequestration and consumption in the placental intervillous space contribute to lower platelet counts during pregnancy. Am J Hematol. 2019;94:E8–E11.

Rönn MM, Mc Grath-Lone L, Davies B, Wilson JD, Ward H. Evaluation of the performance of nucleic acid amplification tests (NAATs) in detection of chlamydia and gonorrhoea infection in vaginal specimens relative to patient infection status: a systematic review. BMJ Open. 2019;9:e022510.

Rose NC, Kaimal AJ, Dugoff L, Norton ME. American College of Obstetricians, Gynecologists' committee on practice bulletins—ObstetricsCommittee on genetics, Society for Maternal-Fetal Medicine. Screening for Fetal chromosomal abnormalities: ACOG practice bulletin, number 226. Obstet Gynecol. 2020;136:e48.

Runkel B, Bein G, Sieben W, Sow D, Polus S, Fleer D. Targeted antenatal anti-D prophylaxis for RhD-negative pregnant women: a systematic review. BMC Pregnancy Childbirth. 2020;20:83.

Sacks V, Balding S. The united states can and should eliminate childhood lead exposure. ChildTrends. 2018. https://www.childtrends.org/publications/united-states-can-eliminate-childhood-lead-exposure.

Sadovsky E, Yaffe H. Daily fetal movement recording and fetal prognosis. Obstet Gynecol. 1973;41:845–50.

Society for Adolescent Health and Medicine (SAHM), American Academy of Pediatrics (AAP), and American College of Obstetrics and Gynecology (ACOG). Confidentiality protections for adolescents and young adults in the health care billing and insurance claims process. J Adolesc Health Care. 2016;58:374–377.

Salomon LJ, Sotiriadis A, Wulff CB, Odibo A, Akolekar R. Risk of miscarriage following amniocentesis or chorionic villus sampling: systematic review of literature and updated meta-analysis. Ultrasound Obstet Gynecol. 2019;54:442–51.

Salvant-Valentine S, Poulin A. Consistency of state statutes and regulations with Centers for Disease Control and Prevention's 2006 perinatal HIV testing recommendations. Public Health Rep. 2018;133:601–5.

Schillie S, Wester C, Osborne M, Wesolowski L, Ryerson AB. CDC recommendations for hepatitis C screening among adults—United States, 2020. MMWR Recomm Rep. 2020;69:1–17.

Seidu S, Khunti K. Non-adherence to diabetes guidelines in primary care—the enemy of evidence-based practice. Diabetes Res Clin Pract. 2012;95:301–2.

Simpson JL. Cell-free fetal DNA and maternal serum analytes for monitoring embryonic and fetal status. Fertil Steril. 2013;99(4):1124–34.

US Preventive Services Task Force, Bibbins-Domingo K, Grossman DC, Curry SJ, Barry MJ, Davidson KW, et al. Screening for preeclampsia: US preventive services task force recommendation statement. JAMA. 2017;317(16):1661–7.

Vounzoulaki E, Khunti K, Abner SC, Tan BK, Davies MJ, Gillies CL. Progression to type 2 diabetes in women with a known history of gestational diabetes: systematic review and meta-analysis. BMJ. 2020;369:m1361.

Wang J, Wang L, Liu H, Zhang S, Leng J, Li W, et al. Maternal gestational diabetes and different indicators of childhood obesity: a large study. Endocr Connect. 2018;7(12):1464–71.

Workowski KA, Bachmann LH, Chan PA, Johnston CM, Muzny CA, Park I, Reno H, Zenilman JM, Bolan GA. Sexually transmitted infections treatment guidelines, 2021. MMWR Recomm Rep. 2021;70(4):1–187.

World Bank. Adolescent fertility rate for high income countries [SPADOTFRTHIC]. 2018a. Retrieved November 22, 2020, from https://fred.stlouisfed.org/series/SPADOTFRTHIC.

World Bank. Adolescent fertility rate for the United States [SPADOTFRTUSA], 2018b. Retrieved November 22, 2020, from https://fred.stlouisfed.org/series/SPADOTFRTUSA.

Wright CF, Wei Y, Higgins JPT, Sagoo GS. Non-invasive prenatal diagnostic test accuracy for fetal sex using cell-free DNA a review and meta-analysis. BMC Res Notes. 2012;5:476.

Yan L, Jin Y, Hang H, Yan B. The association between urinary tract infection during pregnancy and preeclampsia: a meta-analysis. Medicine (Baltimore). 2018;97(36):e12192.

Care of the Newborn

3

**Rita Marie John, Ashley N. Gyura,
Emily R. Harrison, and Bobbie Salveson**

Learning Objectives
After completing the chapter, the learner should
be able to:

1. Identify components of the newborn screening process and common terminology.
2. Recognize the Recommended Uniform Screening Panel (RUSP) of conditions on the newborn screening panel and understand specific state differences.
3. Be aware of potential errors in the newborn screening process and how to avoid them.
4. Acquire resources for the management of positive newborn screening results.
5. Recognize ethical concerns existing in newborn screening.
6. Understand and evaluate different tests done in the newborn period.

7. Characterize the pitfalls of newborn laboratory tests.
8. Synthesize the various clinical presentations of congenital infections and evaluate the proper diagnostic laboratory tests for evaluating the newborn with a possible congenital infection.
9. Understand the limitations of evaluating a newborn with a possible congenital infection.

3.1 Introduction

At the time of delivery, routine laboratory screening tests can vary slightly from institution to institution, and newborn screening can vary from state to state. Laboratory tests are done during the first days of life, depending on the maternal history, the child's gestational, clinical symptoms, and risk factors. The result of newborn screening is critical and must be diligently obtained and followed. In some states, like Washington state, two newborn screenings are done to avoid missing a treatable disease. A complete maternal history and neonatal exam are done routinely based on the American Academy of Pediatrics (AAP) recommendations. A complete history and physical of the newborn should be done within 24 h in a healthy full-term newborn; however, it should be done

R. M. John (✉)
School of Nursing, Columbia University,
New York, NY, USA
e-mail: rmj4@cumc.columbia.edu

A. N. Gyura · E. R. Harrison
Department of Infectious Disease, Children's
Hospitals and Clinics of Minnesota,
Minneapolis, MN, USA

B. Salveson
ARNP - Department of Genetics, Mary Bridge
Children's Health Center/Multicare,
Tacoma, WA, USA

University of Washington, Seattle, WA, USA

© The Author(s), under exclusive license to Springer Nature Switzerland AG 2022
R. M. John (ed.), *Pediatric Diagnostic Labs for Primary Care: An Evidence-based Approach*,
https://doi.org/10.1007/978-3-030-90642-9_3

as soon as possible to help identify any congenital conditions. Bilirubin is assessed by visual inspection, phone applications, transcutaneous devices, and total serum or plasma bilirubin. The total serum or plasma bilirubin remains the gold standard for identification and management to prevent extreme neonatal hyperbilirubinemia. Congenital infections can be symptomatic or asymptomatic, and therefore, close follow-up and maternal education about fever in the newborn period must be emphasized. Even with maternal monitoring of Group B Streptococcus infection, this disease continues to be a source of sepsis in the newborn period.

3.2 The Newborn Period

The pregnant female has routine diagnostic testing done to identify possible conditions the newborn may have, as discussed in Chap. 2. Prenatal tests may be negative, but the mother can still have the condition if she is infected before she seroconverts. Therefore, the mother may have been infected before developing an immune response. Thus, diseases like syphilis and human immunodeficiency may be negative on the antenatal screen. Also, there is a risk of a false-negative test being done at the time of birth. The clinician needs to complete the history and do a physical, even if all the antenatal diagnostic labs are normal.

3.2.1 Overview of Newborn Screening

Newborn screening (NBS) is recognized as one of the most successful public health programs in the United States (Caggana et al. 2013). The goal of NBS is to detect asymptomatic, treatable conditions early enough to intervene and improve outcomes. NBS is not a single test but rather a process that includes blood sample collection, sample transport, sample processing, result review, communicating normal and abnormal results, follow-up of abnormal results, verification of diagnosis, public and providers' education, and continuous quality improvement.

A screening test does not confirm or rule out a condition. Rather, it identifies an individual who *may* have the condition, so definitive diagnostic testing can be performed to determine if the condition is truly present. In NBS, a false positive is defined as a positive screening result for an infant unaffected by the disorder. A false negative would be a negative screening result for an infant who *is* affected. False-negative results would be catastrophic and defeat the goal of the NBS program. Therefore, a screening test must tolerate some false-positive results to minimize or eliminate false-negative results. The screening test's sensitivity must approach 100% to accomplish this (Goldenberg et al. 2016). In NBS, false-positive rates range from 0.07% to 0.33% and positive predictive values from 8% to 18%. When averaged out, there is generally one true positive for every 5–15 false-positive cases (Mak et al. 2019). The rate of false positives underscores the importance of framing a positive NBS result as something requiring follow-up. Until the diagnostic testing is complete, no family should be told their baby has a disorder.

3.2.1.1 Conditions on the NBS Panel
The newborn screening started in the 1960s when Robert Guthrie, MD, Ph.D., developed a blood test that could detect phenylketonuria (PKU), an inherited metabolic condition, in asymptomatic newborns. Since that time, the number of conditions that can be detected on the NBS has expanded to include more than 60 disorders—metabolic, endocrine, hematologic, respiratory, immunologic, and lysosomal/peroxisomal storage disorders (Caggana et al. 2013). Since public health law falls under state governments' jurisdiction, each state determines its own program, and differences exist between

states. The differences between state programs are seen in Box 3.1.

Box 3.1 Areas of Variations between States

- Number of disorders included in the panel.
- Testing methodology.
- Lab reference values for disorders.
- How and to whom results are reported.
- Who is responsible for ordering diagnostic testing.
- Mandatory testing versus parental consent for screening.
- Cost to the patient.
- Parent education.
- The state's method of follow-up.

Adapted from Caggana et al. (2013).

Federal guidelines for evaluating which disorders to include in the newborn screening have been developed by the American College of Medical Genetics (ACMG) Newborn Screening Expert Group and the Secretary's Advisory Committee on Heritable Disorders Newborns and Children. The federal guidelines help address discrepancies in the number of conditions between states. This committee reports to the Health Resources and Services Administration (American College of Medical Genetics Newborn Screening Expert Group [ACMGNSEG] 2006). A rigorous, evidence-based application process was developed, and new conditions are reviewed to determine inclusion on a panel. Currently, 35 primary and 26 secondary disorders are on the Recommended Uniform Screening Panel (RUSP) (Table 3.1). To date, all states screen for at least 30 of the 35 conditions on the RUSP (Recommended Uniform Screening Panel 2020).

Most of the conditions on the RUSP are detected from dried blood spots. These include organic acidemias, amino acid disorders, urea cycle disorders, fatty acid oxidation defects, and others (collectively referred to as inborn errors of metabolism); endocrine disorders, hemoglobinopathies, immunodeficiencies, and lysosomal and peroxisomal disorders (collectively referred to as storage disorders); cystic fibrosis, and spinal muscular atrophy. Two other conditions, hearing loss and congenital heart disease, are detected using point-of-care testing techniques and are not discussed in this chapter.

3.3 Newborn Screening Process

3.3.1 Sample Collection

Blood is collected from the infant on a specific collection card, ordered from the state department of health NBS program. The collection card consists of a demographic/information form attached to five filter paper circles. Blood is typically collected via heel stick, between 24 and 48 h of life at the location of birth. Some states recommend a second sample collected at 7–15 days as well. The filter paper and information form must remain intact, and the form must be accurately completed.

Each circle on the collection card is concave, and care should be taken to collect a single large drop of blood in the circle's center, allowing capillary action to fill the circle. Many state websites have videos and informational posters demonstrating this procedure. Filling the circle with multiple small drops of blood or layering drops may result in errors. The spot should be as uniformly visible on both sides of the collection card as possible. Once all the spots on the card are filled, the card is air-dried for a minimum of 4 h, then sent to the designated NBS lab within 24 h. These spots are collectively referred to as dried blood spots (DBS).

3.3.1.1 Methods Used for Newborn Screening

Before the 1990s, the laboratory methodology for NBS was based on bacterial inhibition methods, which yielded a sensitivity and specificity of

Table 3.1 Disorders in the recommended uniform screening panel (as of July 2018)

Primary	Secondary
Organic acidemias	
Propionic acidemia (PA)	Methylmalonic acidemia with homocystinuria
Methylmalonic acidemia (MMA)	Malonic acidemia
Isovaleric acidemia (IVA)	Isobutyrlglycinuria
Glutaric acidemia type 1 (GA-1)	2-Methylbutyrlglycinuria
3-Methylcrotonyl-CoA carboxylase deficiency (3-MCC)	3-Methylglutaconic aciduria
3-Hydroxyl-3-Methylglutaric aciduria	2-Methyl-3-hydroxybutyric aciduria
Holocarboxylase deficiency	
Beta-ketothiolase deficiency	
Fatty acid oxidation disorders	
Carnitine uptake/carnitine transport defect (CUD/CTD)	Short-chain acyl-CoA dehydrogenase deficiency (SCAD)
Medium-chain acyl-CoA dehydrogenase deficiency (MCAD)	Medium/short-chain L3 hydroxyacyl-CoA dehydrogenase deficiency (M/SCHAD)
Very long-chain acyl-CoA dehydrogenase deficiency (VLCAD)	Glutaric acidemia type II (GA-II)
Long-chain L-3 hydroxyacyl-CoA dehydrogenase deficiency (LCHAD)	Medium-chain ketoacyl-CoA thiolase deficiency
	2,4-Dienoyl-CoA reductase deficiency
	Carnitine palmitoyltransferase deficiency type I (CPT-I)
	Carnitine palmitoyltransferase deficiency type II (CPT-II)
	Carnitine acylcarnitine translocase deficiency (CACT)
Amino acid disorders/urea cycle disorders	
Classic phenylketonuria (PKU)	Benign hyperphenylalaninemia (Hyperphe)
Maple syrup urine disease (MSUD)	Biopterin defect in cofactor biosynthesis
Tyrosinemia type I	Biopterin defect in cofactor regeneration
Homocystinuria (HCY)	Tyrosinemia type II
Argininosuccinic aciduria	Tyrosinemia type III
Citrullinemia type I (CIT)	Hypermethioninemia
	Argininemia
	Citrullinemia type II
Hemoglobinopathies	
Sickle cell disease	Various other hemoglobinopathies
Sickle beta-thalassemia	
Sickle cell hemoglobin C disease	
Endocrinopathies	
Primary congenital hypothyroidism	
Congenital adrenal hyperplasia	
Other disorders	
Biotinidase deficiency	Galactopimerase deficiency
Cystic fibrosis (CF)	Galactokinase deficiency
Classic galactosemia	T cell-related lymphocyte deficiencies
Glycogen storage disorder type II (Pompe disease)	
Severe combined immunodeficiency (SCID)	
Mucopolysaccharidosis type I (MPS I)	
X-linked adrenoleukodystrophy (X-ALD)	
Spinal muscular atrophy (SMA)	
Point-of-care test	
Critical congenital heart disease	
Congenital hearing loss	

Source: United States Health Resources and Services. Retrieved on December 19, 2020, from https://www.hrsa.gov/advisory-committees/heritable-disorders/rusp/index.html

92%and 99.9%, respectively (Mak et al. 2019). In the early 1990s, the adaptation of tandem mass spectrometry (MS/MS) to dried blood spots allowed for the expansion of NBS from 6 conditions to over 35 with a sensitivity and specificity of 99% and 99.995% (Mak et al. 2019). Additionally, MS/MS methodology allows for greater throughput and rapid turnaround time. Other laboratory methods used in NBS analysis include radioimmunoassay, immunofluorescent assay, colorimetric assay, isoelectric focusing, high-performance liquid chromatography, and molecular testing (Caggana et al. 2013). New technologies, like microfluidic techniques, are being developed to include multiple testing methods to be performed simultaneously. These techniques are often referred to as "lab on a chip" and have the potential to increase the speed of results by allowing screening to be done at the hospital's clinical lab (Caggana et al. 2013).

3.4 Notification of NBS Results and Follow-Up of Abnormal Screening

Each state has a standard process for the notification of NBS results. Typically, the results are provided to the person or institution sending the collection card, and the primary care provider (PCP) is included on the collection card. Most states have an online verification system to allow the PCP to check their patients' NBS results. If this is not available, all states offer telephonic result retrieval.

Primary care providers should become familiar with their state's process and learn how to access newborn screening results for their patients. When seeing a newborn, providers can check NBS results and report them to the family. Lack of notification does not indicate a normal screen, as collection cards may have been completed inaccurately or incompletely, making notification difficult.

If an NBS is positive, the PCP should follow the instructions provided for the next steps, either repeating the NBS or assisting the family in pursuing prompt diagnostic testing. When an NBS is

abnormal, diagnostic testing must be completed to confirm or rule out a condition. However, this testing's urgency depends on the disorder; but it should be done quickly, so monitoring and treatment may be initiated if the infant is found to have the disorder (Fabie et al. 2019). If the infant has any concerning symptoms (Table 3.2), this should be communicated to the reporting agency. The PCP may be instructed to send the infant to the nearest emergency department for immediate evaluation.

Many of the concerning symptoms mimic sepsis, making it important to communicate the infant's screened positive disorder for emergency department personnel. Refrain from referring to

Table 3.2 Concerning neonatal symptoms of NBS disorders on the RUSP

Disorder	Concerning symptoms
Organic acidemias Amino acidemias Urea cycle disorders	Poor feeding, lethargy, vomiting, hypotonia, hypothermia, seizures, abnormal urine order
Fatty acid disorders	Poor feeding, hypoketotic hypoglycemia, jaundice, hepatomegaly, hypotonia, muscle weakness, cardiomyopathy, arrhythmia
Hemoglobinopathies	Splenomegaly
Endocrinopathies	Neonatal salt wasting, atypical genitalia, prolonged jaundice, puffy face
Galactosemia	Poor feeding, jaundice, abnormal liver functions, *E. coli* sepsis (in males)
Biotinidase deficiency	Poor feeding, hypotonia, lethargy
Cystic fibrosis	Meconium ileus, poor feeding, wheezing
Pompe disease	Poor feeding, hypotonia, dilated hypertrophic cardiomyopathy, heart failure
Mucopolysaccharidosis type I	Umbilical hernia, diarrhea
Immunodeficiency disorders	Signs of infection
X-linked adrenoleukodystrophy	No symptoms in neonates
Spinal muscular atrophy	Poor feeding, hypotonia, abnormal respiratory breathing pattern— Abdominal breathing

Adapted from Fabie et al. (2019)

the NBS as "the PKU," which implies the infant has screened positive for PKU when the correct diagnostic testing is for a different disorder.

All of the NBS panel conditions have a spectrum of phenotypic presentation, from critical neonatal-onset to milder attenuated. The phenotypic presentation may depend on the genetic mutation(s), other comorbidities, and the amount or quality of enzyme produced. Delaying diagnostic testing because an infant appears normal is not a decision made by the PCP but rather in partnership with the specialty center specific to the disorder. The ACMG has developed ACT sheets and algorithms to help PCPs understand the next steps to take when a newborn has screened positive for a condition on the NBS (ACMG ACT Sheets and Algorithms 2001). The sheets can easily be obtained on the ACMG site. These sheets include additional conditions found on some state panels that are not on the RUSP.

3.4.1   Verification of Diagnosis

Once diagnostic testing results confirm a disorder, a referral for follow-up with a specialist should be made. The specialist type depends on the disorder and may include metabolic (or biochemical) geneticists, genetic counselors, dieticians, endocrinologists, hematologists, immunologists, pulmonologists, and neurologists. Clinicians are not expected to manage care for many rare disorders detected or counsel the family on treatment options. Management of children with rare disorders can be viewed as a team approach, coordinating care between specialists and PCP.

3.4.2   Education of Health Professionals and Public

All state health departments maintain a website dedicated to NBS, and many provide webinars and provider handbooks to assist PCPs in understanding how their process functions. Providers are notified of new conditions being considered and added to the NBS panel and changes in the process, and changes in condition cut-off values.

Education of the public is typically a joint effort between the PCP and the state. Every state has resources available for parent education, including brochures, videos, and other online resources. Many states have this information available in several languages. Parent education about the NBS ideally occurs before delivery, but there is a wide variation in the quality and timing of this education.

3.4.3   Ongoing Quality Improvement

States collect data on each component of the NBS process and publish reports dictated by their state law. Annual reports are typically found on the state NBS website. When new conditions are added to the panel, there is often increased scrutiny to assure the cut-off values can be adjusted to avoid too many false-positive results (Yusuf et al. 2019).

Screening result data are reviewed during the Association of Public Health Laboratories' meetings to examine the NBS process further and make recommendations or changes based on data analysis (American College of Medical Genetics Newborn Screening Expert Group 2006).

3.5   Considerations and Issues Affecting NBS Results

3.5.1   Prematurity and Illness

Premature and very ill infants have a higher chance of false-positive NBS results. Gestational age, exposure to steroids, blood transfusion, birth weight, antibiotics, and nutrition may affect the results.

3.5.2   Maternal Conditions/Diet

Occasionally, a positive newborn screen detects a maternal condition. A positive screen may also be caused by maternal dietary deficiency like B12 or carnitine, resulting from a vegan diet. Maternal medications like steroids, radioactive iodine, or propylthiouracil can result in newborn screenings positive for endocrine disorders (Fabie et al. 2019).

3.5.3 Process Errors

Errors in sample collection result in a delay of screening results and require a repeat screen to be collected. This delay can put an infant at risk if he/she has one of the disorders. Collection errors include insufficient quantity for testing, damaged filter paper, wet specimen, supersaturated specimen, contaminated specimen, serum rings, clotted or layered specimen, and no blood collected on the card. Incomplete or inaccurate completion of the demographic/information form may result in delays in communicating screening results. If cards are not dried correctly or stored in extreme heat or cold, inaccurate results increase. Collection cards should not be held and batched but rather transported every 24 h to expedite processing.

3.6 Ethical Issues

3.6.1 Parental Education and Consent

Unfortunately, parents may be confused about the process of NBS or even unaware their baby has been screened. Early discharge from the hospital, parental exhaustion, and information overload contribute to this lack of knowledge. Parental education about newborn screening varies widely, from a pamphlet included in the discharge materials to obstetricians discussing the NBS as a part of the birth experience.

Newborn screening is mandatory in all states and the District of Columbia. In all states except Nebraska, parents may opt out of screening (Gurian et al. 2006). However, parents must be fully aware that the test is being performed to make that choice. One way to increase parental awareness would be to obtain parental consent. Only Maryland, Wyoming, and the District of Columbia require parental consent before the blood sample collection (Gurian et al. 2006).

3.6.2 Result Ambiguity

For some disorders, the diagnostic tests do not always provide a clear, predictable prognosis. Disorders like X-linked adrenoleukodystrophy (X-ALD) rarely display symptoms until age 3 but require lab monitoring and MRI screening to initiate treatment for maximum effectiveness. Milder or benign forms of a condition may be diagnosed, for example, 3MCC or hyperphenylalaninemia. This can confuse how often to monitor labs, whether the condition will become symptomatic, or if treatment is required (Fabie et al. 2019).

Pseudodeficiency mutations are known to decrease enzyme activity without causing disease. Genetic analysis also discovers mutations or variants of unknown significance, leading to uncertainty and requiring ongoing monitoring for symptoms. A genetics specialist should interpret this information and report to parents (Fabie et al. 2019).

3.6.3 Unintentional Results

The time between receiving an abnormal NBS result and negative diagnostic results can be a source of parental anxiety. Even after parents are informed that the NBS was a false positive, anxiety can persist. Incorrect result reporting occurs when parents are told their baby has a disorder before finalizing diagnostic testing. Some of the disorders include genetic testing, and subsequent parental testing may uncover misattributed paternity. Carrier status may be detected rather than being affected by a disorder. This disclosure contradicts the bioethical value of autonomy or "the right not to know." In NBS, this information becomes a piece of the explanation regarding results (The President's Council on Bioethics 2008).

3.6.4 Consideration for Other Family Members

When a new diagnosis is made, this may have reproductive or health implications for other family members. Parents should be educated on the importance of sharing this information but are not legally obligated to do so. Genetic information is a protected health information, and providers cannot discuss this information with other family members without the patient or guardian's permission.

3.6.5 Storage of Blood Spot Specimens

All states have protocols defining the long-term storage of the dried blood spots once the screening process is completed. Dried blood spots have been de-identified and used for quality control, the development of new tests, and other research. Parental concern about the overuse of their child's blood and fears of genetic profiling prompted some states to require parental consent for any use of the de-identified specimens beyond the original test (Fabie et al. 2019; American College of Medical Genetics Newborn Screening Expert Group 2006).

3.6.6 Resource Inequity

Most states require a fee for newborn screening. This fee is typically included in the billing for birth. Diagnostic testing for positive screening is not always a part of the NBS fee, and laboratory and specialist visits may cost more than some families can afford. If an infant has a disorder, specialist visits, monitoring labs and procedures, special formulas, and treatment medications can be prohibitively expensive without insurance coverage. Even with insurance, determination of coverage is variable and a source of frustration for providers and families (The President's Council on Bioethics 2008).

Despite efforts to decrease the variability of conditions screened for between states, there are still differences in the conditions on state panels. Some states are also involved in pilot studies that allow for expanded screening using new technol-ogies. This variability continues to cause inequity between states (Fabie et al. 2019).

3.7 Specific Information about Screening Tests

3.7.1 Specific Screening Tests

The expansion of newborn tests will vary from state to state. For example, only 36 states screen for spinal muscular atrophy as of this writing, even though there are disease-modifying treatments (CureSMA 2021). Individual states add diseases to their newborn screening from the RUSP by either an executive order or legislative action. Newborn screening for genetic disorders such as cystic fibrosis, spinal muscular atrophy, and severe combined immune deficiency can make a long-term difference in the outcome of a child's life due to the early treatment. Practitioners must be vigilant in their awareness of state differences in newborn screening programs.

3.7.1.1 Congenital Hypothyroidism
Congenital hypothyroidism is done in all 50 states and is found in one out of 2000 births. It is asymptomatic at birth and must be treated early to avoid neurocognitive defects. It is the most common abnormality reported on newborn screening and is discussed in detail in the Endocrine chapter.

3.7.1.2 Hemoglobinopathy Screening
Patients who screen positive for sickle cell disease need confirmatory blood work to start penicillin prophylaxis and family education. Sickle cell screening is universally done in all 50 states and has decreased the mortality in the first 5 years of life from 25% to <3% (Kato et al. 2018). The section on hemoglobinopathies and follow-up is found in Chap. 8.

3.7.2 Real-Life Examples

A 7-day-old breastfed infant was seen in a follow-up visit due to poor weight gain. The neonate was now gaining weight. The clinician noted that the newborn screening was not in the chart and called the state for the newborn screening result. The child was identified with possible hypothyroidism. The child had confirmatory blood work done, and the mother's contact information was obtained. Twelve hours later, the child was started on Levothyroxine to treat the child's hypothyroidism after the laboratory tests confirmed the initial newborn screening result.

A 3-day-old male was discharged home with his mother. On the fifth day of life, the child was seen in the pediatric office, and the clinician called for the newborn screening results. The child was identified as having SMA because it is a genetic test. An immediate appointment was made with a pediatric neuromuscular specialist. A repeat genetic test was done, along with a screen for anti-AAV9 antibodies. The genetic test confirmed a deletion of SMN1, and anti-AAV9 antibodies were negative (Al-Zaidy, Mendel, 2019). The genetic test confirmed SMA. The child was given a prophylactic dose of prednisolone 1 m/kg/day orally 24 h before administering onasemnogene abeparvovec (Zolgensma) via a one-time infusion over 1 h. This gene-modifying therapy was approved for use in 2019. It provides a new copy of the gene responsible for human SMN protein.

Key Learning about Newborn Screening

- Newborn screening programs successfully detect rare diseases in infants to allow for early intervention and treatment.
- These disorders are genetic and require lifelong treatment, managed by a specialist.
- As testing methodologies improved, the number of disorders on the screening panel has increased, from a single test in the 1960s to over 60 conditions in some states.
- Federal guidelines were developed to recommend which conditions to include in the NBS to achieve equity in testing between states.
- As of 2018, all states test for 30 of the 35 recommended conditions.
- Providers are encouraged to become familiar with their state's NBS program and the procedures to retrieve results.

3.7.3 Possible Diagnostic Labs Following Delivery

Routine labs during the early neonatal period will vary between institutions. Blood that is ordered results from possible problems such as hyperbilirubinemia, hypoglycemia, or early-onset sepsis. The AAP recommends universal screening of all infants for bilirubin by either transcutaneous bilirubin or total serum bilirubin (AAP, 2004). This section will discuss the diagnostic lab tests that are ordered to rule out possible health problems.

Newborns need monitoring for problems that can be treated to prevent any complications. A newborn that is LGA is at risk for hypoglycemia, and a newborn that is late preterm or preterm is at higher risk for hyperbilirubinemia. All newborns are at risk for early-onset sepsis, although this is more common in premature infants. Chapter 2 reviewed screening the mother at 35–38 weeks gestation for Group B Streptococcus.

3.7.3.1 CBC

This section will focus on newborn differences in the CBC. RBC disorders in the neonatal period can present with jaundice, polycythemia, and anemia (Watchko 2015). The breakdown of the RBC causes jaundice. Jaundice can result from immune-mediated conditions (see Chap. 2 and Sect. 3.7.3.6), RBC enzyme defects (see Sects. 8.10.4.3 and 8.10.4.4), RBC membrane defects (see Sect. 8.10.1), and hemoglobinopathies (see Sect. 8.11). In the newborn, congenital infections such as parvovirus, cytomegalovirus, toxoplasmosis, and syphilis can cause anemia (Prefumo et al. 2019). Inherited newborn disorders that cause fetal anemia include lysosomal storage disease, Diamond-Blackfan and Fanconi anemia, alpha thalassemia, pyruvate kinase deficiency, glucose-6-phosphate dehydrogenase deficiency, and congenital erythrocyte membrane disorders such as spherocytosis and elliptocytosis (Prefumo et al. 2019).

The newborn CBC varies depending on the gestation age and varies during the first month of life. Alloimmune hemolytic disease of the fetus and newborn is due to transplacental transmission of one of three antigens—ABO, rhesus (Rh), or minor red cell antigens (i.e., Kell, Duffy, Kidd antigens)—leading to hemolysis, jaundice, and anemia. While RhD antigen and the development of anti-D antibodies cause severe anemia, antibodies to Duffy, Kell, and MNS systems are another cause of more severe anemia. It is unusual for ABO hemolytic disease to cause severe anemia (Fasano 2016). The clinician should evaluate the CBC as outlined in Table 8.8. The components are discussed below as it pertains to the newborn CBC.

Hematocrit/hemoglobin. The results of hematocrits and hemoglobin depend on the gestational age of the newborn. For example, the hematocrit in the high 30s in a 27-week-old infant would fall within the normal range but would be abnormal in a term or late preterm infant. The mean reference range for a newborn between 22 and 30 weeks falls in the 40s, whereas the late preterm and term infant have a normal Hct above 50 (Christensen et al. 2009). Polycythemia is defined by a hematocrit >65% in a term newborn. The causes of polycythemia include passive transfusion due to a twin-to-twin transfusion, placental insufficiency, infant of a diabetic mother, and aneuploidies including trisomy 21 (Watchko 2015).

Erythrocyte abnormalities. In newborns with Rh incompatibility, nucleated erythroblasts, polychromatophils, reticulocytes, and schistocytes are seen in the peripheral blood smear and anemia. The presence of schistocytes and the increase in reticulocytes result from the hemolytic process. Blister cells are found in G-6PD deficiency and other red cell enzymopathies. Spherocytosis results from altering the cellular surface-to-volume ratio due to reducing the IgG red cell membrane caused by the reticuloendothelial system (Geaghan 2011).

Erythrocyte indices. The MCV is directly measured using laser optics or aperture-impedance technology (Christensen et al. 2009). The MCHC is calculated using the formula hemoglobin (g/dL/hematocrit L/L. It reflects the concentration of hemoglobin within the average red blood cell (RBC). The MCH measures the average amount of hemoglobin within the circulating RBC and is calculated by taking the hemoglobin/erythrocyte count. In a term newborn, RBC is much larger than the average adult with an average MCV around 105 fL (range of 113 to 97 fL), and in a 26-week-old infant, the MCV is considerably larger, with a range of 133 to 102 fL and a mean around 117 fL. The MCHC does not change during gestation, and an abnormally high MCHC may indicate spherocytosis (Christensen et al. 2009).

Platelet count and size. Thrombopoietin (Tpo) is the regulator of megakaryopoiesis and the production of platelets. The difference depending on gestational age is not seen in that preterm and term infants as they have similar levels of Tpo. A surge in platelet counts is seen in both term and preterm infants between the second and third weeks. Platelet elevations are seen in infection, iron deficiency, and postoperatively due to thrombopoietic factors, including Tpo. The normal platelet count for a term newborn and late preterm is greater than 650,000, much higher than the upper limit of normal of 400,000 in children and adults (Christensen et al. 2009). The MPV rises during the first two postnatal weeks reaching its normal value.

Thrombocytopenia in newborns is rare for healthy newborns but is more common in sick infants in the NICU. The causes are increased destruction, increased loss, and less production. Immune-mediated destruction is the most common cause, and it is the result of alloimmune disorders and auto-immune destruction. Neonatal alloimmune destruction can be severe with platelet counts as low as 1000, which is more common in firstborn children. Autoimmune-mediated thrombocytopenia can result from maternal antibodies due to lupus, maternal immune thrombocytopenia, or another collagen vascular disorder. Fetal and neonatal alloimmune thrombocytopenia (FNAIT) is the most common cause of a low platelet count, and this alloimmune disorder is caused by platelet opsonization from maternal antibodies, leading to platelet destruction (Zdravic et al. 2016).

White blood cells. The neutrophil count increases following delivery in infants over

36 weeks gestation, with lower preterm infants' values. The neutrophil count in infants ≥36 weeks is 2700 μL to 13,000 μL. For infants from 28 weeks to 36 weeks, the range was 1000 μL to 12,500 μL For infants ≤28 weeks, the range was 1300–15,300 μL (Christensen et al. 2009). Immature neutrophils are highest at the time of delivery, with a fall starting at 12 h to 3 days.

Most neonatal cytopenias are transient and result from maternal hypertension, sepsis, immune disorders, and viral infections. However, rare genetic mutations can lead to bone marrow failure with decreased numbers of all three lines of the blood's cellular components as found in amegakaryocytic thrombocytopenia, Fanconi anemia, Shwachman-Diamond syndrome, and dyskeratosis congenita. Single lineage disorders include thrombocytopenia absent radii syndrome and cytopenia absent radii syndrome, as well as severe congenital neutropenia or Kostmann syndrome (Rivers and Slayton 2009). Fortunately, these disorders are rare.

3.7.3.2 Clotting Tests and Coagulation Disorders

Disorders of neonatal coagulation causing bleeding can result from an inherited coagulation disorder. They should be suspected when the family history is positive, or there is continued oozing from the umbilical stump or excessive bleeding from a heel or venipuncture, a cephalohematoma, or a large caput succedaneum without a history of a traumatic delivery. The inherited coagulation disorders include von Willebrand disease, hemophilia, other factor deficiencies, and thrombocytopenia, whereas acquired coagulation disorders include vitamin K deficiency, thrombocytopenia, and disseminated intravascular coagulation (Eberl 2020). Vitamin K deficiency can occur when there is no history of administration of vitamin K at birth, or there is a maternal history of medication use interfering with vitamin K. Acute liver disease can also cause excessive bleeding at birth due to poor utilization of vitamin K, activation of the coagulation and fibrinolytic system, and decreased synthesis of coagulation.

There are significant differences between neonatal and adult coagulation tests. The interpretation of the coagulation tests in the newborn period is difficult as the reference ranges are affected by the laboratory variability of reagents and the type of instruments used (Jaffray et al. 2016). Also, the laboratory usually does a small proportion of coagulation studies on newborn and premature infants, and therefore, there should be good communication between the lab and the clinician (Eberl 2020). False-positive and false-negative values for aPTT and PT tests are common in the neonatal period (Pal et al. 2015). Most coagulation factors are lower than adult levels, and adult levels are not reached until 6 months (Pal et al. 2015). Table 3.3 shows some differences in the neonatal coagulation test results. As a result of all the factors, these tests should be interpreted with a hematologist.

Table 3.3 Neonatal coagulation system differences

Coagulation test	Difference
aPTT (measure of the intrinsic pathway) • Both aPTT and PT can be abnormal due to variations of coagulation factors within normal limits or due to lupus anticoagulants.	Activated by exposed collagen It can be very prolonged by minor decreases in the factors of the intrinsic pathway Term infant >55 is the 95th percentile
PT (measure of the extrinsic pathway)	Activated by tissue factors that are released by damaged cells Sensitive to a mild reduction of procoagulants Term infant 0.15 in the term infant
Fibrinogen (measure of the final common pathway), factor V, VIII, and von Willebrand factor	Close to adult range Fibrinogen range-term infant-1.50 to 3.73
Factors II, VII, IX, X (vitamin K dependent factors) and factors XI, XII, prekallikrein, high-molecular-weight kininogen (contact factors)	50% of adult levels at birth 30% (range of 20%–79%) in 24–29 weeks' gestation infant
Anticoagulants-antithrombin	60%
Anticoagulant-Protein C	36%
Anticoagulant-Protein S	39%

Adapted from Jaffray et al. (2016); Pal et al. (2015)

3.7.3.3 Direct Antigen Test or Direct Coombs

During the first trimester of pregnancy, ABO, Rh (D), and antibody screen is performed on the mother using the indirect antigen test or indirect Coomb's test since the maternal antibodies are unbound or nonagglutinating (Geaghan 2011; Fasano 2016). This test is positive when there is a transplacental transfer of antibodies, a well-known physiologic phenomenon. When the mother's and baby's blood are mixed during the pregnancy or the delivery, the mother's anti-Rh antibodies will adhere to the baby's RhD-positive RBC, causing lysis. Rh isoimmune hemolytic disease (also known as erythroblastosis fetalis, blood group incompatibility, or isoimmunization) is discussed in Chap. 2 and is prevented by anti-D immunoglobulin (Rhogam) prophylaxis. The American College of Obstetricians and Gynecologists (ACOG) gives the mother targeted antenatal anti-D prophylaxis around 28 weeks of gestation and after delivery if the mother is Rh-negative and the baby is Rh-positive (ACOG 2017). However, the clinician must recognize that an Rh-negative mother will carry an RhD-negative fetus about 38–40%. Therefore, the administration of anti-D Ig at 28 weeks may be unnecessary (Fasano 2016). New noninvasive prenatal diagnosis methods involve using fetal DNA extracted from the maternal serum to look for RhD-positive circulating fetal DNA using molecular techniques (Fasano 2016). Alloimmunized RhD mothers are more common in low-income countries where women do not receive this prophylaxis due to a lack of postpartum care. Chap. 2, Sects. 2.6.1.2 and 2.6.1.3, go into this in greater detail.

The most common cause of hemolytic disease of the newborn is ABO incompatibility or heterospecificity (Geaghan 2011). While it is possible to have kernicterus secondary to ABO hemolysis, it is rare. In ABO incompatibility, A or B antigens of the ABO blood group or antigens of one of the other blood group systems cause hemolysis and subsequent jaundice. While 20% of infants have ABO maternal blood group incompatibility, only 1 in 150 to 3000 develop ABO hemolytic disease leading to jaundice. This difference is due to the ability of the fetus's tissue that carries the blood group antigen to bind to maternal antibodies, as well as the weak expression of the blood group antigens A and B that are present on the RBC (Geaghan 2011).

The direct antigen test (DAT) is no longer routinely done on cord blood since ABO incompatibility rarely is the cause of significant hemolytic disease. Also, the DAT is frequently negative in ABO incompatibility, and the cord blood is unreliable and may give a false-positive result. If there is a positive Coombs test, this does not mean that the baby will develop hyperbilirubinemia. The cord blood is usually kept for about 7 days if blood testing is needed. The DAT looks for maternal antibodies that are present in the newborn's red cells. The neonatal erythrocytes are incubated with anti-human (IgG) antibodies. If the newborn has maternal blood group antibodies, the test will be positive. If the DAT test is negative, an eluate test should be done (Van Rossum et al. 2015).

3.7.3.4 Blood Type

Selective blood typing may be done if the mother is O blood type or Rh-negative or it can be done routinely depending on the institution's policy. As noted, the blood group can be O if there is no antigen around the RBC, A if there is A antigen on the RBC, B if there is B antigen on the RBC, and AB if both antigens are present on the RBC. Suppose the mother is type O and the baby has paternally inherited antigen present on their RBC, so the baby is either type A, B, or AB. In that case, the antigen-negative mother may develop antibodies that bind to the RBC, causing hemolysis (Fasano 2016). Keep in mind that if a mother is O negative and the baby is A, B, or AB positive, the ABO setup will predominate, and so the degree of hemolysis will be less than if there was just an RhD incompatibility.

Minor blood group incompatibilities other than RhD can cause neonatal hyperbilirubinemia without any ABO or RhD incompatibility. These minor blood groups include Kell, c, C, E, and e and can be asymptomatic or have a full range of mild anemia with hyperbilirubinemia and reticulosis to fetal hydrops (Agrawal et al. 2020).

3.7.3.5 Genetic Testing for Undiagnosed Perinatal Diseases

A genetic disease can contribute to a perinatal disorder. While karyotyping and chromosomal microarray have helped identify heart, kidney, and nervous system disorders, recent advances in genome sequencing (GS) and exome sequencing (ES) can help identify the critically ill newborn. Testing the sick neonate using these techniques has helped identify over 50% of the diagnoses in these infants (Hays and Wapner 2021). These techniques are discussed in detail in Chap. 12. The benefits of genetic testing include early identification and improved management of the child with a syndrome, helping to decide on end-of-life care if the disorder has a poor prognosis, and promoting family planning. Exome sequencing is less resource-intensive to do and is easier to interpret. While GS may give added details about copy number variants (CNV) and noncopy number variants, the information may not prove that useful in clinical practice (Hays and Wapner 2021).

3.7.3.6 Bilirubin

A neonate may have several blood tests done during the first weeks of life to assess for hyperbilirubinemia. Noninvasive measurements are more commonly used as a screening tool.

The measurement is done by visual inspection, transcutaneous methods, and the gold standard of plasma or serum bilirubin. The AAP recommends that screening for jaundice should be done by transcutaneous methods or by total serum bilirubin, or based on risk factors (Ip et al. 2004). While a total bilirubin ≥95th percentile can be identified, the USPTF failed to find evidence that identifying these infants improved clinical outcomes. There is concern that this may lead to overtreatment (Muchowski 2014). However, the risk of neurodevelopmental problems is a concern of clinicians when the baby appears jaundice. Total serum bilirubin, which is then plotted on bilitool.org, can help determine the need for follow-up.

Jaundice is not normal in the 24 h of life (Anderson and Calkins 2020). In these infants,

direct or conjugated bilirubin and total bilirubin (TB) should be done. If the direct bilirubin is elevated, a referral to a liver specialist should be made. The pathophysiology of bilirubin in liver disease is discussed in detail in Chap. 9. The AAP recommends that infants be assessed for visible jaundice every 8 to 12 h (Ip et al. 2004). The methods of measuring bilirubin include transcutaneous bilirubin (TcB) or direct TB measure, especially when neonatal jaundice is difficult to assess due to darkly pigmented neonates.

Serum bilirubin. Bilirubin is measured from the blood using the diazo method. The analysis reports the direct and total bilirubin. The indirect bilirubin is done by calculating the total minus the direct bilirubin. The direct bilirubin estimates the conjugated bilirubin, and the indirect bilirubin estimates the unconjugated bilirubin. The direct bilirubin can overcalculate the conjugated bilirubin as the diazo reagent interacts with both the bilirubin bound to albumin and the conjugated bilirubin (Anderson and Calkins 2020).

In contrast, the indirect bilirubin will underestimate the unconjugated bilirubin as only a portion will react with a diazo reagent. It is important to get a direct bilirubin to make sure the child does not have biliary atresia. Other quantitative methods including high-performance liquid chromatography, enzymatic assay, and direct spectrophotometry are more accurate but are more expensive.

Transcutaneous bilirubin methods. Transcutaneous methods are quick and reduce the need for blood sampling. Transcutaneous bilirubinometry (TCB) has been studied the most, and it seems more useful in clinical practice. It tends to underestimate the total bilirubin. The results are influenced by postnatal age, the type of TCB device, race/ethnicity, gestational age, and the measurement site. The device is more accurate in the very-low birthweight infant (Fonseca et al. 2012; Bhutani et al. 2000; Nagar et al. 2013, 2016). Several devices are available with a range in sensitivity of 68% to 100% and a specificity of 21–88%. The dev phone applications that take a picture of the baby's skin and estimate the bilirubin are in development but are not available.

Visual inspection. Visual inspection using the Kramer scale assesses jaundice by the clinician pressing on the skin with the fingertip. Jaundice is usually seen when the bilirubin exceeds 5 mg/dL (Anderson and Calkins 2020). There are five dermal zones: the face and neck, chest and upper abdomen, lower abdomen and upper thighs, legs down to the ankles, and palms and soles. Jaundice presenting in the lower abdomen and upper thighs is felt to be ≥11.7, and jaundice that reaches the palms and soles is felt to be ≥14.6 (Kramer 1969). This method has a sensitivity of 70% to 80%. Research suggests that this method is inaccurate (Keren et al. 2009; Moyer et al. 2000). It is better used in the neonate with jaundice that does not extend to the lower abdomen, and it is more accurate in fair-skinned infants. Visual inspection can be used for ruling out jaundice and is never recommended for infants undergoing phototherapy as it causes bleaching (Okwundu and Saini 2021).

Icterometry. Icterometry using the Ingram icterometer, biliruler, and bilistrip has shown to have variable results in studies. The biliruler could miss 10–15% of jaundiced infants, and the biliruler had a sensitivity of 84.5% and a specificity of 83.0% (Lee et al. 2019). The Ingram icterometer showed wide variation and was particularly inaccurate for values ≥15, and it was removed from the market. Bilistrip is newer and more studies are needed (Okwundu and Saini 2021).

For neonates who meet phototherapy thresholds, the bilirubin should be followed and plotted on bilitool.org. A phone application called bilibaby can guide care and uses bilitool.org to guide the need for continued therapy.

Transient indirect hyperbilirubinemia (TIH) occurs when the newborn's production exceeds the newborn's ability to eliminate bilirubin (Anderson and Calkins 2020). Excess bilirubin production can occur due to excess red blood cell (RBC) hemolysis, causing excess bilirubin and/or impaired hepatic conjugation, allowing bilirubin levels to increase. The infant's ability to conjugate bilirubin is based on the amount of bilirubin conjugating enzyme called uridine dephosphoglucuronsyltransferase (UGTA1), which is low in the newborn period (Du et al.

2021). Neonates will develop physiological jaundice after the first 24 h of life (Anderson and Calkins 2020). It is abnormal to see jaundice in the first 24 h or to see the bilirubin increase by more than 5 mg/dL per day or 0.2 mg/dL per hour. A bilirubin that is greater than the 95th percentile on the bilitool would also be considered pathological. Physiologic jaundice should resolve by 2–3 weeks of life and would be considered pathologic if jaundice persists beyond 3 weeks (Anderson and Calkins 2020).

Bilirubin production is from the heme degradation cascade in which heme-containing compounds break down into heme and, in the presence of heme oxygenase, break down into biliverdin. Biliverdin, in the presence of biliverdin reductase, breaks down into unconjugated or indirect bilirubin. Due to the RBC's shortened lifespan in the term newborn, a two- to threefold increase in bilirubin production occurs. Premature infants have a shorter RBC lifespan resulting in higher bilirubin production rates. The breakdown of heme is increased due to stress, cytokines, endotoxin, stress, heavy metals, and UV radiation (Du et al. 2021). Biliverdin and bilirubin are antioxidants that are cellular protective. The increase in bilirubin preload from RBC breakdown and the inability to conjugate the bilirubin to dispose of the bilirubin. IHB is either physiologic or pathologic. The physiological reason for TIH results from increased enterohepatic circulation and increased productions complicated by decreased clearance and impaired conjugation. The pathologic causes of TIH and direct hyperbilirubinemia are discussed further in Chap. 9.

Hemolytic disease of the fetus and the newborn (HDFN) is most commonly caused by the incompatibility of the major blood groups (ABO incompatibility) and can also be caused by minor blood group antigens (Geaghan 2011). The alloimmunization of blood group antigens causes placental transfers of maternal antibodies and results in a spectrum of clinical diseases ranging from anemia, hyperbilirubinemia to kernicterus, fetal hydrops, and death. While Rh incompatibility requires a previous exposure and sensitization for hemolytic disease of the newborn to occur, ABO incompatibility can occur in the firstborn child. While 20% of infants have ABO incompatibility, the incidence of hemolytic disease as a sequela is far lower, only occurring in 1:1150 to 1:3000.

The most common immune cause of severe hemolysis and hyperbilirubinemia is Rh isoimmune hemolytic disease and ABO incompatibility (Geaghan 2011). The nonimmune causes include RBC enzymopathies such as glucose-6-phosphate (G6PD) deficiency and RBC membrane defects such as hereditary spherocytosis and elliptocytosis. Other nonimmune causes include infection, sequestration, and polycythemia. Decreased bilirubin clearance is caused by poor bilirubin uptake and decreased activity of UGTA1 (Anderson and Calkins 2020). Gilbert syndrome is a diagnosis of exclusion that causes mild jaundice in times of stress. When patients have Gilbert syndrome with G6PD, they are at higher risk for severe indirect hyperbilirubinemia. Other causes include congenital hypothyroidism, maternal diabetes, pyloric stenosis, and intestinal obstruction.

The BIND score is used to triage infants with extreme hyperbilirubinemia as total bilirubin ≥25 mg/dL requires timely intervention to avoid acute bilirubin encephalopathy (ABE) or kernicterus. The BIND score uses mental status, muscle tone, and cry pattern to evaluate the infant for ABE (Hameed and Hussein 2021). The adverse neurological outcomes of untreated hyperbilirubinemia are well known, and making sure that neonates are followed closely is critical in preventing these outcomes.

3.7.3.7 Glucose

Some infants are at greater risk for hypoglycemia due to maternal history (maternal diabetes, preeclampsia, eclampsia, or hypertension), birth history (premature or postmature delivery, perinatal stress, birth asphyxia, fetal distress, meconium aspiration), or infant history (large for gestational age, intrauterine growth restriction, symptoms of hypoglycemia, identified genetic symptoms such as Beckwith Wiedemann, Soto syndrome, or abnormal features such as microphallus, or midline facial defects, or family history of a genetic form of hypoglycemia (Thornton et al. 2015;

Thompson-Branch and Havranek 2017). About 6–7% of pregnant women have gestational diabetes using ACOG guidelines, but 18% would have gestational diabetes using the American Diabetes Association. In general, infants who are small for gestational age, large for gestational ages, late preterm infants, and infants of mothers who have diabetes are at risk for low glucose (AAP Committee on Fetus and Newborn and ACOG Committee on Obstetric Practice 2017). These infants will generally respond to treatment and maintain euglycemia by 48 h of life (Tas et al. 2020).

Congenital hyperinsulinism (HI) is the most common reason for persistent hypoglycemia that is nonketotic and results from dysregulated insulin (Tas et al. 2020). A congenital HIN panel includes common genes that cause this. Neonates with growth hormone or cortisol deficiency are also at risk for persistent hypoglycemia. Neonates with inborn errors of metabolism may have persistent neonatal hypoglycemia. The disorders of inborn errors of metabolism include amino acid abnormalities (maple syrup urine disease), disorders of glycogen (hepatic glycogen storage diseases), disorders of glucose metabolism (hereditary fructose intolerance), and disorders of fatty acids (short and medium change acyl-coenzyme dehydrogenase deficiency, galactosemia, carnitine palmitoyltransferase deficiency, types I and II, and long-chain 3-hydroxy and very-long-chain acyl-coenzyme A dehydrogenase deficiency) (Thompson-Branch and Havranek 2017). Endocrinologists and geneticists will be consulted to manage the conditions discussed in this paragraph.

Healthy term infants without any predisposing maternal history do not need routine glucose screening (AAP Committee on Fetus and Newborn and ACOG Committee on Obstetric Practice 2017). There is disagreement in what is considered normal plasma glucose in the neonate. The Pediatric Endocrine Society recommends a cut-off of 50 mg/dL regardless of risk factors, and the AAP recommends a cut-off of 45 mg/dL. The clinical signs are not specific but include the signs and symptoms seen in Table 3.4. Glucose should be measured within minutes on

Table 3.4 Signs and symptoms of hypoglycemia

Symptom	Signs
• Poor feeding	• Tachypnea
• Weak cry	• Apneic episode
• High-pitched cry	• Cyanosis
• Lethargy	• Diaphoresis
	• Weak cry
	• Jittery
	• Floppy
	• Seizures
	• Hemodynamic instability

Adapted from Tas et al. (2020); AAP Committee on Fetus and Newborn and ACOG Committee on Obstetric Practice 2017

any infant with clinical signs of hypoglycemia. The pathophysiology of this hypoglycemia is hyperinsulinism causing low glucose. During the first hours after birth, the mean plasma glucose (PG) concentration in normal newborns is between 55 and 60 mg/dL. After 48 h, the infant has a glucose similar to pediatric levels of 70–100 mg/dL (Adamkin 2011, 2016).

Glucometers are point-of-care testing devices that are the most common way to screen glucose. The glucometer uses glucose oxidase as the reducing to measure capillary blood sugar (Tas et al. 2020). The capillary blood sugar may differ from PG by 11%. Continuous glucose meters in the newborn are problematic due to hemodynamic instability and prematurity; therefore, routine clinical use is not recommended (Tas et al. 2020).

Pitfalls of glucose testing. Technical factors and artifacts may influence the interpretation of a PG value. Whole blood glucose values are about 15% lower than PG concentrations, and due to RBC glycolysis, if there is a delay in processing the specimen, there can be a drop in glucose concentration by as high as 6 mg/dL per hour (Thornton et al. 2015). Point-of-care tests are convenient, but their accuracy can be 10–15 points different when hypoglycemia occurs. In the first 2 days of life, hypoglycemia does not cause hyperketonemia. However, in patients with G6PD, the plasma lactate will rise if the PG is <70, and in patients with defects of fatty acid oxidation, lethargy and tachycardia occur when the PG falls below 70.

3.7.3.8 Apt Test, Kleihauer-Betke Test, Rosette Tests, and Flow Cytometry

The Apt test, Kleihauer-Betke test (acid elution test), and the Rosette test detect fetal RBC. The Apt test is a qualitative test used in newborns that vomit blood in the first few days of life to determine if the blood is from the mother or the baby. The Apt test is done by mixing the emesis with water, spinning it down, and taking the cells to qualitative evaluate the conversion of oxyhemoglobin to hematin. The cells are combined with sodium hydroxide or potassium hydroxide (Chicaiza et al. 2014). Adult hemoglobin is denatured from this process and will turn brown. Fetal hemoglobin is more resistant and will turn pink. The test can be used in a newborn that vomits blood after delivery.

The Rosette test is a quantitative test to detect the amount of fetomaternal blood mixing. The Kleihauer-Betke test is used to adjust the RhoGam based on the amount of mixing that has occurred. When the maternal blood is mixed with citric acid phosphate buffer, the fetal cells will turn pink after acid elution is added, whereas the maternal RBCs will be like ghost cells as the hemoglobin leaves the RBC. The method involves counting fetal cells and using a formula to determine fetomaternal hemorrhage and then determining the amount of Rhogram to be given in the post-partum period (Geaghan 2011).

Flow cytometric methods have been developed to target the RhD blood group on fetal RBC or to use a different method to target fetal hemoglobin. The flow cytometric techniques can be more accurate but are not in widespread use as it is more expensive. The Kleihauer-Betke test is also used to distinguish maternal blood from fetal blood. Fetal hemoglobin is resistant to acid elution, and maternal hemoglobin A is susceptible.

3.7.3.9 C-Reactive Protein (CRP)

The C-reactive protein (CRP) and the erythrocyte sedimentation rate (ESR) are two tests used to evaluate the newborn with possible sepsis. The CRP is an acute-phase protein that will increase before the ESR in response to both acute and chronic inflammatory conditions as part of the innate immune response (Agrawal 2005; Taylor et al. 2020). The CRP activates the classic complement system, promotes the clearance of bacterial lysis products, and prevents immune activation (Taylor et al. 2020). It rises rapidly in response to infection but falls quickly on the resolution of the inflammatory process. A CRP level of <1 mg/dL (10 mg/L) is generally considered normal for clinical predictive purposes, and a CRP < 2 mg/dL can assist with ruling out a serious bacterial infection (SBI) when the duration of the disease is >12 h (Putto et al. 1986; Van den Bruel et al. 2011). Normal CRP ranges for neonates vary within the first 48 h, as noted in Table 3.5. The combination of an elevated procalcitonin of greater than 2 ng/mL and CRP of >10 mg/dL has been shown to increase the likelihood of sepsis in a newborn (Galetto-Lacour et al. 2003).

CRP does not cross the placenta; therefore, its presence in neonates is indicative of de novo production (Weinberg and D'Angio 2016). Consecutive CRP measurements in neonates with concern for infection are useful, as a normal CRP > 24 h after the first clinical suspicion has a high negative predictive value for neonatal SBI (Bhandari 2014; Mathers and Pohlandt 1987). A recent systematic review and meta-analysis concluded that CRP as part of an initial evaluation is not accurate enough to predict late-onset sepsis (Brown et al. 2020); however, the CRP is best if trended or checked after 24 h into illness.

Pitfalls. In neonates, many factors can lead to a transient rise in CRP values, including, but not limited to, meconium aspiration, respiratory distress, and intraventricular hemorrhage. Consecutive CRP measurements are useful in ruling out SBI in these neonates (Stol et al. 2019).

3.7.3.10 Procalcitonin

Procalcitonin (PCT) is a hormone that is the precursor of calcitonin. Procalcitonin is produced in the thyroid to regulate serum calcium concentrations. PCT has utility as a marker of infection, sepsis, and systemic inflammation. It has been identified as having a predictive value in neonatal sepsis (Chiesa et al. 2004; Bhandari 2014),

PCT crosses the placenta, and levels can be high in neonates even after an uncomplicated delivery. PCT levels in neonates fluctuate during the first 48 h of life and by gestational age, requiring careful assessment of normative values and cut-offs (Table 3.5) (Chiesa et al. 2004). The sensitivity and specificity of PCT predictive value change drastically with the varying thresholds that define positivity in current publications, hindering comparisons of PCT across institutions (Woll et al. 2017). PCT elevation occurs within 2–6 h of a trigger, peaking at 12–48 h once the trigger is removed. Compared to CRP, PCT elevations are observed earlier, peaks earlier, and have more rapid normalization after the stimulus has resolved.

3.7.3.11 Blood Cultures

Neonatal sepsis is separated into early and late onset. Early-onset sepsis is typically considered vertical transmission from mother to the newborn, whereas late-onset typically results from environmental exposure. According to recent AAP clinical guidelines, the cut-off between early-onset and late-onset is 72 h (Puopolo et al. 2019). Late-onset sepsis occurs for up to 3 months of life. Obtaining a blood culture is the standard of care before administering antibiotics (Kim et al. 2020). As noted, diagnostic tests such as CRP have low specificity for infection in an infant that appears well (Hooven and Polin 2019; Polin 2012), and procalcitonin, although more sensitive than a CRP, has less specificity (Kim et al. 2020).

Table 3.5 C-reactive protein and procalcitonin upper limit of normal (95th percentile) for term infants

	Birth	24 h	48 h	>72 h
CRP	0.5 mg/dL	1.4 mg/dL	1.2 mg/dL	1.0 mg/dL
PCT	0.7 ng/mL	20 ng/mL	2 ng/mL	<0.1 ng/mL

Adapted from Chiesa et al. (2004); Chiesa et al. (2011)

CRP C-reactive protein, *PCT* procalcitonin, *mg/dL* milligrams per deciliter

In evaluating neonatal sepsis, the standard of care is to collect a blood culture in a pediatric blood culture collection system (Puopolo et al. 2019). Urine cultures are not needed in an infant less than 72 h of age. Modern automated blood culture detection systems are accurate if there are 1–2 viable bacterial colony-forming units which usually mean that 1 mL of blood is needed (Schelonka et al. 1996). Automated blood culture systems are available and can identify most bacterial organisms within a 24-h period.

The time to a positive result is under 24 h using modern blood culture systems (Puopolo et al. 2019). For optimal bacterial isolation, one blood culture bottle should be filled with a minimum of 1–1.5 mL of blood for children less than 11 kg and 7.5 mL for children between 11 and 17 kg (Huber et al. 2020). Contamination of blood cultures occurs between 1% and 3% of the time, resulting in unnecessary treatment (Revell and Doern 2017). Empiric antibiotics should be administered in critically ill infants despite negative cultures (Puopolo et al. 2019). If the clinician wants to optimize isolation of rare strict anaerobic species, one aerobic and one anaerobic culture bottle may be used, although the common anaerobic species. It should be noted that the common neonatal pathogens of Group B Streptococcus, *Escherichia coli*, and *Staphylococcus aureus* will grow under anaerobic conditions (Puopolo et al. 2019). Repeat blood cultures should be done if a neonate develops new symptoms after four days of treatment (Al-Lawama and Badran 2015).

3.7.3.12 Molecular Methods in Possible Septic Infants

The advantages of PCR tests are the need for small blood volumes (usually 1 mL) and the ability to detect intracellular or slow-growing pathogens. PCR results often provide more conclusive results than culture (Blaschke et al. 2012; Banerjee et al. 2015; Salimnia et al. 2016). A positive blood culture can be evaluated with nested multiplex polymerase chain reaction (PCR) testing of positive blood cultures test and can identify not only bacterial pathogens but also antimicrobial resistance genes in a 1-h turn-

around time (Pantell et al. 2021). Similarly, in the same 1-h time, multiplex meningoencephalitis panels can test the CSF for 14 potential CSF pathogens. If HSV signs are present, then do CSF PCR for HSV, surface swabs of the mouth, nasopharynx, conjunctivae, and anus for an HSV culture (Pantell et al. 2021).

PCR tests' disadvantages include high cost, risk of contamination causing false-positive results, limited pathogens that can be detected or tested, and the inability to do resistance testing. The risk of false negative can result from an insufficient blood sample, resulting in a small bacterial load (Huber et al. 2020). A recent meta-analysis on molecular assays and sepsis in neonates reported an average sensitivity of 0.90 and specificity of 0.93 (Pammi et al. 2017). More information about the evaluation of the well-appearing febrile newborn is found in Sect. 3.8.

3.7.4 Real-Life Examples

A Group B strept negative mother delivered an appropriate for gestation age infant at 40 weeks. The mother had an unremarkable prenatal history and labor and delivery. The bottle-fed neonate was in the newborn nursery without any problems until the end of the second day of life. The neonate was noted to have poor feeding with less than 1-ounce intake after 4 h. The mother thought the baby did not look right. The attending examined the infant, and the exam was negative. A sepsis workup was considered 2 h later when the infant was again noted to be feeding poorly. A sepsis workup was done, the child was moved to the ICU, and antibiotics were started. The initial workup showed a CRP of 10.4 mg/dL and a procalcitonin of 8.8 ng/mL. The CBC was remarkable for an elevated WBC count with a left shift. Four hours later, the newborn developed apnea, and resuscitation efforts were unsuccessful.

A first-born, full-term neonate with A-positive blood was born to a mother who was O positive. The direct Coombs test was negative. By 72 h, jaundice was noted to the thighs, and serum bilirubin was 13, which is a lower risk. The hct was 45%. The child was followed, and the bilirubin slowly dropped to a normal level by the beginning of the third week of life. The child was felt to have ABO incompatibility. A subsequent pregnancy was not unaffected, despite having the same blood group.

Key Learning about Newborn Laboratory Tests

- The interpretation of the CBC in the neonate requires an understanding of the changes that occur during the first months of life.
- The interpretation of the coagulation tests in the newborn period is difficult as the reference ranges are affected by the laboratory variability of reagents and the type of instruments used.
- Infants with ABO incompatibility and hyperbilirubinemia may have hemolysis without a positive Coombs test, and not every infant with a positive Coombs test has hyperbilirubinemia.
- The gold standard of accurately diagnosing hyperbilirubinemia remains a serum bilirubin test, and results should be plotted on bilitool.org to determine the risk of severe hyperbilirubinemia.
- A neonate with risk factors such as small for gestational age, large for gestational age, intrauterine growth restriction, and infants of a diabetic mother should be evaluated for hypoglycemia. There are short- and long-term consequences to hypoglycemia or hyperglycemia. Normal glucose levels should be maintained in infants older than 48–72 h of age unless there are underlying health problems.
- The infant with early-onset sepsis cannot be diagnosed by using procalcitonin, CBC, or CRP alone. Positive blood cultures are needed to confirm the diagnosis of sepsis, although, in a sick infant, a negative blood culture would not preclude sepsis. New PCR methods for identifying bacteria are not yet the standard of care.

3.8   Evaluation of the Well Newborn with a Fever

The AAP published new guidelines for the care of the well newborn with fever. Prenatal GBS screening and immunization against *Streptococcus pneumoniae* are two factors that have led to changes in the bacterial causes of neonatal sepsis (Pantell et al. 2021). *Escherichia coli* has evolved as the most common organism causing bacteremia and is the leading or second leading cause of bacterial meningitis in neonates from ages 1 to 60 days. Listeria monocytogenes is now considered a rare cause of neonatal bacterial disease. New guidelines for evaluating the febrile infant were released in 2021 that divide the evaluation of neonates into three categories—ages 8–21 days, ages 22–28 days, and lastly, ages 29–60 days. These guidelines differ from previous practices where the febrile neonate under 30 days would receive a complete evaluation and likely be hospitalized pending culture results. The infant between 30 and 90 days who was well-appearing would receive IM ceftriaxone pending culture results of blood, urine, and CSF. The guidelines are meant for the infant who has the characteristics seen in Box 3.2.

Box 3.2 Characteristics of Well Febrile Infants for Use with 2021 Guidelines

- The febrile infant should be well appearing.
- Have a history of a rectal temperatures ≥38.0 °C or 100.4 °F in the home within 24 h or a clinical setting.
- Have a gestational age between 37 and under 42 weeks.
- Age is between 8 and 60 days from discharge from a newborn nursery or home delivery.

The guidelines do not apply to infants in the following categories.

It should be kept in mind that the difference between a well-appearing or sick neonate is not as easy as writing it. The evaluation of the febrile newborn is even more challenging if the infant does not yet have a social smile (McCarthy et al. 1982). There is a risk that 1–2.1% of neonates will have viral and bacterial infections (Pantell et al. 2021).

While WBC, absolute neutrophil counts, band count, and the neonate's appearance were previously used to evaluate the infant, the new guidelines emphasize the importance of C-reactive protein and procalcitonin as inflammatory markers in neonatal sepsis. As previously discussed in the point-of-care testing, C-reactive protein is available as a point-of-care test. Procalcitonin is the most effective laboratory test for risk stratification but may not be available around the clock. Table 3.6 summarizes the workup of the well-appearing neonate who presents with fever in primary care.

Table 3.6 Work-up of the well-appearing neonate with fever

Age	Diagnostic workup	Comments
8–21 days of age	• Urine and blood culture • CSF for cell count, gram stain, glucose, protein, bacterial culture, and enterovirus PCR if a seasonal increase in enterovirus or pleocytosis in CSF • May get inflammatory markers (IM) including procalcitonin, C-reactive protein and CBC (for evaluation of WBC, ANC and band count) • HSV culture should be done if maternal history or physical exam is positive for vesicles, seizures	• Elevation of inflammatory markers include the following: • Procalcitonin >0.5 ng/mL, • CRP > 20 mg/L • ANC > 4000 to 5200/mm
22 to 28 days of age	• Urinalysis first and if positive do urine culture obtained via suprapubic or catheterization • If the urine culture is positive, there is no need to do CSF in a well-appearing infant • Blood culture • IM as outlined in the above row. If abnormal, consider lumbar puncture for CSF	If the IM is abnormal, do CSF. Abnormal IM includes fever and the markers above
29 to 60 days	• Urinalysis • Blood culture • IM (procalcitonin along with ANC or CRP) • Can do urine culture via catheterization or suprapubic if urinalysis is positive • HSV is rare but should be done if the signs of HSV are present (see Box 3.4)	

Adapted from Pantell et al. (2021)

3.9 Congenital Infection

3.9.1 Herpes Simplex Virus

Both HSV 1 and HSV 2 cause disease in the neonate (Pinninti and Kimberlin 2018). HSV in the neonate will present in one of three ways: (1) skin, eye, and mucous membrane disease (SEM), (2) disseminated disease with or without CNS involvement, or (3) CNS disease. SEM and disseminated disease present in the first 2 weeks of life, with CNS disease, typically presenting between the second and third weeks of life (AAP 2018). Regardless of maternal history of HSV, testing should be considered in neonates presenting with sepsis syndrome; fever, particularly in the first 3 weeks of life; a vesicular rash, although the rash may look atypical in neonates; or seizures of unknown etiology.

The recommendations for a newborn with possible HSV infection include (1) cerebral spinal fluid for indices and HSV DNA PCR; (2) swab for viral culture or PCR from the base of the vesicles; (3) swab from the mouth, nasopharynx, conjunctiva, and rectum for viral culture or PCR; and (4) whole blood for HSV DNA PCR. Alanine aminotransferase levels (ALT) are often elevated in disseminated disease and can be a helpful adjuvant test (Pinninti and Kimberlin 2018). The tests for HSV are discussed in Sect. 6.4.5, and the ALT is discussed in both the well-child chapter and liver section in the GI chapter.

Box 3.4 Signs of Possible HSV in the Neonate

- Genital HSV lesions in the mother.
- Maternal history of fevers from 2 days before to 2 days after delivery.
- Neonate has vesicles or mucous membrane ulcers.
- Neonate has seizures or hypothermia.
- Neonate has CSF pleocytosis but a negative Gram stain.
- CBC has leukopenia or thrombocytopenia.
- Neonate has elevated alanine aminotransferase levels.

Adapted from Pantell et al. (2021).

3.9.2 Congenital Cytomegalovirus (CMV)

Congenital CMV (cCMV) infection is the most common congenital infection in the developed world. It is estimated to occur in ~0.5 to 0.7% of all live births in the United States (Dollard et al. 2007; Kenneson and Cannon 2007). Although symptomatic infection is only evident in approximately 10% of cCMV infections, cCMV remains the leading infectious cause of neurodevelopmental disability and congenital hearing loss (AAP 2018). Even if the child is asymptomatic, hearing loss can occur during the child's early years, with the average age of late-onset hearing loss being 44 months. Approximately 50% of either symptomatic or asymptomatic infants have progressive sensorineural hearing loss (Fowler and Boppana 2018). Recent reviews showed that infection with CMV in the neonate could occur with maternal reactivation of CMV or reinfection with a different CMV strain during pregnancy (Wang et al. 2011; deVries et al. 2013). Mass testing of all neonates for CMV is not recommended (Fowler and Boppana 2018). Term and preterm infants can acquire CMV peri- and postnatally due to exposure to maternal cervicovaginal secretions during delivery and the ingestion of breast milk after delivery and may present with a sepsis-like syndrome (Hodinka 2015).

Serology may be helpful in pregnancy to determine whether the pregnant woman is susceptible to CMV. Infants with a sepsis-like syndrome without evidence of other bacterial, fungal, or viral causes (such as HSV) may also have CMV testing performed. CMV testing should be performed within the first 3 weeks of life for newborns who present with any of the following: signs and symptoms consistent with cCMV not explained by other causes, abnormal neuroimaging consistent with CMV, documented sensorineural hearing loss, infants born to mothers with known or suspected primary or reactivation CMV during pregnancy, and immunocompromised newborns (Luck et al. 2017; Rawlinson et al. 2017).

3.9.2.1 Urine and/or Saliva for CMV

The diagnosis of congenital cytomegalovirus-infected neonates includes PCR of saliva, urine, or both within the first 3 weeks of life, although ideally as soon as possible after suspicion develops (Luck et al. 2017; Rawlinson et al. 2017). In one multicenter study, CMV PCR in urine had a sensitivity of 100% and specificity of 99% (de Vries et al. 2012). Another study of saliva PCR showed a sensitivity >97% and specificity of 99% (Boppana et al. 2010). Positive urine or saliva PCR establishes the diagnosis for cCMV when performed before 21 days of life (Luck et al. 2017). Importantly, saliva samples for PCR testing should be taken immediately before or at least 1 h after feeding in breastfed newborns, as false-positive results have been reported due to contamination with CMV from breastmilk (Koyano et al. 2013). PCR assay of newborn dried blood spots (DBS) has also been studied and is available at select research laboratories. However, the test has variable sensitivity depending on the laboratory, and therefore a negative test cannot definitively rule out cCMV (Wang et al. 2015; Boppana et al. 2011). Serologic testing is not useful in diagnosing cCMV as a positive CMV IgG may represent a maternal passive transfer of antibody, and CMV IgM is highly insensitive in neonates (Britt 2016).

Early post-natal infection. Post-natal infection can be acquired through saliva and breastmilk. CMV excretion typically begins 3–12 weeks after exposure. A positive CMV PCR within the first 3 weeks of life is considered evidence of congenitally acquired infection; a positive CMV PCR after the first 3 weeks of life may be considered postnatally acquired. However, a negative CMV result during the first 3 weeks of life is necessary to diagnose post-natal infection and exclude cCMV. Early post-natal CMV infection diagnosis may be made utilizing PCR of saliva, urine, or both. Retrospectively, a positive DBS PCR could confirm cCMV in infants with a positive CMV PCR after 3 weeks of life. Still, a negative DBS PCR cannot rule out cCMV in these infants due to variable sensitivity (Wang et al. 2015; Boppana et al. 2011). Serologic testing in these infants has the same limitations described for infants with cCMV.

3.9.3 Syphilis

Maternal-to-child transmission occurs due to in utero transplacental passage of infection or possibly due to neonatal exposure to infected secretions during birth (AAP 2018; Soreng et al. 2014). There has been a steady increase in congenital syphilis in the United States, with 1870 cases reported in 2017 (CDC 2021b). All neonates born to women with reactive serologic tests for syphilis need a physical exam looking for intrauterine growth restriction, jaundice, snuffles (rhinitis), cataracts, seizures, hepatosplenomegaly, skin rash, pseudoparalysis of Parrot (paralysis of an extremity), or nonimmune hydrops fetalis (Cooper and Sanchez 2018). However, at birth, 50% of infants with congenital syphilis may be asymptomatic. Untreated infants will often have clinical manifestations by 3 weeks to 6 months (Larsen et al. 1995).

Given the non-specific symptoms of active syphilis, known latency periods, and the importance of identifying pregnant women with syphilis, the primary care clinician should have a high clinical suspicion to screen for syphilis in pregnancy. Pediatric clinicians care for infants born to mothers with syphilis, so they should be familiar with testing in these children.

3.9.3.1 VDRL and RPR

Serologic testing in infants measures passively transferred antibodies from mother to infant, so nontreponemal and treponemal antibodies partially reflect maternal serology. Venous blood from mother and infant should be sent for the same nontreponemal test; cord blood should not be tested. The VDRL and the RPR are nontreponemal serological tests for congenital syphilis. The same nontreponemal test must be sent on the mother and the infant (Cooper and Sanchez 2018). When the nontreponemal test is fourfold higher (2 dilutions higher) than the mother's titer, congenital syphilis should be considered (CDC 2021b); however, a lack of this increase in an infant with positive exam findings or an infant with a positive darkfield test or PCR of lesions or body fluid does not exclude syphilis. Only 22% of infants with congenital syphilis have a nontreponemal titer higher than their mother's, so lower titers do not exclude congenital syphilis (Larsen et al. 1995; Peeling, Ye 2004). A comprehensive clinical approach, including consideration of maternal treatment and risk for reinfection plus infant examination, should guide the diagnosis of congenital syphilis (AAP 2018). Any infant with syphilis should also be evaluated for HIV as there is an increase in HIV infections in patients with syphilis (Cooper and Sanchez 2018).

3.9.4 HIV

Children born to known HIV-infected mothers acquire passive maternal antibodies; therefore, immunoassays are not recommended to diagnose HIV infection in perinatally exposed infants or children <18 months.

3.9.4.1 HIV DNA and HIV RNA PCR Assays

Diagnostic testing for HIV-exposed infants with HIV DNA or RNA PCR assays is recommended at 14–21 days of age. If these results are negative, repeat testing should be performed at 1–2 months of age and 4 to 6 months. Infants with a higher risk of perinatal HIV transmission may be tested at birth (0 to 2 days) and 2 to 6 weeks after discontinuing antiretroviral prophylaxis (Panel on Antiretroviral Therapy and Medical Management of Children Living with HIV 2020). If a woman presents in labor and her HIV status is unknown, she should undergo expedited HIV screening with a combined HIV antigen/antibody test (Chadwick et al. 2020).

An infant with perinatal HIV exposure is considered infected if two samples from two different time points test positive by HIV DNA or RNA PCR assay. Testing requirements for excluding HIV in nonbreastfed infants born to HIV-infected mothers are reviewed in Chap. 6, Box 6.3. For infants who have met definitive exclusion with two or more negative DNA or RNA PCR tests, an HIV immunoassay collected at 18 to 24 months may be performed to confirm the loss of passively acquired maternal antibody to HIV (AAP 2018).

To completely exclude HIV in nonbreastfed infants <12 months born to HIV-infected mothers, there must be two separate negative HIV DNA or RNA PCR assays obtained when the infant is ≥1 month and again at ≥4 months. Another way to exclude HIV in an infant born to HIV-infected mother is to do two negative antibody tests at least 1 month apart when the infant is ≥6 months. There should be no evidence of HIV infection in both these instances, either clinical or laboratory evidence (AAP 2018).

3.9.5 ZIKA Virus

Infants born to mothers with possible ZIKV exposure during pregnancy should be tested for ZIKV if they are (1) symptomatic or (2) asymptomatic with laboratory evidence of possible maternal ZIKV infection during pregnancy. Clinical findings consistent with congenital ZIKV syndrome include severe microcephaly, decreased brain tissue, ocular abnormalities, congenital contractures, and hypertonia (Mlakar 2016).

For symptomatic pregnant patients with possible exposure to ZIKV and/or DENV, sample collection should occur within 12 weeks of symptom onset and is reviewed in Fig. 3.1. The exact timing of infection cannot be determined from serologic testing alone; infants born to women with positive serology during pregnancy should have ZIKV testing to determine the risk for congenital ZIKV (Sharp et al. 2019). Dengue virus (DENV) and chikungunya virus (CHIKV) evaluations should also be initiated in patients with suspected ZIKV as these viruses have similar clinical manifestations and geographic distributions (Miller et al. 2018).

3.9.5.1 PCR Testing for Infants with Possible ZIKV Exposure

For asymptomatic pregnant women with ongoing possible ZIKV exposure, PCR testing should be offered three times during pregnancy as part of routine obstetric care. The optimal timing and frequency of testing are unknown. Serologic testing is not recommended for asymptomatic

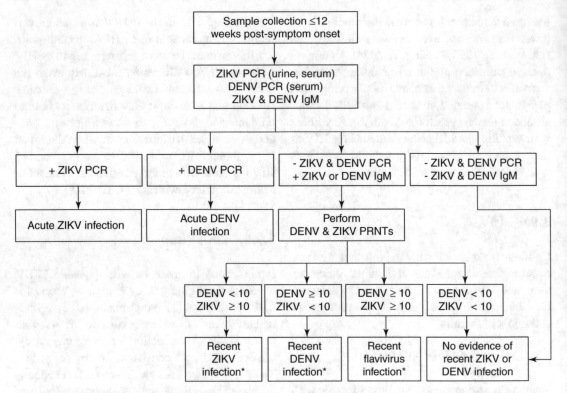

Fig. 3.1 Zika and dengue virus testing algorithm for symptomatic, pregnant patients with risk for both viruses. *The exact timing of infection cannot be determined from serologic testing. Infants born to mothers with laboratory evidence of acute or recent ZIKV infection or unspecified *Flavivirus* infection should undergo testing for congenital ZIKV. *ZIKV* zika virus, *DENV* dengue virus, *PCR* polymerase chain reaction, *IgM* immunoglobulin M, *PRNTs* plaque reduction neutralization tests. Adapted from Sharp et al. (2019). Source: CDC, MMWR

pregnant women, as IgM results cannot reliably determine when ZIKV exposure occurred due to the potential for persistently positive IgM antibodies (Oduyebo et al. 2017).

All infants suspected of congenital ZIKV syndrome should have ZIKV testing initiated as soon as possible after birth. Figure 3.2 reviews testing for an infant with possible ZIKV infection in utero. ZIKV PCR and IgM in CSF should be considered for all infants with symptoms consistent with congenital ZIKV infection. CSF testing may also be considered in asymptomatic infants born to women with possible ZIKV exposure who have negative initial testing or if CSF is obtained for other reasons. Infants with clinical indications for testing, who were not tested near birth, can have ZIKV PRNTs sent at age ≥ 18 months to confirm or exclude congenital ZIKV infection (Adebanjo et al. 2017).

3.9.6 Hepatitis B

The primary care clinician may care for infants born to HBsAg-positive mothers. These infants should receive HBV vaccine and hepatitis B immune globulin at birth or within 12 h of birth to reduce HBV transmission. Infants should then receive a follow-up HBV vaccine at 1 to 2 months and 6 months, followed by post-immunization testing for HBsAg and anti-HBs at 9–12 months (AAP 2021). Testing for hepatitis B is discussed in detail in Chap. 6, Sect. 6.5.2.1.

3.9.7 Hepatitis C

Infants born to HCV-positive mothers are at risk of perinatal transmission of HCV. All children born to HCV-positive mothers should have HCV

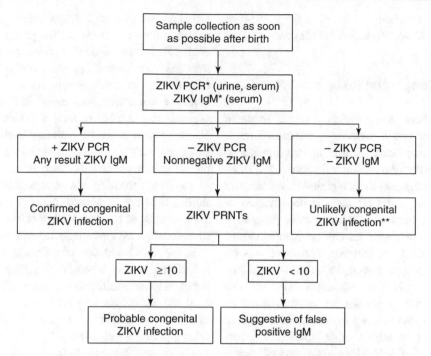

Fig. 3.2 Testing for infants with possible zika virus exposure in utero. * Consider CSF testing for ZIKV PCR and IgM in infants who (1) have possible ZIKV exposure and have symptoms consistent with congenital ZIKV infection, regardless of maternal results, or (2) are asymptomatic with negative ZIKV PCR in urine/serum and negative ZIKV IgM in serum but born to a mother with laboratory evidence of possible maternal ZIKV infection during pregnancy. **Unlikely if specimens are collected within the first few days after birth, and the clinical evaluation is normal; clinicians should remain alert for new findings of congenital ZIKV infection. *ZIKV* zika virus, *PCR* polymerase chain reaction, *IgM* immunoglobulin M, *PRNTs* plaque reduction neutralization tests. Adebanjo et al. (2017). Source: CDC, MMWR

antibody testing at 18 months when maternal antibody has waned (AAP 2018; AASLD-IDSA 2018). Earlier testing is typically not indicated as the risk of maternal-to-child transmission is relatively low. Children often remain asymptomatic, and there is currently no approved therapy for HCV in children younger than 3 years (AAP 2021).

3.9.7.1 HCV RNA PCR

HCV RNA PCR testing can be considered as early as 2 months; however, the benefit is debated (AASLD-IDSA 2018). Some perinatally HCV-infected infants can spontaneously clear HCV infection in infancy (Ceci et al. 2001; Ketzinel-Gilad et al. 2000; Shebl et al. 2009), making an early positive HCV RNA PCR result of unclear utility. Children with perinatally acquired HCV infection can also have fluctuations in viremia, so

an early negative HCV RNA PCR may not definitively exclude infection (Polywka et al. 2006).

New HCV RNA PCR assays may have improved sensitivity and specificity for diagnosing perinatally acquired HCV infection in the first 6 months of life (Gowda et al. 2020). All HCV perinatally exposed infants who have HCV RNA PCR testing, regardless of results, should have definitive HCV antibody testing at 18 months (AASLD-IDSA 2018). Many infants born to mothers with HCV are never appropriately screened (Chappell et al. 2018; Epstein et al. 2018; Kuncio et al. 2016; Watts et al. 2017), so clinicians must remember to perform HCV testing in these infants. An HCV RNA PCR can be sent at 2 to 6 months, especially when there is concern a child may be lost to follow-up, if the family prefers early testing, or if antiviral therapy becomes available for younger children (AASLD-IDSA 2018; AAP 2021).

3.9.8 Congenital Toxoplasmosis

Transplacental transmission of the parasite *Toxoplasma gondii* resulting in congenital toxoplasmosis can occur during the acute phase of acquired primary maternal infection. A full laboratory investigation for congenital toxoplasmosis should occur when (1) there is documented or suspected maternal infection during pregnancy and/or (2) a newborn has clinical manifestations of congenital toxoplasmosis, and there was no maternal serologic testing for toxoplasmosis during pregnancy. Notably, 80 to 90% of infants with congenital toxoplasmosis are asymptomatic at birth, and those that are symptomatic may have symptoms that mimic other congenital infections, such as CMV. The classic triad of hydrocephalus, intracerebral calcification, and chorioretinitis is only seen in a small number of infected newborn infants (Peyron et al. 2016).

All neonatal samples with concern for congenital toxoplasmosis should be sent to a toxoplasma reference lab for testing specific panels with high diagnostic accuracy (Montoya 2002).

3.9.9 Chagas Disease

Chagas disease is caused by a protozoan, *Trypanosoma cruzi*. The parasite is endemic in Central and South America, with an estimated 5–6 million persons infected (Bern 2015). It is estimated that 40,000 women of childbearing age are infected and have chronic Chagas disease (Edwards et al. 2018; Edwards et al. 2019). This means that between 63 and 315 infected neonates are born every year in the US (CDC 2021b). Congenital Chagas disease is symptomatic in 10–40% of neonates and can present with anemia, thrombocytopenia, hepatosplenomegaly, prematurity, and jaundice (Bern and Montgomery 2009; Edwards et al. 2019). The disease can be transmitted by vector via the reduviid insect or kissing bug (*Triatominae* subfamily) since the feces left on the skin after a blood meal can cross

the skin and mucosa barriers entering the lymphatic system and infecting the patient (Wagner et al. 2016). It can also be acquired by eating food infected with Reduviidae feces, and this method of transmission is an emerging route of infection. While transmission via blood transfusion or organ transplantation occurs, it is less common. Vertical transmission from mother to child occurs in approximately 5%, depending on the degree of parasitemia in the mother (Wagner et al. 2016).

Healthy appearing but congenitally infected infants may not be symptomatic in infancy, but 20% to 40% of children will develop fatal heart disease after asymptomatic infection (Edwards et al. 2019). Conduction abnormality is an early manifestation, but a progressive dilated cardiomyopathy can manifest as sudden death (Edwards et al. 2018). Infants with congenital Chagas disease are missed due to a lack of disease knowledge and disease awareness. The diagnosis must be considered in infants born to immigrants from Latin America (Edwards et al. 2018). Diagnostic testing in the newborn is discussed below, but a clinical examination is important along with direct blood microscopic exam (Wagner et al. 2016). If the mother has tested positive for Chagas disease during prepregnancy, the CDC (2021a) advised using whole blood from the infant or cord blood if there was no maternal blood contamination. Three tests could be done: (1) microscopic examination of blood (Giemsa stain for *T. cruzi* trypomastigotes), (2) PCR, or if the mother was not tested during pregnancy, but there is suspicion of Chagas disease, Chagas disease serology to detect maternal antibody.

3.9.9.1 Direct Microscopic Examination

The Giemsa stain is a gold standard staining technique used for thin and thick smears of blood. During an acute infection, the trypanosomes can be seen with thick-thin smears or concentration techniques.

3.9.9.2 PCR

In the acute phase or during early reactivation, blood PCR is highly sensitive. The use of PCR in patients with chronic disease has a sensitivity of 60–90%. With quantitative PCR, an elevated parasite count indicated an increased risk of transmission to the neonate. PCR may help detect newborns with congenital infection. Still, it is limited due to false-positive results from nonviable parasites and lack of availability in most diagnostic labs outside of tertiary centers (Wagner et al. 2016). If PCR and Giemsa staining are negative at birth, the CDC recommends repeating the Giemsa stain and the PCR at 4–6 weeks. If the results are negative at 4 to 6 weeks, serology should be done at 9 to 12 months (CDC 2021a).

3.9.9.3 Serology

Serological methods include enzyme-linked immunosorbent assay, indirect hemagglutination assays and indirect immunofluorescence. Due to cross-reactivity, two different serological tests are advised (Wagner et al. 2016). Pregnancy women from endemic areas should be screened with serologic testing. A child over 9 months can be screened with serology, but this test is not recommended as the sole test in the newborn period (Gomes et al. 2019). Whole family screening is advised once an index case is identified (Wagner et al. 2016). If the serology is negative at 9 to 12 months, Chagas disease is excluded (CDC 2021b).

3.9.10 Real-Life Examples

A 4-year-old female who lived in an inner city was seen for a well-child visit. The 19-year-old mother reported no significant history. The physical exam was normal. Table 3.7 shows the result of the hearing screen was during the visit.

An audiological exam confirmed moderate sensorineural hearing, and the child was fitted for hearing aids. An ENT referral and genetic referral were initiated, which failed to reveal the source of the child's hearing loss. Based on the high inci-

dence of CMV infections among adolescents in the community, it was presumed that this child had an asymptomatic neonatal CMV infection.

Key Learning about Congenital Infections

- Congenital neonatal infections may be asymptomatic at birth, and screening must be considered depending on the maternal history, the neonatal exam, and the community incidence of infectious diseases.
- Congenital CMV is best identified by PCR of saliva, urine, or both within the first 3 weeks of life.
- At birth, 50% of infants with congenital syphilis are asymptomatic and untreated infants will often have clinical manifestations by 3 weeks to 6 months.
- Neonates exposed to HIV need to be followed closely. Diagnostic testing for HIV-exposed infants with HIV DNA or RNA PCR assays is recommended at 14–21 days of age. If these results are negative, repeat testing should be performed at 1–2 months of age and 4–6 months.
- Neonates born to women with positive serology during pregnancy should have ZIKV testing to determine the risk for congenital ZIKV.
- Neonates exposed to hepatitis B in utero should be treated within 12 h with HBIG and hepatitis B vaccine, with follow-up vaccines at 1 and 6 months. Following immunization, testing for HBsAg and anti-HBs is recommended 1–2 months after the last vaccine.
- Congenital toxoplasmosis is asymptomatic in 80–90% of neonates, and those that are symptomatic may have symptoms that mimic other congenital infections.
- Chagas disease tends to be a missed diagnosis. While universal screening of mothers who come from Central or South America is not yet recommended, the disease should be considered in a neonate with anemia, thrombocytopenia, hepatosplenomegaly, prematurity, and jaundice.

Table 3.7 Hearing screen results

HZ	Decibels
500	20
1000	40
2000	50
4000	65

Questions

1. A mother asks if she can opt-out of the PKU test. Which of the following is the best response?
   - (a) The PKU test and NBS test are interchangeable.
   - (b) The PKU test is one of many tests done during the newborn screening to identify treatable disorders.
   - (c) The PKU test identifies babies with a PKU deficiency, and the baby will be symptomatic within a few days of birth.
   - (d) The PKU test must be done.
2. An African American male has prolonged jaundice. He has normal direct bilirubin and elevated total bilirubin. The mother is A+, and the child is 0+. What is the most likely diagnosis?
   - (a) Physiologic jaundice.
   - (b) ABO setup.
   - (c) RhD incompatibility.
   - (d) G6PD deficiency.
3. When is the optimal timing for a newborn metabolic screening to be done in a full-term infant?
   - (a) 6–11 h after the first feeding
   - (b) 12–23 h after birth
   - (c) 24 h after the first feeding
   - (d) At the time of birth.
4. A newborn has a positive Coombs test and anemia. What is the most likely diagnosis?
   - (a) Diamond-Blackfan anemia.
   - (b) Hemorrhage.
   - (c) Isoimmune hemolytic anemia.
   - (d) Aplastic anemia.
5. You receive the results of a CBC on a newborn. It shows the following—decreased hemoglobin level, normal reticulocyte count, negative Coombs' test, and decreased MCV. What is the most likely cause of this anemia?
   - (a) Alpha thalassemia.
   - (b) Hereditary spherocytosis.
   - (c) Rh incompatibility.
   - (d) G6PD deficiency.
6. What test distinguishes fetal RBCs from maternal RBCs?
   - (a) Direct antiglobulin test.
   - (b) Hemoglobin electrophoresis.
   - (c) Kleihauer-Betke test.
   - (d) Reticulocyte count.
7. You are seeing a newborn for a well visit, and the mother tells you that the older sibling was diagnosed with fifth disease (parvovirus B19) while she was pregnant. What would you expect on a CBC in a newborn exposed to parvovirus in utero?
   - (a) Anemia due to decreased RBC production.
   - (b) Anemia due to increased RBC destruction.
   - (c) Anemia due to blood loss.
   - (d) Anemia due to a fetomaternal transfusion.
8. Who is responsible for communicating normal newborn screening results to the family?
   - (a) The primary care provider.
   - (b) The genetics department.
   - (c) The state where the child was born.
9. What is usually part of the management of neonates with ABO incompatibility?
   - (a) Phototherapy.
   - (b) Serial monitoring of bilirubin and hemoglobin levels.
   - (c) Administration of Rhogam.
   - (d) Partial exchange transfusion.
10. Which of the following is a *non-treponemal test* for syphilis?
    - (a) VDRL.
    - (b) FPT-ABS.
    - (c) FTA-ABS.
    - (d) TRUST.
11. A healthy full-term 72-hour-old infant has indirect bilirubin of 18.2 and a direct of 0.1 (normal 0.1–0.8). Using bilitool.org as a guide, what is the next step?
    - (a) Order an abdominal ultrasound.
    - (b) Do a CBC.
    - (c) Do an exchange transfusion.
    - (d) Initiate phototherapy.
12. A neonate has type O-negative blood, and the mother has type B-negative blood. Which of the following is the most likely scenario?

(a) The neonate will develop mild hemolysis.

(b) The neonate will develop moderate hemolysis.

(c) The neonate will develop severe hemolysis.

(d) The neonate will have no problems.

13. Infants diagnosed with a disorder on the NBS panel are always symptomatic.

(a) True.

(b) False.

14. A 40-week pregnant mother arrives via airplane from Peru. She delivers a 4-pound, five-ounce neonate with hepatosplenomegaly, anemia, and thrombocytopenia. Which of the following diagnostic laboratory tests should be done to evaluate the child?

(a) A Giemsa stain with a PCR for Trypanosoma cruzi DNA in blood.

(b) A VDRL.

(c) An HIV.

(d) All of the above.

15. A well-appearing 34-day-old neonatal male presents with a fever of 101.6 to the primary care office. The mother reports that his older sibling had a viral infection lasting 24 h, 2 days ago. The mother states that she had no infection during the pregnancy and was Group B Streptococcus negative. There was no history of maternal fever or antibiotic use. The physical exam is normal. Based on the new guidelines, what is the next step?

(a) Blood, urine, and CSF cultures along with a chest X-ray.

(b) Blood, urine and CSF cultures along with inflammatory markers.

(c) Blood culture, urinalysis, and inflammatory markers.

(d) Blood culture and inflammatory markers.

Rationale

1. Answer: B

In this case, the mother needs more knowledge about the purposes of newborn screening and would need extensive education. B is the best answer as it is the only correct statement. The PKU test is one part of the newborn screening. Newborn screening identifies children with treatable disorders before they become symptomatic. Newborn screening is an opt-out test that a mother can opt-out of, but clinicians must explore why they declined the test and educate them about newborn screening benefits.

2. Answer: D

There is no ABO setup nor RhD incompatibility in this patient as the mother is A+ and the infant is O+. Physiologic jaundice is not usually prolonged. G-6PD deficiency is the correct answer to this question.

3. Answer: C

The best time to do a newborn screening is after the baby has been fed for 24 h. If a newborn screening is done at the time of birth or on the first day after a feeding, certain PKU tests can give a false-negative result.

4. Answer: C

Isoimmune hemolytic anemia is the correct answer as hemorrhage, aplastic anemia, and Diamond-Blackfan syndrome may cause anemia but not a positive Coombs' test.

5. Answer: A

Only alpha thalassemia will cause a decreased MCV, anemia with a normal reticulocyte count. The other three choices should cause an elevated reticulocyte count due to the body's attempt to raise the blood count by releasing premature RBCs or reticulocytes.

6. Answer: C

The Kleihauer-Betke test or acid elution test is one test to determine the amount of fetal RBC. It is a quantitative test. None of the other tests will determine fetal RBCs.

7. Answer: A

Parvovirus causes a red cell aplasia following infection. Fetuses infected with parvovirus during the pregnancy can develop severe anemia leading to heart failure and hydrops fetalis. Parvovirus does not cause red cell destruction or blood loss.

8. Answer: A

The primary care provider is responsible for following up on the newborn screening. They must make sure that the child receives the appropriate care after a positive newborn screening is done. Treatment with levothyroxine can be initiated for the neonate with a positive screen for hypothyroidism. Treatment can involve emergency room care and hospital admission for a baby with urea cycle disorder. The clinician must educate the family about the importance of follow-up and ensure that appropriate care is carried out. Social services must be contacted when the mother refuses to go to the appropriate provider.

9. Answer: B

Newborns with ABO incompatibility need close follow-up to avoid the complications of extremes of indirect hyperbilirubinemia. The neonate needs close follow-up to monitor the bilirubin level and to evaluate for resultant anemia. While it is unlikely the newborn will need exchange transfusions, the neonate does need close follow-up.

10. Answer: A

The only nontreponemal test listed is a VDRL.

11. Answer: D

According to bilitool.org, a bilirubin above 17.7 will put a full-term infant in the high-risk category, and phototherapy should be initiated.

12. Answer: D

This mother-child unit does not have an ABO incompatibility set up, so no hemolysis should occur based on the information given.

13. Answer: B

Most neonates who ultimately have a positive screening are not symptomatic at the time of birth. The advantage of newborn screening is that the neonate can be identified and treated before they become symptomatic.

14. Answer: D

All of the above is the correct answer. An HIV screen should be done since the mother has no records from her country. In this case,

Chagas disease should be ruled out (CDC 2021a), and a VDRL would also be important to rule out congenital syphilis.

15. Answer: C

Blood cultures, urinalysis, and inflammatory markers would be the initial workup in a child from 29 to 60 days.

References

AASLD-IDSA. HCV in children. Recommendations for testing, managing, and treating hepatitis C. 2018 [https://www.hcvguidelines.org/unique-populations/children

ACMG ACT Sheets and Algorithms. [Internet]Newborn screening ACT sheets and algorithms. Bethesda (MD): American College of Medical Genetics and Genomics; 2001.

Adamkin DH. Neonatal hypoglycemia. Curr Opin Pediatr. 2016;28(2):150–5.

Adamkin DH, et al. Clinical report—postnatal glucose homeostasis in late-preterm and term infants. Pediatrics. 2011;127:575–9.

Adebanjo T, Godfred-Cato S, Viens L, et al. Update: interim guidance for the diagnosis, evaluation, and management of infants with possible congenital Zika virus infection—United States, October 2017. MMWR Morb Mortal Wkly Rep. 2017;66:1089–99.

Agrawal A. CRP after 2004. Mol Immunol. 2005;42(8):927–30.

Agrawal A, Hussain KS, Kumar A. Minor blood group incompatibility due to blood groups other than Rh(d) leading to hemolytic disease of the fetus and newborn: a need for routine antibody screening during pregnancy. Intractable Rare Dis Res. 2020;9(1):43–7.

Al-Lawama M, Badran E. Clinical value of repeat blood cultures in neonatal patients receiving antibiotic treatment. J Int Med Res. 2015;43(1):118–24.

Al-Zaidy SA, Mendell JR. From Clinical Trials to Clinical Practice: Practical Considerations for Gene Replacement Therapy in SMA Type 1. Pediatr Neurol. 2019;100:3–11.

American Academy of Pediatrics. Summaries of infectious diseases. In: Kimberlin DW, Brady MT, Jackson MA, Long SS, editors. Red book: 2018 report of the committee on infectious diseases. American Academy of Pediatrics; 2018. p. 235–901.

American Academy of Pediatrics. Summaries of infectious diseases. In: Kimberlin DW, Brady MT, Jackson MA, Long SS, editors. Red book: 2021 Report of the Committee on Infectious Diseases. American Academy of Pediatrics; 2021:Section 3.

American Academy of Pediatrics Committee on Fetus and Newborn and ACOG Committee on Obstetric Practice. In: Kilpatrick SJ, Papile L, Macones GA,

Watterberg K, editors. Guidelines for Perinatal Care. 8th ed. Elk Grove Village, Illinois: American Academy of Pediatrics; 2017.

American College of Medical Genetics Newborn Screening Expert Group. Newborn screening: toward a uniform screening panel and system—executive summary. Pediatrics. 2006;117(5 Pt 2):S296–307.

American College of Obstetricians and Gynecologists. Prevention of Rh D Alloimmunization. ACOG Practice Bulletin, Number 181. Obstet Gynecol. 2017;130:e57–70.

Anderson NB, Calkins KL. Neonatal indirect hyperbilirubinemia. NeoReviews. 2020;21(11):e749–60.

Banerjee R, Teng CB, Cunningham SA, Ihde SM, Steckelberg JM, Moriarty JP, et al. Randomized trial of rapid multiplex polymerase chain reaction-based blood culture identification and susceptibility testing. Clin Infect Dis. 2015;61(7):1071–80.

Bern C. Chagas' disease. N Engl J Med. 2015;373:456–66.

Bern C, Montgomery SP. An estimate of the burden of Chagas disease in the United States. Clin Infect Dis. 2009;49:e52–4.

Bhandari V. Effective biomarkers for diagnosis of neonatal sepsis. J Pediatr Infect Dis Soc. 2014;3(3):234–45.

Bhutani VK, Gourley GR, Adler S, Kreamer B, Dalin C, Johnson LH. Noninvasive measurement of total serum bilirubin in a multiracial predischarge newborn population to assess the risk of severe hyperbilirubinemia. Pediatrics. 2000;106(2):E17.

Blaschke AJ, Heyrend C, Byington CL, Fisher MA, Barker E, Garrone NF, et al. Rapid identification of pathogens from positive blood cultures by multiplex polymerase chain reaction using the FilmArray system. Diagn Microbiol Infect Dis. 2012;74(4):349–55.

Boppana SB, Ross SA, Novak Z, Shimamura M, Tolan RW Jr, Palmer AL, et al. Dried blood spot real-time polymerase chain reaction assays to screen newborns for congenital cytomegalovirus infection. JAMA. 2010;303(14):1375–82.

Boppana SB, Ross SA, Shimamura M, et al. Saliva polymerase-chain-reaction assay for cytomegalovirus screening in newborns. N Engl J Med. 2011;364(22):2111–8.

Britt W. Cytomegalovirus. In: Wilson CB, Nizet V, Maldonado YA, Remington JS, Klein JO, editors. Remington and Klein's infectious diseases of the fetus and newborn infant. 8th ed. Philadelphia, PA: Elsevier Saunders; 2016. p. 724–65.

Brown JVE, Meader N, Wright K, Cleminson J, McGuire W. Assessment of C-reactive protein diagnostic test accuracy for late-onset infection in newborn infants: a systematic review and meta-analysis. JAMA Pediatr. 2020;174(3):260–8.

Caggana M, Jones EA, Shahied SI, Tanksley S, Hermerath CA, Lubin IM. Newborn screening: from Guthrie to whole-genome sequencing. Public Health Rep. 2013;128(Suppl 2):14–9.

Ceci O, Margiotta M, Marello F, Francavilla R, Loizzi P, Francavilla A, et al. Vertical transmission of hepatitis C virus in a cohort of 2,447 HIV-seronegative pregnant women: a 24-month prospective study. J Pediatr Gastroenterol Nutr. 2001;33(5):570–5.

Centers for Disease Control. Congenital chagas disease. Retrieved May 6, 2021, 2021a. https://www.cdc.gov/parasites/chagas/health_professionals/congenital_chagas.html

Centers for Disease Control. (2021b). Congenital syphilis. Retrieved on April 15, 2021, at https://www.cdc.gov/std/tg2015/congenital.htm

Chadwick EG, Ezeanolue EE, Committee on Pediatric AIDS. Evaluation and management of the infant exposed to HIV in the United States. Pediatrics. 2020;146(5):e2020029058.

Chappell CA, Hillier SL, Crowe D, Meyn LA, Bogen DL, Krans EE. Hepatitis C virus screening among children exposed during pregnancy. Pediatrics. 2018;141:6.

Chicaiza H, Hellstrand K, Lerer T, Smith S, Sylvester F. Potassium hydroxide: an alternative reagent to perform the modified apt test. J Pediatr. 2014;165(3):628–30.

Chiesa C, Natale F, Pascone R, Osborn JF, Pacifico L, Bonci E, De Curtis M. C reactive protein and procalcitonin: reference intervals for preterm and term newborns during the early neonatal period. Clin Chim Acta. 2011;412(11–12):1053–9.

Chiesa C, Panero A, Osborn JF, Simonetti AF, Pacifico L. Diagnosis of neonatal sepsis: a clinical and laboratory challenge. Clin Chem. 2004;50(2):279–87.

Christensen RD, Henry E, Jopling J, Wiedmeier SE. The CBC: reference ranges for neonates. Semin Perinatol. 2009;33(1):3–11.

Cooper JM, Sanchez PJ. Congenital syphilis. Semin Perinatol. 2018;42:176–84.

CureSMA, Newborn screening for SMA. Retrieved April 17, 2021., from https://www.curesma.org/newborn-screening-for-sma/

de Vries JJ, van der Eijk AA, Wolthers KC, et al. Real-time PCR versus viral culture on urine as a gold standard in the diagnosis of congenital cytomegalovirus infection. J Clin Virol. 2012;53(2):167–70.

deVries JJ, van Zwet EQ, Dekker FW, Kroes AC, Verkerk PH, Vossen AC. The apparent paradox of maternal seropositivity as a risk factor for congenital cytomegalovirus infection; a population-based prediction model. Rev Med Virol. 2013;23:241–8.

Dollard SC, Grosse SD, Ross DS. New estimates of the prevalence of neurological and sensory sequelae and mortality associated with congenital cytomegalovirus infection. Rev Med Virol. 2007;17(5):355–63.

Du L, Ma X, Shen X, Bao Y, Chen L, Bhutani VK. Neonatal hyperbilirubinemia management: clinical assessment of bilirubin production. Semin Perinatol. 2021;45(1):15135.

Eberl W. Diagnostic challenges in newborns and infants with coagulation disorders. Hamostaseologie. 2020;40(1):84–7.

Edwards MS, Abayie FA, Montgomery SP. Survey of pediatric infectious disease society members about congenital Chagas disease. Pediatr Infect Dis J. 2018;37(1):e24–7.

Edwards MS, Stimpert KK, Bialek SR, Montgomery SP. Evaluation and management of congenital Chagas disease in the United States. J Pediatr Infect Soc. 2019;8(5):4961–469.

Epstein RL, Sabharwal V, Wachman EM, Saia KA, Vellozzi C, Hariri S, et al. Perinatal transmission of hepatitis C virus: defining the cascade of care. J Pediatr. 2018;203:34–40. e1

Fabie NAV, Pappas KB, Feldman GL. The current state of newborn screening in the United States. Pediatr Clin N Am. 2019;66(2):369–86.

Fasano RM. Hemolytic disease of the fetus and newborn in the molecular era. Semin Fetal Neonatal Med. 2016;21(1):28–34.

Fonseca R, Kyralessa R, Malloy M, Richardson J, Jain SK. Covered skin transcutaneous bilirubin estimation is comparable with serum bilirubin during and after phototherapy. J Perinatol. 2012;32(2):129–31.

Fowler KB, Boppana SB. Congenital cytomegalovirus infection. Semin Perinatol. 2018;42:149–54.

Galetto-Lacour A, Zamora SA, Gervaix A. Bedside procalcitonin and C-reactive protein tests in children with fever without localizing signs of infection seen in a referral center. Pediatrics. 2003;112(5):1054–60.

Geaghan SM. Diagnostic laboratory technologies for the fetus and neonate with isoimmunization. Semin Perinatol. 2011;35(3):148–54.

Goldenberg A, Green NS, Kemper AR, Botkin JR, Ojodu J, Prosser LA, et al. Evaluating harms in the assessment of net benefit: a framework for newborn screening condition review. Matern Child Health J. 2016;20(3):693–700.

Gomes C, Almeida A, Rosa A, Araujo PF, Teixeira A. American typanosomiasis and Chaga disease: sexual transmission. Int J Infect Dis. 2019;81:81–4.

Gowda C, Smith S, Crim L, Moyer K, Sanchez PJ, Honegger JR. Nucleic acid testing for diagnosis of perinatally-acquired hepatitis C virus infection in early infancy. Clin Infect Dis. 2020:ciaa949.

Gurian EA, Kinnamon DD, Henry JJ, Waisbren SE. Expanded newborn screening for biochemical disorders: the effect of a false-positive result. Pediatrics. 2006;117(6):1915–21.

Hameed NN, Hussein MA. BIND score: a system to triage infants readmitted for extreme hyperbilirubinemia. Semin Perinatol. 2021;45(1):151354.

Hays T, Wapner RJ. Genetic testing for unexplained perinatal disorders. Curr Opin Pediatr. 2021;33:195–202.

Hodinka RL. Human Cytomegalovirus. In: Jorgenson JH, Pfaller MA, Carroll KC, Funke G, Landry ML, Richter SS, et al., editors. Manual of clinical microbiology. 11th ed. Washington, DC: ASM Press; 2015. p. 1718–38.

Hooven TA, Polin RA. Neonatal bacterial infections. In: Martin GL, Rosenfield W, editors. Common problems in the newborn nursery; an evidence and case-based guide. Switzerland: Springer; 2019.

Huber S, Hetzer B, Crazzolara R, Orth-Höller D. The correct blood volume for paediatric blood cultures: a conundrum? Clin Microbiol Infect. 2020;26(2):168–73.

Ip S, Chung M, Kulig J, O'Brien R, Sege R, Glicken S, et al. American Academy of Pediatrics Subcommittee on hyperbilirubinemia. An evidence-based review of important issues concerning neonatal hyperbilirubinemia. Pediatrics. 2004;114(1):e130–53.

Jaffray J, Young G, Ko RH. The bleeding newborn: a review of presentation, diagnosis, and management. Semin Fetal Neonatal Med. 2016;21(1):44–9.

Kato GJ, Piel FB, Reid CD, Gaston MH, Ohene-Frempong K, Krishnamurti L, et al. Sickle cell disease. Nat Rev Dis Primers. 2018;4:18010.

Kenneson A, Cannon MJ. Review and meta-analysis of the epidemiology of congenital cytomegalovirus (CMV) infection. Rev Med Virol. 2007;17(4):253–76.

Keren R, Tremont K, Luan X, Cnaan A. Visual assessment of jaundice in term and late preterm infants. Arch Dis Child Fetal Neonatal Ed. 2009;94:F317–22.

Ketzinel-Gilad M, Colodner S, Hadary R, Granot E, Shouval D, Galun E. Transient transmission of hepatitis C virus from mothers to newborns. Eur J Clin Microbiol Infect Dis. 2000;19(4):267–74.

Kim F, Polin RA, Hooven TA. Neonatal sepsis. BMJ. 2020;371:m3672.

Koyano S, Inoue N, Nagamori T, Moriuchi H, Azuma H. Newborn screening of congenital cytomegalovirus infection using saliva can be influenced by breastfeeding. Arch Dis Child Fetal Neonatal Ed. 2013;98(2):F182.

Kramer LI. Advancement of dermal icterus in the jaundiced newborn. Am J Dis Child. 1969;118:454–8.

Kuncio DE, Newbern EC, Johnson CC, Viner KM. Failure to test and identify perinatally infected children born to hepatitis C virus-infected women. Clin Infect Dis. 2016;62(8):980–5.

Larsen SA, Steiner BM, Rudolph AH. Laboratory diagnosis and interpretation of tests for syphilis. Clin Microbiol Rev. 1995;8(1):1–21.

Leber AL, Everhart K, Balada-Llasat JM, Cullison J, Daly J, Holt S, et al. Multicenter evaluation of BioFire FilmArray meningitis/encephalitis panel for detection of bacteria, viruses, and yeast in cerebrospinal fluid specimens. J Clin Microbiol. 2016;54(9):2251–61.

Lee AC, Folger LV, Rahman M, Ahmed S, Bably NN, Schaeffer L, et al. A novel Icterometer for hyperbilirubinemia screening in low-resource settings. Pediatrics. 2019;143(5):e20182039.

Luck SE, Wieringa JW, Blazquez-Gamero D, Henneke P, Schuster K, Butler K, et al. Congenital cytomegalovirus: a European expert consensus statement on diagnosis and management. Pediatr Infect Dis J. 2017;36(12):1205–13.

Mak CM, Hencher- Lee HC, Chan AYW, Lam CW. Inborn errors of metabolism and expanded newborn screening: review and update. Crit Rev Clin Lab Sci. 2019;50(6):142–62.

Mathers NJ, Pohlandt F. Diagnostic audit of C-reactive protein in neonatal infection. Eur J Pediatr. 1987;146(2):147–51.

McCarthy PL, Sharpe MR, Spiesel SZ, Dolan TF, Forsyth BW, DeWitt TG, Fink HD, Baron MA, Cicchetti DV. Observation scales to identify serious illness in febrile children. Pediatrics. 1982;70(5): 802–9.

Miller JM, Binnicker MJ, Campbell S, Carroll KC, Chapin KC, Gilligan PH et al. A Guide to Utilization of the Microbiology Laboratory for Diagnosis of Infectious Diseases: 2018 Update by the Infectious Diseases Society of America and the American Society for Microbiologya. Clin Infect Dis. 2018;67(6):e1–e94.

Mlakar J, Korva M, Tul N, Popović M, Poljšak-Prijatelj M, Mraz J, et al. Zika Virus Associated with Microcephaly. N Engl J Med. 2016;374(10):951–8.

Montoya JG. Laboratory diagnosis of toxoplasma gondii infection and toxoplasmosis. J Infect Dis. 2002;185(Supplement_1):S73–82.

Moyer VA, Ahn C, Sneed S. Accuracy of clinical judgment in neonatal jaundice. Arch Pediatr Adolesc Med. 2000;154:391–4.

Muchowski KE. Evaluation and treatment of neonatal hyperbilirubinemia. Am Fam Physician. 2014;89(11):873–8.

Nagar G, Vandermeer B, Campbell S, Kumar M. Reliability of transcutaneous bilirubin devices in preterm infants: a systematic review. Pediatrics. 2013;132(5):871–81.

Nagar G, Vandermeer B, Campbell S, Kumar M. Effect of phototherapy on the reliability of transcutaneous bilirubin devices in term and near-term infants: a systematic review and meta-analysis. Neonatology. 2016;109(3):203–12.

Oduyebo T, Polen KD, Walke HT, et al. Update: interim guidance for health care providers caring for pregnant women with possible Zika virus exposure—United States (including U.S. territories), July 2017. MMWR. 2017;66(29):781–93.

Okwundu CI, Saini SS. Noninvasive methods for bilirubin measurements in newborns: a report. Semin Perinatol. 2021;45(1):151355.

Pal S, Curley A, Stanworth SJ. Interpretation of clotting tests in the neonate. Arch Dis Child Fetal Neonatal Ed. 2015;100(3):F270–4.

Pammi M, Flores A, Versalovic J, Leeflang MMG. Molecular assays for the diagnosis of sepsis in neonates. Cochrane Database Syst Rev. 2017;2:CD011926. https://doi.org/10.1002/14651858.

Panel on Antiretroviral Therapy and Medical Management of Children Living with HIV. Guidelines for the Use of Antiretroviral Agents in Pediatric HIV Infection 2020 December 2020 http://aidsinfo.nih.gov/contentfiles/lvguidelines/pediatricguidelines.pdf.

Pantell RH, Roberts KB, Adams WG, Dreyer BP, Kuppermann N, O'Leary ST, Okechukwu K, Woods CR Jr; SUBCOMMITTEE ON FEBRILE INFANTS. Evaluation and Management of Well-Appearing Febrile Infants 8 to 60 Days Old. Pediatrics. 2021;148(2):e2021052228.

Peeling RW, Ye H. Diagnostic tools for preventing and managing maternal and congenital syphilis: an overview. Bull World Health Organ. 2004;82(6):439–46.

Peyron F, Wallon M, Kieffer F, Garweg J. Toxoplasmosis. In: Wilson CB, Nizet V, Maldonado YA, Remington JS, Klein JO, editors. Remington and Klein's infectious diseases of the fetus and newborn infant. 8th ed. Philadelphia, PA: Elsevier Saunders; 2016. p. 949–1024.

Pinninti S, Kimberlin DW. Herpes simplex infection in the neonate. Semin Perinatol. 2018;42:168–75.

Polin RA. Committee on Fetus and Newborn. Management of neonates with suspected or proven early-onset bacterial sepsis. Pediatrics. 2012;129(5):1006–15. https://doi.org/10.1542/peds.2012-0541. Epub 2012 Apr 30. PMID: 22547779.

Polywka S, Pembrey L, Tovo PA, Newell ML. Accuracy of HCV-RNA PCR tests for diagnosis or exclusion of vertically acquired HCV infection. J Med Virol. 2006;78(2):305–10.

Prefumo F, Fichera A, Fratelli N, Sartori E. Fetal anemia: diagnosis and management. Best Pract Res Clin Obstet Gynaecol. 2019;58:2–14.

Puopolo KM, Lynfield R, Cummings JJ; American Academy of Pediatrics, Committee on Fetus and Newborn, Committee on Infectious Diseases. Management of Infants at Risk for Group B Streptococcal Disease. Pediatrics. 2019;144(2):e20191881.

Putto A, Ruuskanen O, Meurman O, Ekblad H, Korvenranta H, Mertsola J, et al. C reactive protein in the evaluation of febrile illness. Arch Dis Child. 1986;61(1):24–9.

Rawlinson WD, Boppana SB, Fowler KB, Kimberlin DW, Lazzarotto T, Alain S, et al. Congenital cytomegalovirus infection in pregnancy and the neonate: consensus recommendations for prevention, diagnosis, and therapy. Lancet Infect Dis. 2017;17(6):e177–e88.

Recommended Uniform Screening Panel. [Internet] Official website of the U.S. Health Resour Serv Administration. 2020; [cited 2020Nov24]. https://www.hrsa.gov/advisory-committees/heritable-disorders/rusp/index.html

Revell P, Doern C. Pediatric blood cultures. In: Dunne Jr WM, Burnham C, editors. The dark art of blood cultures. Washington, DC: ASM Press; 2017. p. 151–62.

Rivers A, Slayton WB. Congenital cytopenias and bone marrow failure syndrome. Semin Perinatol. 2009;33:20–8.

Salimnia H, Fairfax MR, Lephart PR, Schreckenberger P, DesJarlais SM, Johnson JK, et al. Evaluation of the FilmArray blood culture identification panel: results of a multicenter controlled trial. J Clin Microbiol. 2016;54(3):687–98.

Schelonka RL, Chai MK, Yoder BA, Hensley D, Brockett RM, Ascher DP. Volume of blood required to detect common neonatal pathogens. J Pediatr. 1996;129(2):275–8.

Sharp TM, Fischer M, Muñoz-Jordán JL, Paz-Bailey G, Staples JE, Gregory CJ, et al. Dengue and Zika virus diagnostic testing for patients with a clinically compatible illness and risk for infection with both viruses. MMWR. 2019;68(1):1–10.

Shebl FM, El-Kamary SS, Saleh DA, Abdel-Hamid M, Mikhail N, et al. Prospective cohort study of mother-to-infant infection and clearance of hepatitis C in rural Egyptian villages. J Med Virol. 2009;81(6):1024–31.

Soreng K, Levy R, Fakile Y. Serologic testing for syphilis: benefits and challenges of a reverse algorithm. Clin Microbiol Newsl. 2014;36(24):195–202.

Stol K, Nijman RG, van Herk W, van Rossum AMC. Biomarkers for infection in children: current clinical practice and future perspectives. Pediatr Infect Dis J. 2019;38:6S.

Tas E, Garibaldi L, Muzumdar R. Glucose homeostasis in newborns: an endocrinology perspective. NeoReviews. 2020;21(1):e14–29.

Taylor MD, Allada V, Moritz ML, Nowalk AJ, Sindhi R, Aneja RK, Torok K, Morowitz MJ, Michaels M, Carcillo JA. Use of C-reactive protein and ferritin biomarkers in daily pediatric practice. Pediatr Rev. 2020;41(4):172–83.

The President's Council on Bioethics. The changing moral focus of newborn screening: An ethical analysis by the President's Council on Bioethics. [Transcript available on the Internet]. Washington DC: The President's Council on Bioethics; 2008 [cited 2020 December 12]. https://bioethicsarchive.georgetown.edu/pcbe/reports/newborn_screening/index.html

Thompson-Branch A, Havranek T. Neonatal Hypoglycemia. Pediatr Rev. 2017;38(4):147–57.

Thornton PS, Stanley CA, De Leon DD, Harris D, Haymond MW, et al. Pediatric Endocrine Society. Recommendations from the pediatric endocrine society for evaluation and management of persistent hypoglycemia in neonates, infants, and children. J Pediatr. 2015;167(2):238–45.

Van den Bruel A, Thompson MJ, Haj-Hassan T, Stevens R, Moll H, Lakhanpaul M, et al. Diagnostic value of laboratory tests in identifying serious infections in febrile children: systematic review. BMJ. 2011; 342:d3082.

Van Rossum HH, de Kraa N, Thomas M, Holleboom CAG, Castel A, van Rosssum. Comparison of the direct antiglobulin test and the eluate technique for diagnosing hemolytic disease of the newborn. Pract Lab Med. 2015;3:17–21.

Wagner N, Jackson Y, Chappius F, Posfay-Barbe KM. Screening and management of children at risk for Chagas disease. Pediatr Infect Dis J. 2016;35(3): 335–7.

Wang C, Zhang X, Bialek S, Cannon MI. Attribution of congenital cytomegalovirus infection to primary versus nonprimary maternal infection. Clin Infect Dis. 2011;52:e11–3.

Wang L, Xu X, Zhang H, Qian J, Zhu J. Dried blood spots PCR assays to screen congenital cytomegalovirus infection: a meta-analysis. Virol J. 2015;12:60.

Watchko JF. Common hematologic problems in the newborn nursery. Pediatr Clin N Am. 2015;62:509–24.

Watts T, Stockman L, Martin J, Guilfoyle S, Vergeront J. Increased risk for mother-to-infant transmission of hepatitis C virus among transmission of hepatitis C virus among medicaid recipients—Wisconsin, 2011–2015. MMWR. 2017;66(42):1136–9.

Weinberg GA, D'Angio CT. Laboratory aids for diagnosis of neonatal sepsis. In: Wilson CB, Nizet V, Maldonado YA, Remington JS, Klein JO, editors. Remington and Klein's infectious diseases of the Fetus and newborn infant. 8th ed. Philadelphia, PA: Elsevier Saunders; 2016. p. 1132–43.

Woll C, Neuman MI, Aronson PL. Management of the febrile young infant: update for the 21st century. Pediatr Emerg Care. 2017;33(11):748–53.

Yusuf C, Sontag MK, Miller J, Kellar-Guenther Y, McKasson S, Shone S, et al. Development of national newborn screening quality indicators in the United States. Int J Neonatal Screen. 2019;5:34.

Zdravic D, Yougbare I, Vadasz B, Li C, Marshall AH, Chen P, Kjeldsen-Kragh J, Ni H. Fetal and neonatal alloimmune thrombocytopenia. Semin Fetal Neonatal Med. 2016;21(1):19–27.

Additional Reading for Specific Conditions in the Newborn Screening

Bodamer OA, Scott CR, Giugliani R. And on behalf of the Pompe disease Newborn screening working group. Newborn screening for Pompe disease. Pediatrics. 2017;140(Supplement 1):S4–S13.

King JR, Hammarström L. Newborn screening for primary immunodeficiency diseases: history, current and future practice. J Clin Immunol. 2018;38(1):56–66.

Matern D, Gavrilov D, Oglesbee D, Raymond K, Rinaldo P, Tortorelli S. Newborn screening for lysosomal storage disorders. Semin Perinatol. 2015;39(3):206–16.

Moser AB, Fatemi A. Newborn screening and emerging therapies for X-linked adrenoleukodystrophy. JAMA Neurol. 2018;75(10):1175–6.

Rosenfeld M, Sontag MK, Ren CL. Cystic fibrosis diagnosis and newborn screening. Pediatr Clin N Am. 2016;6:599–615. https://doi.org/10.1016/j.pcl.2016.04.004.

Sharer JD. An overview of biochemical genetics. C P Hum Genet. 2016;89:17.1.1–17.16.

The Well Pediatric Primary Care Visit and Screening Laboratory Tests

4

Rita Marie John

Learning Objectives

After completing the chapter, the learner should be able to:

1. Evaluate different tests recommended when seeing a child during a well-child visit.
2. Characterize the pitfalls of screening tests used during a well-child visit.
3. Synthesize screening that is fundamental to caring for a child with obesity.
4. Summarize the screening recommendation for adolescents.

Screening during well childcare is based on the principles that the early identification of the child at risk for diseases will prevent and/or treat illness. For example, in a toddler at risk for lead poisoning, early identification of a slightly elevated lead level can prevent further adverse outcomes from lead poisoning. Despite the value of early screening and intervention services, many practices fail to screen pediatric patients at significant risk for the problem (Wakai et al. 2018). The goal of primary prevention is to remove lead from the home before the child is exposed. In contrast, secondary prevention includes lead testing and follow-up to identify a child who has already been exposed to lead (Ettinger et al. 2019). The AAP has a periodicity table outlining the timing of well visits and the screening schedule. This chapter will review standard screening as well as common issues that arise during a well visit.

4.1 Introduction

Well-child visits are the foundation of pediatric care. The clinician has the opportunity to evaluate the child's growth and development, give anticipatory guidance, address the guardian's concerns, evaluate the child's mental and physical health, and order screening tests as indicated by the AAP periodicity table. Routine labs should not be done without a reason. Diagnostic stewardship points to the need to have a reason for ordering the test, and there are several guidelines to help the clinician order the right test. Choosing Wisely is another initiative that addresses laboratory test stewardship (Baird 2019). The Choosing Wisely initiative was started in the United States to avoid overutilization of healthcare. There is a phone application as well as a website to help clinicians stay current with evidence-based guidelines.

R. M. John (✉)
School of Nursing, Columbia University,
New York, NY, USA
e-mail: rmj4@cumc.columbia.edu

4.2   The Newborn Visit

A family bringing a newborn home experiences stress related to the transition of having a new baby and learning how to care for the infant. New mothers experience significant hormone changes and have to recover from childbirth. Families with children already in the home must learn to adjust their schedules and help children adjust to a new sibling's presence.

Bright Futures and the American Academy of Pediatrics [AAP] recommend visits 3–5 days and again by 1 month (AAP 2021; Hagan et al. 2017). Also, if the mother is breastfeeding, the recommendation is that the child is seen at 2–3 days following hospital discharge to make sure the weight is appropriate, answer the mother's concerns, and see how the baby is doing. The priority for the first visit must be the concerns of the parents. Meeting the parent's needs helps the parents meet the child's needs (Hagan et al. 2017). If there are concerns about the newborn or the parental adjustment, the clinician should see the family before the 1-month visit. If the newborn has hyperbilirubinemia, the newborn should be seen for a follow-up visit based on the recommendation of bilitool.org. Detailed information about hyperbilirubinemia will be discussed in Chap. 3.

4.2.1   Newborn Screening Follow-Up

It is the responsibility of the clinician to follow up on the newborn screening. While the AAP recommends visits at 3–5 days and again by 1 month, the results may not be available for a few days following a visit at 3 days. A clinician needs to develop a system for follow-up on the newborn screen following any newborn visit or visit during the first month of life. Clinicians may also see patients from countries where newborn screening is limited or not done. It is important to consider diseases that normally would have been picked up at a newborn screening but may not have been done in the country of origin. Newborn screening is discussed in detail in Chap. 3.

4.2.1.1 HIV Screening

HIV screening is done during pregnancy and repeated as part of the newborn care as clinically indicated. The test may still be negative as the mother may be infected and has not yet seroconverted. A positive HIV newborn screen and the needed follow-up will be discussed in Chap. 3, and general information about HIV is reviewed in Sect. 6.4.6.

4.2.1.2 Newborn Bilirubin

Newborns need to be screened for hyperbilirubinemia before the nursery discharge or at the first newborn visit if they are born in a birthing facility or home (Hagan et al. 2017). While follow-up for hyperbilirubinemia will be discussed in Chap. 3, the clinician must ensure normal direct bilirubin was done in the nursery. Any newborn with persistent hyperbilirubinemia should have both the direct (conjugated) and total bilirubin repeated. The bilirubin should be plotted for risk on bilitool.org.

> **Key Learning about Newborn Well Visits**
> - Meeting the needs of the newborn guardians is important for them to meet the newborn's needs.
> - All newborn screening must be followed up. States may require repeat newborn screening on all newborns. Hypothyroidism is the most common endocrine problem found on newborn screens and should be followed up within 24 h whenever possible.
> - Hyperbilirubinemia must be followed carefully. All newborns with persistent hyperbilirubinemia must have a total and direct bilirubin obtained, and it should be repeated based on plotting the results on bilitool.org.

4.2.2   Real-Life Example

A one-week-old came for a well check 3 days after the original visit. The newborn screen was obtained and was positive for hypothyroidism. Repeat blood was drawn after a complete explanation was given. The mother gave two phone numbers to reach her. The follow-up lab obtained on the day of the visit was consistent with hypothyroidism. The mother failed to answer the phone despite calling several times a day. It was decided that the police would be sent to the home to assure that she came in for medication. The mother came into the clinic accompanied by the police officers. A social work consult was obtained after a complete explanation was given. The mother reported that she did not want anything to be wrong with her child. The child was started on Synthroid, an endocrine follow-up appointment was given, and the follow-up in the clinic was also given for 1 week. The labs returned to normal, and the mother was excellent in giving the medication and keeping all follow-up appointments. The mother ultimately thanked the provider for her diligence in making sure that the child was treated.

4.3   Anemia Screening

Iron deficiency is a global problem and a common nutritional deficiency with a prevalence among 1–3-year-olds of 8%–14%. Full-term infants deplete their iron stores by 6–9 months, with iron deficiency occurring by 9–12 months. Children under 24 months are at risk for iron deficiency due to rapid growth and the change to whole milk from iron-fortified formula and breast milk (Wood and Sperling 2019). There are two periods where iron deficiency is more common—in toddlerhood and for female adolescents. The recommendations from the various organization stem from the changes mentioned above.

The American Academy of Pediatrics (AAP) and the World Health Organization (WHO) recommend screening for anemia with hemoglobin (Hb) at 1 year of age; however, the US Preventive Task Force (USPTF) did not find any evidence to recommend any universal screening. The AAP does recommend that at 4 months and every recommended well visit, a nutrition history should be done looking for risk factors for anemia. Table 4.1 outlines

Table 4.1 Recommendations for anemia screening

Organization	Age of screening	Screen-based on risk factors
AAP periodicity table	• 12 months	All children are screened at 12 months regardless of risk factors with a hematocrit or hemoglobin Take nutrition history as well as history for blood loss
Bright futures	A screen with hematocrit or hemoglobin at ages below based on risk factors: • 9–12 months • 15–18 months (six months after initial screen) • Annually from ages 2–5 years	Risk factors: Children from families who have: • Low income • Eligible for WIC • All recently arrived refugees • Infants and children who are migrants
	A screen before six months based on risk factors	Risk factors: Preterm and low-birth-weight infants fed infant formula without iron
	Only screen based on risk factors • Screen all children from 5 to 10 • Screen adolescent children from 12 to 18	Risk factors: • History of low iron intake • Special healthcare needs • Previous history of iron deficiency
	Adolescent females 12–18	Screen every 5–10 years during well visits
	Adolescent females 12–18 years	An annual screening if they have risk factors • Extensive menstrual or other blood loss • Low iron intake, a previous diagnosis of iron-deficiency anemia Screen every 5–10 years during routine health examinations

Adapted from: Hagan et al. (2017), Committee on Practice and Ambulatory Medicine; Bright Futures Periodicity Schedule Workgroup [CPAM-BF] [2019]

the recommendation for screening based on risk as outlined by Bright Futures and the AAP (Hagan et al. 2017).

The AAP periodicity table does recommend a screening history for iron deficiency throughout adolescence (CPAM-BF 2019). Due to rapid growth, menstruation, and overall lower body iron, adolescent females are at increased risk of iron-deficiency anemia (Sekhar et al. 2015). As a result, the Centers for Disease Control and Prevention [CDC] recommends anemia screening for repro-ductive-age females every 5–10 years and annu-ally for those with risk factors. This is consistent with Bright Futures' 2017 recommendation to annually screen females with extensive blood loss from menstrual bleeding, low iron intake, or iron deficiency history. Bright Futures also recom-mends that screening for iron deficiency be done every 5–10 years during routine exams (Hagan et al. 2017). An analysis of the National Health and Nutrition Examination Survey confirms a higher prevalence of iron-deficiency anemia in women (Sekhar et al. 2015). None of the guide-lines recommend a complete CBC but rather rec-ommend a Hb as an initial screening.

4.3.1 Real-Life Examples

A 12-month-old presented for a well visit. The child was very pale, although active and not ill-appearing. The mother's history was unremark-able, and she reported switching to whole milk at 11 months of age. The physical exam was normal except for pallor. A Hb was ordered and reported as 4.1. A stat CBC showed marked microcytosis with a low RBC and MCV. The mother was que-ried again about the child's formula intake. She later admitted to changing formula at 4 months of age, thus accounting for the iron deficiency severity.

4.4 Lead Screening and Testing

Lead is a common environmental hazard and can lead to significant neurological effects as infants and children's brains absorb lead easily from the gastrointestinal tract (Wang et al. 2019). Whether in small or large concentrations, exposure to lead exposure has adverse effects on the central ner-vous system, hematopoietic system, and skeletal, renal, and reproductive systems (Mitra et al. 2017). The effect of lead on the brain leads to cognitive and behavioral effects. At lead levels of ≤ 5 µg/dl, the child will have lower academic achievement, lower IQ scores, and attention-related behavioral problems. At lead levels of ≤ 10 µg/dl, there are also delays in puberty, decreased postnatal growth, and decreased hearing. There is limited evidence regarding decreased kidney function. Therefore, there is no safe level of lead (Council on Environmental Health 2016; Wood and Sperling 2019). Lead toxicity may also be a factor involved in antisocial behaviors. From 1980 to 2010, there was a decline in blood lead levels over 10 in chil-dren from 1 to 5 years, decreasing from 88.2% to 0.9% (CDC 2011). The CDC's National Surveillance Data from 2016 reported that approximately 3% of children still have lead lev-els ≥ 5 µg/dL and 1% of children still have lead levels ≥ 10 µg/dL (CDC 2020).

Different bodies have different recommenda-tions, including contradictory recommendations from the USPSTF, the AAP, and the CDC. The clinical guidelines from the AAP endorse tar-geted testing of children of 12–24 months of age who live in communities where $\geq 25\%$ of housing was built before 1960, or there is a prevalence of children's blood lead concentrations ≥ 5 mcg/dL (≥ 50 ppb) in $\geq 5\%$ of the population (Council on Environmental Health 2016). The Centers for Medicare and Medicaid Services (CMS) requires blood lead tests for 1–2-year-old children cov-ered by Medicaid. CMS recommends performing a capillary or venous blood lead test (not the questionnaire). If there has been no previous lead screen and the child is between 24 and 72 months, a lead test must be done regardless of the verbal lead screening questionnaire results (Medicaid. gov 2021). Lead screening involves using a ques-tionnaire, whereas lead testing is blood testing by either capillary or venous blood (Council on Environmental Health 2017). If there has been no previous lead screen and the child is between 24 and 72 months, a lead test must be done regardless of the verbal lead screening questionnaire results (Medicaid.gov 2021). Lead screening involves using a questionnaire, whereas lead testing is blood testing by either capillary or venous blood (Council on Environmental Health 2017).

The USPSTF found evidence for using questionnaires or other clinical prediction tools to identify pediatric patients who might be at risk but not pregnant women. The USPSTF also found adequate evidence that capillary blood testing accurately identifies patients with elevated blood levels. Still, they did not find sufficient evidence to screen for elevated leads in patients 5 years and younger and pregnant women (US Preventive Services Task Force 2019a, 2019b). Aside from the federal guideline differences, the clinician may also note differences in state and local recommendations (Michel et al. 2020). The basics of a good history and knowledge of risk factors may help the clinician determine who needs lead screening. All federal bodies agree that high-risk children between 1 and 2 years of age need to be screened (Weitzman 2019).

In contrast, the CDC has developed a schedule for screening refugees and pregnant women, summarized in Table 4.2. To complicate the varying differences around the guidelines, the clinician needs to take a good history, screen for risk factors, and decide on the most appropriate action to minimize lead poisoning risk. The real-life examples at the end of the section below may provide insight into the importance of history.

Lead testing is done in young children due to their pica behavior and exposure to environmental risks of lead from the soil, dust, air, food, and water. Lead is found more commonly in children that live near manufacturing facilities; in older housing with lead-based paint, old toys, or toys that have entered the marketplace with lead paint on them; in drinking water with contaminated pipes; and parental occupations with take-home lead and mining lead (Dignam et al. 2019). Children who live in older housing are at increased risk of having a lead ≥ 5 µg/dL. There are no treatments that will alleviate the effects of lead toxicity, so preventing lead toxicity is very important. Identification and elimination of sources of lead

Table 4.2 CDC recommendations for screening all newly arrived refugee infants, children, adolescents, and pregnant and lactating women and girls

Recommended screening	Population
Initial lead exposure screening with a blood test	1. All refugee infants and children ≤16 years of age 2. Refugee adolescents >16 years of age if there is a high index of suspicion or clinical signs/symptoms of lead exposure 3. All pregnant and lactating women and girls[a]
Follow-up testing with a blood test, 3–6 months after initial testing	• All refugee infants and children ≤6 years, regardless of the initial screening result • Children and adolescents 7–16 years with EBLL at initial screening • Consider repeat testing in adolescents >16 years of age with risk factors

Department of Health and Human Services, Centers for Disease Control (CDC) Retrieved on December 14, 2020, from https://www.cdc.gov/immigrantrefugeehealth/guidelines/lead-guidelines.html
[a] All newly arrived pregnant or breastfeeding women should be prescribed a prenatal or multivitamin with adequate iron and calcium. Referral to a healthcare provider with expertise in high-risk lead exposure treatment and management may indicate EBLLs

exposure is the optimal strategy. Lead ingestion and absorption are higher in the first 3 years of life, with a peak between 18 months and 36 months of age. Taking a history of possible environmental hazards and pica behaviors is important. Lead paint in houses varies by the age of the house. A house built between 1978 and 1998 contains about 2.8% lead paint hazards, but a house built from 1960 to 1977 has an 11.4% risk of lead paint hazards. In older housing built from 1940 to 1959, lead paint risk is 39%, but in houses built before 1940, there is a 67% risk of lead hazards (United States Department of Health and Human Services 2011). Household dust, water contamination, and residential soil also are areas of concern (Council on Environmental Health 2016).

Screening questionnaires used in primary care may fail to identify children who have elevated blood lead levels (Ossiander 2013). However, they may help identify lead poisoning sources in the house (Council on Environmental Health 2016). Screening for lead must be accompanied by explaining the results and nutrition counseling about the importance of iron-rich foods and calcium-containing foods. Children with a diet deficient in lead and calcium absorb more lead from their GI tract into their blood (Kordes 2017). Similarly, diets with adequate calcium and iron may allow the child to excrete more lead (Schmidt 2017). It should also identify household hazards, screen for iron adequacy, and screen with developmental tests to identify delays (Council on Environmental Health 2016). The longer the child has lead toxicity, the longer the lead levels' decline will take since lead accumulates in the bones (Schmidt 2017). Oral chelation is considered once the child's lead level is ≥45 mcg/dL. Chelation therapy used to treat lead levels may need to be repeated if the lead rises again. It is important to closely follow patients at risk for lead poisoning and initiate dietary and household measures to avoid further lead contact. Table 4.3 reviews risk factors for lead poisoning.

4.4.1 Lead Screening Techniques

4.4.1.1 Capillary Lead Screening

In many private practices, blood lead is done on capillary samples using a point-of-service machine called LeadCare. LeadCare is approved for both capillary and venous samples. Capillary samples are less expensive and easier to perform and eliminate the need to send out the sample.

Pitfalls of capillary lead screening. Due to lead dust in the environment, there is an increased risk of false positive using a finger stick. The acceptable margin of error in point-of-care lead tests is the greater of ±4 µg/dL or ± 10% for proficiency testing programs approved under the Clinical Laboratory Improvement Amendments of 1988. Also, testing variability across laboratories may contribute to false readings (Parsons et al. 2001).

Wang et al. reported a sample of 3898 children screened by capillary samples for the lead between 2011 and 2017. In that study, 2330 or 55% were identified as false positives. They urged that providers obtain a venous sample for confirmatory testing,

Table 4.3 Risk factors for lead poisoning

Risk factors for lead poisoning	
House	The child lives in or frequently visits houses built before 1950
	The child lives in or frequently visits a house built before 1978 that is undergoing renovations in the past six months
Folk remedies	Ask about the use of any medications from the native countries
	Ayurvedic medications may be formulated with mercury, arsenic, and lead (Bissell et al. 2015)
Child characteristics	A child with a developmental delay or an older child with an intellectual impairment. An older child or adolescent with a neurodevelopmental disorder that presents with oral behaviors or pica
Imported candy, toys, jewelry	Be cautious about toys from China, Mexico, and South America
Imported cosmetics	Eye cosmetics such as kohl (eyeliner used in the Middle East, India, Africa) Surma (powder used in the eyes is from India)
Household hazards	Pottery, ceramics, dishware,
	Paint chips from lead-based paint
	Tea kettle
	Vinyl miniblinds
	Water from lead solder, pipes, valves, and fixtures
	Outdoor soil
Parental occupations	Painter
	Ceramic workers
	Construction workers
	Furniture refinishers
	Radiator repair workers
Sibling or playmate	Does a sibling or playmate have lead poisoning?

Adapted from Bissell et al. (2015), Council on Environmental Health (2016), Department of Health and Human Services, Centers for Disease Control and Prevention (2020); Mayans (2019), Obeng-Gyasi (2019)

4.4.1.2 Venous Lead Screening

A venipuncture avoids the risk of contamination from lead dust when the venipuncture site is properly cleaned. The blood is analyzed using atomic absorption spectrometry, anodic stripping voltammetry, or inductively coupled plasma mass spectrometry. If an elevated lead is found after the first venous screen, the child must be seen back based on the schedule outlined by the CDC (see Table 4.4). After the second screen is positive, the patient's follow-up with an elevated lead will need further lead testing as outlined by the CDC and included in Table 4.5.

4.4.2 Other Markers of Lead Toxicity

All of the other markers of lead toxicity are not specific or sensitive and cannot be used to diagnose lead toxicity.

Table 4.4 Follow-up of venous lead screening for levels ≥5

Blood lead level (µg/dL)	Time to confirmation testing
≥5–9	1–3 months
10–44	1 week–1 month*
45–59	48 h
60–69	24 h
≥70	Urgently as emergency test

Department of Health and Human Services, CDC. Retrieved on December 14, 2020, from https://www.cdc.gov/nceh/lead/advisory/acclpp/actions-blls.htm

Table 4.5 Schedule for follow-up blood lead testing after confirmation testing[a]

Venous blood lead levels (µg/dL)	Early follow-up testing (2–4 tests after identification)	Later follow-up testing after BLL declining
≥5–9	3 months[b]	6–9 months
10–19	1–3 months[b]	3–6 months
20–24	1–3 months[b]	1–3 months
25–44	2 weeks–1 month	one month
≥45	As soon as possible	As soon as possible

Department of Health and Human Services, CDC. Retrieved on December 14, 2020, from https://www.cdc.gov/nceh/lead/advisory/acclpp/actions-blls.htm
[a] Seasonal variation of BLLs exists and may be more apparent in colder climate areas. Greater exposure in the summer months may necessitate more frequent follow-ups
[b] Some clinicians may choose to repeat blood lead tests on all new patients within a month to ensure that their BLL level is not rising more quickly than anticipated

4.4.2.1 Elevated Zinc Protoporphyrin and Free Erythrocyte Protoporphyrin

Elevated zinc protoporphyrin (ZP) levels or free erythrocyte protoporphyrin (FEP) levels are present in moderate to severe lead poisoning but can be elevated iron-deficiency anemia. In the case of FEP, the level may not be elevated until the blood level is over 25–35.

Free erythrocyte protoporphyrin is elevated in iron deficiency and will be elevated in lead toxicity. Zinc protoporphyrin is directly measured using hematofluorometry but is considered a secondary by-product and, therefore, not as accurate in the confirmation of lead toxicity (Harada, Miura 1984).

4.4.2.2 Delta Aminolevulinic Acid (ALAD)

ALAD is a nonspecific marker of lead intoxication. A recent study looked at an inverse relationship between lead exposure and low levels of delta-aminolevulinic acid (ALAD) in pregnant women. In this study, ALAD activity was significantly lower in pregnant women with lead levels ≥5 (La-Llave-León et al. 2017). The effects of lead in bone marrow arise mainly from lead interaction with some enzymatic processes involved in heme syntheses, such as the inhibition of ALAD and ZP variations.

4.4.2.3 CBC

It should be noted that with lead levels ≥20 µg/dL, a workup for iron deficiency, including a Hct or Hb, should be initiated. Children with significant lead poisoning may have neither anemia nor microcytosis, although mild anemia with basophilic stippling on a peripheral smear can be seen.

4.4.3 Real-Life Examples

A breastfeeding Pakistani newborn was seen in follow-up at the 1-month visit. She was noted to be mildly irritable and did not respond to the clinician's usual techniques of calming the baby. Black staining was noted around the eye. When questioned about the source, the mother responded that it was a substance from her country put in the eye to ensure the baby's normal vision. She was unable to identify the name of the substance.

Further research was done, and it was determined that the child had kohl put into her eye. A lead level drawn and repeated showed the infant's lead level was 16. Counseling was initiated, and a kohl substitute was agreed on. The child's lead returned to <5 by the four-month visit.

A 14-year-old female with an intellectual impairment presented acutely with status epilepticus. The child had no history of seizures in the past. The lab studies were normal except for significant microcytic anemia consistent with IDA. A careful history revealed significant risk factors for lead poisoning, including living in housing built in 1940, pica behavior, restrictive dietary behavior, and sibling with lead poisoning. A stat venous lead showed a lead level of 79. The child was admitted for chelation therapy. Discharge planning included moving the family to newer housing and educating them about improving dietary intake. Aside from chelation therapy, the child was started on multivitamins and therapeutic iron.

Key Learning about Anemia and Lead Screening

- A dietary history is important in identifying pediatric patients that may need screening for IDA or lead.
- Lead levels should be done on all patients receiving Medicaid between ages one and two.
- Evaluating risk factors for both IDA and lead helps identify at-risk children.
- A venous blood lead must confirm an elevated capillary lead.
- An elevated venous blood lead must be confirmed within a set time based on the degree of elevation.
- Based on history, adolescents with developmental disabilities or neurodevelopmental disorders should be screened for anemia and/or lead.

4.5 Routine Dyslipidemia Screening

Promoting cardiovascular health is important, but clinicians are faced with several things to do during a primary care visit. Screen for dyslipidemia may not be a priority. It should be recognized that identifying a child with dyslipidemia has the added benefit of identifying a parent with this problem. There is a 50% chance that a parent will be recognized when a child is identified with a familial hyperlipidemia disorder (Blackett et al. 2018). The National Cholesterol Education Program (NCEP) and the AAP promote a low-fat diet in childhood to establish a healthy, lifelong diet and to lower lipids across the population. The prevention of adult cardiovascular disease is important for the long-term health of our children. The reasons for the lack of screening in children is clinician's lack of knowledge about lipid disorders, disagreement with the guidelines, and uncertainty about the treatment approaches (Dixon et al. 2014; Herrington et al. 2019; Blackett et al. 2018).

The 2018 guidelines from the American Heart Association and American College of Cardiology (ACC) stated that universal lipid screening at 9–11 years and again at 17–21 years of age was given a B-nonrandomized (B-NR) level of evidence (LOE) and a IIb strength of recommendation. The B-NR LOE is a moderate quality of evidence from observational studies. The class IIb recommendation is weaker but may be reasonable (Writing Committee, Cholesterol Clinical Practice Guidelines 2018). The AAP regularly revises its recommendations for screening for dyslipidemia. At present, it has been updated to occur once between 9 and 11 years of age and once between 17 and 21 years of age. Targeted screening should be done in children 2–8 and 12–16 if there is dyslipidemia or early CVD in first-degree family members, smoking history, or hypertension. The presence of risk conditions such as type 1 or type 2 diabetes mellitus, chronic renal disease, post-orthotopic cardiac or renal transplantation, nephrotic syndrome, HIV, a history of Kawasaki disease, or chronic inflammatory disease is also a reason to target screen patients (NHLBI 2011). Approximately one in five children are believed to have dyslipidemia (Kit et al. 2015), and identifying those children may also help identify parental dyslipidemia.

The American Association of Clinical Endocrinologists and the American College of Endocrinology recommend that children at risk for familial hyperlipidemia due to a family history of early cardiovascular disease or early elevated cholesterol should be screened at 3 years, ages 9–11 years, and again at age 18. They further recommend that adolescents older than 16 years be screened every 5 years and more frequently if they have one of the risk factors for hyperlipidemia. A lipid profile is the recommended screening and includes total cholesterol (TC), high-density lipoprotein cholesterol (HDL-C), low-density lipoprotein cholesterol (LDL-C), triglycerides (TG), very low-density lipoprotein cholesterol (VLDL-C), and non-HDL-C. The USPTF (2016) does not recommend any routine screening for lipidemia in asymptomatic pediatric patients under 20, citing a lack of evidence. They agree that intensive dietary interventions are safe but of uncertain clinical significance.

There are primary disorders of lipid metabolism that result from genetic defects in lipid synthesis and metabolism. Familial hypercholesterolemia is an autosomal dominant disorder and the most common primary dyslipidemia (Viigimaa et al. 2018). Primary TG in children and adolescents usually presents in adulthood, but in the face of obesity and insulin resistance, it can present in adolescence. A parental history may be helpful, but on physical exams, eruptive, palmer, or tuberoeruptive xanthomas may be present (Shah and Wilson 2015). Box 4.1 lists some examples of genetic dyslipidemia.

Box 4.1 Examples of Types of Genetic Dyslipidemia

Familial hypercholesterolemia.
  Homozygous.
  - ↑↑ LDL-C
  Heterozygous.
  - ↑ LDL-C
Familial defective apolipoprotein.
  - ↑ LDL-C
Familial combined hyperlipidemia*.
  - Type IIa: ↑ LDL-C, autosomal dominant, tendon xanthoma.
  - Type IV: ↑ VLDL-C, ↑ TG, autosomal dominant.
  - Type IIb: ↑ LDL-C, ↑ VLDL-C, ↑ TG, polygenic, early CVD in family members.
  - Types IIb and IV (autosomal dominant) often with ↓ HDL-C.
Polygenic hypercholesterolemia.
  - ↑ LDL-C
Familial hypoalphalipoproteinemia.
  - ↓ HDL-C
Dysbetalipoproteinemia.
  - TC:250–500 mg/dL.
  - ↑ IDL-C,
  - ↑ Chylomicron remnants
  - TG: 250–600 mg/dL.

Retrieved from: Expert Panel on Integrated Guidelines for Cardiovascular Health and Risk Reduction in Children and Adolescents, National Heart, Lung, and Blood Institute [NHLBI] (2011) (https://www.nhlbi.nih.gov/files/docs/peds_guidelines_sum.pdf).

Hypertriglyceridemia results from either increased production or reduced clearance of triglycerides. While the etiology can be primary or secondary hypertriglyceridemia, it is likely to be mixed. Hypertriglyceridemia is complicated by a high-fat and high-carbohydrate diet, sedentary lifestyle, obesity, and type 2 diabetes (Valaiyapathi et al. 2017). A high TG is associated with decreased HDL-C, increased non-HDL levels, increased apoB, and higher low-density lipoprotein levels (Valaiyapathi et al. 2017). Table 4.6 is a brief review of the primary and secondary hypertriglyceridemia.

In a recent survey study of 548 subjects, 34% performed no screening, 50% screened selectively, and only 16% performed universal screening. The perceived barriers included a lack of comfort in addressing lipid disorders in 43% and unfamiliarity with the guidelines in 57%. The majority of the participants were uncomfortable in managing lipid disorders, and 57% were against the use of lipid-lowering agents (Dixon et al. 2014). The identification of children with dyslipidemia and management can reduce future cardiovascular risk. In a retrospective cohort study of children from 2009 to 2013 that evaluated 1,736,032 children from ages 2 to 18 years to see if they had been screened for dyslipidemia, only 6.6% of well children were screened with an increase in screening if the patient had known risk factors of hypertension, diabetes mellitus, or another endocrine disorder. Still, fewer than 10% of children with parental dyslipidemia or overweight BMI were screened (Herrington et al. 2019).

4.5.1 Lipid Screening Tests

The initial screening is allowed to be fasting or nonfasting. If the child is nonfasting, a TC and HDL-C should be ordered as these are stable in the nonfasting state. From these measures, the non-HDL-C is calculated. If the non-HDL-C is greater than 145, a fasting lipid profile should be done (Kavey 2015). A repeat fasting screening should be done whenever the results are elevated, and the two results should be averaged. The repeat lipid screen should be done two weeks later but not more than three months apart (NHLBI 2011). The usual abnormal findings

Table 4.6 Primary and secondary hypertriglyceridemia

Primary hypertriglyceridemia	Secondary hypertriglyceridemia
Primary hypertriglyceridemia	Endocrinopathies
• Incidence of 1 in 500	• Uncontrolled type 1 and 2 diabetes mellitus
• TG 200–1000 mg/dL	• Obesity
• Associated with very increased VLDL	• Metabolic syndrome
• ↑ TG	• Hypothyroidism
Severe hypertriglyceridemia (≥ 1000 mg/dL)	• Hypercortisolism
• ↑ chylomicrons	Medications
• ↑ VLDL-C	• Second-generation antipsychotics
• ↑TG	• Sirolimus
Lipoprotein lipase deficiency	• Antiretroviral therapy–protease inhibitors
• Autosomal recessive	• Beta-blockers
• Incidence 1:500,000 to 1:1000,000	• Bile acid sequestrants
• TG > 10,000 mg/dL	• Estrogen and anabolic steroids
• Associated with very high chylomicrons	• Retinoids
Mixed hypertriglyceridemia	• Antidepressants
Familial combined hyperlipoproteinemia	• Anabolic steroids
• One of the most common	Pregnancy
• 0.5%–1% of population	Liver diseases
• 3 X more common than familial hypercholesterolemia	• Acute hepatitis
• Also, elevated LDL and low HDL	Excessive alcohol intake
Dysbetalipoprotemia	
• Incidence of 1/5000	
• Increased chylomicrons and VLDL	
Increased total cholesterol	

Retrieved from Blackett et al. (2015), Shah and Wilson (2015), NHLBI (2011)

on screening are low HDL and high triglycerides. Table 4.8 outlines acceptable values for lipids. Again, it cannot be stressed enough that the current guidelines recommend that an abnormal result be repeated a second time before any diagnosis of dyslipidemia (Daniels 2015).

4.5.1.1 Cholesterol

Overview. TC and lipoprotein carriers of cholesterol—LDL, VLDL, and HDL—relate to cardiovascular risk factors. Prevention of heart disease should start in childhood, and therefore screening for risk factors is important. LDL-C is considered the "bad" cholesterol as it is the dominant form of atherogenic cholesterol. VLDL-C is also a problem as it is the main carrier of triglycerides. VLDL cholesterol (VLDL-C) has atherogenic qualities, while HDL is not atherogenic. The combination of LDL-C and VLDL-C is called non-HDL-C and is considered more atherogenic than either substance alone. Within LDL and VDL is a protein called apolipoprotein B (apoB). Similar to non-HDL-C, apoB has more atherogenicity than LDL-C alone (Grundy et al. 2019). An elevation of the TG causes an increase in high-density lipoprotein and low-density lipoproteins, causing HDL degradation and LDL particle formation (Blackett et al. 2015).

Cholesterol plays an important role in cell membranes and makes fat-soluble vitamins, hormones, and bile acids. Animal-based foods are the primary source of cholesterol in the body. Cholesterol elevations can be secondary to diabetes, renal and cardiac transplant, chronic kidney disease, nephrotic syndrome, Kawasaki disease, HIV infection, thyroid disorders, other endocrine disorders, or oral contraceptive drugs (Herrington et al. 2019; Sundjaja and Pandey 2020).

4.5.1.2 Low-Density Lipoprotein Cholesterol (LDL-C)

LDL-C can be indirectly or directly measured. When it is indirectly measured, it is calculated using the Friedewald formula (see Table 4.7). However, there are limitations to this formula as it assumes that the ratio of the cholesterol to the triglycerides is constant. The formula is not accurate when the triglycerides are either too low or too high, and the formula cannot be used with a triglyceride greater than 400. When the triglycerides are over 400 mg/dL, the direct method of measuring TG will be higher, and the indirect method will be lower. The formula cannot be used in TG > 400 when there are chylomicrons in the plasma and if the patient has type III familial hypercholesterolemia (Sundjaja and Pandey 2020).

4.5.1.3 Non-high-Density Lipoprotein Cholesterol (Non-HDL-C)

Non-HDL cholesterol and HDL cholesterol are better tools for risk assessment for cardiovascular disease than LDL-C (Sacks, Jensen 2018). Non-HDL-C is calculated by using the formula in Table 4.7.

4.5.1.4 High-Density Lipoprotein Cholesterol (HDL-C)

High-density lipoprotein cholesterols (HDL-C) are biological cholesterols protecting humans against atherosclerosis and cardiovascular dis-

Table 4.7 Formula to calculate the LDL-C and non-HDL cholesterol

LDL-C	= [Total cholesterol] – [high-density lipoprotein-cholesterol] – [triglyceride]/5
Non-HDL cholesterol	= Total cholesterol – HDL cholesterol

Adapted from Sundjaja and Pandey (2020)

Table 4.8 Evaluating lipid results

Type of lipid	Acceptable	Borderline	High
Total cholesterol	<170	170–199	>200
HDL cholesterol	<40	40–45	>60
LDL-C	<110	110–129	>130
Non-HDL-C	<120	120–144	>145
ApoB	<90	90–109	>110
Apolipoprotein A-1	<115	>120	
Apolipoprotein A-1	<115	>120	115–120
TG 0–9 years	<75	75–99	>100
TG 10–19 year	<90	90–129	>130

National Heart, Lung, and Blood Institute (2011); National Institutes of Health; U.S. Department of Health and Human Services (2011) Retrieved from https://www.ncbi.nlm.nih.gov/pmc/articles/PMC4536582/

ease (CVD). HDL is not only a carrier of cholesterol for redistribution and removal from humans but is a more complex protein and phospholipids with many functions (Sacks, Jensen 2018). When the HDL cholesterol is low, there is an increased risk for CHD. CVD risk significantly increases when HDL decreases from 40 to 30 mg/dL.

If a cell has more cholesterol than it needs for optimal cell function, it transfers the excess cholesterol by cholesterol efflux. HDL is the main player for this movement, along with apoB lipoprotein, VLDL, and LDL (Sacks, Jensen 2018). HDL, which is identified by the presence of apoA1, circulates for 2–4 days. HDL serves as a mover of cholesterol. The cholesterol taken up by the HDL is delivered to the liver, where it is excreted in the bile, organs to make steroid hormones, and the intestine for transintestinal cholesterol efflux. As a result of HDL's role in cellular cholesterol extraction and the role in reverse cholesterol transport, HDL is anti-atherogenic. A low HDL cholesterol concentration is considered to be a value below 35 mg/dL and high HDL >60 mg/dL. HDL cholesterol values are also used in the calculation of LDL cholesterol. Table 4.8 outlines how to evaluate lipid results.

4.5.1.5 Lipoprotein A

Lipoprotein A is a low-density lipoprotein (LDL) particle in which apolipoprotein(a) (apo[a]) attaches to the apolipoprotein(b) (apo[b]) component of the LDL particle via a disulfide bridge. Elevated Lp(a) is causally implicated in CVD. There is a lack of standardization, so optimal cutoffs are a subject of intense debate. Lp(a) structure is highly heterogeneous due to many different apo(a) isoforms within the population. An individual's Lp(a) level is about 80–90% genetically determined and is fully expressed by 1–2 years of age, with adult levels by 5 years. It is inherited in an autosomal codominant inheritance pattern.

4.5.1.6 ApoA1

Apolipoprotein A1 (ApoA1) is a primary protein associated with HDL particles playing an important role in reverse cholesterol transport. High HDL-C and ApoA1 significantly lower CVD risk (Sacks, Jensen 2018). The pattern of the association between HDL and CVD is not linear as it plateaus when the HDL cholesterols reach >75 mg/dL (men) and >90 mg/dL (women). The AMORIS (Apolipoprotein-related Mortality Risk) study done in adults showed that patients with increased levels of apoB had increased CVD risk. Increased ApoA1 was protective against CVD in men and women (Waldius et al. 2001). ApoA1 and apoB 100 are separate tests and are not included in most lipid panels.

4.5.1.7 ApoB 100

ApoB 100, also known as Apo B, is used if there is a family history of early CVD to determine individual risk. Apo B is the main protein constituent of lipoproteins, especially LDL and VLDL. It would not be ordered in pediatrics but might be ordered by a lipid specialist. Cholesterol-rich apoB-containing lipoproteins' central role in causing atherosclerotic cardiovascular disease (CVD) is now fully understood. LDL is the principal force in the formation of atherosclerotic plaques. The confirmation of a direct cause between plasma cholesterol sitting on apoB-containing lipoproteins to atherosclerosis led to statins development (Shapiro and Fazio 2017).

4.5.1.8 Triglycerides (TG)

Approximately 10.7% of adolescents have a TG level over 150 mg/dL. Secondary TG elevations are primarily the result of obesity, diabetes, renal disease, and liver disease (Jacobson 2020). Primary TG elevations can result from a lipoprotein lipase deficiency or type V hyperlipoproteinemia, but these are rare diseases accounting for less than 6% of patients with elevated TG. An elevation of the triglyceride level of about 500 mg/dL puts the patient at risk for pancreatitis (Blackett et al. 2015).

The Bogalusa study reported an increase in the blood vessel's intima-media thickness when the TG is elevated between 150 and 499 mg/dL. However, the LDL and the VLDL, represented in the non-HDL-C, predict cardiovascular risk better than TG (Blackett et al. 2015).

Pitfalls of lipid testing. Lipids and lipoproteins only change minimally in response to normal food intake. Avoiding the fasting states improves the likelihood that the screen will be done since it avoids the need for the blood draw to be done early in the day and avoid hypoglycemia in patients with diabetes (Langsted and Nordestgaard 2019). The postprandial state is the usual state of the patient. Therefore, the lipids done when the patient is not fasting reflects what the patient is doing most of the day. Drawing a lipid profile at any time also makes it much easier for the lab to schedule the test (Scartezini et al. 2017). The TC, HDL-C, non-HDL-C, and LDL-C do not change significantly if the patient does not fast. The TG levels may not change significantly if a regular meal is consumed. If the TG level is >400, the test should be repeated after a 12-h fast (Scartezini et al. 2017).

4.5.1.9 Genetic Testing when Familial Dyslipidemia Is Identified

In their 2018 consensus panel report, the ACC advised that FH genetic testing should be the standard of care for patients and their relatives with a possible or definitive FH diagnosis. The genetic testing should include looking at the genes for low-density lipoprotein receptor (LDLR), proprotein convertase subtilisin/kexin 9 (PCSK9) and apolipoprotein B (apoB) (Grundy et al. 2019). Other possible genes should be added depending on the results of lipid profile and physical exam. Genetic testing is discussed in Chap. 7.

4.5.2 Real-Life Example

A 12-month-old was seen for a well-child visit. A finger-stick Hct was done, and the serum was noted to be turbid in appearance. A repeat sample confirmed the turbid serum. A lipid panel was ordered, and the results showed elevated cholesterol and a triglyceride level over 10,000. The toddler was referred for further diagnosis and management to a lipid specialist and a pediatric cardiologist. A diagnosis of a lipoprotein lipase deficiency was made.

Key Learning about Dyslipidemia

- Children and adolescents should be screened for dyslipidemia once between ages 9 and 11 and once between ages 17 and 21.
- Targeted screening should be done in children 2–8 and 12–16 if there is dyslipidemia or early CVD in first-degree family members, smoking history, or hypertension.
- The presence of risk conditions such as type 1 or type 2 diabetes mellitus, chronic renal disease, post-orthotopic cardiac or renal transplantation, nephrotic syndrome, HIV, a history of Kawasaki disease, or chronic inflammatory disease is also a reason to target screen patients.
- If the lipids' results are elevated, a repeat lipid screen should be done two weeks later, but not more than three months apart.

4.6 Screening for Tuberculosis Infection (LTBI)

Tuberculosis is a leading cause of death from an infectious disease worldwide (Walzi et al. 2018). Screening for mycobacterium tuberculosis exposure is no longer done annually and is done as risk assessment. Risk assessment includes screening for TB after exposure in a household, school, daycare center, or closed setting. The CDC recommends that screening for LTBI focus travel, birth, previously living outside of the United States and close contact with an infectious individual. The Bright Futures Guidelines ask the following three questions to do a risk assessment for tuberculosis:

- Was your child or any household member born in or has the child traveled to a country where tuberculosis is common (including

Africa, Asia, Latin America, and Eastern Europe)?

- Has your child had recent contact with an adult who has tuberculosis or had a positive tuberculosis test?
- Is your child infected with HIV? (Hagan et al. 2017).

The child with a TB infection (exposure to TB or latent TB infection) must be identified and treated to avoid active TB disease. The World Health Organization states that a tuberculin skin test is recommended in children younger than 5 years exposed to an adult with tuberculosis. The American Thoracic Society, the Infectious Diseases Society, and the CDC (2020a) endorse TB skin testing over TB blood tests for children less than 5 years old (Holmberg et al. 2019). An interferon-γ release assay (IGRA) (either QuantiFERON TB Gold [QFT] or T-SPOT) is used in children 5 years and over. The QFT measures the IFN-γ secreted by the patient's T lymphocyte, whereas the T-SPOT measures the number of IFN-γ-secreting lymphocytes. Both IGRAs utilize a positive and negative control, and if either control fails, the results are reported as indeterminate (QFT) or invalid (T-SPOT). For the T-SPOT, an invalid result is borderline. There is no risk quantification based on the patient's risk factors (Dunn et al. 2016). The economic advantages of using IGRA rather than TST have yet to be determined (Auguste et al. 2016).

4.6.1 IGRA Versus TST

IGRAs have higher specificities than a TST. TST is less specific for latent tuberculosis infection, especially in children who have been vaccinated with BCG. IGRAs and TST have similar sensitivities, but the IGRA in a BCG vaccinated child or adult is 85–95% versus 45–60% for TST. Neither IGRA nor TST is sensitive in immunocompromised children with severe tuberculosis. Neither blood test can differentiate TB infection from TB as a disease.

There is controversy regarding IGRA performance in children under 5 years, which is why the CDC or WHO is not recommending using an IGRA in children younger than 5 years of age (Carvalho et al. 2018; CDC 2020a); however, many experts now use IGRAs to test for tuberculosis infection down to 2 years of age (Lamb and Starke 2017). While there is increasing evidence that an IGRA may be an adequate test in children from two to five, at present, all guidelines state that an individual is at risk for LTBI if either the TST or IGRA is positive (Hasan et al. 2018). Tuberculosis is discussed in depth in Sect. 6.4.2.

4.7 Urinalysis

There are no longer any recommendations for routine urinalysis as part of the well-child visit; however, screening is recommended for high-risk children for renal disease. A urinalysis is recommended for children with diabetes following acute trauma to the abdomen, including the flank, or a history of hemolytic uremic syndrome, postglomerulonephritis, or Henoch-Schonlein purpura. The urinalysis should be followed in patients with these conditions until negative (Hains and Spencer 2017).

4.8 The Child Who Is Overweight or Obese

The AAP recommends screening for pediatric obesity at every well-child visit (Barlow and Expert Committee 2007). Obesity is associated with insulin resistance, which, in turn, drives hypertension, glucose intolerance, and dyslipidemia (Blackett et al. 2018). The US Preventive Task Force [USPTF] recommended screening for obesity starting at age six (2017). Both groups cite significant obesity complications, including psychological issues, asthma, adverse cardiometabolic effects, orthopedic problems, and endocrine problems. The clinical guidelines for caring for the child who is overweight or obese comes from the AAP, the Pediatric Endocrine Society, and the North American Society of Pediatric Gastroenterology,

Hepatology, and Nutrition (Barlow and Expert Committee 2007; Krebs et al. 2007; Magge et al. 2017; Styne et al. 2017; Vos et al. 2017). There is fairly good agreement on the recommended diagnostic screening evaluating for complications for the child with overweight (body mass index [BMI] > 84th to 94th percentile) or obesity (>95th percentile). Screening for risk factors of diabetes, hypertension, and dyslipidemia should be done in all children with obesity (Chung et al. 2018). This chapter will focus on the diagnostic screening tests needed when evaluating a child who is overweight or obese.

4.8.1 Diabetic Screening

The AAP has recommended that children over 10 years of age with a BMI >84th percentile or a BMI over the 95th percentile with any of the risk factors seen in Box 4.2 be evaluated for prediabetes or type 2 diabetes.

Box 4.2 Risk Factors for Screening for Prediabetes or Type 2 Diabetes

- Family history of type 2 diabetes.
- Signs of insulin resistance or conditions associated with insulin resistance (dyslipidemia, small-for-gestational-age, hypertension, acanthosis nigricans, polycystic ovarian disease).
- Race/ethnicity (Black American, Native American. Latino, Asian American, Pacific Islander).
- Use of atypical antipsychotic medications.
- Maternal history of gestational diabetes or a history of diabetes during the pregnancy.

Adapted from Styne et al. (2017)

The Pediatric Endocrine Society has recommendations for specific screening in the child with obesity. They recommend screening for prediabetes and dyslipidemia (Styne et al. 2017). The recommendations for dyslipidemia follow the expert panel report (NHLBI 2011). According to the Pediatric Endocrine Society, screening for prediabetes using a HbA1c, as recommended by the American Diabetes Association, is unpredictable in pediatrics since there is an ethnic variation that is not well understood (Styne et al. 2017). Iron-deficiency anemia (Christy et al. 2014), sickle cell disease, and other hemoglobinopathies (Lacy et al. 2017) may alter the results of the HbA1c. Due to poor performance of A1C, an oral glucose tolerance test (OGTT) is the recommended screening test for cystic fibrosis-related diabetes (Moran et al. 2010). A HbA1c also will miss acute type 1 diabetes. The advantages of a HbA1c include no fasting, less variability than glucose, less subject to acute changes, and increased screening by clinicians when they order HbA1c.

The Endocrine Society points out that HbA1c is a poor predictor since it underestimates the rate of prediabetes and diabetes in children. It is also poorly correlated with blood glucose in certain ethnic groups and therefore not an optimal diagnostic tool. A fasting or random glucose or an oral glucose tolerance test is needed in high-risk children based on the medical history, family history, race/ethnicity, or any other risk factors for diabetes. The Endocrine Society points out that the best test for a patient with dysglycemia is the 2-h glucose tolerance test. This test is 100% effective and is cost-efficient at $390 per case. A HbA1c as an initial screen is the least effective with a range of 7–32% and most expensive with the cost of testing and follow-up, ranging from $938 to $3370 per case. Since the HbA1c leads to several additional tests and misses children with obesity and prediabetes/diabetes, it is not a good first-line test in children with obesity. It should not be used in patients with a hemoglobin variant, including SCT (Lacy et al. 2017). Table 4.9 shows how to evaluate the results of diagnostic lab tests done to evaluate for diabetes.

Table 4.9 Diagnostic lab test, prediabetes, and diabetes

Diagnostic lab test	Prediabetes	Diabetes[a]	Comments
Fasting morning glucose	100–125 mg/dL	≥125 mg/dL	Fasting for at least 8 h without calorie intake
2-h plasma glucose	140–199 mg/dL	≥200 mg/dL	Use a loading dose of 1.75 g/kg of body weight of glucose to a maximum of 75 gm
Random plasma glucose	Not applicable	≥200 mg/dL	In patients with classic symptoms of hyperglycemia such as polydipsia or polyuria or patients with a hyperglycemic crisis
Hemoglobin A1c	5.7–6.4%		Screening

Adapted from Styne et al. (2017), Lacy et al. (2017), Christy et al. (2014), Moran et al. (2010)
[a]Diagnosis is confirmed if two or more of these tests are above the threshold or if the same test is above the threshold twice

4.8.2 Dyslipidemia Screening

In a child with obesity, there are excess free fatty acids (FFA) to the liver from high-fat diets and the excess adipose tissue release of FFA (Valaiyapathi et al. 2017). As a result, hepatic TG production and secretion of TG-rich VLDL increase. Consumption of a high-carbohydrate diet causes chronic stimulation of VLDL overproduction. Lipoprotein lipase is stimulated by insulin, and this results in postprandial TG excursions. A child with obesity is at a higher risk of abnormal lipid screening. Children with obesity and an average of two abnormal lipid screening should be counseled extensively following the NHLBI guidelines with a repeat lipid rescreen in 6 months.

4.8.3 Polycystic Ovarian Syndrome (PCOS)

PCOS is the most common endocrine problem in females (Azziz et al. 2018). The discussion of this is outlined in the endocrine section. It is associated with hyperinsulinemia and insulin resistance, but insulin levels are not recommended as a screening test for insulin resistance (Azziz et al. 2018).

4.8.3.1 Evaluation of Elevated Androgen

Total and free testosterone levels and SHBG are recommended to evaluate elevated androgen levels. This topic is discussed in detail in the endocrine section.

4.8.4 Nonalcoholic Fatty Liver Disease (NAFLD)

NAFLD is the most common liver disorder, with possible hepatomegaly and splenomegaly present on the exam. NAFLD incidence increases with increasing weight and male children (Shah et al. 2018). The spectrum of disease activity ranges from NAFLD to hepatic steatosis to NASH and, finally, fibrosis and cirrhosis. In patients with obesity and elevation of liver enzymes, the disease can be thought of as two different subtypes: (1) nonalcoholic fatty liver (hepatic steatosis without inflammation) and (2) NASH. Patients with NASH have hepatocyte injury with inflammation, resulting in fibrosis resulting in a greater risk of cirrhosis and, later, hepatocellular carcinoma (McDaniel 2019). Patients with NASH typically have mildly elevated AST and ALT (usually less than 4 times normal), with a De Ritis ratio usually less than 1.0. The range can occur through childhood, and there is an increasing number of liver transplants related to obesity and liver disease. Children may be asymptomatic, and clinicians need to be aware of the importance of screening (Shah et al. 2018). If the child is symptomatic with significant ALT elevation, they should be referred to a pediatric gastroenterologist or hepatologist (Koot & Nobili 2017).

Children with increased adiposity are at increased risk for NAFLD (Barlow and Expert Committee 2007; Vos et al. 2017). NAFLD is higher among children with obstructive sleep apnea, obesity, diabetes, prediabetes, obstructive sleep apnea, and panhypopituitarism. Caucasian,

Asian, and Hispanic children are at greater risk, but Hispanics are at the greatest risk with a four-fold prevalence (Shakir et al. 2018). The recommendation from both the NASPGHAN and the AAP is to start screening for NAFLD at age 9–11 years.

4.8.4.1 ALT and AST

The Vos et al. (2017) recommends all obese children and overweight children with other risk factors (insulin resistance, central adiposity, prediabetes or diabetes, dyslipidemia, sleep apnea, or a family history of nonalcoholic steatohepatitis [NASH or NAFLD]) should be screened for NAFLD with alanine aminotransferase (ALT) every 2–3 years. This recommendation has the highest strength of recommendation backed by good level evidence. They recommend screening the child before age 10 when the child has severe obesity, a family history of NAFLD/NASH, or hypopituitarism with a strength of evidence ranked at two.

The NASPGHAN recommends the upper limit of normal in children is 22 U/L for girls and 26 U/L for boys rather than lab normal. If the ALT is more than twice the upper limit for more than three months, the child should be referred for other chronic hepatitis causes. However, if the ALT is over 80, the child should be referred for evaluation. The child with aspartate aminotransferase (AST)/ALT greater than 1 or with ALT levels greater than 80 and splenomegaly needs further evaluation by specialists. The NASPGHAN also recommends that if the obesity increases or the child develops risk factors for NAFLD such as OSA or type 2 diabetes, the child will be rescreened earlier (Vos et al. 2017). They do not recommend routine ultrasound imaging. However, new ultrasound modalities need more study and may be incorporated into future guidelines combining ultrasound and ALT testing (Koot & Nobili 2017).

In contrast, the AAP (Barlow and Expert Committee 2007) recommends screening using ALT and AST every 2 years starting at age 10. If the ALT or AST is twice the normal, specialty consultation is advised. Clinicians must remember that NAFLD is a diagnosis of exclusion, and the persistent elevation of liver enzymes needs further evaluation to rule out other causes of the elevation.

Of interest, the European Society of Pediatric Gastroenterology and Nutrition recommends screening with an ALT and ultrasound imaging. Despite these clear guidelines from several specialty groups, a recent study found that even in a pediatric weight management clinic with 1312 patients, only 64.5% had liver enzymes in their management (Ferguson et al. 2018). Screening for NAFLD is not uniformly performed in clinical practice (Koot & Nobili 2017). It is important to do ALT routinely when seeing patients with obesity or patients with overweight and risk factors. Follow-up in 3 months is needed to evaluate for the persistently elevated liver enzyme. Any child with elevation for more than twice the upper limit for 3 months should be referred to a pediatric hepatologist or gastroenterologist (Shakir et al. 2018). In a study reported by Shakir et al. 2018, there was an association between NASH and diabetes, pointing to the importance of screening for diabetes in obese children or children with overweight and risk factors who have elevated liver enzymes.

AST

AST is found in the heart, kidney cells, muscles, and liver, unlike ALT, primarily from the liver (McDaniel 2019). It is also found in the RBC. An increase in AST without an increase in ALT suggests a cause other than the liver. These enzymes are located in the liver's hepatocytes; thus, an elevation suggests liver damage (Kwo et al. 2017). Since ALT is found in the hepatocyte cytoplasm (cytosol), it is released first when there is damage to the liver (Agrawal et al. 2016). AST is found in both the cytosol and the mitochondria, and there is a delayed release of AST during liver disease. The elevation of the liver enzymes may not reflect the extent of liver damage, and, in some cases, very high ALT can be seen in acute hepatitis with complete resolution (Agrawal et al. 2016).

The De Ritis ratio is the ratio of AST to ALT that can help determine the cause of the liver damage. For example, in a patient with acute hepatitis, the De Ritis ratio is <1 due to ALT's outpouring from the hepatocyte. In patients with

NAFLD, the ratio is elevated but generally not over 2 (McDaniel 2019). In patients with hepatic steatosis, hepatitis, and cirrhosis, the ratio is generally equal to or greater than 2 with an AST that rarely exceeds 300 IU/dL. Further workup for the child with persistently elevated AST ≥ 80 or the symptomatic child will be discussed in the liver section but will include alkaline phosphatase (ALP) and GGT.

The R ratio has been included in the (Kwo et al. 2017) to calculate whether the injury is cholestatic, hepatocellular, or mixed using the following formula: R = (ALT value/ALT upper limit of normal)/(ALP value/ALP upper limit of normal).

If the R ratio is >5, the liver injury is hepatocellular, whereas an R ratio of less than 2 identifies the liver injury as cholestatic. If the R ratio is between 2 and 5, this indicates a mixed pattern. A detailed discussion of other liver functions will be found in the section on liver disease in the GI chapter.

Pitfalls of these AST and ALT. As discussed in Chap. 1, minor elevations of a few points do not always mean liver disease. The results should be repeated when there are minor elevations in the AST/ALT before further workup. Since AST is also found in RBCs, hemolysis (either pathogenic or hemolyzed from the blood draw itself) causes elevations in the AST. Usually, if the reason for the elevation is hemolysis from the blood draw, the potassium is also similarly elevated.

Key Learning about the Child with Obesity
- The asymptomatic child with obesity needs to be screened for prediabetes and diabetes.
- Children with obesity and an average of two abnormal lipid screening should be counseled extensively following the NHLBI guidelines with a repeat lipid rescreen in 6 months.
- The NASPGHAN (2017) recommends that all obese children and overweight children with other risk factors (insulin resistance, central adiposity, prediabetes or diabetes, dyslipidemia, sleep apnea, or a family history of nonalcoholic steatohepatitis [NASH] or [NAFLD]) should be screened for NAFLD with alanine aminotransferase (ALT) every 2–3 years.
- The AAP (Barlow and Expert Committee 2007) recommends screening using ALT and AST every two years starting at age 10.

4.8.5 Real-Life Example

A 15-year-old female presented for a well visit for the first time. Her weight was three standard deviations above the 95th percentile, and her height was on the 50th percentile. Her BMI was over the 95th percentile. Her fasting glucose was 95, her cholesterol was 224, her triglycerides were 155, and her HDL cholesterol was 35. A screen for fatty liver disease was done, and her ALT was 267, and her AST was 275. The rest of her comprehensive metabolic profile was normal. Due to the marked elevation, a complete workup for other liver disease was done and was negative. The child was referred to a liver specialist who felt her increased BMI was the cause of the abnormal diagnostic tests. She advised intensive lifestyle changes, and after six months of follow-up, the child's ALT and AST were dropping, and she lost 15 pounds. A year later, her diagnostic laboratory tests were normal, and her BMI was in the overweight range.

4.9 Special Adolescent Issues

4.9.1 Screening for Sexually Transmitted Infection (STI)

The rate of STIs is about one in four adolescents (Shafii and Levine 2020). The AAP recommends routine screening for sexually transmitted infections as part of the adolescent well-child visit. Screening for STIs is also recommended by the CDC, USPTF, the American Academy of Family Physicians, and the American Academy of Obstetricians and Gynecologists. The screening rate for STIs among adolescents is well below STI incidence in adolescents (Shafii and Levine 2020). Chlamydia (CT) and gonorrhea (GC) are the most common STIs in adolescence. Box 4.3 lists risk factors for an STI with CR or GC. CT and GC can lead to pelvic inflammatory disease and scarring with subsequent infertility. CT is more common in adolescents due to the nature of the cervical mucosa. A survey of pediatricians reported 46% did routine STI screening, and 27% reported HIV routine screening (Henry-Reid et al. 2010). Adolescents less than 15 years of age are less likely to be screened. Lack of time, cultural barriers, discomfort with sexual subjects, and adolescent concerns about confidentiality all play a role in why STI screening is not part of routine care. Table 4.10 reviews the needs for routine screening in special populations as recommended by the AAP.

Table 4.10 Screening for sexually transmitted infections in special populations

	Screen for GC and CT	Screen for syphilis	Screen for HIV	Screen for trichomonas
Females 35 and younger entering juvenile detention or jails	Yearly	• If risk factors	Annual screen from 13 to 64 (CDC 2015) Screen adolescents once between 16 and 18 in high-prevalence communities (AAP 2021) (opt-out screening)	Consider screening (CDC 2015)
Females who have been exposed to CT and/or GC	Yearly	If risk factors	Annual screen and repeat as indicated by history or symptoms	Consider screening
Females who are pregnant	First trimester with a repeat in the final trimester at increased risk	First prenatal visit Retest early in the third trimester Retest at delivery if at high risk	First prenatal visit and retest if high-risk behavior, symptoms, or history of partner with HIV	Consider screening (CDC 2015)
HIV-positive females	Yearly	Annually or more frequently if local prevalence is high or risk factors	N/A	
Sexually active males in juvenile detention facilities, jails, national job training programs, STI clinics High school clinics Adolescent clinics	Yearly	Consider screening	N/A	
Men having sex with other men (MSM)	Yearly Urine, rectal, pharyngeal	• Annually for MSM (Centers for Disease Control and Prevention 2015) • Repeat every three to six months if at increased risk	N/A	
HIV positive	Yearly Urine, rectal, pharyngeal	Annually or more frequently if local prevalence is high or risk factors	N/A	

Adapted from Department of Health and Human Services, Centers for Disease Control and Prevention 2015; AAP (2018); Levy et al. (2019)

Box 4.3 Risk Factors for CT, GC, and Syphilis
With risk factors

- Prior GC, CT infection in the past year.
- Partner with multiple other partners.
- Sex worker or transactional sex.
- IV drug use and/or partners who are drug users.
- High prevalence population.
- More than one sex partner in the past year.

Adapted from Department of Health and Human Services, Centers for Disease Control and Prevention (2015) and Levy et al. (2019)

The most common STIs in order of incidence are human papillomavirus (HPV), chlamydia (CT), trichomoniasis, gonorrhea (GC), and genital herpes (Levy et al. 2019). Adolescents are at higher risk for sexually transmitted infections due to unprotected sex and greater biological susceptibility (AAP red Book 2021). The importance of having time to discuss confidential issues during a well-child adolescent visit remains a barrier to delivering reproductive care. The clinician must clarify the type of sexual activity (oral, vaginal, anal) and partner gender. There are several ways of evaluating the adolescent for STIs, including NAAT, culture, and POC NAAT such as GeneXpert (Cepheid). BINX 10 was approved March 2021 by the FDA as a point-of-care test to give results in 30 min (Mybinxhealth 2021). The CDC has published a mnemonic called the 5 P's seen in Box 4.4:

Box 4.4 The Five P's: Partners, Practices, Prevention of Pregnancy, Protection from STDs, and Past History of STDs
1. Partners
   - "Do you have sex with men, women, or both?"
   - "In the past two months, how many partners have you had sex with?"
   - "In the past 12 tmonths, how many partners have you had sex with?"
   - "Is it possible that any of your sex partners in the past 12 months had sex with someone else while they were still in a sexual relationship with you?"
2. Practices
   - "To understand your risks for STDs, I need to understand the kind of sex you have had recently."
   - "Have you had vaginal sex, meaning 'penis in vagina sex'?" If yes, "Do you use condoms: never, sometimes, or always?"
   - "Have you had anal sex, meaning 'penis in rectum/anus sex'?" If yes, "Do you use condoms: never, sometimes, or always?"
   - "Have you had oral sex, meaning 'mouth on penis/vagina'?"
   - For condom answers:
   - If "never": "Why don't you use condoms?"
   - If "sometimes": "In what situations (or with whom) do you use condoms?"
3. Prevention of pregnancy
   - "What are you doing to prevent pregnancy?"
4. Protection from STDs
   - "What do you do to protect yourself from STDs and HIV?"
5. Past history of STDs
   - "Have you ever had an STD?"
   - "Have any of your partners had an STD?"

Additional questions to identify HIV and viral hepatitis risk include:

- "Have you or any of your partners ever injected drugs?"
- "Have you or any of your partners exchanged money or drugs for sex?"
- "Is there anything else about your sexual practices that I need to know about?"

Department of Health and Human Services, CDC. Retrieved from: https://www.cdc.gov/std/tg2015/clinical.htm

All states allow minors to give their consent for testing for sexually transmitted diseases. Forty-five states allow clinicians to treat partners of the adolescents they are treating (CDC 2020b). Expedited partner therapy can stop the chain of transmission to other sexual partners (AAP Red Book: Report of the Committee on Infectious Diseases (AAP red Book 2021).

4.9.1.1 Nucleic Acid Amplification Tests for Chlamydia (CT) and Gonorrhea (GC)

All adolescent females less than 25 should be screened annually for STIs. There is a clear recommendation to screen asymptomatic female adolescents annually (<25 years) for CT and gonorrhea (GC) (Shafii and Levine 2020; Workowski et al. 2021). For adolescents of both sexes who have HIV, annual screening for CT and GC should be done. If an adolescent female is pregnant, they should have a CT and GC screening in the first trimester and, depending on risk, have it repeated in the third trimester. Urogenital infection with CT is diagnosed by different methods including vaginal swabs, cervical swabs, or first-void urine (Workowski et al. 2021).

There is no specific recommendation for screening adolescent males (Workowski et al. 2021). If an adolescent male has sex with another male (MSM), they should have annual urine and rectal screening for GC and a GC pharyngeal screening. MSM should be screened annually for syphilis. Adolescent males with a CT urethral infection are diagnosed by either testing a first-void urine or doing a urethral swab, with the former being preferred and just as accurate. Routine screening of asymptomatic adolescents is also not recommended for syphilis, herpes simplex, trichomoniasis, or hepatitis. More frequent screening can be done based on risk factors such as a history of an STI within the past 24 months, new partners, multiple partners in the past year, a partner with an STI, inconsistent condom use, use of IV drugs, transactional sex, or being incarcerated (Levy et al. 2019; Workowski et al. 2021).

NAATs are the most sensitive tests for these specimens and are the recommended test for detecting *C. trachomatis* infection. GC and CT testing's gold standard is the nucleic acid amplification test (NAAT) since it has the highest sensitivity and specificity (Levy et al. 2019; Workowski et al. 2021). Screening with a urine sample is preferred in males and has the same sensitivity and specificity as a urethral swab without the discomfort. Self-collected vaginal swabs are preferred for female patients as they are preferred among female adolescents with higher sensitivity than clinician-collected swabs (Shafii and Levine 2020). Urine collection can be done, but self-collected vaginal swabs have a high sensitivity and specificity. Self-collection can be easily taught using CDC educational material. NAATs are acceptable for detection of CT in either vaginal or urine specimens from pre-pubescent girls (Centers for Disease Control and Prevention 2015). There are no recommendations for test of cure for CT testing unless there is a question about adherence, if there are persistent symptoms, or reinfection is suspected (Workowski et al. 2021). However, adolescent females and males treated for gonorrhea should have a retest 3 months following treatment whether their sex partners were treated or not. It is important to schedule the follow-up visit at the time of treatment. When retesting at 3 months is not a possibility, clinicians should retest at the next visit, preferably <12 months after initial treatment (Workowski et al. 2021).

The advantage of point-of-care technology or near the point of care technology is to allow the patient to be treated while they are being seen in the healthcare system. The field of point-of-care technology for CT and GC tests is constantly changing, and newer technologies are being developed that will need to be studied in a population that is not at high risk of CT and GC. At present, many of the studies of the devices for point of care or near the point of care have specificities and sensitivities done in research studies on high-risk populations (Herbst de Cortina et al. 2016; Murtagh 2019). These tests will be discussed in detail in Chap. 5.

4.9.1.2 Culture for CT and GC

Cultures are not routinely used as they are more expensive and require considerable technical expertise. However, culture for CT from rectal specimens in girls and boys is recommended in prepubescent children suspected of being sexually assaulted. The meatal swab should be cultured in males, and in females, nonurogenital sites should be cultured for CT. Vaginal cultures can be done in prepubescent girls suspected of being sexually assaulted.

4.9.1.3 Complement Fixation for CT

CT serology using complement fixation is hampered by a lack of standardization and a high level of experience to interpret. It is not a recommended way to screen for CT. The presence of a particular antigen or antibody in the patient serum is confirmed based on whether complement fixation is present.

4.9.1.4 Point-of-Care Tests for CT

Point-of-care testing minimizes the lack of follow-up in that the patient received the results while still being seen. The rapid POC tests have high specificity regardless of specimen types (range 97–100%); however, the pooled sensitivity is much lower (36–62%). For chlamydia, the USA-made tests include ACON Chlamydia (ACON Laboratories, USA), BINX 10, Clearview Chlamydia (Abbott, USA), HandiLab-C (HandiLab, USA), and QuickVue (Quidel, USA). These tests will be discussed in detail in Chap. 5.

4.9.2   HIV Screening

The AAP recommends HIV screening during the well adolescent should occur at least once in a healthcare setting starting at age 15 (Hsu and Rakhmanin 2021). Take out in contrast. the CDC advises annual HIV screening from age 13–64 in all healthcare settings. There is no longer any recommendation for consent, but the adolescent should be informed that an HIV test will be done. The patient can be offered the option of opting out of the testing (Centers for Disease Control and Prevention 2015). The CDC also advises that testing for HIV be done when an adolescent is being treated for a sexually transmitted infection, even if they had a recent test. All pregnant teens should be screened for HIV as part of their routine prenatal care (Centers for Disease Control and Prevention

2015). The United States Preventive Services Task Force recommends that clinicians screen all adolescents aged 15 years and older and younger adolescents at increased risk of infection for HIV (US Preventive Services Task Force 2019b). Most patients with a positive screening test need further testing to confirm the presence of the disease. HIV is discussed in detail in Sect. 6.3.5, and point-of-care testing is discussed in Chap. 5.

4.9.3   Syphilis

The testing for syphilis is discussed in detail in Sect. 6.4.1.

4.9.4   Trichomonas Vaginalis

The three most common vaginitis types are bacterial vaginosis, vulvovaginal candidiasis, and trichomonas vaginalis (TV). Traditionally, the Amsel criteria or Nugent score determined bacterial vaginosis (see Box 4.5). In contrast, candidiasis was diagnosed by looking for budding yeast on a wet mount or getting back a positive culture. Clinical symptoms or physical exam findings were the reason for doing the culture or wet mount (Schwebke et al. 2018). Patient self-diagnosis is wrong 50–66% of the time (Sobel 2007; Powell et al. 2014), and up to 40% of women do not get the correct diagnosis at the initial office visit using the methods above (Carr et al. 2005). Today DNA targets can be used for the direct detection of the bacterial associated with bacterial vaginosis. The BD MAX vaginal panel is an automated assay used for this purpose (Kawa et al. 2021). Aptima® Bacterial Vaginosis and Aptima BV/CV are two NAAT tests for identifying the three most common vaginitis causes approved by the FDA in 2019.

Trichomoniasis is thought of as the most prevalent nonviral STI around the world (Workowski et al. 2021). TV infection is associated with an increased risk of HIV (Mavedzenge et al. 2010) and a prolonged HPV infection (Shew et al. 2006). It also leads to a higher risk of other STIs and, if left untreated during pregnancy, leads to 1.4 times higher rate of premature delivery of low-birth-weight babies, small for gestational age, and premature rupture of membranes (Donders et al. 2009; Workowski et al. 2021). Seventy to eighty-five percent of patients with TV have minimal or no genital symptoms. This means that untreated infections can linger from months to years (Workowski et al. 2021). The classic presentation is greenish, frothy, malodorous vaginal discharge with an inflamed cervix termed strawberry cervix (AAP, 2018). The incubation period can start after 5 days and last as long as 28 days. There are several diagnostic tests used to diagnose the condition. While TV can be found on wet mount, this method is far less reliable than biochemical detection, with a reported sensitivity of 51–63% (AAP, 2018) to 44–68% (Workowski et al. 2021). Microscopy is no longer recommended (Kawa et al. 2021). The three methods for detecting trichomonas vaginalis are antigen-based, nucleic acid hybridization, or nucleic acid amplification-based assays or nucleic acid hybridization (Schwebke et al. 2018). The CDC 2015 guidelines recommended NAAT as the preferred method to diagnose TV infection (Centers for Disease Control and Prevention 2015). The point-of-care tests include the Aptima *T. vaginalis* assay (Beckton Dickinson), OSOM lateral flow test, AmpliVue test, the Solana test, and the GeneXpert test (Gaydos et al. 2017; Workowski et al. 2021). Solana trichomonas assay (Quidel) is a rapid test for the qualitative detection of *T. vaginalis* DNA yielding results in around 40 min (Workowski et al. 2021). Retesting is recommended for all sexually active adolescents at <3 months after initial treatment (Workowski et al. 2021).

> Nugent score involved a quantitative estimate of the concentration of the following bacteria noted in a Gram stain
>
> 1. *Lactobacillus*.
> 2. Small Gram-negative and Gram-variable rods (e.g., *G. vaginalis*, *Bacteroides*, *Prevotella*, *Porphyromonas*, *Peptostreptococcus*)
> 3. Curved Gram-variable rods (e.g., *Mobiluncus*).
>
> Adapted from Amsel et al. (1983); Nugent et al. (1991)

4.9.4.1 Antigen-Based Testing for TV Using Immunochromatographic Capillary Flow

OSOM Rapid Test can give results in 10–15 min with a sensitivity of 82–95% and specificity of 97–100%, compared with wet mount, culture, and transcription-mediated amplification. It is only approved in females. OSOM test is a point-of-care test, is equipment-free, and has Clinical Laboratory Improvement Amendments (CLIA) waiver. Tests for TV will be discussed in Chap. 5.

4.9.4.2 DNA Hybridization Probe

Affirm VPIII can give results in 45 min using vaginal swab specimen in either a point-of-care testing or laboratory testing. The test is not approved in males.

4.9.4.3 Nucleic Acid Amplification Test (NAAT)

DNA probe technology finds target organisms based on their genetic DNA. The APTIMA CV/TV assay and the BD Probe Tec TV Q amplified DNA assay are commercially available tests with FDA approval for testing vaginal swage, urine specimens, and endocervical samples. These tests cannot be used for treatment success as nucleic acids from TV are persistent in genital cultures. The BD probe has a

> **Box 4.5 Ansel Criteria and Nugent Score for Bacterial Vaginosis**
> Amsel criteria (3 of 4 signs or symptoms for positive diagnosis)
>
> 1. Thin, homogenous vaginal discharge.
> 2. Presence of clue cells (vaginal epithelial cells studded with adherent coccobacilli on microscopic examination)
> 3. Vaginal pH >4.5.
> 4. Positive whiff test results.

sensitivity of 93.1–93.2% depending on whether the specimen is self-collected versus clinician-collected, respectively. The specificity is 99.3 whether the specimen is self-collected or clinician-collected (Kara et al. 2021). The APTIMA CV/TV assay tests for candida vaginalis and TV. The AmpliVue and the Solana tests are molecular amplified assays and must be done in a lab with a one-hour completion time.

4.9.4.4 Culture of T Vaginalis

Cultures of TV using Diamond media or the InPouch system (BioMed Diagnostics) had been the most sensitive method for TV detection before the different molecular methods were available. The sensitivity of culture ranges from 75% to 96% and the specificity is under 100% (Workowski et al. 2021).

4.9.5 Real-Life Example

A 17-year-old female presented with a 2-week history of vaginal discharge but no abdominal pain or discomfort. She reported having vaginal sex only with three different male sexual partners in the past year. All of her partners were her age, and she had sex willingly without any pressure. She reported that she had been dating each of the boyfriends at different times. She reported consistent condom use. She is previously healthy, and there is no previous screening done for any sexually transmitted diseases, including HIV.

Her physical exam is unremarkable. There is some mildly yellow vaginal discharge seen on the external exam. Based on the AAP recommendations, a molecular test for STIs using a patient-obtained vaginal sample and a point-of-care HIV test was done. The adolescent lived in a low-risk area for HIV, and her HIV test was negative. The NAAT test was negative for GC and CT. A point-of-care test for trichomonas was positive, and the child was treated.

Key Learning about STI
- Screening for STIs is recommended by the AAP, CDC, USPTF, the American Academy of Family Physicians, and the American College of obstetricians and Gynecologist.
- There are similar outcomes with vaginal obtained or provider-obtained vaginal samples once the patient is taught how to do it.
- Expedited partner therapy can stop the chain of transmission to other sexual partners.
- Point-of-care testing will increase, and a recent CLIA-waived POCT test was approved for GC and CT.
- While the number and age of starting screening for HIV tests may vary, it is clear that if an adolescent has a positive screen for an STI, an HIV screen should be done. These tests are opt-out tests. This means the adolescent should be told the provider wants to do the test but that the adolescent has an option to refuse testing.
- Seventy to eighty percent of patients with TV are asymptomatic. New POCT testing for trichomonas is more accurate than using microscopy.
- Females, unlike males, commonly present asymptomatically with STI, pointing to the need to routinely screen for these infections to avoid complications of infertility and pelvic inflammatory disease.

4.9.5.1 Drug Screening

Children and adolescents are at risk for substance abuse disorders. The problem of substance abuse in pediatric patients over 12 is not rare. In 2017, the rate of nonmedical use of psychotherapeutic drugs was 2.2%, whereas in adolescents 12 and over, 11.2% admitted to any illicit drug use for the previous month (National Center for Health

Statistics 2020). The nonmedical use of prescription drugs, along with designer drugs, has caused overdose deaths, fueling concerns among clinicians and parents alike. Overdose deaths involving synthetic opioids such as fentanyl and tramadol (not including methadone) continued to increase in 2018 (rate of 9.9/100,000). Cocaine and psychostimulants with abuse potential accounted for 4.5/100,000 deaths in 2018, increasing from 2017's rate of 4.3/100,000. The age-adjusted rate of drug overdose deaths involving psychostimulants with abuse potential increased fivefold from 2012 to 2018 (Hedegaard et al. 2020). Clinicians need to be aware of abuse potential when prescribing psychostimulants to adolescents, and therefore screening all adolescents for drug use by use of approved screening tools is critical. Screening for tobacco, alcohol, or drug use is recommended yearly from 11 to 21 years.

A clinician must decide how to handle a guardian's request to do a drug screening when doing an adolescent exam. In some school districts, the school is allowed to screen the child without the adolescent's permission. If the drug test is positive, disciplinary action can follow without regard for the test's sensitivity and specificity. It would not be uncommon for the adolescent to be brought in by the guardian after the testing is done since the adolescent has been suspended from school. In emergency rooms, adolescents may present with bizarre behavior, and a urine drug screen is ordered to evaluate for possible drug use. Clinicians need to understand the variety of toxidromes (how the drugs present clinically) for illicit drugs. Adolescents and children with chronic pain may be screened to ensure that they are taking the drugs and that the medication is not being diverted for money. Aside from obtaining the adolescent's permission to screen, the clinician must consider the false-positive and false-negative drug testing results.

4.9.5.2 Screening Tools

The AAP and the National Institute on Drug Abuse recommended two tools: Brief Screener for Tobacco, Alcohol, and other Drugs (BSTAD) and Screening to Brief Intervention (S2BI). The tools can be administered to the patient in the waiting room or administered by any healthcare professional. The S2BI asks one question about various commonly abused substances, including designer drugs and prescription drugs. It is a complete screening, and the online version decides the patient's level of risk for substance abuse based on the response. The BSTAD is a shorter version and focuses on smoking, alcohol, and marijuana but does not ask for a wider variety of commonly abused substances. The AAP and the National Institute on Drug Abuse have online versions of both the BSTAD and the S2BI, which are available at https://www.drugabuse. gov/nidamed-medical-health-professionals/ screening-tools-prevention/screening-tools- adolescent-substance-use/adolescent-substance- use-screening-tools. Despite this, parents or schools will ask for drug screening.

4.9.5.3 Immunoassay Urine Drug Testing

When ordered, urine drug testing (UDT) is usually done by immunoassay as a first-line screening. UDT can be done in a clinical laboratory or using a point-of-care device. Point-of-care (POC) devices, both using a strip or a urine cup, offer the advantages of quick turnaround and detection of several classes of drugs. Immunoassay tests employ the use of antibodies to detect a drug's presence. POC within an office setting is quick, but the reliability depends on the user's skill and understanding of the results. The common traditional drug classes in a screen include barbiturates, benzodiazepines, cocaine (metabolite benzoylecgonine), methadone, cannabinoids (tetrahydrocannabinol), opiates (codeine, hydrocodone, hydromorphone, morphine), phencyclidine (PCP), and methadone (Krasowski et al. 2020). Positive immunoassay results must be confirmed by confirmatory testing utilizing techniques of gas chromatography-mass spectrometry (GC-MS), liquid chromatography-mass spectrometry (LC-MS), or high-performance liquid chromatography (HPTLC) (Mahajan 2017).

Drug testing can be done on urine, blood, hair, sweat, nail clipping, meconium, and saliva

(Moeller et al. 2017). Urine screening is the most common method as urine is available in large amounts, involves no invasive procedures, is inexpensive, and contains the drug and drug metabolites in higher concentrations than serum equivalents (Kapur & Aleksa 2020, Mahajan 2017). The disadvantages of urine screening include ease of adulteration, short to an intermediate window of detection, patients feeling like criminals when a witnessed urine collection is required, and difficulty to provide a spontaneous specimen. While blood, hair, sweat, and saliva are available methods, the use of these methods is limited by short windows of detection (blood, saliva), ease of detection (hair), high cost (hair), low concentration (saliva), lack of data on cross-reactivity (saliva), invasive testing (blood), and two visits (sweat) (Mahajan 2017).

Immunoassay is used as first-line testing since it is quick, can be done using point-of-care testing, and is inexpensive. It can help the clinician make initial treatment decisions providing the clinician recognizes the weaknesses that result in both false-positive and false-negative results. UDT using urine is limited by drug-drug interactions, drug-disease interactions, dilution, urine pH, a lag time between ingestion and urinary excretion, and genetics. It is limited as it only provides a snapshot of the drug present when the sample is collected (Kapur & Aleksa 2020). A morning sample tends to be more concentrated and is recommended (Mahajan 2017). The patient can make a diluted sample look more yellow by ingesting Vitamin B or niacin or several products (Stealth, Urine Luck, Instant Clean, Klear, Whizzles, UrinAid) available over the Internet to get a negative drug screening (Kapur & Aleksa 2020). The labs now can detect some but not all of the adulterants used by adolescents (Kapur & Aleksa 2020). There may be signs of residue in the sample. There is reasonable agreement between urine drug tests and an adolescent report of drug use (Gignac et al. 2005).

While positive results on an immunoassay require confirmation of the positive result, a negative result is not sent out for further testing despite the risk of it being a false negative. The risk of false negative stresses the importance of combining drug screening with history, physical examination, and pertinent past medication records and reviewing the prescription drug-monitoring program (PDMP).

Each state has its PDMP. The PDMP is an electronic database that monitors the prescription of controlled substances in the state. The pharmacist will enter the information about a prescription into the database so that providers will know whether a patient has been to multiple clinicians seeking a drug. However, states have varying regulations about whether a clinician must check the database before prescribing a controlled substance (CDC 2020c).

Enzyme immunoassays. Enzyme immunoassays (EIA) involve using chemically linked antibodies or antigens that detect the drug. There are three main types of immunoassays used (Moeller et al. 2017); however, the two most common immunoassays used are enzymatic and fluorescent. In talking about drug screening, competitive binding is used, and the patient's sample competes with the labeled drug for the specific binding sites on the antibody. When binding occurs, it causes a color change in the solution, fluoresce under light, or induction of radiation or light signal that can be measured (Kapur & Aleksa 2020). Immunoassays are fast and automated and can be done with small values; however, they lack specificity and can only be used for certain drug classes. Some laboratories will provide information on how to interpret the test results. The clinician can also contact the laboratory if they have a concern or question about the test results.

Pitfalls of immunoassay urine drug testing by immunoassay (UDT). While urine drug screen is used in primary care, the clinician must recognize they lack the specificity and sensitivity and therefore are plagued with inappropriate results. Parents will request a drug screen for the adolescent, but the clinician must understand that a common urine drug screening panel does not screen for designer drugs and has a limited panel of drugs. The majority of IASs look for amphetamine, cocaine, marijuana, PCP, and a limited number of opiates (codeine, morphine, and the by-product of heroin 6-monoacetylmorphine).

The test will only report a positive opiate screen, but it will not distinguish between the three substances. There is an inconsistent or lack of ability to detect the semisynthetic opioids (oxycodone, hydromorphone, oxymorphone, buprenorphine) and synthetic opioids (meperidine, fentanyl, methadone) (Mahajan 2017). The difficulty is that opioids and benzodiazepines have extensive steps before their conjugated metabolites can be detected (Kapur & Alesksa 2020). These substances are common prescriptions and are frequent sources of abuse and overdose in the United States. Many adolescents also use designer drugs, herbal drugs of abuse, and synthetic cannabinoids such as "spice" or "K2" (Moeller et al. 2017). While there are immunoassays or POCT to detect the known substances, the designer drugs are always altered to avoid detection. Certain designer drugs such as salvia require GC-MS, LC-MS, or HPTLC to detect them (Moeller et al. 2017). The laboratory establishes the cutoffs, but if the patient has only a small amount of a particular drug, they may be reported as negative as the results fall below the cutoff.

The cost of testing is linked to the number of drugs analyzed (Mahajan 2017). Insurances may not cover the cost of random testing of adolescents or frequent screening as they may limit the number of times a patient can be tested in a year.

The clinician needs to be aware of the pitfalls before ordering the test. The first step is to point out to the parent the limitations of the testing and the possibility that the adolescent could be using drugs and the test could be negative. The next step is to get permission from the adolescent to do a urine drug screen. Immunoassays suffer significant limitations, including cross-reactivity with other drugs and substances, resulting in false positives. An immunoassay screen results cannot distinguish between opiates when a positive result is reported. If an adolescent is taking dextromethorphan, diphenhydramine, fluoroquinolones, quinine, or rifampin, the result for opiates will be positive due to false-positive results (Mahajan 2017). Amphetamine screens can also be positive if the adolescent takes pseudoephedrine, ranitidine, amantadine, bupropion, fluoxetine, or L-methamphetamine (nasal decongestant). The laboratory may report cross-reactivity. The immunoassay is inconsistent or unable to detect semisynthetic (hydrocodone, oxymorphone, buprenorphine) and synthetic opioids (fentanyl, methadone, pentazocine, and meperidine) (Mahajan 2017). Medications such as proton pump inhibitors and nonsteroidal anti-inflammatory drugs can cross-react with cannabinoid immunoassays (Moeller et al. 2017). A higher threshold of detection can miss the patient who is using the drug. Finally, the immunoassay cannot distinguish between the parent drug and its active metabolite (Saitman et al. 2014).

The clinician needs to know what immunoassay the laboratory uses as not all labs use the same immunoassay detection method or threshold values. Asking the clinical laboratory sciences for more information about the test is very important before interpreting any urine immunoassay drug screen (Nelson et al. 2016). A working relationship with the lab helps discuss the results (Moeller et al. 2017).

Laboratory error, rapid metabolism of the drug, mislabeling of the specimen, and faulty equipment can result in a false-negative result. A negative result occurs if the opioid or its metabolite falls below the test's threshold of detectability. A pseudo false positive occurs due to cross-reactivity with another drug during the immunoassay. Drug testing using immunoassay needs to be backed up with chromatographic methods.

4.9.5.4 Chromatographic Methods (CM)

The confirmatory drug screen is done by chromatographic methods (Moeller et al. 2017). Chromatographic techniques do not require a drug-specific reagent and can detect multiple drugs in a single analysis. The main chromatographic methods (CM) used in toxicological drug evaluation are thin-layer chromatography (CM-TLC), high-performance liquid chromatography (HPTLC), and gas chromatography. The drugs are separated and then detected using several techniques—ultraviolet, fluorescent, flame ionization, and mass spectrometry. Chromatographic techniques with mass spectrometry are commonly used to confirm drugs of abuse (Kapur & Alesksa 2020). Federal cutoff concentrations for CM for the workplace are higher to avoid false positives (Moeller et al. 2017). Urine is the most common way to detect drugs due to concentrations about 100 times greater than blood samples (Ahadi et al. 2011).

Pitfalls of chromatographic methods. Due to potential false-positive and false-negative UDT immunoassay testing, confirmatory testing with GC-MS and LC-MS/MS should be done to avoid the legal consequences and possible school dismissal (Moeller et al. 2017). These tests have high specificity and sensitivity to detect the particular substance. However, there is always a possibility of laboratory error, mislabelling, or the sample being adulterated.

4.9.6   Real-Life Example

A 16-year-old female presented for a well visit. She was interviewed separately from the parents. While the child was filling out a Patient Health Questionnaire for Adolescents and Drug Abuse–Brief Screener for Tobacco, Alcohol, and other Drugs (BSTAD), the single mother was interviewed separately to elicit her concerns. The mother was adamant about doing a drug screening without the child's knowledge, just in case. The mother was asked about specific symptoms for depression and drug use, and the review of symptoms was negative. The clinician explained to the mother that drug screening was not done without the adolescent permission. The adolescent screenings were reviewed and scored, and the results were unremarkable. With the adolescent's permission, the results were shared with the mother, but she insisted she wanted the test done.

The adolescent was also asked about drug use and reported that her best friend had used marijuana at a party. Based on her friend's experience, she reported that she did not want to use any drugs. She did report tasting beer at a party and thought it was disgusting. The adolescent gave the clinician permission to do the drug screening to satisfy her mother's unrelenting request.

The mother's concern was addressed in a follow-up interview after the history and physical were complete. The limitations of the test were explained to the mother. The adolescent was willing to satisfy her mother. A drug screening was returned as negative.

> **Key Learning about Drug Screening**
>
> - Due to the limitations of drug screening, the use of a screening questionnaire should be done.
> - Immunoassays are commonly done as first-line screening for urine drug testing (UDT).
> - UDT can be done in a clinical laboratory or using a point-of-care device. The clinician needs to understand the limitation of immunoassays.
> - Chromatographic methods must be done to confirm a positive drug screen.

Questions

1. Which of the following is recommended by the American Academy of Pediatrics?
   (a) Start to screen children for dyslipidemia between 9 and 11 years of age.
   (b) Children should not be screened for dyslipidemia unless they have a family history of CVD or hyperlipidemia.
   (c) Lipid screening should only be done fasting.
   (d) All children should have an initial screen for dyslipidemia between 2 and 8 years.
2. A 5-year-old developmentally delayed child is observed frequently putting objects in his mouth. His previous lead levels were all below 10, and there is no history of housing changes. He started Kindergarten three months ago. The mother reports that she does not know the building's age, but it is not new. What is the best approach to the management of this child?
   (a) Do a lead screening.
   (b) Do **a** free erythrocyte protoporphyrin (FEP).

(c) Do nothing as his lead has been normal.

(d) Encourage the child to stop putting things in his mouth.

3. A 7-year-old male presents for a well visit. The history and physical are unremarkable except that his 39-year-old father had a myocardial infarction 1 month ago. Which of the following screening laboratory tests are indicated for the child?

   (a) Anemia screen.

   (b) Lipid panel.

   (c) Lipoprotein A.

   (d) Liver function test.

4. A 10-year-old African American male with sickle cell trait presents for a well visit. His weight is at least two standard deviations above the 95th percentile, and his height is following his curve on the 75th percentile. What screening would be appropriate for this child?

   (a) Lead screening, total cholesterol (TC), high-density lipoprotein (HDL), CBC, AST, and serum insulin level.

   (b) TC, HDL, aspartate aminotransferase (AST), alanine aminotransferase (ALT).

   (c) Fasting glucose, lipid panel, AST, ALT.

   (d) CBC, hemoglobin A1c, TC.

5. A newborn is seen for the two-week visit during the morning session. What should be done if the newborn screen is not in the chart?

   (a) Assume that if the history and physical is normal and the newborn screen was done.

   (b) Remind the staff to call for the newborn screen, and move on to the next patient.

   (c) Call the state's newborn screening office, and have the mother wait until you have the result.

   (d) Ask the mother if the newborn screen was received at home and if it was normal.

6. When should an 11-year-old with two abnormal lipid panel screens done four weeks apart come back for a repeat screen?

   (a) One month

   (b) Three months

   (c) Six months

   (d) One year

7. A mother brings a 16-year old into the office due to a positive drug screen done in school. The child denies any drug use, and the Brief Screener for Tobacco, Alcohol, and other Drugs (BSTAD) is negative. The mother shows you the result of urine immunoassay, which is positive for opiates. The mother reports the child is taking diphenhydramine for allergies. What is the next step?

   (a) Tell the mother that the child is taking opiates since the screening is positive.

   (b) Ask the mother to stop giving the child diphenhydramine for 1 month and repeat the urine immunoassay.

   (c) Tell the mother the positive opiate result is from the ingestion of diphenhydramine.

   (d) Do a high-performance liquid chromatography urine specifically looking at an extended opiate panel.

8. A 17-year-old female denies any form of sexual activity in the past year during a well visit. She reports having multiple boyfriends before this past year but denies any male or female partners for the last year. She has never been screened with a lipid panel, HIV screen, or any STD. What is the best approach to her care?

   (a) She is due for a lipid panel this visit.

   (b) Do a lipid panel and HIV screen at this visit.

   (c) Do a lipid panel, HIV screen, and a pelvic exam for STD screening.

   (d) Do a lipid panel, HIV screen, and nucleic acid amplification tests (NAATs) for *C. trachomatis* and *Neisseria gonorrhoeae*.

Rationale

1. Answer: A

   The AAP recommends screening for dyslipidemia between 9 and 11 years of age and between 17 and 21 years. There is no need to fast for an initial screening for dyslipidemia, including total cholesterol and an HDL-C. Children who have a significant family history of CVD should be screened between 2 and 8 years.

2. Answer: A

In this patient, the best approach is to screen the child for lead poisoning. An FEP is not specific enough to evaluate the lead level. Given the child's developmental status, just telling him to stop putting things in his mouth is not the most effective choice. Given the mother's uncertainty about the building's age and the child's behavior in the office, it would be best to do the lead test.

3. Answer: B

Cardiovascular disease before the age of 55 years should warrant more investigation. It is recommended that all children above the age of 2 years should be screened if they have a family history of premature cardiovascular disease. Familial hypercholesterolemia can manifest at a very early age. Therefore, a family history of such a disease should raise suspicion and is an indication for screening.

4. Answer: C

In this patient, a lead screening is not needed. A serum insulin level is a research test and is not recommended by the Endocrine Society's guidelines on obesity. Choice B does not screen for prediabetes or diabetes. Answer C is the best answer. If the patient is fasting for the glucose level, a lipid panel should be done, especially given obesity. Screening for fatty liver disease with an ALT and AST is the recommendation of the AAP. A hemoglobin A1c is unreliable in a patient with inherited hemoglobin variants and should not be done in a patient with SCT (Lacy et al. 2017).

5. Answer: C

You must make sure you have the newborn screen results before the mother leaves. While the mother may have given you contact information, the phone number can change between the time she leaves and you have the results. Moving on to the next patient can be done if the mother is waiting for the results. Make sure you have the screening results in the chart before the end of the day. You can never assume that someone else will follow up. If you see a patient after the hours that the newborn screening office is open, do get several ways to contact the mother. Remember, hypothyroidism is asymptomatic at this age, and it is very important to treat these infants (Wassner 2018).

6. Answer: C

The child should return for a repeat lipid panel at 6 months or as soon as possible after six months. Lifestyle changes take time to initiate and carry through. This is the earliest the lipid panel should be done.

7. Answer: D

In this patient, the result should be repeated with a chromatographic method. The use of diphenhydramine may be the cause of the positive result on the opiate screen. Positive results from an immunoassay test need to be repeated with gas chromatography/mass spectrometry or high-performance liquid chromatography (Standridge et al. 2010).

8. Answer: D

Shafii and Levine (2020) recommended screening for HIV and sexually transmitted diseases using NAAT technology to screen for *C. trachomatis* and *Neisseria gonorrhoeae*. The STD guidelines (Workowski et al. 2021) recommend NAAT testing. While this 17-year-old is not reporting current sexual activity, she has not been previously screened. It is important to remember that the AAP recommends a repeat lipid screen between 17 and 21 years.

Websites

https://www.brightfutures.org/wellchildcare/04_labs/resources/BFN_Anemia.pdf

https://www.ncbi.nlm.nih.gov/pmc/articles/PMC4348148/#R2

https://pediatrics.aappublications.org/content/pediatrics/137/6/e20160714A.full.pdf

https://www.nhlbi.nih.gov/files/docs/peds_guidelines_sum.pdf

https://choosingwisely.org

References

Agrawal S, Dhiman RK, Limdi JK. Evaluation of abnormal liver function tests. Postgrad Med J. 2016;92(1086):223–34.

Ahadi A, Partoazar A, Abedi-Khorasgani MH, Shetab-Boushehri SV. Comparison of liquid-liquid extraction-thin layer chromatography with solid-phase extraction-high-performance thin layer chromatography in detection of urinary morphine. J Biomed Res. 2011;25(5):362–7.

American Academy of Pediatrics. Summaries of infectious diseases. In: Kimberlin DW, Brady MT, Jackson MA, Long SS, editors. Red book: 2021 report of the committee on infectious diseases. American Academy of Pediatrics; 2021. Section 3.

Amsel R, Totten PA, Spiegel CA, Chen KC, Eschenbach D, Holmes KK. Nonspecific vaginitis. Diagnostic criteria and microbial and epidemiologic associations. Am J Med. 1983;74(1):14–22.

Auguste P, Tsertsvadze A, Court R, Pink J. A systematic review of economic models used to assess the cost-effectiveness of strategies for identifying latent tuberculosis in high-risk groups. Tuberculosis (Edinb). 2016;99:81–91.

Azziz R. Polycystic Ovary Syndrome. Obstet Gynecol. 2018;132(2):321–36.

Baird GS. The choosing wisely initiative and laboratory test stewardship. Diagnosi. 2019;6(1):15–23.

Barlow SE, Expert Committee. Expert committee recommendations regarding the prevention, assessment, and treatment of child and adolescent overweight and obesity: summary report. Pediatrics. 2007;120(Suppl 4):S164–92.

Bissell DM, Lai JC, Meister RK, Blanc PD. Role of delta-aminolevulinic acid in the symptoms of acute porphyria. Am J Med. 2015;128(3):313–7.

Blackett P, George M, Wilson DP. Integrating lipid screening with ideal cardiovascular health assessment in pediatric settings. J Clin Lipidol. 2018;12(6):1346–57.

Blackett PR, Wilson DP, McNeal CJ. Secondary hypertriglyceridemia in children and adolescents. J Clin Lipid. 2015;9:S29–40.

Carr PL, Rothberg MB, Friedman RH, Felsenstein D, Pliskin JS. "Shotgun" versus sequential testing. Cost-effectiveness of diagnostic strategies for vaginitis. J Gen Intern Med. 2005;20(9):793–9.

Carvalho I, Goletti D, Manga S, Silva DR, Manissero D, Migliori G. Managing latent tuberculosis infection and tuberculosis in children. Pulmonology. 2018;24(2):106–14.

Centers for Disease Control and Prevention [CDC]. Ten great public health achievements—United States, 2001–2010. Morb Mortal Wkly Rep MMWR. 2011;60(19):619–23.

CDC. Tuberculosis in children. 2020a. Retrieved on December 15, 2020, https://www.cdc.gov/tb/topic/populations/TBinChildren/#:~:text=TB%20skin%20testing%20is%20considered,than%205%205years%20of%20age.&text=All%20children%20with%20a%20positive,should%20undergo%20a%20medical%20evaluation

CDC. Legal status of expedited partner therapy (EPT). 2020b. Retrieved December 15, 2020, https://www.cdc.gov/std/ept/legal/default.htm

CDC. CDC promising features of PDMPs. (2020c). Retrieved November 20, 2020, https://www.cdc.gov/drugoverdose/pdmp/states.html

Centers for Disease Control and Prevention. Sexually transmitted infection treatment guidelines. Retrieved on November 30, 2020, 2015. https://www.cdc.gov/std/tg2015/hiv.htm#a1

Centers for Disease Control and Prevention. CDC national childhood blood lead surveillance data. 2020. Retrieved on November 10, 2020, https://www.cdc.gov/nceh/lead/data/national.htm

Christy AL, Manjrekar PA, Babu RP, Hegde A, Rukmini MS. Influence of iron deficiency anemia on hemoglobin A1c levels in diabetic individuals with controlled plasma glucose levels. Iran Biomed J. 2014;18(2):88–93.

Chung ST, Onuzuruike AU, Magge SN. Cardiometabolic risk in obese children. Ann N Y Acad Sci. 2018;1411(1):166–83.

Committee on Practice and Ambulatory Medicine; Bright Futures Periodicity Schedule Workgroup. 2019 recommendations for preventive pediatric health care. Pediatrics. 2019;143(3):e20183971.

Council on Environmental Health. Prevention of childhood lead toxicity. Pediatrics. 2016;138(1):e20161493.

Council on Environmental Health. Prevention of childhood Lead toxicity update. Pediatrics. 2017;140(2):e20171490. Retrieved December 14, 2020, from https://pediatrics.aappublications.org/content/140/2/e20171490

Daniels SR. Pediatric guidelines for dyslipidemia. J Clin Lipidol. 2015;9(5 Suppl):S5–S10.

Dignam T, Kaufmann RB, LeStourgeon L, Brown MJ. Control of lead sources in the United States, 1970-2017: public health progress and current challenges to eliminating Lead exposure. J Public Health Manag Pract. 2019;25(Suppl 1) Lead Poisoning Prevention(Suppl 1 LEAD POISONING PREVENTION):S13–22.

Dixon DB, Kornblum AP, Steffen LM, Zhou X, Steinberger J. Implementation of lipid screening guidelines in children by primary pediatric providers. J Pediatr. 2014;164(3):572–6.

Donders GG, Van Calsteren K, Bellen G, Reybrouck R, Van den Bosch T, Riphagen I, Van Lierde S. Predictive value for preterm birth of abnormal vaginal flora, bacterial vaginosis and aerobic vaginitis during the first trimester of pregnancy. BJOG. 2009;116(10):1315–24.

Dunn JJ, Starke JR, Revell PA. Laboratory diagnosis of mycobacterium tuberculosis infection and disease in children. J Clin Microbiol. 2016;54(6):1434–41.

Ettinger AS, Leonard ML, Mason J. CDC's Lead poisoning prevention program: a long-standing responsibility and commitment to protect children from lead exposure. J Public Health Manag Pract. 2019;25(Suppl 1) Lead Poisoning Prevention(Suppl 1 LEAD POISONING PREVENTION):S5–S12. https://doi.org/10.1097/PHH.0000000000000868.

Expert Panel on Integrated Guidelines for Cardiovascular Health and Risk Reduction in Children and Adolescents, National Heart, Lung, and Blood Institute Expert Panel on Integrated Guidelines for Cardiovascular Health and Risk Reduction in Children and Adolescents: summary report. Pediatrics. 2011;128. https://www.nhlbi.nih.gov/files/docs/peds_guidelines_sum.pdf.

Ferguson AE, Xanthakos SA, Siegel RM. Challenges in screening for pediatric nonalcoholic fatty liver disease. Clin Pediatr (Phila). 2018;57(5):558–62.

Gaydos CA, Klausner JD, Pai NP, Kelly H, Coltart C, Peeling RW. Rapid and point-of-care tests for the diagnosis of Trichomonas vaginalis in women and men. Sex Transm Infect. 2017;93(S4):S31–S35.

Gignac M, Wilens TE, Biederman J, Kwon A, Mick E, Swezey A. Assessing cannabis use in adolescents and young adults: what do urine screen and parental report tell you? J Child Adolesc Psychopharmacol. 2005;15(5):742–50.

Grundy SM, Stone NJ, Bailey AL, Beam C, Birtcher KK, Blumenthal RS, et al. 2018 AHA/ACC/AACVPR/AAPA/ABC/ACPM/ADA/AGS/APhA/ASPC/NLA/PCNA Guideline on the management of blood cholesterol: a report of the American College of Cardiology/American Heart Association Task Force on clinical practice guidelines. J Am Coll Cardiol. 2019;73(24):e285–350.

Harada K, Miura H. Free erythrocyte protoporphyrin (FEP) and zinc protoporphyrin (ZnP) as biological parameters for lead poisoning. Int Arch Occup Environ Health. 1984;53(4):365–77.

Hagan DM, Shaw JS, Duncan PM, editors. Bright futures: guidelines for health supervision of infants, children, and adolescents. 4th ed. Elk Grove Village, Il: Am Acad Pediatr; 2017.

Hains D, Spencer JD. Use of urinalysis and urine culture in screening. In: McInerny TK, Adam HM, Campbell DE, DeWitt TG, Foy JM, Kamat DM, editors. American Academy of Pediatrics Textbook of Pediatric Care. 2nd ed. Elk Grove Village, Il: American Academy of Pediatrics; 2017.

Hasan T, Au E, Chen S, Tong A, Wong G. Screening and prevention for latent tuberculosis in immunosuppressed patients at risk for tuberculosis: a systematic review of clinical practice guidelines. BMJ Open. 2018;8(9):e022445.

Hedegaard H, Miniño AM, Warner M. Drug overdose deaths in the United States, 1999–2018. NCHS data brief, no 356. Hyattsville, MD: National Center for Health Statistics; 2020.

Henry-Reid LM, O'Connor KG, Klein JD, Cooper E, Flynn P, Futterman DC. Current pediatrician practices in identifying high-risk behaviors of adolescents. Pediatrics. 2010;125:4. www.pediatrics.org/cgi/content/full/125/4/e741

Herbst de Cortina S, Bristown CC, Davey DJ, Klausner JD. A systematic review of point of care testing for chlamydia trachomatis, Neisseria gonorrhoeae, and trichomonas vaginalis. Infect Dis Obstet Gynecol. 2016; article ID 4386127

Herrington L, Susi A, Gorman G, Nylund CM, Hisle-Gorman E. Factors affecting pediatric dyslipidemia screening and treatment. Clin Pediatr (Phila). 2019;58(5):502–10.

Hsu KK, Rakhmanina NY. Adolescents and Young Adults: The Pediatrician's Role in HIV Testing and Pre- and Postexposure HIV Prophylaxis. Pediatrics. 2022;149(1):e2021055207.

Holmberg PJ, Temesgen Z, Banerjee R. Tuberculosis in children. Pediatr Rev. 2019;40(4):168–78.

Jacobsen A, Duffy E, Blumenthal R, Martin S. Clinical Review on Triglycerides. Retrieved January 25, 2022 from: https://www.acc.org/latest-in-cardiology/articles/2020/03/03/15/08/clinical-review-on-triglycerides.

Kapur BM, Aleksa K. What the lab can and cannot do: clinical interpretation of drug testing results. Crit Rev Clin Lab Sci. 2020;57(8):548–85.

Kavey RE. Combined dyslipidemia in childhood. J Clin Lipidol. 2015;9(5 Suppl):S41–56.

Kawa D, Paradis S, Yu JH, LeJeune M. Elevating the Standard of Care for Women's Health: The BD MAX™ Vaginal Panel and Management of Vaginal Infections. Retrieved February 6, 2021. https://moleculardiagnostics.bd.com/wp-content/uploads/2017/08/MAX-Vaginal-Panel-Whitepaper.pdf

Kit BK, Kuklina E, Carroll MD, Ostchega Y, Freedman DS, Ogden CT. Prevalence of and trends in dyslipidemia and blood pressure among US children and adolescents 1999–2012. JAMA Pediatr. 2015;169:272–9.

Koot BGP, Nobili V. Screening for non-alcoholic fatty liver disease in children: do guidelines provide enough guidance? Obes Rev. 2017;18(9):1050–60.

Kordes K. The "lead diet". Can dietary approaches prevent or treat lead exposure? J Pediatr. 2017;185:224–31.

Krasowski MD, McMillin GA, Melanson SEF, Dizon A, Magnani B, Snozek CLH. Interpretation and utility of drug of abuse screening immunoassays: insights from laboratory drug testing proficiency surveys. Arch Pathol Lab Med. 2020;144(2):177–84.

Krebs NF, Himes JH, Jacobson D, Nicklas TA, Guilday P, Styne D. Assessment of child and adolescent overweight and obesity. Pediatrics. 2007;120(Suppl 4):S193–228.

Kwo PY, Cohen SM, Lim JK. ACG clinical guideline: evaluation of abnormal liver chemistries. Am J Gastroenterol. 2017;112:18–35.

Lacy ME, Wellenius GA, Sumner AE, Correa A, Carnethon MR, Liem RI, et al. Association of sickle cell trait with hemoglobin A1c in African Americans. JAMA. 2017;317(5):507–15.

La-Llave-León O, Méndez-Hernández EM, Castellanos-Juárez FX, et al. Association between blood lead levels and Delta-Aminolevulinic acid dehydratase in pregnant women. Int J Environ Res Public Health. 2017;14(4):432.

Lamb GS, Starke JR. Tuberculosis in infants and children. Microbiol Spectr. 2017;5:2.

Langsted A, Nordestgaard BG. Nonfasting versus fasting lipid profile for cardiovascular risk prediction. Pathology. 2019;51(2):131–41.

Levy SB, Gunta J, Edemekong P. Screening for sexually transmitted diseases. Prim Care. 2019;46(1):157–73.

Magge SN, Goodman E, Armstrong SC, Committee on Nutrition, Section on Nutrition, Section on Endocrinology. The metabolic syndrome in children and adolescents: shifting the focus to cardiometabolic risk factor clustering. Pediatrics. 2017;140(2):e20171603.

Mahajan G. Role of urine drug testing in the current opioid epidemic. Anesth Analg. 2017;125(6):2094–104.

Mavedzenge SN, Pol BV, Cheng H, Montgomery ET, Blanchard K, de Bruyn G, Ramjee G, Av S. Epidemiological synergy of trichomonas vaginalis and HIV in Zimbabwean and south African women. Sex Transm Dis. 2010;37(7):460–6.

Mayans L. Lead poisoning in children. Am Fam Phys. 2019;100(1):26–30.

McDaniel MJ. Hepatic function testing. Phys Asst Clin. 2019;4(3):541–50.

Medicaid.gov. Lead screening. Retrieved on February 7, 2021., https://www.medicaid.gov/medicaid/benefits/early-and-periodic-screening-diagnostic-and-treatment/lead-screening/index.html

Michel JJ, Erinoff E, Tsou AY. More guidelines than states: variations in US lead screening and management guidance and impacts on shareable CDS development. BMC Public Health. 2020;20(1):127.

Mitra P, Sharma S, Purohit P, Sharma P. Clinical and molecular aspects of lead toxicity: an update. Crit Rev Clin Lab Sci. 2017;54(7-8):506–28.

Moeller KE, Kissack JC, Atayee RS, Lee KC. Clinical interpretation of urine drug tests: what clinicians need to know about urine drug screens. Mayo Clin Proc. 2017;92(5):774–96.

Moran A, Brunzell C, Cohen RC, Katz M, Marshall BC, Onady G, et al. Clinical care guidelines for cystic fibrosis-related diabetes: a position statement of the American Diabetes Association and a clinical practice guideline of the Cystic Fibrosis Foundation, endorsed by the Pediatric Endocrine Society. Diabetes Care. 2010;33(12):2697–708.

Murtagh M. The point-of-care diagnostic landscape for sexually transmitted infections (STIs). Retrieved on February 8, 2019. https://www.who.int/reproductivehealth/topics/rtis/Diagnostic-Landscape-for-STIs-2019.pdf?ua=1.

MyBINXhealth. https://mybinxhealth.com/point-of-care on August, 18, 2021.

National Center for Health Statistics, Illicit drug use, 2020. Retrieved on November 20, 2020, https://www.cdc.gov/nchs/fastats/drug-use-illicit.htm

Nelson ZJ, Stellpflug SJ, Engebretsen KM. What can a urine drug screening immunoassay really tell us? J Pharm Pract. 2016;29(5):516–26.

Nugent RP, Krohn MA, Hillier SL. Reliability of diagnosing bacterial vaginosis is improved by a standardized method of gram stain interpretation. J Clin Microbiol. 1991;29(2):297–301.

Obeng-Gyasi E. Sources of lead exposure in various countries. Rev Environ Health. 2019;34(1):25–34.

Ossiander EM. A systematic review of screening questionnaires for childhood lead poisoning. J Public Health Manag Pract. 2013;19(1):E21–9.

Parsons PJ, Reilly AA, Esernio-Jenssen D, Mofenson HC, Stanton NV, Matte TD. Evaluation of blood lead proficiency testing: comparison of open and blind paradigms. Clin Chem. 2001;47(2):322–30.

Powell AM, et al. Recurrent vulvovaginitis. Best Pract Res Clin Obstet Gynaecol. 2014;28(7):967–76.

Sacks FM, Jensen MK. From High-Density Lipoprotein Cholesterol to Measurements of Function: Prospects for the Development of Tests for High-Density Lipoprotein Functionality in Cardiovascular Disease. Arterioscler Thromb Vasc Biol. 2018;38(3):487–99.

Saitman A, Park HD, Fitzgerald RL. False-positive interferences of common urine drug screen immunoassays: a review. J Anal Toxicol. 2014;38(7):387–96.

Scartezini M, Ferreira CEDS, Izar MCO, Bertoluci M, Vencio S, Campana GA, et al. Positioning about the flexibility of fasting for lipid profiling. Arq Bras Cardiol. 2017;108(3):195–7.

Schmidt CW. After the screening: what happens next for children with elevated blood Lead? Environ Health Perspect. 2017;125(10):102001.

Schwebke JR, Gaydos CA, Nyirjesy P, Paradis S, Kodsi S, Cooper CK. Diagnostic performance of a molecular test versus clinician assessment of vaginitis. J Clin Microbiol. 2018;56(6):e00252–18.

Sekhar DL, Murray-Kolb LE, Wang L, Kunselman AR, Paul IM. Adolescent anemia screening during ambulatory pediatric visits in the United States. J Community Health. 2015;40(2):331–8.

Shafii T, Levine D. Office-based screening for sexually transmitted infections in adolescents. Pediatrics. 2020;145(Suppl 2):S219–24.

Shah A, Wilson DP. Primary hypertriglyceridemia in children and adolescents. J Clin Lipid. 2015;9:S20–8.

Shah J, Okubote T, Alkhouri N. Overview of updated practice guidelines for pediatric nonalcoholic fatty liver disease. Gastroenterol Hepatol (N Y). 2018;14(7):407–14.

Shakir AK, Suneja U, Short KR, Palle S. Overview of pediatric nonalcoholic fatty liver disease: a guide for general practitioners. J Okla State Med Assoc. 2018;111(8):806–11.

Shapiro MD, Fazio S. Apolipoprotein B-containing lipo-proteins and atherosclerotic cardiovascular disease. F1000Res. 2017;6:134.

Shew M, Fortenberry JD, Tu W, Juliar BE, Batteiger BE, Qadadri B, Brown DR. Association of condom use, sexual behaviors and sexually transmitted infections with the duration of genital human papillomavirus infection among adolescent women. Arch Pediatr Adolesc Med. 2006;160(2):151–6.

Sobel JD. Vulvovaginal candidosis. Lancet. 2007;369(9577):1961–71.

Standridge JB, Adams SM, Zotos AP. Urine drug screening: a valuable office procedure. Am Fam Physician. 2010;81(5):635–40.

Styne DM, Arslanian SA, Connor EL, Farooqi IS, Murad MH, Silverstein JH, Yanovski JA. Pediatric obesity-assessment, treatment, and prevention: an Endocrine Society Clinical Practice Guideline. J Clin Endocrinol Metab. 2017;102(3):709–57.

Sundjaja JH, Pandey S. Cholesterol Screening. [Updated 2020 Jul 10]. In: StatPearls [Internet]. Treasure Island (FL): StatPearls Publishing; 2020. https://www.ncbi. nlm.nih.gov/books/NBK560894/

United States [US] Department of Health and Human Services. American healthy homes survey. Lead and arsenic findings. Office of healthy homes and lead hazard controls. Washington, DC: US Depart of Health and Human Services; 2011. Retrieved December 14, 2020, https://www.hud.gov/sites/documents/AHHS_ REPORT.PDF

US Preventive Services Task Force. Screening for lipid disorders in children and adolescents US Preventive Services Task Force Recommendation Statement. 2016;316:525–33. file:///C:/Users/jimandrita/Down-loads/lipidscreening_children-recstatement.pdf

US Preventive Services Task Force. Screening for elevated blood Lead levels in children and pregnant women: US preventive services task force recommendation statement. JAMA. 2019a;321(15):1502–9.

US Preventive Services Task Force. Screening for HIV infection: US preventive services task force recommendation statement. JAMA. 2019b; https://doi. org/10.1001/JAMA.2019.6587.

US Preventive Services Task Force, Grossman DC, Bibbins-Domingo K, Curry SJ, Barry MJ, Davidson KW, Doubeni CA, Epling JW Jr, Kemper AR, Krist AH, Kurth AE, Landefeld CS, Mangione CM, Phipps MG, Silverstein M, Simon MA, Tseng CW. Screening for obesity in children and adolescents: US Preventive Services Task Force Recommendation Statement. JAMA. 2017;317(23):2417–26.

Valaiyapathi B, Sunil B, Ashraf AP. Approach to hypertriglyceridemia in the pediatric population. Pediatr Rev. 2017;38(9):424–34.

Viigimaa M, Heinsar S, Lovie D, Katsimardou A, Piperidou A, Duishvili D. New horizons in the pathogenesis, pathophysiology and treatment of familial hypercholesterolemia. Curr Pharm Des. 2018;24: 3599–604.

Vos MB, Abrams SH, Barlow SE, Caprio S, Daniels SR, Kohli R, Mouzaki M, Sathya P, Schwimmer JB, Sundaram SS, Xanthakos SA. NASPGHAN Clinical Practice Guideline for the diagnosis and treatment of nonalcoholic fatty liver disease in children: recommendations from the Expert Committee on NAFLD (ECON) and the North American Society of Pediatric Gastroenterology, Hepatology and Nutrition (NASPGHAN). J Pediatr Gastroenterol Nutr. 2017;64(2):319–34.

Wakai T, Simasek M, Nakagawa U, Saijo M, Fetters MD. Screenings during well-child visits in primary care: a quality improvement study. J Am Board Fam Med. 2018;31(4):558–69.

Waldius G, Jungner I, Holme I, Aastveit AH, Kolar W, Steiner E. High apolipoprotein B, low apolipoprotein A-I, and improvement in the prediction of fatal myocardial infarction (AMORIS study): a prospective study. Lancet. 2001;358: 2026–33.

Walzi G, McNerney R, duPleasis N, Bates M, McHugh TD, Chegou N, Zumla A. Tuberculosis: advances and challenges in development of new diagnostics and biomarkers. Lancet. 2018;18:e199–209.

Wang A, Rezania Z, Haugen K, Baertlein L, Yendell SJ. Screening for elevated blood leads; false-positive rates of tests on capillary samples, Minnesota, 2011–2017. JPHMP. 2019;25(1):S44–50.

Wassner AJ. Congenital hypothyroidism. Clin Perinatol. 2018;45(1):1–18.

Weitzman M. Blood Lead screening and the ongoing challenge of preventing children's exposure to Lead. JAMA Pediatr. 2019;173(6):517–9.

Wood SK, Sperling R. Pediatric screening: development, anemia, and lead. Prim Care. 2019;46(1): 69–84.

Workowski KA, Bachmann LH, Chan PA, Johnston CM, Muzny CA, Park I, Reno H, Zenilman JM, Bolan GA. Sexually transmitted infections treatment guidelines, 2021. MMWR Recomm Rep. 2021;70(4): 1–187.

Writing Committee, Cholesterol Clinical Practice Guidelines. AHA/ACC/AACVPR/AAPA/ABC/ACPM/ ADA/AGS/APhA/ASPC/NLA/PCNA guideline on the Management of Blood Cholesterol: executive summary. A report of the American College of Cardiology/American Heart Association Task Force on Clinical Practice Guidelines. Circulation. 2019. 2018;139:e1046–81.

Further Reading

American Academy of Pediatrics. Periodicity Table 2021. Retrieved January 25, 2022 from https://downloads. aap.org/AAP/PDF/periodicity_schedule.pdf.

Point-of-Care Testing in Primary Care

5

Laura Britton Stace

Learning Objectives After completing the chapter, the learner should be able to:

1. Discuss POCT and use this knowledge to assess the test result.
2. Comprehend the potential limitations of POCT and know the appropriate gold standard test for the medical condition where indicated.
3. Differentiate the CLIA-waived POCT versus tests that are not CLIA-waived.
4. Identify children with strep pharyngitis signs and symptoms and avoid strep testing children with a viral presentation.
5. Identify the need for COVID-19 testing and order and interpret COVID-19 testing for symptomatic or asymptomatic exposed children.
6. Correctly recommend the need for influenza testing and understand the limitations of rapid influenza diagnostic tests (RIDTs).
7. Discriminate when to use POCT HIV, glucose, HbA1c, and hCG tests in pediatric primary care and understand the pitfalls of each test.
8. Synthesize the limitation of POCT CRP and its potential future uses in the United States.

5.1 Introduction

Point-of-care testing (POCT) in pediatric primary care is essential for primary care clinicians to make a timely and accurate diagnosis. POCT is even more important in rural and underserved settings where access to hospital laboratories may be less available. During the current COVID-19 pandemic, the combined use of telemedicine and drive-through POCT can aid pediatric primary care clinicians in determining a diagnosis and treatment plan. If an in-person exam is necessary, rapid POCT may determine what personal protective equipment (PPE) and cleaning protocols are required. However, for POCT to be beneficial, it also has to be accurate. Although there are many different POCTs that can be employed in the pediatric primary care setting, this chapter will focus on the following rapid tests: Group A streptococcus (GAS), influenza A & B, SARS-CoV-2 (COVID-19), human immunodeficiency virus (HIV), C-reactive protein (CRP), human chorionic gonadotropin (hCG), and hemoglobin A1c (HbA1c). The emergence of the novel coronavirus, COVID-19, has highlighted the importance of rapid testing in the primary care setting and highlighted the importance of accurate testing.

L. B. Stace (✉)
Valley Health Page Memorial Hospital, Luray, VA, USA

James Madison University, Harrisonburg, VA, USA
e-mail: Lstace@valleyhealthlink.com

© The Author(s), under exclusive license to Springer Nature Switzerland AG 2022
R. M. John (ed.), *Pediatric Diagnostic Labs for Primary Care: An Evidence-based Approach*,
https://doi.org/10.1007/978-3-030-90642-9_5

5.2 Overview of Point-of-Care Testing

POCT should be cost-effective, have sufficient diagnostic accuracy and reliability, impact the patient outcome, have clinical benefit, be user-friendly and rapid (ideally less than 15 min), and have adequate operational technology geared to the environment of the application (Keitel et al. 2018). There are many benefits to pediatric primary care POCT. POCT avoids specimen transportation and processing (Patel and Suh-Lailam 2019). The shorter turnaround improves medical decision-making and can improve patient care, leading to improved patient satisfaction. The POCT techniques only need a small specimen volume, which is ideal for pediatric settings.

Most ambulatory pediatric primary care clinicians have access to at least one, if not several, POCT options to help diagnose and manage different common pediatric illnesses and conditions. Onsite testing greatly reduces the turnaround time for results and adds to a clinician management plan. An additional benefit of POCT is distinguishing between viral and bacterial infections, which is important for antibiotic stewardship and may decrease antibiotic prescribing. During the COVID-19 pandemic, quick identification of COVID-19 will lead to better patient outcomes and decrease the spread of COVID-19 in communities. The COVID outbreak has confirmed the importance of doing POCT tests in nontraditional testing sites. For a POCT to make a meaningful difference, the test must be easy to perform by a non-laboratorian, and it must be accurate enough not to need confirmation (Samuel 2020).

5.2.1 POCT and CLIA Regulations

POCT in pediatric primary care has benefits and risks associated with POCT use. Federal regulations such as the Clinical Laboratory Improvement Amendments of 1988 (CLIA '88) are minimum standards regarding validation and quality control for a laboratory test. There are different levels of CLIA approval for diagnostic lab tests. The levels include (1) high complexity, (2) moderate complexity, and (3) CLIA-waived. The latter is for use in primary care offices. POCT must be CLIA-waived, which means they have US Food and Drug Administration (FDA) clearance for home or office use. A CLIA-waived test should not require the specimen's processing before it is tested (Samuel 2020). It is important to note that a CLIA test of moderate or high complexity must be done in the clinical laboratory. Still, the turnaround time for these tests is quicker, so the patient could wait for the results and receive treatment during the visit. There are three kinds of POCT tests at present. Box 5.1 outlines them.

Box 5.1 Types of Point-of-Care Tests
- Direct detection of antigen.
  - Detects antigen-antibody complex typically by using lateral flow assay or a variant of this technology.
- Detection of antibody.
  - Finger-stick assays for detection of antibody to a specific pathogen.
- Direct detection of pathogen's RNA/DNA.
  - Current nucleic acid amplification tests (NAAT) directly detect the pathogen's genomic material in the patient's sample (i.e., PCR for COVID-19, influenza, or Group A strep).

CLIA-waived POCT must employ simple methodologies so that inaccurate results are negligible and pose no harm if the test is employed incorrectly (Nichols 2007). Trained, experienced laboratory clinicians run moderate- to high-complexity CLIA-approved POCT in hospital laboratories, but clinical staff performs CLIA-waived POCT. Therefore, training and ongoing testing of competency for clinical staff who perform POCT testing are needed. Competency should be initially checked with repeat testing at 6 and 12 months. The College of American Pathologists and Joint Commission regulations require observation of technique when doing POCT tests, along with written exams. The office must record quality control and test results, including demonstrating problem-solving skills (Nichols 2007).

POCT should be properly stored and should have timely quality control checks as determined. Some outpatient locations performing CLIA-waived POCT are part of their hospital systems laboratory certification, and other freestanding clinician offices could hold their certificate of waiver (CoW). Federal law states the laboratories and freestanding offices that hold CoW do not have to adhere to CLIA regulations dealing with quality management and proficiency testing (PT), leading to concerns about quality issues (Babady et al. 2019). CoW laboratories make up about 71% of all CLIA laboratories (Babady et al. 2019). Quality concerns in early 2000 lead to CMS initiating a program to visit 2% of CoW laboratories every year; however, the program was discontinued in 2016 (Scott 2021). Therefore, there are potential problems for CoW laboratories in clinician offices, and the importance of quality checks and proficiency training among staff is stressed to ensure the reliability of POCT in primary care pediatrics.

A physician, nurse practitioner, or physician assistant can be an acting laboratory director for CLIA waiver of an outpatient practice POCT. Nurse practitioners and nurses may be responsible for other clinical staff competency checks, POCT quality checks, documentation, and review. Clinicians should evaluate the positive and negative predictive values of the test. As a general reminder, the positive predictive value is if the test is positive, what is the probability that the patient does have the disease. If the test is negative, the negative predictive value is the probability that the patient does not have the disease. Test sensitivity is a test's ability to correctly identify those with the disease or the true positive rate. Test specificity is a test's ability to identify those without the disease or the true negative rate. When deciding which test to use and correctly interpret the significance of a test result, the clinician should be aware of the positive and negative predictive values and the disease prevalence in the community. Pre-test probability and post-test probability for a diagnosis add to sensitivity and specificity and help determine pre- and post-test likelihood ratios (Akobeng 2007a, b). A manufacturer may publish data regarding their test sensitivity and specificity or publish data regarding the positive and negative predictive values. If a positive or negative predictive value was listed instead of sensitivity and specificity, it is noted in the text. The pros and cons of the POCT are seen in Table 5.1.

5.2.2 Collection Sites for POCT

The collection sites for POCT vary according to the test. Certain tests are not approved for certain collection sites. This must be considered when using POCT. The clinician must be sure that the POCT can be used for that site. For example, in bullous impetigo, a POCT test for strep throat is not an approved use for the test.

Table 5.1 Pros and cons of POCT tests

Pros	Cons
1. Alleviate waiting and anxiety	6. Negative POCT antigen-based testing has limited value due to inadequate sensitivity (Samuel 2020)
2. Allows clinician to initiate therapy immediately	7. Patients do not understand POCT testing and need further explanation about the need for backup
3. Reduces need for follow-up with test results	8. Costs of POCT and lack of insurance reimbursement
4. Optimal use of healthcare resources	9. A negative result does not necessarily mean the child does not have the disease
5. Improves care of patients who do not come back for follow-up	10. Patients still want treatment despite negative tests
	11. The staff has difficulty integrating POCT into their workflow, citing time constraints
	12. The staff may be reluctant to do POCT

Adapted from Samuel (2020), Kozel and Burnham-Marusich (2017)

5.2.2.1 Throat Specimen Collection

The clinician should have the correct swab that correlates with the rapid POCT. The clinician should perform hand hygiene and don gloves before specimen collection. During the COVID-19 pandemic, particularly if there is a concern for COVID-19 coinfection, the clinician should consider additional protection such as mask (surgical loop mask or N95), face shield or eye protection, and gown following PPE requirements of the facility. Simultaneous throat culture collection should be done to avoid repeat throat swabbing, if the POCT needs a backup throat culture if negative. The rapid test should be nearby and ready to run following the specimen collection. The patient should be correctly identified with two patient identifiers and the swab labeled correctly with patient information.

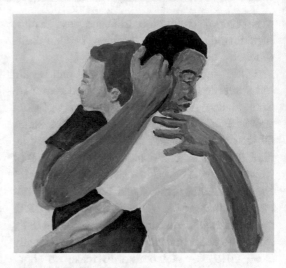

Fig. 5.1 Shoulder hug

The clinician should instruct the child to open wide and say "ahh" "ha, ha" or ask the child to "roar like a lion" while sticking out their tongue and opening their mouth. It may be preferable for some children to use a comfort holding technique such as a shoulder hug or supine hold. Figures 5.1 and 5.2 shows different positions that can be used to obtain the specimen securely. A supine hold is also best for face or head procedures in young children. The parents recline on the exam table with the child in their lap facing away in this hold. The parent secures the child's arms by giving a hug and wraps their legs over the child's ankles (Nationwide Children's 2016).

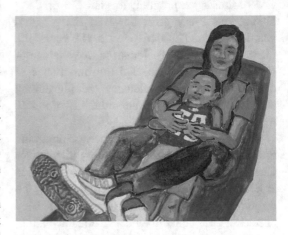

Fig. 5.2 Supine hold

A tongue depressor can be used to depress the tongue. The clinician should direct the swab's tip to the back of the child's pharynx and rub the swab across the posterior pharynx to include bilateral tonsils. Avoid touching the swab to the tongue, buccal surfaces, or lips. The rapid test should be run as soon as possible following the swab. Clinicians working with children may use distraction techniques such as music, iPhone/iPad video, and reward techniques such as stickers, popsicles, or treasure box toys. Staff should hand out treasure or toys; do not allow the patient

to take a toy directly from the treasure box due to infection control concerns.

5.2.2.2 Nasal Swab (NS), Mid-Turbinate Specimens (MTS), and Nasopharyngeal Specimen Collection

POCT influenza and COVID testing specimen sites include nasal swab (NS), nasopharyngeal swab (NPS), or nasopharyngeal wash or aspirate (Shulman 2016). The anterior nasal swab is a commonly used collection site for RIDT in pediatric primary care since it is an easier sample collection method in children. Anterior nasal swabs appear to be as accurate as nasal washes in the pediatric population for RIDTs. Therefore, this method is preferred to requiring less time, technical experience, and decreased risk for aerosol formation (Cruz et al. 2010).

Nasopharyngeal wash or aspirate is typically not CLIA-waived for the primary care office. A more recent study conducted in 2017, conducted with both children and adults, compared nasopharyngeal swab to mid-turbinate swab and nasal swab for accuracy and discomfort on laboratory run RT-PCR. They found that mid-turbinate specimens (MTS) were more comfortable than nasopharyngeal and nearly as sensitive (Frazee et al. 2018). This study did not compare the accuracy of RIDT using molecular methods and specimen collection location. Figure 5.3 shows the varying location of nasal collection sites.

Clinicians may choose to use distractors such as iPad video or music before, during, and after the test. Comfort positioning or holds depend on the patient's age, and an area test will be obtained. For infants, ask the parent to hold the infant in their arms; consider swaddling as illustrated in Fig. 5.4.

Alternatively, swaddle the infant, and place the infant on a safe, firm surface with the parent standing alongside. For toddlers, consider using the back-to-chest hold, in which the child sits on the

caregiver's lap, facing out, and instruct the parent to hug the child from behind to hold the arms down. Instruct the caregiver to cross their legs over the child's legs to prevent the child from kicking (Nationwide Children's 2016; Morgan et al. 2020).

For preschool-aged and young school-aged children, consider using the back-to-chest, shoulder hug, or supine hold (refer to Figs. 5.5 and 5.6 back-to-chest, Fig. 5.1 shoulder hug, and Fig. 5.2 supine hold). For other POCT requiring capillary blood, the clinician may consider chest-to-chest

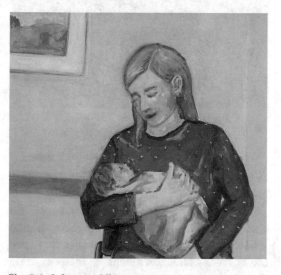

Fig. 5.4 Infant swaddle

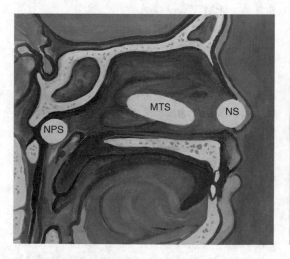

Fig. 5.3 Nasal specimen collection site

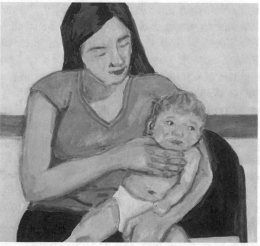

Fig. 5.5 Back-to-chest hold

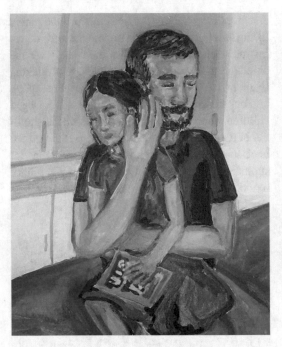

Fig. 5.6 Back-to-chest hold

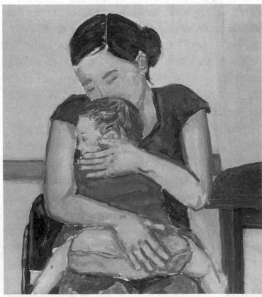

Fig. 5.7 Chest-to-chest hold

or back-to-chest hold (refer to Fig. 5.7 chest-to-chest and Figs. 5.5 and 5.6 back-to-chest).

Clinicians should follow the guidelines for specimen collection outlined in their specific influenza or COVID-19 kit. However, an example of nasal collection technique includes using the nasal swab that is provided in your POCT kit: gently insert the sterile swab in the nares until resistance is met at the level of the turbinates (less than once inch into the nostril, shorter distance in younger children), rotate the swab a few times against the nasal wall, and remove from a nostril. The sample should be tested as soon as possible. Some tests require the sample to be obtained from both nostrils, and others only require unilateral collection. Less often used is the nasopharyngeal collection technique for POCT influenza or COVID-19. In this collection technique, the child's head should be tilted back 70 degrees. The swab should be inserted into the nostril, keeping the swab near the nose's septum floor while gently pushing the swab into the posterior nasopharynx. Stop when resistance is met. The anatomical reference for depth is the length from the patient's nostril to the ear. The

patient's eye tearing is common. Leave the swab in place for several seconds, then rotate it, and remove it from the nares. The sample should be tested as soon as possible. Nasal wash and aspirate collection techniques will not be discussed, as they are atypical for collection methods for pediatric primary care POCT (Morgan et al. 2020).

5.3 POCT for Group A Streptococcal Infection

Sore throat is one of the most common pediatric complaints. Although viral infections are the main reason for pediatric sore throats, it is important to rule out Group A streptococcus (GAS) to avoid this infection's sequela. The most common cause of bacterial pharyngitis in pediatrics is Group A streptococcus (GAS). The gold standard for the diagnosis of streptococcal pharyngitis is throat culture. However, throat cultures are limited since they take 24–48 h to result. Therefore, in children with symptoms consistent with strep pharyngitis, rapid POCT strep testing is often employed in the primary care setting. Table 5.2 is

Table 5.2 Differential diagnosis of acute sore throat in pediatrics

Organisms	Clinical syndrome	Common additional symptoms or history
Infectious causes		
Bacterial		
Group A streptococcus	Pharyngitis, tonsillitis, scarlet fever	Tender lymphadenopathy, HA, fever, abdominal discomfort
Group C and G streptococcus	Pharyngitis, tonsillitis	Similar symptoms as GAS
Arcanobacterium haemolyticum	Scarlatiniform rash, pharyngitis	More common in adolescents, resembles EBV infection, pruritus, fever, cough
Neisseria gonorrhoeae	Tonsillopharyngitis	Cervical lymphadenopathy, fever, high-risk sexual behavior or history of sexual assault
Corynebacterium diphtheriae	Diphtheria pharyngitis with gray pseudomembrane	Fever, malaise, loss of appetite, swollen neck, trouble breathing
Mixed anaerobes	Vincent's angina, gingival ulcerations	Halitosis, bleeding gums, cervical adenopathy
Fusobacterium necrophorum	Lemierre's syndrome, peritonsillar abscess, tonsillitis	High fever, trouble breathing or swallowing, cervical lymphadenopathy, hemoptysis
Francisella tularensis	Tularemia (oropharyngeal), tonsillitis	Fever; mouth ulcers; cervical, parotid, or retropharyngeal lymphadenopathy; a recent history of eating or drinking possibly contaminated food or water (i.e., hunting, hiking, camping, handling sick or dead animals, eating undercooked game meat such as rabbits)
M. pneumoniae and *C. pneumoniae*	Pharyngitis	Cough, fever, bronchitis, pneumonia
Haemophilus influenzae type b (Hib)	Epiglottitis (drooling, open mouth)	Otitis media, high fever, cough, pneumonia, bacteremia, meningitis Under-vaccinated or unvaccinated child
Viral		
Adenovirus	Pharyngitis	Conjunctivitis, fever, upper respiratory symptoms such as rhinorrhea or cough, diarrhea, vomiting, nausea, and stomach pain
Herpes simplex virus 1 and 2	Gingivostomatitis, anterior mouth lesions	Fatigue, fever, decreased appetite, dehydration
Coxsackievirus	Herpangina, vesicles posterior pharynx	Fever; additional vesicles on hands, feet, and occasionally buttocks/upper thighs (hand, foot and mouth disease); irritability; decreased appetite; dehydration; most common summer and fall
Rhinovirus	Nasopharyngitis, upper respiratory infection or common cold (URI)	Common cold symptoms such as rhinorrhea, congestion, low-grade fever, sneezing, clear eye discharge
Coronavirus	Nasopharyngitis, URI	Common cold symptoms such as rhinorrhea, congestion, cough, low-grade fever, sneezing, clear eye discharge
Novel COVID-19 SARS-CoV-2	Nasopharyngitis, URI	Common cold symptoms as above; some children may have a more severe course to include high fever, headache, myalgias, diarrhea, vomiting, nausea, loss of taste and smell, bronchitis/pneumonia, tachypnea, respiratory distress; sequelae include multisystem inflammatory syndrome in children (MIS-C)
Influenza A & B	Nasopharyngitis, pharyngitis	Cough, fever, myalgias, fatigue, congestion, rhinorrhea, pneumonia, respiratory distress, bronchitis, bronchiolitis (infants)
Parainfluenza	Cold, croup, mild sore throat	Rhinorrhea, cough, fever, stridor, croupy/barking cough that is worse at night

(continued)

Table 5.2 (continued)

Organisms	Clinical syndrome	Common additional symptoms or history
Epstein-Barr virus (EBV)	Infectious mononucleosis, exudative pharyngitis, tonsillitis	Most common viral cause of mono. Symptoms include fever, myalgia, lymphadenopathy including posterior cervical, fatigue, malaise, headache, abdominal pain, hepatosplenomegaly, prolonged course, maculopapular exanthem following beta-lactam antibiotic use
Cytomegalovirus (CMV)	Infectious mononucleosis, mild pharyngitis	Has a similar presentation to EBV, usually not accompanied by posterior cervical lymphadenopathy, less likely to have exudative tonsillitis, less common in pediatrics, prominent liver involvement and elevated transaminases
Human immunodeficiency virus (HIV)	Primary acute HIV infection, sore throat, tonsillitis	Flu-like symptoms including fever, fatigue, lymphadenopathy, arthralgia and myalgia, diarrhea, rash
Non-infectious		
Allergic rhinitis	Mild sore or itchy throat due to environmental allergies	Congestion, rhinorrhea, sneezing, itchy eyes, cough, seasonal or exposure-related, no fever, on physical exam may include cobblestone appearance on the pharynx, pale boggy nasal mucosa, allergic shiners, conjunctivitis with clear watery discharge
Accidental ingestion of caustic chemical	Oropharyngeal burns, mouth pain	Drooling, swelling of the pharynx, breathing difficulty, abdominal pain, bloody vomiting, history of a known or suspected ingestion
Gastroesophageal reflux	Sore throat	Heartburn worsened after acid food ingestion, history of reflux following eating, abdominal pain

Adapted from John (2019), Shulman (2015)

a review of the common causes of pharyngitis in children and adolescents.

5.3.1 Clinical Indications for Strep Testing

Clinical indications for strep testing can include acute onset of symptoms, including sore throat, fever, tender or swollen lymph nodes, and absence of cough or significant nasal symptoms. GABHS is most common in children 5–13 years of age (Kalra et al. 2016). Children may have a headache and abdominal discomfort or nausea. GABHS is more common in late winter or early spring.

While the modified Centor Score is used in adults, it is not recommended in children. The Centor scoring system uses five criteria to judge whether the adult needs to test for strep. The criteria are a fever >38 degrees Celsius, absence of cough, swollen tender anterior cervical nodes, tonsillar swelling, and age between 3 and 14 years. The American Academy of Pediatrics (AAP) and the Infectious Diseases Society of America (IDSA) only recommend antibiotic treatment for confirmed strep pharyngitis based on rapid antigen detection test (RADT) or throat culture (Shapiro et al. 2017; McIsaac et al. 1998). In adults, the American Academy of Family Physicians (AAFP) supports testing or empiric treatment for a Centor score greater than or equal to 4 (Centor Score 2021; Kalra et al. 2016; McIsaac et al. 1998. Shephard et al. 2015) reported a sensitivity of 27.5% and a specificity of 79.7% when using clinical assessment (CAST) alone. CAST also had poor predictive accuracy, and as a result, 86.9% of patients would take unnecessary antibiotics if CAST alone was used to diagnose GAS (Shephard et al. 2015). The low sensitivity of clinical exam means that either POCT for strep or culture is advised in children aged 3 years or more (Shulman et al. 2012).

5.3.2   Differential Diagnosis of Throat Symptoms

The diagnosis of sore throat is a common presenting complaint. Table 5.2 reviews the differential diagnosis around complaints of throat pain.

5.3.3   Types of Rapid Antigen Detection Tests

The older RADT has a sensitivity of 85.6% and a specificity of 95.4% (Cohen et al. 2016). Based on the RADT's sensitivity, a clinician will detect 86 of 100 children with strep pharyngitis, and 14 of 100 children would be missed and not receive antibiotic treatment, thus explaining the reason for backup testing with a culture (Cohen et al. 2016).

5.3.3.1 Latex Agglutination (LA) Assays

Latex agglutination (LA) assays are no longer used in clinical practice: the sample is placed in the presence of latex beads coupled with GAS-specific antibodies; the result is determined by observing the agglutination of the beads if they are related to the specific antigen in the sample. The first-generation tests should not be used in clinical practice. Latex agglutination assay has a range of sensitivities from 53% to 92% and has a specificity below 90% (Miceika et al. 1985; White et al. 1986).

5.3.3.2 Second-Generation Tests

Enzyme immunoassay. Enzyme immunoassays (EIA) are second-generation tests where the throat swab is mixed with reagent and then placed in a well at the end of a nitrocellulose strip. As it migrates, it forms an antigen-antibody complex. They are the most widespread and most used RADTs in clinical practice. Clinicians should use caution with RADT. RADT should be used for children with acute symptoms consistent with GAS. The clinician should avoid testing in children with overtly viral presentations to avoid false-positive tests on children who are strep carriers (Shapiro et al. 2017). The RADT is performed by obtaining a throat swab, and then typically, the antigen test is run by nursing or other clinical support staff. The test typically takes about 5 min, and most employed in primary care settings are optical antigen tests.

With this test, the throat swab specimen particles are mixed with the reagent and then move along the test strip to a test line coated with a GAS carbohydrate cell wall antigen. If GAS is present in the sample, it will create a colored line, indicating a positive result. The absence of color along the test line indicates a negative result (Thompson and McMullen 2020). There also must be a control line; without this line, the test is invalid. Several new devices are CLIA-waived for rapid strep detection. The manufacturers report a sensitivity and specificity of >95%. There is a review that reported a lower sensitivity of 85% (Lean et al. 2014).

5.3.3.3 Third-Generation Tests

Optical immunoassay (OIA). Third-generation tests are less commonly used due to their cost, but the test's sensitivity and specificity are higher. OIA tests involved placing the sample mixed with a reagent on a silicon membrane. If there is an antigen-antibody complex present, there is a change in the optical properties of the inert membrane. A systematic review reported the summary estimates of several OIA tests as 86.2% sensitivity and 93.7% specificity (Cohen et al. 2016; Thompson and McMullen 2020). The authors concluded that optical immunoassays and enzyme immunoassays have similar accuracy (*P*-value equal to 0.23).

Combination POCT for strep. Some of these new devices, such as the BD Veritor System, combine lateral flow assay with an optical reader to increase accuracy. Another example of a device for rapid strep is the Sofia Strep A FIA (fluorescent immunoassay). While the devices may be slightly more accurate than the traditional simple lateral flow assay, they are also more expensive.

5.3.3.4 Molecular Methods

There are newer rapid POCTs that use polymerase chain reaction (PCR) tests or isothermal nucleic amplification. These tests have improved sensitivity compared to the RADT. As a result, some authors feel they do not require backup when negative (Pritt et al. 2016), but the guidelines do not clearly state this (Shulman et al. 2012). The tests include the Roche cobas strep A assay with a sensitivity of 95% and a specificity of 94.2%, Abbott strep A and strep A2 assay with a sensitivity of 98.5% and a specificity of 93.4%, and the Cepheid Xpert Xpress strep A assay with a sensitivity of 99.4% and a specificity of 94.1% (Thompson and McMullen 2020). However, there is considerable concern about Group A strep carriage when the PCR is weakly positive (Cohen et al. 2016). For molecular tests, the time for the result ranges from 2 to 18 min, depending on the test. Table 5.3 is a sample of rapid strep tests and their differences.

5.3.4 Barriers and Pitfalls to POCT Strep Tests

Clinicians working with children know that one pitfall of an accurate test is the actual test collection. Not all children are cooperative for specimen collection, i.e., throat swab. Therefore, improper technique or an uncooperative child could lead to poor specimen collection and false-negative results.

Occasionally, specimen collection may be so difficult that the result's accuracy is questionable. In these instances, clinicians should use their clinical judgment regarding test interpretation, diagnosis, and management. If another care team member obtained the test, they should inform the clinician that the specimen collection was difficult. Researchers found that the posterior pharynx swab was superior to the oral swab in children. The RADT sensitivity and specificity were 80.6% and 100%, respectively, from the posterior pharynx swab but dropping when an oral specimen was obtained to 19.4% sensitive and 100% specific (Fox et al. 2006).

Additional pitfalls of using POCT strep tests include swabbing children with symptoms consistent with a viral illness such as cough, oral vesicles, conjunctivitis, coryza, diarrhea, and viral exanthem. If a patient has overt viral features, a rapid test should not be done as 5–21% of asymptomatic children are GAS carriers, resulting in overuse of antimicrobial therapy (Shapiro et al. 2017). Due to COVID, children may present with a sore throat but have predominant viral features such as cough and rhinorrhea. If they are inappropriately tested for strep pharyngitis, there is a risk of inappropriately treating a child with a virus with antibiotics. There is an increase in the possible risk of missing COVID-19 diagnosis by not testing for COVID. Unfortunately, this

Table 5.3 Sample of rapid strep tests with times and statistics

Test	Type/platform	Time	Sensitivity	Specificity
QuickVue Dipstick Strep A Test	Lateral flow immunoassay/ none	5 min	92%	98%
QuickVue In-Line Strep A Test	Lateral flow immunoassay/none	5 min	92%	99%
BD Veritor System Strep	Lateral flow and optical reader/BD Veritor reader	5 min	96.6%	95.5%
Quidel Sofia Strep A FIA	Immunofluorescence-based lateral flow/Sofia	5 min	90.6%	96.1%
Alere i Strep A	Molecular/Alere i	8 min	95.9% (culture) 98.7%[a] (PCR)	94.6% (culture) 98.5%[a] (PCR)

Information for this table is based on the manufacturer package insert
[a]Alere i Strep A manufacturer insert lists sensitivity and specificity based on comparison to throat culture. However, an independent study compared Alere i Strep A to Strep A laboratory PCR and found higher sensitivity and specificity (Cohen et al. 2015)

clinical misstep has implications for the child's diagnosis and management and poses a public health risk.

Key Learning about POCT Strep Pharyngitis

- Backup cultures are needed in children who test negative for RADT but have symptoms of strep pharyngitis.
- Know the sensitivities and specificities of the POCT strep test you are using and whether a backup culture is required.
- Do not be pressured into the screening with a RADT for a child with overtly viral symptoms.
- Children that are carriers of strep may have a weakly positive PCR test for strep.

5.3.5 Real-Life Example

A six-year-old presented with a 12-h onset of sore throat, fever, abdominal pain, and anorexia. There was tonsillar erythema and exudate with palatal petechiae and anterior cervical nodes of 1.5 cm on the exam. The guardian was concerned about COVID-19, but the child was without upper respiratory symptoms, cough, nausea, vomiting, or loss of smell or taste. There was no known COVID-19 exposure in the past 2 weeks; however, there was a known strep pharyngitis exposure recently. A RADT was negative, and a throat culture was sent out. The child was given supportive treatment and told to stay home from school pending send out testing. Due to high community prevalence of COVID-19, testing for COVID 19 was obtained and was negative. Two days later, the backup culture was positive, and the child was started on amoxicillin.

5.4 Rapid Influenza Diagnostic Tests (RIDTs)

During the COVID-19 pandemic, RIDT is important. Influenza and COVID-19 may likely have similar features to include fever and cough in children. RIDT is particularly important for infants and toddlers aged 2 years and younger and older children with underlying risk factors for severe flu illness. In the absence of testing, clinicians relied on clinical diagnosis and prompt treatment with antiviral if indicated for high-risk groups. With the new onset of COVID-19, RIDT is particularly important.

5.4.1 Overview of Influenza and co-Pathogens

Influenza often presents in children as acute-onset illness with high fever, headache, rhinorrhea, sore throat, dry cough, and body aches. Some children may present with gastrointestinal symptoms in addition to the more commonly listed symptoms above. Very young children under 2 years are more likely to become very sick and require hospitalization. Although the most common cause of bronchiolitis is respiratory syncytial virus (RSV), influenza may also cause bronchiolitis in infants. POCT flu testing can reduce antibiotic use (Lee et al. 2019). Other than RSV and influenza, other differential diagnoses for viral respiratory infection include the common cold, parainfluenza, and mycoplasma pneumonia (John 2019). COVID-19 is an important differential to rule out, given the risk of transmission to high-risk populations.

5.4.2 Clinical Indications for Influenza Testing

Generally, COVID-19 has a more gradual onset than influenza, but COVID-19 testing may also be indicated for children presenting with flu-like symptoms. Children may commonly have viral coinfections with both flu and COVID; a positive flu test does not rule out COVID-19. Reassuringly, social distancing and masking measures seem to have decreased the spread of other common pediatric viral respiratory infections such as influenza and respiratory syncytial virus. Therefore, coinfection does not seem to be prevalent thus far in the 2020–2021 winter season in the United States.

5.4.3 Differential Diagnosis of Influenza

The child who presents with influenza-like symptoms may have another virus that can present with similar symptoms. However, it is important to recognize that fever and cough in a sick-appearing child can present as community-acquired pneumonia or a coinfection of pneumonia with influenza. While the winter season is the most common season to see influenza infection, the H1N1 epidemic was from April through September 2009. The CDC stresses the importance of considering COVID-19 and other differentials such as influenza and community-acquired pneumonia (CDC 2020a).

5.4.4 Types of Rapid Influenza Diagnostic Tests (RIDTs)

5.4.4.1 Influenza RIDT Using Influenza Antigen

As of August 2020, there were 16 CLIA-waived rapid influenza diagnostic tests (RIDTs) detect influenza antigen (CDC 2020a). RIDTs detect influenza viral antigen in 10–15 min, and the sensitivity ranges from 50% to 70% and the specificity greater than 90% (CDC 2020b). Sensitivity for Influenza B is lower than sensitivity for Influenza A. Some rapid tests can differentiate between A and B. Rapid tests cannot differentiate between seasonal influenza A and novel influenza A. Table 5.4 lists examples of CLIA-waived rapid antigen tests for influenza.

5.4.4.2 Influenza Rapid Molecular Tests

Recently there have been developments in FDA-cleared nucleic acid detection-based tests for influenza that are CLIA-waived. In 2015, the first CLIA-waived molecular test for influenza was approved (Babady et al. 2019). As of August 2020, there are 7 CLIA-waived rapid nucleic acid tests, shown in Table 5.5. The technology used is an isothermal amplification-based technology that eliminated the need for hardware with temperature cycling capabilities (Samuel 2020).

There are additional POCT molecular flu tests that include testing for other viruses to include

Table 5.4 Examples of CLIA-waived rapid antigen influenza diagnostic tests

Test	Platform	Specimen	Time	Sensitivity flu A/B	Specificity flu A/B
Abbott BinaxNOW Influenza A & B Card 2	DIGIVAL	Nasopharyngeal or nasal swab direct	15 min	A 84.3% B 89.5%	A 94.7% B 99.4%
Becton Dickinson Veritor Flu A + B	BD Veritor reader or BD Veritor plus Analyzer	Nasopharyngeal or nasal swab direct	11 min	PPA A 81.3% B 77.8%	NPA A 95.6% B 100%
Quidel Corp Sofia Influenza A + B FIA	Sofia FIA Analyzer and Sofia 2 FIA Analyzer	Nasopharyngeal or nasal swab direct (nasopharyngeal wash and aspirate samples are of moderate complexity, not for office use)	Sofia: 15 min Sofia 2: 3–15 min	Nasal A 90% B 89%	Nasal A 95% B 96%
Quidel Corp QuickVue Influenza A + B	None	Nasal or nasopharyngeal swab direct	10 min or less	PPA A 81.5% B 80.9%	NPA A 97.8% B 99.1%
Sekisui OSOM Ultra Plus Flu A&B Test	None	Nasal or nasopharyngeal swab direct	10 min	A 90.3% B 88%	A 96.7% B 99.2%

Table partially adopted from CDC (2020a). Rapid influenza diagnostic tests (RIDTs) Table 2: Available FDA-cleared rapid influenza diagnostic tests (antigen detection only) (Frazee et al. 2018)

Not an exhaustive list of all tests

[a]Sensitivity/specificity or positive predictive agreement (PPA)/negative predictive agreement (NPA) is based on manufacturer package inserts and nasal swab data when available

Table 5.5 CLIA-waived nucleic acid influenza detection tests

Test	Platform	Sample	Time	Sensitivity A/B	Specificity A/B
Abbott ID NOW Influenza A & B 2	ID NOW Platform	NPS, NS direct or NPS and NS in VTM	<15 min	A 96.3% B 100%	A 97.4% B 97.1%
Xpert Xpress Flu	GeneXpert Xpress	NPS, NS in VTM	30 min	PPA A 98.9% B 98.4%	NPA A 97.6% B 99.3%
Mesa Biotech Accula Flu A/Flu B	Accula Dock	NS direct	<30 min	A 97% B 94%	A 94% B 99%
Roche cobas Influenza A/B Assay	cobas Liat Analyzer	NPS in VTM	<30 min (approximately 22 min) Samuel 2020	A 100% B 100%	A 96.8% B 94.1%
Sekisui Silaris Influenza A&B	Silaris Dock	NPS direct	<30 min	A 97% B 94%	A 94% B 99%

Adapted from CDC Table 3: FDA-cleared nucleic acid detection-based tests for influenza (CDC 2020a) Samuel 2020, and Babady et al. 2019. Sensitivity/specificity or positive predictive agreement (PPA)/negative predictive agreement (NPA) is based on manufacturer package inserts and based on nasal swab data if applicable

RSV such as the Roche cobas Influenza A/B and RSV Assay. There is also dual viral POCT for influenza and COVID-19. These include the Quidel Sofia 2 Flu + SARS Antigen FIA. A rapid POC CR platform, cobas Liat, Roche Diagnostics, was approved to detect COVID-19 and influenza A and B in November 2020 (Tran et al. 2020). This test is a PCR and more accurate than antigen testing. PCR is still considered the gold standard for both influenza and COVID-19. This test is CLIA-waived. The point-of-care cobas SARS-CoV-2 & Influenza A/B Assay uses a nasopharyngeal sample and takes 20 min to run. For SARS-CoV-2 detection, the POCT cobas Liat is highly accurate; in one study, PPA was 100%, and NPA was 97.4% (Hansen et al. 2021). Given this high sensitivity and specificity of rapid PCR testing, follow-up laboratory testing is not required.

Guidelines for interpretation of the test. Influenza POCTs are specific >98%, but rapid antigen detection tests (RADTs) have low sensitivity compared with nucleic acid amplification tests (53–54% versus 92–95%) (Lee et al. 2019). Therefore, a negative result should not determine treatment. If the clinician has a strong clinical suspicion for influenza in a high-risk patient, it is appropriate to initiate antiviral treatment. Interestingly manufacturer package inserts for

RIDT indicate a higher sensitivity than the reviewed published studies. Influenza POCT changed clinician management in ambulatory care, reducing the use of routine blood tests (20%), reducing blood cultures (18%), and reducing chest radiography (19%) (Lee et al. 2019). These results suggest POCTs have a role in reducing diagnostic uncertainty for children with ILI [influenza-like illness], but the impact on patient outcomes remains unclear. Antibiotic prescribing was not affected by testing, but prescriptions for antiviral medication more than doubled. POCTs did not affect the time in the emergency department or the number of patients returning for care (Lee et al. 2019). In children under 2 years, the sensitivity for influenza POCT is the highest likely due to higher viral load in young children (Cruz et al. 2010).

5.4.5 Barriers and Pitfalls of Influenza RIDT Testing

The pitfalls of influenza RIDT include a greater false-negative rate when the influenza burden is high in the community. False negatives can also occur if an adequate sample is not obtained or if testing occurs too late in the illness.

Conversely, false positives are not very common, but they can occur during low influenza activity, such as in the summer months when the influenza burden is low. If the clinician suspects a false-negative result, it can be confirmed with the more accurate laboratory molecular assay. Testing is most accurate within 3–4 days of onset of illness (CDC 2020c).

RIDTs previously were antigen tests with molecular tests exclusively done in laboratories. The low sensitivity of the antigen tests causes cases to be missed. The new CLIA-waived rapid molecular influenza tests are more sensitive, but there are concerns about environmental or amplicon contamination from broken pouches or cartridges (Babady et al. 2019). RIDT is less expensive and may be more sensitive early in illness due to the high viral load (Cruz et al. 2010).

5.4.6 Real-Life Example

In January, a six-year-old presented to the primary care office 6 h after being in the ED. The child's history included a 2-day history of fever, persistent dry cough, anorexia, running nose, headache, sore throat, and body aches. The child who had no risk factors for severe influenza was diagnosed with a viral illness after an RIDT was negative. The guardian brought him to the office since she felt he "was sicker than he usually gets." The physical exam was remarkable for decreased breath sounds on the right base, tachypnea between 56 and 62, mild intercostal retractions, and suprasternal retractions. The child also had a 2 cm spleen tip palpable. The RIDT in the office was positive, but the child was sicker than expected, and a bacteria coinfection was suspected. The child was admitted via the ED to the PICU after a chest X-ray confirmed a lung abscess, later identified as *Staphylococcus aureus*, one of the three common coinfections *with influenza (*Morris et al. 2017*). In this case, the clinical presentation was more important than whether the child had a positive or negative RIDT.*

Key Learning about Influenza
- Children at high risk for more severe influenza include the following:
  - Ages under 5 years with particular caution in children less than 2 years or a history of prematurity.
  - Children with chronic illnesses including asthma, heart disease, kidney disease, liver disease, diabetes, obesity, compromised immune systems.
  - Unvaccinated children.
- Influenza is characterized by an acute onset of illness in a sick child with a high fever, headache, cough, sore throat, and dry cough symptoms.
- Most POCT in ambulatory care is rapid antigen tests, which have lower sensitivity than molecular influenza tests.
- If the clinician has strong clinical suspicion, treat with antiviral if appropriate, regardless of test results. Testing is most accurate within 3–4 days of onset of illness.

5.5 POCT for SARS-CoV-2 or COVID-19

Initially, children were thought to be less likely to acquire and transmit COVID-19 and were less likely to become severely ill with COVID-19. Therefore, when test availability was scarce, tests were initially reserved for healthcare workers and hospitalized patients, predominately adults. However, as our knowledge of COVID-19 has expanded, clinicians recognize that most children do not become severely ill with COVID-19 rather have mild COVID-19 infections. Adolescents may be just as likely as adults to spread COVID-19 (Park et al. 2020). Several notable outbreaks occurred as children across the United States returned from summer camps, schools, and universities (Szablewski et al. 2020, Wilson et al. 2020).

5.5.1 Clinical Indications for COVID-19 Testing

Clinical symptoms that warrant COVID-19 testing can include fever, chills, cough, shortness of breath or difficulty breathing, sore throat, fatigue, muscle or body aches, headache, the new loss of taste or smell, congestion or runny nose, nausea or vomiting, abdominal pain, and diarrhea (Patel 2020). Unlike adults, children may not be able to confirm or deny loss of taste or smell. The child or parent may describe that their child has a decrease in appetite or that their favorite food or drink "tastes different." Neurological symptoms and signs include anosmia, and less commonly, Guillain-Barré syndrome, acute flaccid myelitis, and febrile seizures (Christy 2020).

5.5.2 Differential Diagnosis of COVID-19

The differential diagnosis for COVID-19 includes influenza; respiratory syncytial virus (RSV); upper respiratory infection (URI) from different viruses including rhinovirus and regular coronaviruses; croup due to a variety of different viruses, including adenovirus; strep pharyngitis; acute bacterial sinusitis; acute otitis media; mycoplasma pneumonia; bacterial pneumonia; pertussis; viral or bacterial gastroenteritis; foreign body ingestion/aspiration pneumonia; and allergic rhinitis/environmental allergies. Whether in person or via telehealth, a complete history and exam may help narrow the differential diagnosis. COVID-19 is covered in the pediatric infectious disease Chap. 6, Section 6.4.10.

While the disease is generally milder in children, it can present a similar presentation to adults, especially in children with underlying pulmonary diseases (Christy 2020). The new delta variant seems to be making children sicker and has caused an increase in hospitalizations (Fiore 2021). Children can present with MIS-C in a clinical presentation that is similar to Kawasaki disease.

5.5.3 Types of POCT COVID-19 Tests

POCT COVID-19 testing and evidence are rapidly evolving. A low threshold for testing a child with COVID-19 like symptoms has public health implications and household contact implications. Current CDC guidelines recommend that people exposed to a contact with COVID-19 should quarantine regardless of initial COVID-19 testing results unless they are up-to-date on COVID-19 vaccinations or have a confirmed history of COVID-19 in the past 90 days. Current CDC guidelines offer new guidelines that allow the patient to quarantine for 5 days and if asymptomatic, may come off of quarantine on days 6-10 as long as they wear a well fitting mask. It is recommended to obtain testing at least 5 days after the exposure and to continue to monitor for symptoms. If symptoms develop, immediate isolation is required. https://www.cdc.gov/coronavirus/2019-ncov/your-health/quarantine-isolation.html. According to the AAP, asymptomatic exposures should be tested at least 4 days after exposure (2020). The CDC states that a positive antigen test is likely reliable. Still, a negative antigen test should be confirmed with PCR if the pre-test probability is high or the patient has symptoms or a known exposure (CDC 2020e). For asymptomatic exposures, only PCR testing should be used. The FDA has approved Emergency Use Authorization (EUA) for many tests. Tables 5.6 and 5.7 illustrate several tests along with the manufacturer's sensitivity, specificity, time to run the test, and whether it is CLIA-waived. As this chapter goes to print, many new COVID-19 antigen home and self-test kits are now available over the counter. The focus of this chapter is POCT in the office setting and therefore home-testing will not be addressed in depth. However, generally speaking, a positive home COVID antigen test is very likely a true positive and isolation should begin. A negative home Covid test should be repeated in 24–36 hours, or a confirmation COVID-19 PCR should be obtained, or consultation with a healthcare provider regarding clinical scenario and interpretation of test results should occur prior from ending isolation.

5.5.3.1 COVID Antibody Tests

The antibody testing is unlikely to help screen or diagnose symptomatic infections early in infection. Still, it may help determine the immune status of asymptomatic patients, epidemiology, or diagnosing patients presenting with possible COVID-19 sequela (Hanson et al. 2020). When used in COVID-19 outbreaks, rapid antibody tests can be a reliable screening tool (Mathur and Mathur 2020). Antibody tests may also be helpful in patients presenting late in illness with negative molecular tests. Rapid antibody tests can use rapid lateral flow immunoassay, with an example being COVID-19 IgG/IgM rapid test cassette (whole blood/serum/plasma). Still, this test is run in a clinical laboratory but not in the office. Rapid lateral flow immunoassays identify IgM and IgG antibodies to help identify recent COVID-19 infections. Seroconversion occurs after 7 days of symptomatic infection in 50% and 14 days in all patients (Tang et al. 2020). Recent treatment guidelines recommended against the use of serologic testing for the sole basis of a diagnosis of SARS-CoV-2 (National Institutes of Health (NIH) 2021). The guidelines recommend that a molecular or antigen test be used with the knowledge that a repeat test should be considered in patients with a high likelihood of COVID-19 based on exposure and clinical presentation (NIH 2021).

5.5.3.2 POCT COVID-19 Antigen Tests

Currently, antigen testing for COVID-19 identifies target proteins. The rapid COVID-19 antigen tests are the most commonly used for POCT that are newly available under emergency use authorization. Primary care clinicians need to be aware of the sensitivity and specificity and negative and positive predictive values of the test they use in their office. A reflex molecular diagnostic test should be collected if a child presents clinically with signs of SARS-CoV-2 infection but has a negative antigen test (NIH 2021).

Examples of POCT COVID-19 antigen tests. Following a super spreader event, the Abbott BinaxNOW was distributed to nursing homes, schools, and the White House. The Abbott BinaxNOW is the only self-contained POCT test that does not require additional machinery currently on the market as of November 2020. It is inexpensive, takes 15 min to run, and is highly sensitive and specific, as outlined in the table. It can also be paired with a mobile app called NAVICA, enabling the results to be scanned like a boarding pass when entering an event (Abbott 2021).

The Quidel Sofia and Sofia 2 SARS Antigen Fluorescent Immunoassay use immunofluorescence-based lateral flow to detect nucleocapsid protein from SARS-CoV-2. The kit comes with a self-contained test cassette, reagent tubes, reagent solution, pipettes, and nasal swab, although alternatively, the purchaser can request a nasopharyngeal swab. The specimen is run quickly on a nearby Sofia machine, and it takes 15 min for the machine to give results. The Sofia machine can also run additional POCT such as influenza and RSV. The positive predictive value for SARS-CoV-2 is 96.7%, and a negative predictive value is 100% per manufacturer.

A new combo Sofia test Quidel Sofia 2 Flu + SARS Antigen FIA includes testing for both COVID-19 and influenza with one swab. Table 5.6 is a review of some of the currently approved rapid antigen tests.

5.5.3.3 SARS-CoV-2 PCR

The gold standard for diagnosing acute COVID-19 infection is still the SARS-CoV-2 PCR run from a nasopharyngeal sample. However, initially, the PCR tests were laboratory-based only. Even more recently, rapid molecular PCR tests have been waived for use in a primary care setting.

Most rapid COVID-19 tests can be run with a nasal swab, which young children better tolerate than NP swabs. Self-swabbing for older school-aged children and adolescents may be feasible for nasal swabs but should be directly observed by the clinician to ensure an adequate specimen is obtained (AAP 2020). For direct respiratory testing in the era of COVID-19, the clinician wears PPE to include facemask (N95 preferred), face shield or goggles, gown, and gloves. Appropriate precautions should be used to limit aerosolization for in-office swabbing, and the room must be thoroughly cleaned between patients (Pondaven-Letourmy et al. 2020).

Table 5.6 Examples of COVID-19 rapid antigen tests

Test	PPA/NNA	Time to run the test
Abbott BinaxNOW COVID-19 Ag Card	84.6%/98.5%	15 min (no instrumentation required)
Quidel Sofia SARS Antigen FIA	96.7%/100%	15 min
Quidel Sofia 2 Flu + SARS Antigen FIA	SARS 95.2%/ 100% Flu A 90%/ 95% Flu B 89%/ 96%	15 min
BD Veritor System for Rapid Detection of SARS-CoV-2	84%/100%	15 min
Access Bio CareStart COVID-19 Antigen Test	87.2%%/100%	10 min
LumiraDx SARS-CoV-2 Ag Test	97.6%/96.6%	12 min

Table adapted from Fiore 2020, FDA 2021, Tang et al. 2020, manufacturer's inserts and is based on nasal swab when applicable. Since the creation of this table, many additional COVID-19 Home Tests have become available

Table 5.7 Examples of molecular COVID-19 tests

Test	PPA/PNA	Time to run the test (does not include transport time)	CLIA-waived/ POCT
Abbott ID NOW	100%/100%	13 min	Yes
Roche cobas SARS-CoV-2	100%/100%	3.5 h	No
Roche cobas SARS-CoV-2 Nucleic Acid Test for use on cobas Liat System	COVID 100%/100% Flu A 98.4/96.5% Flu B 97.9%/ 99.4%	20 min	Yes
Panther Fusion SARS-CoV-2 Assay	100%/100%	3 h	No
Cepheid Xpert Xpress SARS-CoV-2 Test	97.8%/95.6%	45 min	Yes
Cepheid Xpert Xpress SARS-Cov-2/Flu/RSV	COVID 97.9%/100% Flu A 100%/100% Flu B 100%/99% RSV 100%/100%	36 min	Yes
Thermo Fisher TaqPath	100%/100%	4 h	No
Labcorp COVID-19 RT-PCR Test	100%/100%	24 h	No

Information for table obtained from FDA (2021). Additional sensitivity and specificity as well as positive and negative predictive values from the manufacturer package insert

Example of molecular tests. Molecular testing is more sensitive for SARS-CoV-2 than rapid antigen testing. Current guidelines, as discussed previously, recommend reflex PCR if rapid antigen testing is negative. However, there has been recent development of CLIA-waived rapid SAR-CoV-2 tests to alleviate the need for confirmation testing. Table 5.7 outlines examples of some of the molecular COVID-19 tests along with information about timing to result and whether the test is CLIA-waived.

5.5.4   Barriers and Pitfalls of POCT COVID-19 Tests

Despite rapid innovation in COVID-19 testing, there are still many pitfalls and barriers to testing.

The clinician should be prepared to explain and answer all of these questions and concerns before ordering and obtaining testing. It may help remind parents that we use a similar rapid test with secondary confirmation testing for strep pharyngitis. If a parent seems likely to decline two tests, it may be preferable to offer only the more accurate PCR. Some families disbelieve or downplay the danger of COVID-19, whereas others may mistrust the test itself. Parental refusal of the COVID-19 test does occur for various reasons, including concerns about any pain or discomfort associated with the test or that the child will be "exposed" to the virus during the testing. Other barriers include lack of transportation to the testing site, lack of clinicians comfortable with obtaining samples from young infants, and parental concern regarding the cost. The child may be uncooperative for the test, and the family may not want to subject their child to any restraints.

The rapid nasal antigen test is attractive to many parents due to nasal specimen collection with less associated discomfort. Due to the lower sensitivity of the rapid antigen tests, it is recommended to repeat testing with COVID-19 PCR tests if the rapid antigen is negative. Many parents have difficulty understanding the need for two tests and seem satisfied with an initial negative rapid test and, as a result, refuse to follow up PCR.

Pitfalls include a possible lower sensitivity and specificity of the antigen testing. There is considerable variation in the results depending on the test used. The molecular COVID-19 can pick up residual viral nucleic acid fragments that may be present due to a previous infection. If a child has had confirmed COVID-19 in the past 90 days and symptoms resolved completely, and then new symptoms present, the clinician should attempt to find an alternative diagnosis and use caution with repeat COVID-19 PCR as it may be difficult to interpret the results. caution with repeat COVID-19 PCR as it may be difficult to interpret results.

The emergency use approval for a particular SARS-CoV-2 diagnostic test varies. Some tests have been authorized for screening, and other tests can only be used if the clinician suspects COVID-19 infection, whether the child is asymptomatic, pre-symptomatic, or symptomatic (Food and Drug Administration (FDA) 2021). As a rule of thumb, antigen tests should only be used in symptomatic patients suspected of COVID-19. Typically molecular tests can be used for asymptomatic and pre-symptomatic patients exposed to COVID-19 and symptomatic patients suspected to have COVID-19. Table 5.8 gives specific examples of when to use.

5.5.5 Respiratory Multiplex Tests

BioFire Respiratory Panel 2.1 EZ is a multiplex molecular test available for POCT, CLIA-waived testing for 19 different respiratory viruses. The

Table 5.8 COVID-19 "who, what, when" test guidance

Who to test	When to test	What test to order
Symptomatic child with or without known exposure with any of the following symptoms: Fever, chills, cough, congestion, runny nose, loss of taste or smell, shortness of breath or difficulty breathing, body aches, fatigue, headache, sore throat, nausea, vomiting, or diarrhea	Suspicion is high Immediate testing	SARS-CoV-2 NAAT 1. Rapid COVID Antigen Test if available, with reflex to SARS-CoV-2 NAAT (PCR) if rapid test negative 2. Alternatively only obtain a SARS-CoV-2 NAAT (PCR)
Asymptomatic exposed child: In close contact with a confirmed or suspected COVID-19 contact. Close contact is defined as less than 6 feet for 15 min cumulatively. Clinicians may consider testing for exposures of shorter duration or greater distance on a case-by-case basis	Per AAP, delayed testing at least 4 days after exposure. Further testing after the initial negative test should be guided by symptomatology. A negative test after exposure does not negate the need to quarantine Newer CDC guidelines suggest a negative test on day 5 may assist for early release from quarantine	SARS-CoV-2 NAAT preferred for asymptomatic exposed patient
Indirectly exposed child: Indirect exposure to an exposed contact and not directly with an infected person, child asymptomatic	No test is needed unless the child becomes symptomatic, exposed contact becomes symptomatic/tests positive, avoidance of exposed contact while they quarantine	No test needed
Child needing test to return to school after confirmed infection	No test is needed; the child may return to school based on CDC guidelines regarding quarantine	No test is needed; the clinician may write a letter

Table 5.8 (continued)

Who to test	When to test	What test to order
The parent thinks the child may have had COVID-19 infection previously but is now recovered	Minimum of 2 weeks since the infection has passed, IDSA guidelines recommend antibody test 3–4 weeks after symptom onset	Either SARS-CoV-2 IgG or total antibody (IgM, IgG)
Pediatric patient presenting to ambulatory setting or ED with signs of MIS-C	Immediate testing and admission	Both nucleic acid amplification test (SARS-CoV-2 NAAT) and antibody testing to provide evidence on current or past COVID-19 infection
A child with confirmed COVID-19 infection who needs a return to sports clearance	N/A	No COVID-19 test needed; children with mild to moderate COVID-19 should contact PCP for return to sports guidance once the criteria to come off of quarantine are met; if cardiac screening questions or abnormal exam, additional evaluation to include EKG and referral to a cardiologist may be needed. Children with severe COVID-19 should be restricted from exercise for 3–6 months postinfection and cleared by cardiology
Infant perinatally exposed to confirmed or suspected COVID-19 mother	At 24 h of age, and again at 48 h (in hospital), if negative and discharged home and becomes symptomatic, the clinician should retest. Otherwise, infant and guardian stay on quarantine with continued use of hand hygiene and masking. If initially positive at 24 h, consider follow-up testing at 48–72-h intervals to see if the infant has cleared the virus from mucosal sites	PCR, single swab nasopharynx or single swab throat followed by nasopharynx or two separate swabs from both sites submitted as 1 test; some centers use anterior nasal swabs

Adapted from AAP (2020), Hanson et al. (2020), Jenco (2021), CDC (2020k). https://www.cdc.gov/coronavirus/2019-ncov/your-health/quarantine-isolation.html

BioFire Respiratory Panel 2.1 EZ tests for SARS-CoV-2; adenovirus; coronavirus 229E; coronavirus HKU1; coronavirus NL63; coronavirus OC43; human metapneumovirus; human rhinovirus/enterovirus; influenza A, including subtypes H1, H3, and H1–2009; influenza B; parainfluenza virus; respiratory syncytial virus; *Bordetella parapertussis*; *Bordetella pertussis*; *Chlamydia pneumoniae*; and *Mycoplasma pneumoniae* (BioFire 2021). Four types of parainfluenza virus (PIV1, PIV2, PIV3, and PIV4) can be detected and reported as parainfluenza virus detected. The BioFire RP2.1 EZ is authorized as a POCT and has a CLIA Certificate of Waiver, Certificate of Compliance, or Certificate of Accreditation. Diagnostic stewardship points to the need for clinicians to use these tests for a specific reason.

Routine care of an otherwise healthy child should not merit the use of these tests (Baird 2019).

5.5.6 Real-Life Example

An eight-year-old presented to the office two and one-half weeks after a positive COVID rapid PCR test. The child's symptoms included fever, abdominal pain, diarrhea, conjunctivitis, polymorphous rash, and shortness of breath. By the mother's history, the child had an uneventful recovery from COVID but developed his present symptoms 24 h ago. Based on the mother's history and how ill the child appeared, multisystem inflammatory syndrome in children (MIS-C) was considered along with Kawasaki disease. The child was admitted to the hospital. Laboratory testing was consistent with MIS-C since the child had elevated serum ferritin, CRP, D-dimer, alanine aminotransferase, aspartate aminotransferase, creatine kinase, blood urea nitrogen, and serum creatinine levels. The child was successfully treated for MIS-C.

Key Learning about POCT for COVID-19

1. Making sure that the test specimen is properly obtained is key to getting the best possible results.
2. POCT antigen testing is not as accurate as PCR testing. In a child who you suspect has COVID, a PCR test should be done.
3. There are over 340 tests that received emergency authorization for use in the United States. The test's sensitivity and specificity vary greatly, and the clinician should evaluate the results of the tests based on each test's sensitivity and specificity.
4. Antibody testing can be done at a minimum of 2 weeks after an illness, with the IDSA recommending 3–4 weeks.

5.6 POCT C-Reactive Protein (CRP)

An overview of C-reactive protein (CRP) is discussed in Chap. 6, Section 6.3.2. CRP is a protein produced in the liver and rises in response to infection or inflammation. CRP should be higher in bacterial infection than in viral infection; however, the cutoff value to differentiate viral versus bacterial is somewhat disputed. CRP and PCT (procalcitonin) are often used together and are helpful to detect pneumonia and meningitis in children (Tsao et al. 2020).

5.6.1 Clinical Indications for POCT CRP Testing

Due to an earlier rise in CRP when a child is ill, a POCT CRP can be used to determine a possible cause of the patient's complaint. POCT CRP is new and is employed in a variety of ambulatory and inpatient settings. POCT CRP is currently used most frequently in limited-resource communities where access to other testing is limited. A benefit of POCT CRP is it has been shown to decrease antibiotic prescribing in children with acute viral respiratory illnesses (Tsao et al. 2020; Keitel et al. 2017). A study performed in the neonatal intensive care unit found that POCT CRP compares favorably to laboratory CRP with POCT results coming back on average 4 min. In contrast, laboratory results took over 4 h (Prince et al. 2019).

5.6.2 Types of POCT CRP Diagnostic Tests

ProciseDx applied for FDA approval for its Precise CRP assay in July 2021. ProciseDx is a POCT for C-reactive protein that gives a CRP result in 2–5 min (Westlake 2020). FebriDx is a POCT multiplex lateral flow assay that gives results in 10 min. It has a sensitivity and specificity of 80–95% (Tsao et al. 2020). This test is indicated for use in patients presenting with acute respiratory infections and detects CRP and myxoma resistance protein 1 (MxA). MxA is a marker for viral infection, whereas CRP is a marker for bacterial infection. FebriDx is an all-in-one test that uses a finger-stick blood sample. This test is currently available in Europe, Canada, the United Kingdom, Pakistan, Singapore, and Malaysia.

Additional POCT CRP includes NycoCard and Afinion. A French study conducted in 2017 evaluated the use of a POCT CRP Afinion in a pediatric emergency department in children presenting with fever (Roulliaud et al. 2018). They reported a decrease in average emergency room time and decreased other lab tests and imaging due to using the test (Roulliaud et al. 2018).

The use of POCT CRP in this study indicated there might be an economic benefit. A Thailand study reported that POCT CRP testing reduced antibiotic resistance's economic costs with POCT CRP test that costs $1 (Althaus et al. 2019).

5.6.3 Pitfalls of POCT CRP Testing

POCT CRP tests are not readily available for use in the United States. A systemic review and meta-analysis of POCT in pediatric ambulatory care found that POCT CRP may be beneficial in low- to middle-income countries in reducing antibiotic prescribing for acute respiratory illnesses but not in high-income countries (Van Hecke et al. 2020). As discussed in Chap. 6, one of the pitfalls of POCT CRP is the large range of CRP values (Tsao et al. 2020). While some evidence points to a higher CRP in bacterial illness, the cutoff is unclear since there is a wide range of normal. According to the CDC, about 30% of antibiotics prescribed in the United States primary care are unnecessary (CDC 2020f). While CRP levels may be higher in bacterial illness than in viral illness and a higher value of >8–10 mg/L is more likely to be a bacterial cause, the test is not perfect (Andreola et al. 2007; Lee et al. 2020). CRP does not adequately differentiate between viral and bacterial pneumonia and therefore is not recommended for immunized children treated outpatient (Tsai et al. 2020).

CRP is highly sensitive and moderately specific at identifying bacterial illness. A Southeast Asia study of children and adults presenting febrile to primary care reported a CRP sensitivity of 86% and specificity of 67% with a threshold of 20 mg/L (Althaus et al. 2019). While POCT CRP alone may not be enough to diagnose bacterial pneumonia in the United States and other developed countries, a recent study performed in three pediatric emergency departments in Switzerland used CRP as a three-step process to identify children at high risk for community-acquired pneumonia (CAP) (Alcoba et al. 2017). The first step was evaluating for clinical signs indicating pneumonia to include two out of three of the following: unilateral hypoventilation, grunting, and absence of wheezing. If two out of three clinical signs were positive, the second step was to obtain a CRP. By adding CRP as a second step with a cutoff of 40 mg/L, the investigators could rule out pneumonia with a 92% sensitivity rate and a negative predictive value of 87% for pneumonia with consolidation and 94% for complicated pneumo-

nia (Alcoba et al. 2017). The investigators in this study felt these two steps could decrease the need for antibiotic coverage and chest radiographs in pediatric emergency departments. This study did not specifically list POCT CRP but stated the CRP test was rapidly available (Alcoba et al. 2017).

Key Learning about POCT for CRP

1. A POCT for CRP is not readily available for use in the United States.
2. May provide additional ancillary data and assist with diagnosis in a resource-poor or rural setting and serve to decrease antibiotic prescribing.
3. A large range of CRP values make it difficult to determine cutoff between viral and bacterial infection.
4. The technology or platforms for using POCT tests for CRP are widely used. For example, the Alere Afinion™ platform for running POCT used for HbA1c is used in primary care clinics.

5.7 POCT Human Immunodeficiency Virus (HIV) Testing

Rapid POCT HIV testing allows patients to be tested and receive their results in the same office visit. The rapid test can be performed in the clinic instead of being sent to a lab. Most rapid tests identify antibodies to HIV in the blood or, less frequently, sputum instead of identifying the virus itself. Therefore, rapid tests are screening tests. Initial testing could be nonreactive; however, if the potential exposure were within 3 months, another test may be indicated. If the rapid test is positive, this should be considered a preliminary positive, and confirmation laboratory testing should be done (Broeckaert and Challacombe 2015). Some newer POCT molecular tests identify RNA and are used in other countries, but these tests are not currently FDA approved in the United States. There are three types of HIV tests available today—the nucleic acid tests to detect HIV ribonucleic acid (RNA), the antibody tests to detect HIV IgM and/or IgG antibodies, and the confirmatory antigen/antibody combination test that detect HIV IgM, HIV IgG, and HIV p24 antigen (CDC 2020g).

5.7.1 Clinical Indications for POCT HIV Testing

Clinical indications for testing include known exposure to HIV, including possible perinatal exposure, high-risk behavior such as unprotected sexual activity or intravenous illicit drug use, routine preventative care screening to identify asymptomatic patients, and the patient presenting with symptoms suspicious for HIV.

According to the American Academy of Pediatrics Bright Futures and the United States Preventative Services Task Force, adolescents should be screened for HIV once between 15 and 18 years of age (Hagan et al. 2017; United States Preventive Services Task Force et al. 2019). Adolescents at increased risk of HIV infection should be tested annually along with other sexually transmitted diseases (STD) testing. Those at high risk for HIV who should be screened at least annually include people who inject substances and their sexual partners, people who exchange sex for money or illicit substances, sexual partners of people with HIV, sexually active men who have sex with men (MSM), heterosexuals who themselves or their partners have had greater or equal to one sexual partner since their most recent HIV test, and those receiving treatment for hepatitis, tuberculosis, or other sexually transmitted diseases (CDC 2020h).

Perinatal transmission in the United States and other developed countries is rare due to universal antenatal testing, antiviral medications, cesarean births, and abstaining from breastfeeding (CDC 2021, 2022). In underdeveloped countries where access to safe water to make formula is limited, breastfeeding is still encouraged regardless of the HIV status of the mother. In the United States, perinatally exposed infants are tested within the first 48 h of life with HIV DNA PCR or HIV qualitative RNA, and then follow-up testing is done at 1–3 months of life and 4–6 months of life (CDC 2016). If all three tests are negative, the infant is considered HIV-negative. If two positives on any of these tests, then the infant is considered HIV-positive. HIV culture, HIV p24 antigen assay, and immune complex-dissociated p24 antigen assay are not recommended for infants less than 1 month of age (NIH 2019). HIV antibody assay should not be used in cases of perinatal exposure in children less than 18 months of age, as it could result in a false-positive result (NIH 2019). If a newborn is delivered and maternal HIV status is unknown, the newborn may also undergo rapid HIV testing. However, in known prenatal exposures, rapid POCT is not recommended as a testing method for infants in the United States.

5.7.2 Differential Diagnosis of HIV

Children who present with symptoms such as lymphadenopathy, hepatosplenomegaly, failure to thrive, chronic or recurrent diarrhea, pneumonia, recurrent bacterial or fungal infections such as oral candidiasis and other opportunistic infections, chronic parotid swelling, and progressive neurological deterioration should be considered for HIV testing (NIH 2019). The differential diagnosis of HIV includes influenza-like illnesses caused by a virus, immunodeficiency disorders, and mononucleosis-like illnesses caused by viruses, including CMV and EBV.

5.7.3 Differential Diagnosis for HIV in Pediatric Patients

Pediatric HIV diagnosis is relatively rare in most areas in the United States. There are certain areas and patient populations that are at higher risk. Due to HIV testing in pregnancy, very few infants are born to mothers whose HIV status is unknown. The availability of rapid testing of mothers at delivery decreases this likelihood even further. Other than perinatal transmission, older children rarely contract HIV through sexual abuse and accidental puncture wound from a discarded needle, bite wound, physical fight, or sports activity. However, these transmission methods are relatively rare (CDC 2016; NIH 2019). Adolescents may contract HIV through high-risk sexual behavior or the use of intravenous substances.

The primary care clinician needs to review the newborn discharge summary at first well-baby check to verify the mother was tested and was HIV-negative. If a child previously thought to be HIV-negative with no known exposure begins to exhibit signs or symptoms of HIV, HIV should promptly be ruled out. In a child over 18 months of age, if HIV is suspected, HIV screening should be done with HIV antibody assays plus confirmation antibody test or virologic detection test (NIH 2019). As previously discussed, antibody testing may be negative in acute early infection, and follow-up virologic testing is necessary. The differential diagnosis could include immunodeficiency due to immunosuppressive therapy, congenital immunodeficiency, inflammatory bowel disease, DiGeorge syndrome, chronic allergies, cystic fibrosis, graft-versus-host disease, congenital newborn infections, or ataxia-telangiectasia (King and Hammarström 2018.

5.7.4   Types of Diagnostic Tests for POCT HIV

The benefits of using rapid POCT HIV include: results are available within minutes, and the person receives results at the time of visit. Alternatively, laboratory tests sent out to a lab can take several days to complete, and studies have shown that sometimes patients cannot be reached to relay results (Pai et al. 2015). Additional benefits include: rapid testing may increase access to testing, thereby increasing the likelihood of early diagnosis. Outside the United States, where the burden of HIV-positive mothers delivering infants is higher such as in South Africa, the birth and 10 weeks HIV-PCR presents challenges, including loss of follow-up and delayed results (Spooner et al. 2019). A study by

Spooner et al. researched using a new POCT called Alere q HIV-1/2 Detect, which detects HIV RNA from a finger stick or, in the case of infants, a heel stick with results in 50 min (2019). This study found that mothers and healthcare clinicians preferred HIV POCT since it decreased the likelihood of delayed results or lack of follow-up. All infants testing positive could be started quickly on antiviral medication. The study found POCT HIV testing for early infant diagnosis is an accurate and acceptable test that allowed early ART for all infants who tested positive and were born in birth facilities (Spooner et al. 2019). By using a POCT HIV, there was a threefold increase in initiating antiretroviral therapy within 60 days in a child who was newly diagnosed with HIV (Van Hecke et al. 2020).

5.7.4.1 Antibody Tests

Several antibody CLIA-waived rapid tests include DPP HIV 1/2 Assay, HIV 1/2 STAT-PAK, INSTI HIV-1/HIV-2 Antibody Test, OraQuick Advance Rapid HIV-1/2 Antibody Test, SURE CHECK HIV 1/2 Assay, and Uni-Gold Recombigen HIV-1/2. These tests are single-use, with test results back within 2–25 min. These tests are used with whole blood, although some can also be run from saliva. One test, Determine HIV-1/2 Ag/Ab Combo Test, is an antigen and antibody rapid test. It is a single-use test that detects IgM, IgG antibodies and reports Ag and Ab separately. It is CLIA-waived and uses whole blood specimens such as a finger stick. Different types of CLIA-waived rapid HIV POCT tests are found in Table 5.9.

5.7.5   Barriers and Pitfalls for POCT HIV

Pai et al. researched barriers to implementing rapid and POCT tests for HIV across patients, clinicians, and health systems (2015). The study found that patient-level barriers to POCT HIV include lack of awareness of accuracy, time constraints, privacy concerns, fear of receiving the result in the clinic setting, and costly confirmation testing. In the study, some patients preferred

Table 5.9 CLIA-waived rapid HIV POCT

Test	Detection	Sensitivity/specifically (finger-stick whole blood when available)	Specimen types	Time for blood results
Chembio DDP HIV-1/2	Antibodies HIV-1 and 2	99.8%/100%	Finger-stick or whole venous blood or oral fluid	10 min
Chembio SURE CHECK HIV 1/2 Assay	Antibodies HIV-1 and 2	99.7%/99.9%	Finger-stick or whole blood	15 min
Clearview HIV 1/2 STAT-PAK	Antibodies HIV-1 and 2	99.7%/ 99.9%	Finger-stick or whole venous blood	15 min
Determine HIV-1/2 Ag/Ab Combo Test	Antibodies HIV-1 and 2, HIV-1 p24 Antigen	99.9%/ 100% (low risk pt.) or 99.7% (high risk pt.)	Finger-stick whole blood	20 min
INSTI HIV-1/HIV-2 Antibody Test	Antibodies HIV-1 and 2	99.8%/99.5%	Finger-stick whole blood	<2 min
OraQuick advance Rapid HIV-1/2 Antibody Test	Antibodies HIV-1 and 2	99.6%/100%	Finger-stick or whole venous blood or oral fluid	20 min
Uni-Gold Recombigen HIV-1/2	Antibodies HIV-1 and 2	100%/99.7%	Finger-stick or whole venous blood	10 min

Partially adapted from CDC 2020i, and manufacturer package insert

time to prepare for the result, so they preferred traditional laboratory testing instead of rapid POCT. Barriers on the clinician level included challenges integrating POCT into clinical workflow, time, cost, attitude, and staff reluctance to do POCT. Barriers at the healthcare level included implantation, cost, and concerns with accuracy. POCT HIV testing was one of the first POCT for sexually transmitted diseases (STDs), and therefore initial POCT was not as accurate as they are today. Unfortunately, this concept continues to linger in both the medical community and patients alike. In high-prevalence areas, HIV POCT can have an accuracy of 98–99%. However, in lower prevalence settings, there can be an increase in false results.

There have been concerns that certain rapid POCT HIV tests are not as accurate as other laboratory tests for HIV. However, the INSTI HIV-1/HIV-2 has a sensitivity of 99.6% and a specificity of 99.3% (Broeckaert and Challacombe 2015). The Determine HIV-1/2 Ag/AB Combo has a sensitivity of 99.9% and a specificity of 99.8% (Broeckaert and Challacombe 2015). These values verify slightly from manufacturer-reported data; however, as you can see, based on the table

and study, these tests are highly sensitive and specific.

Pitfalls to rapid POCT HIV tests include that when used with finger-stick whole blood, they are not as sensitive near the time of infection as antigen or antibody tests performed on plasma (CDC 2020i).

5.7.6 Real-Life Example

A five-month-old comes for his first visit to the office. There are no previous medical records available. The mother reports two hospitalizations for sepsis at 1 and 4 months. The child's birth weight was 8 pounds. Today, you note that the child is small for age and is growing on the fifth percentile for weight and height and the 25th percentile for head circumference. The exam is remarkable for small 1 cm anterior cervical nodes and a spleen tip. Based on the history, you consider a complement disorder. You decide to do a CBC with differential, HIV DNA PCR, immunoglobulins, and total complement (C50) as well as C3 and C4. HIV testing was negative. The child's C50 was low, and an immunologist's further diagnostic workup showed a complement component 2 deficiency.

> **Key Learning about POCT for HIV**
> 1. Detect intracellular HIV-1 nucleic acids typically present 10–14 days after HIV exposure, either in the form of viral RNA in plasma or proviral DNA in peripheral blood mononuclear cells.
> 2. The oral fluid testing device that measures HIV antibody in mucosal transudate. It is well accepted and used in many outreach settings (Committee on Pediatric Aids et al. 2011 reaffirmed 2016, COVID-19 2021).
> 3. A positive rapid HIV test is considered a "preliminary positive," and confirmation HIV screening should be performed with a fourth-generation antibody/antigen test.
> 4. Western blot is no longer recommended.
> 5. Detects HIV-1 and HIV-2 antibodies and the HIV-1 p24 antigen, with supplemental testing after a reactive assay to differentiate between HIV-1 and HIV-2 antibodies.

5.8   POCT Pregnancy Screening

Many pediatric clinicians continue to care for adolescents through at least 18 years of age, while some continue care until 21 years. Adolescent pregnancy is on the decline in most areas of the United States; however, rapid, discreet pregnancy testing is still needed in primary care. Unfortunately, the United States still has one of the highest adolescent pregnancy rates compared to other developed countries (Hornberger 2017). According to the CDC, adolescent pregnancy is declining due to increased availability and use of birth control and abstinence. The most current statistics from the CDC show a birth rate of 18.8 per 1000 teens. The birth rates fell 10% for teens 15–17 years and 6% for teens 18–19 years of age (CDC 2020j).

5.8.1   Clinical Indications for POCT Pregnancy Tests

Adolescent reported history may be vague and can sometimes be purposely misleading due to privacy or safety concerns. The pediatric clinician should have a low threshold to test for pregnancy in adolescent females. An adolescent patient may present to primary care for confirmation of a positive pregnancy test at home. Early pregnancy signs such as breast tenderness, lower back pain, abdominal cramping, nausea or vomiting, or missed menstruation may be reported. Irregular menstruation or amenorrhea and urinary tract symptoms may be other clinical indications to obtain POCT pregnancy testing. Also, initiation of contraception or reporting recent unprotected intercourse may be other reasons to employ rapid pregnancy screening. A POCT urine hCG should be performed in all female adolescents that present with amenorrhea, even if the patient denies previous sexual intercourse. If the parent is involved in the visit and depending on state law, the clinician may wish to explain to the parent and patient that a baseline POCT urine hCG is standard of care in all women of childbearing age presenting with amenorrhea. Lower abdominal pain may indicate a tubal or normal pregnancy, and a POCT urine hCG test can help rule out pregnancy as the cause.

5.8.2   Types of POCT Pregnancy Tests

POCT qualitative urine hCG used in most clinic settings can identify pregnancy by the first day of the missed period. POCT urine hCG can typically detect hCG at a level of 25 IU/L (Hornberger 2017). POCT serum hCG tests are also on the market but are less commonly used in a clinical setting as they are moderate complexity and more invasive due to the need for venipuncture. The result on either qualitative urine or serum hCG is positive or negative.

5.8.2.1 Rapid Urine Immunoassay

Overall, POCT hCG tests are accurate and easy to use. However, certain circumstances increase the risk for false results. Suppose the pediatric clinician has a strong suspicion of false results on POCT. In that case, the POCT hCG could be repeated in several days, or a serum hCG could be sent to the laboratory. As with other POCT tests, the benefit to POCT is rapid results within minutes; the patient can be informed of the positive result during the visit, allowing the appropriate education and referral to take place within the office visit. POCT for pregnancy is typically a lower-cost test.

The pediatric clinician should have access to rapid urine immunoassays that test for the presence of human chorionic gonadotropin (hCG). HCG is a chemical created by trophoblast tissue found in early embryos, eventually becoming part of the placenta (Betz and Fane 2020). Most POCT urine hCG tests use hCG monoclonal antibodies specific to hCG beta-subunit to detect hCG in the specimen. Typically, several drops of a urine sample are added to the test well, and after several minutes, a control line will appear. The additional appearance of a test line indicates a positive result. The urine sample can be random; however, a first-morning sample may be more concentrated in early pregnancy and increase the likelihood of a true positive.

Office-based tests can detect concentrations ranging from 12 to 50 mIU/L, and some home pregnancy tests can detect concentrations as low as 5.5 mIU/L (Latifi et al. 2019). POCT urine hCG has a sensitivity of 90–97% and specificity of 99.2% in the first weeks following missed menstruation (Latifi et al. 2019).

5.8.2.2 Nonpoint of Service Pregnancy Tests

The most accurate pregnancy test is the laboratory-based quantitative serum hCG, which measures and provides an hCG value. This test is used less often than its counterparts and takes longer to perform. However, the quantitative serum hCG is preferred when the clinician suspects pregnancy and the POCT is negative; or the clinician wants the most accurate test to confirm or rule out pregnancy (Furtado et al. 2012) quantitative hCG can also help clinician to estimate how far along a pregnancy is. Laboratory quantitative serum hCG is more sensitive and can detect hCG at 1 IU/L. The negative predictive value of both laboratory qualitative and quantitative serum hCG is 99.9% (Furtado et al. 2012).

In the adolescent population specifically, caution should be used in confidential send-out testing, as contacting the adolescent at home may be more difficult without parental knowledge, particularly if adolescents don't have access to their own telephone. Cost comparison from 2019, the reimbursement rate for POCT urine hCG was $8.61, and quantitative serum hCG testing was $16.73 (Latifi et al. 2019).

5.8.3 Barriers and Pitfalls of POCT Pregnancy Tests

The most common reason for a false-negative result is human error, particularly at home tests (Hornberger 2017). The clinician should observe the test for a control line (typically blue) and a test line (typically pink/red). The test is only considered accurate if the control line appears. A faint test line is still considered a positive. However, this should not be confused with an evaporation line, and a colorless streak may appear in the test line area if read after the recommended time as the urine dries on the test strip. It is important to read the test result at the exact time recommended by the manufacturer. Suppose there is reported unprotected sexual activity in the past 3 weeks and a POCT urine hCG is negative at the time of visit. In that case, a repeat test in 2 weeks is warranted, or a laboratory hCG test could be obtained.

False-negative could occur due to testing too early but also due to testing late in the first trimester due to the hook effect. The hook effect can occur when the urine has an excess of hCG, which prevents the necessary antibody-antigen-antibody sandwich formation, causing a false-negative result (Latifi et al. 2019). False negatives are most likely to occur between 8 and 14 weeks gestation but can occur as early as 6 weeks. It can also occur with dilute urine specimens (Betz and Fane 2020).

False-positive results are less likely and differ based on whether serum or urine specimen. Serum false positives can be due to recent or subclinical abortions, gestational trophoblastic disease, malignancies, heterophile antibodies, rheumatoid factors, and IgA deficiency (Betz and Fane 2020). Other rare causes of false-positive serum hCG may include renal failure on hemodialysis, recent blood transfusion from donor blood with hCG, and medications for weight loss or fertility that contain exogenous hCG (Betz and Fane 2020). False-positive results on POCT urine hCG may include blood or protein in the urine, human error in result interpretation, ectopic production or exogenous hCG, and certain medications such as anticonvulsants, hypnotics, and tranquilizers (Betz and Fane 2020). Testing too soon after a recent delivery or miscarriage could also result in a false-positive result. In an older population, menopause can sometimes trigger a false-positive hCG result.

5.8.4 Real-Life Example

A 16-year-old had a chief complaint of right lower quadrant pain for 3 days duration. The child denies fever and has a good appetite. She does complain of the new onset of heartburn over the past 2 weeks. The child has a normal exam. Rovsing sign, Markle heel jar test, and rebound were all negative. A POCT urine pregnancy test was positive. An ultrasound of the pelvis confirmed the patient was 8 weeks pregnant.

Key Learning about POCT Pregnancy Tests

1. POCT HCG is very accurate. If there is strong clinical concern and POCT is negative, the clinician may reflex to laboratory serum hCG or repeat POCT urine hCG in 2 weeks.
2. False negative most commonly early (due to low HCG levels) or late (due to hook effect) in the first trimester.

3. POCT urine hCG should be performed in all cases of adolescent amenorrhea regardless of reported sexual activity.
4. POCT urine hCG should be read promptly per manufacturer time recommendation.

5.9 POCT for Hemoglobin A1C

Hemoglobin A1C (HA1C) measures the mean blood glucose levels in red blood cells for the past 3 months. A POCT for hemoglobin A1C can provide real-time results to the clinician enabling efficient and effective management decisions. The majority of POCT HA1C uses a drop of whole capillary blood. The different analytical methods used in POCT HA1C include cation exchange chromatography, immunoassay, affinity chromatography and enzymatic assay (English et al. 2020). However, studies show a significant difference with POCT HbA1c being lower than laboratory-based HbA1C, especially in pediatric (0–13 years) and female patients (Clark and Rao 2017). The authors point out that the difference may be related to differences in pediatric and female there is some physiological difference in pediatric and female subcutaneous capillary beds. Moffett's et al. 2011 study pointed out that 14% of patients did not follow up on laboratory referrals after being seen by the clinician, pointing to the value of POCT.

5.9.1 Clinical Indication for POCT HbA1c

Clinical indications for HbA1c include concern for signs or symptoms indicating diabetes and the management of prediabetic patients or confirmed diabetic patients. POCT HbA1c may be used in clinical settings to manage known diabetics but should not be used for a new diagnosis of diabetes (O'Brien and Sacks 2019). The majority of studies have been in adults. The pediatric primary care clinician is a likely member of the care team to diagnose pediatric diabetes with either a POCT or laboratory glucose or a laboratory HbA1c or both. However, most likely pediatric diabetes will be managed in pediatric endocrinology clinics, and therefore POCT HbA1c is more likely to be utilized in this setting.

Screening for type 2 diabetes mellitus in the obese child is found in the well-child chapter, and the use of HbA1c is also found in the section on diabetes in the endocrine chapter.

5.9.2 Types of POCT HbA1c

The FDA approved the handheld AC1Now and the DCA Vantage Analyzer for POCT HbA1c as CLIA-waived devices. These devices are approved for monitoring but not diagnosing diabetes. In contrast, the FDA approved the Afinion HbA1c Dx assay for both monitoring and diagnosing diabetes. However, the Afinion HbA1c must be used in a clinical laboratory since it is a moderately complex device. The National Glycohemoglobin Standardization Program (NGSP) certified all three POCT HA1C for use (Whitley et al. 2015).

The DCA Vantage Analyzer is a multiparameter POCT with a CLIA-waived for HbA1c using 1 microliter finger stick with results in 6 min. The platform also may provide albumin, creatinine, and albumin-to-creatine ratio, although these tests are of moderate complexity. A potential downfall of this system is the expensive platform.

The handheld AC1Now is a CLIA-waived portable device with reported 99% accuracy with results in 5 min using a five-microliter blood sample. The Afinion HbA1c is a benchtop model that is CLIA-waived. It requires 1.5 microliter blood volume of capillary blood or anticoagulated venous blood and takes 3 min to run.

The FDA approved the Afinion HbA1c Dx assay (Abbott) as the first rapid point-of-care test to diagnose diabetes and assess a patient's risk of developing the disease. The new clearance for the expanded diagnostic indication is specific to laboratories with CLIA certification to perform tests that are of moderate or higher complexity and does not extend to those that can only perform CLIA-waived tests. Unlike the AC1Now, the Afinion system states there is no influence from common Hb variants like HBC, HbD, HbE, and HbS.

A HA1c of 6.5% or higher on two separate occasions is diagnostic for diabetes in adults. As stated, the use of HA1C for diagnosis in children is still somewhat controversial, particularly for type 2 diabetes (Atteih and Ratner 2020). Normal HbA1c in the non-diabetic patient is 4–5.6%. Prediabetes is considered from 5.7% to 6.4%. For children with T1DM, the A1c goal is less than 7.5%, higher than the adult goal of less than 7%, due to concern for increased risk for hypoglycemia in children. For children with T2DM, the goal is less than 7% if on metformin alone (Atteih and Ratner 2020).

5.9.3 Barriers and Pitfalls of POCT HbA1c

The evidence is conflicting on the accuracy of POCT HbA1c. O'Brien and Sacks found a wide variability of POCT HbA1c (2019). However, other studies have found that POCT HbA1c is comparable to laboratory HbA1c when the value is 9–13.9% (Agrawal et al. 2018). POCT HbA1c is unreliable in levels of 14% and greater, and therefore children with known marked elevations should only have laboratory HbA1c. Nathan et al. compared the POCT Alere Afinion assay to the laboratory Premier Affinity assay and found that the two tests performed similarly (Afinion HbA1c 2019). However, there was a difference in the performance of the POCT and whether the operator was a physician or a medical assistant (Nathan et al. 2019).

There is a paucity of literature regarding primary care pediatrics and POCT HbA1c. However, in adult patients in primary care practices without POCT, HbA1c were nearly four times more likely to miss follow-up HbA1c labs than practices with POCT HbA1c (Crocker et al. 2020). Interestingly, while rapid testing seems to increase glycemic control in adults, it does not seem to affect pediatric control (Agrawal et al. 2018; Agus et al. 2010). Despite that, both these studies found that POCT HbA1c is more convenient for families, and children often report that a finger stick is less painful than venipuncture. Evidence indicates that continuous glucose monitors or an insulin pump is more likely to reduce HbA1c levels in newly diagnosed children with type 1 diabetes mellitus (Patton et al. 2019). Another benefit of POCT HbA1c was less frequent clinician-patient communication between visits, resulting in time saved for the clinician (Van Hecke et al. 2020; Agus et al. 2010). Thus, the clinician will have real-time results and will be able to make medication modifications based on those results instead of the traditional laboratory method where the clinician must wait on the lab and follow up after the visit with a telephone call. Pitfalls of using HbA1c include the test may be unreliable in patients with abnormal red cell life span or morphology, such as sickle cell disease and spherocytosis (Atteih and Ratner 2020). POCT HbA1c may also be less reliable than laboratory tests with higher HbA1c, particularly above 14% (Agrawal et al. 2018).

Key Learning about POCT HbA1c

- A CLIA-waived POCT HbA1c is designed to assist in the management of diabetes and not for use in the initial diagnosis.
- One of the major benefits of POCT HbA1c is the decreased need for the pediatric patient to have venipuncture and go to the lab. It also decreases the need for clinician follow-up telephone calls regarding labs.
- The POCT HbA1c may be less reliable than laboratory tests if HA1C is above 14%.
- The use of this technology is more practical in the pediatric endocrinology office than in the primary care pediatric office.

5.10   Conclusion

In conclusion, POCT in the primary care setting continues to be an important resource for clinicians. When used appropriately, POCT can be incredibly helpful in providing safe, timely, and accurate patient care. Certain POCTs, when used properly, can help maintain antibiotic stewardship. Other POCTs can help diagnose or manage chronic disease processes directly from the clinic. In the age of the COVID-19 pandemic and the continued threat of new pathogens, correctly identifying the cause of the illness is important for the treatment and management of the pediatric patient. As previously discussed, positive and negative predictive values and an awareness of disease prevalence in the community may help determine pre- and post-test probability for an individual, then sensitivity and specificity alone. The likelihood ratios using Fagan's nomogram may provide additional data on the accuracy of a test for a specific patient and are discussed in Chap. 1 (Akobeng 2007a, b). As a clinician ordering and utilizing POCT in primary care, it is critical to evaluate the test for cost, diagnostic accuracy and reliability, patient outcome, ease of use, timeliness, and operational technology suiting clinics' environment (Keitel et al. 2018).

Questions

1. You are the acting laboratory director for your pediatric clinic's CLIA waiver. What do your responsibilities include in this role?
   (a) To make sure that you are using the CLIA-waived tests in the office.
   (b) To make sure the entire staff understands how to run the tests.
   (c) To make sure that the billing is done correctly.
   (d) To make sure quality checks are done and the staff is fully competent.
2. The clinician orders a rapid antigen strep test, and the result is negative. What additional tests should be ordered?
   (a) No further testing is needed.
   (b) Do a backup throat culture.

(c) Treat the child with antibiotics since you suspected strep tonsillitis.

(d) Do a streptozyme.

3. Which of the following would be the best test to do for confirming COVID-19 in a pediatric patient?

(a) A COVID-19 antibody test.

(b) A COVID-19 antigen test.

(c) A COVID-19 PCR test.

4. A mother is at the clinic wanting to know if her child is still contagious 1 month after the child had a positive PCR test. The child has clinically recovered. She wants another PCR test for COVID-19 done. What is the best approach to her request?

(a) Repeat the PCR test for COVID-19.

(b) Explain that there is no need to do a follow-up test.

(c) Explain that the PCR test might be falsely positive.

(d) B & C.

5. If the clinician has strong suspicion for influenza in a high-risk pediatric patient, but the antigen RIDT is negative, what is the next best step?

(a) Reassure the family that the child does not have influenza.

(b) Treat the child with antiviral medication.

(c) Repeat the antigen RIDT test.

6. What is the preferred test for SARS-CoV-2 (COVID-19) in an asymptomatic individual?

(a) A COVID-19 antibody test.

(b) A COVID-19 antigen test.

(c) A COVID-19 molecular test.

7. The clinician sees a 17-year-old for well-child check and orders a rapid HIV test. The POCT HIV is positive. What is the next step?

(a) Tell the adolescent that the test is positive and he is infected with HIV.

(b) Confirm that the test is positive, and order a repeat rapid HIV.

(c) Confirm that the preliminary results are positive, and order a fourth-generation antibody/antigen test.

(d) Confirm that the preliminary results are positive, and order a Western Blot.

8. What is the most appropriate indication for the clinicians to use POCT HbA1c?

(a) It should be used to make management decisions in a pediatric patient with known diabetes.

(b) It should be used on all pediatric patients for diagnosing type 1 and type 2 diabetes.

(c) It should be used on pediatric patients over 10 for diagnosing type 2 diabetes.

(d) It has no place in the management of pediatric patients.

9. It is June, and you see a 5-year-old with tachypnea, retractions, and a pulse oxygen of 95%. There are decreased breath sounds on the right base. Which of the following diagnostic tests would be the most helpful?

(a) POCT CRP.

(b) POCT for strep.

(c) POCT for COVID-19.

(d) POCT for influenza.

10. What is a potential cause of a false-negative POCT hCG at the end of the first trimester of pregnancy?

(a) The hook effect.

(b) Concentrated urine sample.

(c) Following the manufacturer's instructions.

Rationale

1. Answer: D

The laboratory director for a CoW laboratory is responsible for competency checks of other clinical staff, POCT quality checks, documentation, and review (Nichols 2007, Babady et al. 2019, Nichols et al. 2020).

2. Answer: B

A negative rapid antigen strep test should be confirmed with laboratory throat culture (Shapiro et al. 2017; Shulman 2015; Shulman et al. 2012).

3. Answer: C

The test with the highest sensitivity and specificity is the molecular test for COVID-19.

4. Answer: D

A molecular COVID-19 will pick up viral nucleic acid that is present due to a previous infection, and there is no need to do follow-up testing in a well-appearing child.

5. Answer: B

Due to the limited sensitivity and predictive values of antigen RIDT, the clinician should treat the child with an antiviral if influenza infection is strongly suspected (John 2019; Lee et al. 2019).

6. Answer: C

As a general rule, the PCR test is preferred for asymptomatic individuals. Potential symptoms of COVID-19 include fever, chills, cough, shortness of breath or difficulty breathing, sore throat, fatigue, muscle or body aches, headache, the new loss of taste or smell, congestion or runny nose, nausea or vomiting, and diarrhea. Children may have very mild or even asymptomatic infections. Therefore, clinicians should have a low threshold to test if high community prevalence or known exposure. If a rapid antigen test is negative in a symptomatic child, the reflex to SARS-CoV-2 PCR testing should be considered (NIH 2021; AAP 2020).

7. Answer: C

If the rapid HIV test is positive, this should be considered a preliminary positive, and confirmation HIV screening should be performed with a fourth-generation antibody/antigen test (CDC 2020h).

8. Answer: A

POCT HbA1c may be used in clinical settings to manage known diabetics but should not be used for new diagnoses of diabetes (O'Brien and Sacks 2019).

9. Answer: C

While an elevated POCT CRP may indicate acute bacterial illness in pediatrics, specifically community-acquired pneumonia (CAP) and bacterial meningitis (Tsao et al. 2020; Alcoba et al. 2017), it is a non-specific test. Influenza is usually seasonal and unlikely to cause disease in June. COVID-19 is the most likely organism to present as

pneumonia. A POCT for strep is unlikely to be a true positive in June, and strep would not present in this way.

10. Answer: A

The hook effect occurs when there is an excess hCG in the urine, causing antibody saturation and preventing the formation of an antibody-antigen-antibody sandwich. This would cause a false-negative result (Latifi et al. 2019). This is most likely to occur between 8 and 14 weeks' gestation but can occur as early as 6 weeks. Other causes of a false negative on urine POCT HCG include dilute urine specimens (Betz and Fane 2020).

Acknowledgement Figures 5.1–5.7 were contributed by Lieselotte Elliehausen.

References

AAP. FAQs: Management of infants born to mothers with suspected or confirmed COVID-19. 2020 Retrieved on January 30, 2021, http://services.aap.org/en/pages/2019-novel-coronavirus-covid-19-infections/clinical-guidance/faqs-management-of-infants-born-to-covid-19-mothers/

Abbott. Taking COVID-19 testing to a new level | Abbott U.S. Retrieved January 20, 2021., https://www.abbott.com/BinaxNOW-Test-NAVICA-App.html

Afinion HbA1c. 2019. https://www.globalpointofcare.abbott/en/product-details/afinion-hba1c.html. Accessed 31 Jan 2021

Agrawal S, Reinert SE, Baird GL, Quintos JB. Comparing HbA1C by POC and HPLC. R I Med J. (2013). 2018;101:43–6.

Agus MS, Alexander JL, Wolfsdorf JI. Utility of immediate hemoglobin A1c in children with type I diabetes mellitus. Pediatr Diabetes. 2010;11(7):450–4.

Akobeng AK. Understanding diagnostic tests 2: likelihood ratios, pre- and post-test probabilities and their use in clinical practice. Acta Paediatr. 2007a;96:487–91.

Akobeng AK. Understanding diagnostic tests 1: sensitivity, specificity and predictive values. Acta Paediatr. 2007b;96(3):338–41.

Alcoba G, Keitel K, Maspoli V, Lacroix L, Manzano S, Gehri M, Tabin R, Gervaix A, Galetto-Lacour A. A three-step diagnosis of pediatric pneumonia at the emergency department using clinical predictors, C-reactive protein, and pneumococcal PCR. Eur J Pediatr. 2017;176:815–24.

Althaus T, Greer RC, Swe MMM, Cohen J, Tun NN, Heaton J, Nedsuwan S, et al. Effect of point-of-care C-reactive protein testing on antibiotic prescription in febrile patients attending primary care in Thailand and Myanmar: an open-label, randomised, controlled trial. Lancet Glob Health. 2019;7(1):e119–31.

Andreola B, Bressan S, Callegaro S, Liverani A, Plebani M, Da Dalt L. Procalcitonin and C-reactive protein as diagnostic markers of severe bacterial infections in febrile infants and children in the emergency department. Pediatr Infect Dis J. 2007;26(8):672–7.

Atteih S, Ratner J. Endocrinology. In: Kleinman K, McDaniel L, Molloy M, editors. Harriet lane handbook. 22nd ed. Philadelphia: Elsevier Health Sciences; 2020.

Babady NE, Dunn JJ, Madej R. CLIA-waived molecular influenza testing in the emergency department and outpatient settings. J Clin Virol. 2019;116:44–8.

Baird GS. The choosing wisely initiative and laboratory test stewardship. Diagnosi. 2019;6(1):15–23.

Betz D, Fane K. Human chorionic gonadotropin. In: StatPearls [internet]. Treasure Island (FL): StatPearls Publishing; 2020.

Broeckaert L, Challacombe L. Rapid point-of-care HIV testing: a review of the evidence. 2015. Retrieved January 31, 2021, https://www.catie.ca/en/pif/spring-2015/rapid-point-care-hiv-testing-review-evidence.

CDC. HIV testing for pregnant women and newborns. 2016. Retrieved on March 7, 2021, https://www.cdc.gov/stophivtogether/library/one-test-two-lives/fact-sheets/cdc-lsht-ottl-factsheet-hiv-testing-for-pregnant-women-and-newborns.pdf

CDC. Rapid influenza diagnostic tests (RIDTs). 2020a. Retrieved on January 21, 2021 https://www.cdc.gov/flu/professionals/diagnosis/clinician_guidance_ridt.htm#:~:text=Rapid%20influenza%20diagnostic%20tests%20(RIDTs,of%20RIDTs%20are%20commercially%20available.

CDC. Overview of influenza testing methods. 2020b Retrieved on January 29, 2021, https://www.cdc.gov/flu/professionals/diagnosis/overview-testing-methods.htm

CDC. Table 3. Nucleic acid detection based tests. 2020c Retrieved on January 29, 2021, from https://www.cdc.gov/flu/professionals/diagnosis/table-nucleic-acid-detection.html

CDC. Options to reduce quarantine for contacts of persons with SARS-CoV-2. In: Centers for disease control and prevention; 2020d. https://www.cdc.gov/coronavirus/2019-ncov/more/scientific-brief-options-to-reduce-quarantine.html. Accessed 30 Jan 2021.

CDC. Labs. In: Centers for Disease Control and Prevention. 2020e Accessed January 20, 2021, https://www.cdc.gov/coronavirus/2019-ncov/lab/resources/antigen-tests-guidelines.html

CDC. Antibiotic use in the United States, 2017: progress and opportunities | Antibiotic Use | CDC. 2020f Accessed February 6, 2021, https://www.cdc.gov/antibiotic-use/stewardship-report/2017.html

CDC. Diagnostic tests: newer, improved HIV tests allow for earlier HIV detection. 2020g. Accessed March 5, 2021, https://www.cdc.gov/hiv/clinicians/screening/diagnostic-tests.html

CDC. Benefits of routine screening | screening for HIV | Clinicians | HIV | CDC. 2020h. Accessed Jan 31, 2021, from https://www.cdc.gov/hiv/clinicians/screening/benefits.html.

CDC. Advantages and disadvantages of FDA-approved HIV assays used for screening, by test category. 2020i. [pdf] https://www.cdc.gov/hiv/pdf/testing/hiv-tests-advantages-disadvantages_1.pdf Accessed 31 January 2021

CDC. About teen pregnancy. 2020j Accessed March 5, 2021, https://www.cdc.gov/teenpregnancy/about/index.htm#:~:text=In%202017%2C%20a%20total%20of,drop%20of%207%25%20from%202016.&text=Birth%20rates%20fell%2010%25%20for,women%20aged%2018%E2%80%9319%20years.

CDC. Healthcare workers. In: Centers for Disease Control and Prevention. Retrieved October 25, 2020, 2020k. https://www.cdc.gov/coronavirus/2019-ncov/hcp/pediatric-hcp.html.

CDC. HIV and pregnant women, infants, and children. 2021. Retrieved on March 7, 2021, https://www.cdc.gov/hiv/group/gender/pregnantwomen/index.html

CDC. Quarantine and isolation. 2022. Retrieved 29 January 2022, from: https://www.cdc.gov/coronavirus/2019-ncov/your-health/quarantine-isolation.html

Centor Score (Modified/McIsaac) for Strep Pharyngitis. In: MDCalc. https://www.mdcalc.com/centor-score-modified-mcisaac-strep-pharyngitis. Accessed 24 Jan 2021.

Christy A. COVID-19: a review for the pediatric neurologist. J Child Neurol. 2020;35(13):934–9.

Clark J, Rao LV. Retrospective analysis of point-of-care and laboratory-based hemoglobin A1c testing. J Appl Lab Med. 2017;1(5):502–9.

Cohen DM, Russo ME, Jaggi P, Kline J, Gluckman W, Parekh A. Multicenter clinical evaluation of the novel Alere i Strep A isothermal nucleic acid amplification test. J Clin Microbiol. 2015;53(7):2258–61.

Cohen JF, Bertille N, Cohen R, Chalumeau M. Rapid antigen detection test for group A streptococcus in children with pharyngitis. Cochrane Database Syst Rev. 2016;7(7):CD010502.

Committee on Pediatric AIDS, Emmanuel PJ, Martinez J. Adolescents and HIV infection: the pediatrician's role in promoting routine testing. Pediatrics. 2011;128(5):1023–9.

COVID-19 Testing Guidance. Retrieved on January 29, 2021, from: http://services.aap.org/en/pages/2019-novel-coronavirus-covid-19-infections/clinical-guidance/covid-19-testing-guidance

Crocker JB, Lynch SH, Guarino AJ, Lewandrowski K. The impact of point-of-care hemoglobin A1c testing on population health-based onsite testing adherence: a primary-care quality improvement study. J Diabetes Sci Technol. 2020; 1932296820972751

Cruz AT, Demmler-Harrison GJ, Caviness AC, Buffone GJ, Revell PA. Performance of a rapid influenza test in children during the H1N1 2009 Influenza A outbreak. Pediatrics. 2010;125:e645–50.

English E, Schaffert L, Lenters-Westra E. Point-of-care testing for HbA1c: clinical need and analytical quality. Retrieved January 31, 2020, from Clinical Laboratory Int. https://clinlabint.com/point-of-care-testing-for-hba1c-clinical-need-and-analytical-quality/.

FDA. In vitro diagnostics EUAs. 2021. Retrieved January 21, 2021, from https://www.fda.gov/medical-devices/coronavirus-disease-2019-covid-19-emergency-use-authorizations-medical-devices/vitro-diagnostics-euas#individual-molecular.

FilmArray Respiratory Panel EZ | In-Clinic Diagnostic Testing Solution. In: BioFire Diagnostics. https://www.biofiredx.com/products/the-filmarray-panels/filmarray-respiratory-panel-ez/. Accessed 30 Jan 2021.

Fiore K. What are the most popular COVID-19 Tests? 2020 Retrieved January 31, 2021, https://www.medpagetoday.com/infectiousdisease/covid19/89348.

Fiore K. Is delta variant more severe in children. 2021. Retrieved August 15, 2021, https://www.medpageto-day.com/special-reports/exclusives/93979

Food and Drug Administration (FDA). COVID-19 test uses: FAQs on testing for SARS-CoV-2. 2021. Retrieved February 18, 2021, from https://www.fda.gov/medical-devices/coronavirus-covid-19-and-medical-devices/covid-19-test-uses-faqs-testing-sars-cov-2

Fox JW, Marcon MJ, Bonsu BK. Diagnosis of streptococcal pharyngitis by detection of Streptococcus pyogenes in posterior pharyngeal versus oral cavity specimens. J Clin Microbiol. 2006;44(7):2593–4.

Frazee BW, Rodríguez-Hoces de la Guardia A, Alter H, Chen CG, Fuentes EL, et al. Accuracy and discomfort of different types of intranasal specimen collection methods for molecular influenza testing in emergency department patients. Ann Emerg Med. 2018;71:509–517.e1.

Furtado LV, Lehman CM, Thompson C, Grenache DG. Should the qualitative serum pregnancy test be considered obsolete? Am J Clin Pathol. 2012;137:194–202.

Hagan JF, Shaw JS, Duncan PM, editors. Bright futures: guidelines for health supervision of infants, children, and adolescents. 4th ed. Elk Grove Village, IL: Bright Futures/American Academy of Pediatrics; 2017.

Hansen G, Marino J, Wang ZX, Beavis KG, Rodrigo J, Labog K, et al. Clinical performance of the point-of-care cobas Liat for detection of SARS-CoV-2 in 20 minutes: a multicenter study. J Clin Microbiol. 2021;59(2):e02811–20.

Hanson KE, Caliendo AM, Arias CA, Englund JA, Hayden MK, Lee MJ, Loeb M, Patel R, Altayar O, El Alayli A, Sultan S, Falck-Ytter Y, Lavergne V, Morgan RL, Murad MH, Bhimraj A, Mustafa RA. Infectious Diseases Society of America Guidelines on the Diagnosis of COVID-19:Serologic Testing. Clin Infect Dis. 2020 Sep 12:ciaa1343. https://doi.org/10.1093/cid/ciaa1343. Epub ahead of print. PMID: 32918466; PMCID: PMC7543294.

Hanson KE, Caliendo AM, Arias CA, Hayden MK, et al. Infectious Diseases Society of America Guidelines on the Diagnosis of COVID-19: Molecular Diagnostic Testing. Infectious Diseases Society of America 2020; Retrieved on April 25, 2021, https://www.idsociety.org/practice-guideline/covid-19-guideline-diagnostics/

Hornberger LL. Committee on adolescence. Diagnosis of pregnancy and providing options counseling for the adolescent patient. Pediatrics. 2017;140(3): e20172273.

Jenco M. AAP: Wear face coverings during most sports. AAP News. 2021. Retrieved February 15, 2021, https://www.healthychildren.org/English/health-issues/conditions/COVID-19/Pages/Why-Cloth-Face-Coverings-are-Needed-in-Youth-Sports-During-COVID-19.aspx

John R. Respiratory disorders. In: Maaks DL, Starr NB, Brady MA, Gaylord NM, Driessnack M, Duderstadt KG, editors. Burns' pediatric primary care. 7th ed. St. Louis, MO: Elsevier, Inc; 2019.

Kalra MG, Higgins KE, Perez ED. Common questions about streptococcal pharyngitis. Am Fam Physician. 2016;94(1):24–31.

Keitel K, Kagoro F, Samaka J, et al. A novel electronic algorithm using host biomarker point-of-care tests for the management of febrile illnesses in Tanzanian children (e-POCT): a randomized, controlled non-inferiority trial. PLoS Med. 2017;14:e1002411.

Keitel K, Lacroix L, Gervaix A. Point-of-care testing in pediatric infectious diseases. Pediatr Infect Dis J. 2018;37:108–10.

King JR, Hammarström L. Newborn screening for primary immunodeficiency diseases: history, current and future practice. J Clin Immunol. 2018;38(1):56–66.

Kozel TR, Burnham-Marusich AR. Point-of-care testing for infectious diseases: past, present, and future. J Clin Microbiol. 2017;55(8):2313–20.

Latifi N, Kriegel G, Herskovits AZ. Point-of-care urine pregnancy tests. JAMA. 2019;322:2336–7.

Lean WL, Arnup S, Danchin M, Steer AC. Rapid diagnostic tests for group A streptococcal pharyngitis: a meta-analysis. Pediatrics. 2014;134(4):771–81.

Lee JJ, Verbakel JY, Goyder CR, Ananthakumar T, Tan PS, Turner PJ, et al. The clinical utility of point-of-care tests for influenza in ambulatory care: a systematic review and meta-analysis. Clin Infect Dis. 2019;69:24–33.

Lee TG, Yu ST, So CH. Predictive value of C-reactive protein for the diagnosis of meningitis in febrile infants under 3 months of age in the emergency department. Yeungnam U J Med. 2020;37(2):106–11.

Mathur G, Mathur S. Antibody testing for COVID-19: can it be used as a screening tool in areas with Low prevalence? Am J Clin Pathol. 2020;154:1–3.

McIsaac WJ, White D, Tannenbaum D, Low DE. A clinical score to reduce unnecessary antibiotic use in patients with sore throat. CMAJ. 1998;158:75–83.

Miceika BG, Vitous AS, Thompson KD. Detection of group A streptococcal antigen directly from throat swabs with a ten-minute latex agglutination test. J Clin Microbiol. 1985;21(3):467–9.

Moffet HH, Parker MM, Sarkar U, Schillinger D, Fernandez A, Adler NE, et al. Adherence to laboratory test requests by patients with diabetes: the Diabetes Study of Northern California (DISTANCE). Am J Manag Care. 2011;17(5):339–44.

Morgan M, Perez K, Cavanaugh M. Tips for COVID 19 specimen collection for pediatric patients. 2020. https://www.advocatehealth.com/covid-19-info/_assets/documents/ambulatory-physician-office/covid-19-specimen-collection-for-pediatric-patients.pdf. Accessed 30 Jan 2021.

Morris DE, Cleary DW, Clarke SC. Secondary bacterial infections associated with influenza pandemics. Front Microbiol. 2017;23(8):1041.

Nathan DM, Griffin A, Perez FM, Basque E, Do L, Steiner B. Accuracy of a point-of-care Hemoglobin A1c assay. J Diabetes Sci Technol. 2019;13:1149–53.

Nationwide Children's. Comfort hold techniques 2016. Retrieved on January 29, 2021, https://www.nationwidechildrens.org/family-resources-education/health-wellness-and-safety-resources/helping-hands/comfort-hold-techniques.

Nichols JH, Alter D, Chen Y, Isbell TS, Jacobs E, Moore N, Shajani-Yi Z. AACC Guidance Document on Management of Point-of-Care Testing. J Appl Lab Med. 2020;5(4):762–87. https://doi.org/10.1093/jalm/jfaa059. PMID: 32496555.

Nichols JH. Point-of-care testing. Clin Lab Med. 2007;27:893–908.

NIH. Panel on antiretroviral therapy and medical management of children living with HIV. (2019) Guidelines for the Use of Antiretroviral Agents in Pediatric HIV Infection. Retrieved January 31, 2021, http://aidsinfo.nih.gov/content- les/lvguidelines/pediatricguidelines.pdf

NIH. SARS-CoV-2 testing. In: COVID-19 treatment guidelines (2021). Retrieved January 29, 2021, https://www.covid19treatmentguidelines.nih.gov/overview/sars-cov-2-testing

O'Brien MJ, Sacks DB. Point-of-care hemoglobin A1c. JAMA. 2019;322:1404–5.

Pai NP, Wilkinson S, Deli-Houssein R, Vijh R, Vadnais C, Behlim T, et al. Barriers to implementation of rapid and point-of-care tests for human immunodeficiency virus infection. Point Care. 2015;14:81–7.

Park Y, Choe Y, Park O, Park S, Kim Y, Kim J, et al. Contact tracing during coronavirus disease outbreak, South Korea, 2020. Emerg Infect Dis. 2020;26(10):2465–8.

Patel K, Suh-Lailam BB. Implementation of point-of-care testing in a pediatric healthcare setting. Crit Rev Clin Lab Sci. 2019;56(4):239–46.

Patel NA. Pediatric COVID-19: systematic review of the literature. Am J Otolaryngol. 2020;41(5):102573.

Patton SR, Noser AE, Youngkin EM, Majidi S, Clements MA. Early initiation of diabetes devices relates to improved glycemic control in children with recent-onset type 1 diabetes mellitus. Diabetes Technol Ther. 2019;21(7):379–84.

Pondaven-Letourmy S, Alvin F, Boumghit Y, Simon F. How to perform a nasopharyngeal swab in adults and children in the COVID-19 era. Eur Ann Otorhinolaryngol Head Neck Dis. 2020;137:325–7.

Prince K, Omar F, Joolay Y. A comparison of point of care C-reactive protein test to standard C-reactive protein laboratory measurement in a neonatal intensive care unit setting. J Trop Pediatr. 2019;65:498–504.

Pritt BS, Patel R, Kim TJ, Thomson RB. Point-counterpoint: a nucleic acid amplification test for streptococcus pyogenes should replace antigen detection and culture for detection of bacterial pharyngitis. J Clin Microbiol. 2016;54(10):2413–9.

Roulliaud M, Pereira B, Cosme J, Mourgues C, Sarret C, Sapin V, et al. Evaluation of the capillary assay of C-reactive protein (CRP) through the length of consultation in pediatric emergencies and its economic impact. Ann Biol Clin (Paris). 2018;76:545–52.

Samuel L. Point-of-care testing in microbiology. Clin Lab Med. 2020;40(4):483–94.

Scott K. The labs no one inspects | AACC.org. Retrieved January 18, 2021., https://www.aacc.org/cln/articles/2019/janfeb/the-labs-no-one-inspects. Accessed 18 Jan 2021.

Shapiro DJ, Lindgren CE, Neuman MI, Fine AM. Viral features and testing for streptococcal pharyngitis. Pediatrics. 2017;139:e20163403.

Shephard A, Smith G, Aspley S, Schachtel BP. Randomised, double-blind, placebo-controlled studies on flurbiprofen 8.75 mg lozenges in patients with/without group A or C streptococcal throat infection, with an assessment of clinicians' prediction of 'strep throat'. Int J Clin Pract. 2015;69:59–71.

Shulman AJ. Office rapid strep tests: state of the art. Contemp. Pediatr. 2015: Retrieved January 25, 2021, https://www.contemporarypediatrics.com/view/office-rapid-strep-tests-state-art.

Shulman AM. POC influenza testing: state of the art. Contemp Pediatr. 2016; Retrieved January 29, 2021, https://www.contemporarypediatrics.com/view/poc-influenza-testing-state-art

Shulman ST, Bisno AL, Clegg HW, Gerber MA, Kaplan EL, Lee G, et al. Infectious Diseases Society of America. Clinical practice guideline for the diagnosis and management of group A streptococcal pharyngitis: 2012 update by the Infectious Diseases Society of America. Clin Infect Dis. 2012;55(10):e86–102.

Spooner E, Govender K, Reddy T, Ramjee G, Mbadi N, Singh S, Coutsoudis A. Point-of-care HIV testing best practice for early infant diagnosis: an implementation study. BMC Public Health. 2019;19:731.

Szablewski CM, Chang KT, Brown MM, Chu VT, Yousaf AR, Anyalechi N, et al. SARS-CoV-2 transmission and infection among attendees of an overnight Camp—Georgia, June 2020. MMWR Morb Mortal Wkly Rep. 2020;69(31):1023–5.

Tang YW, Schmitz JE, Persing DH, Stratton CW. Laboratory diagnosis of COVID-19: current issues and challenges. J Clin Microbiol. 2020;58(6):e00512–20.

Thompson TZ, McMullen AR. Group A streptococcus testing in pediatrics: the move to point-of-care molecular testing. J Clin Microbiol. 2020;58(6): e01494–19.

Tran NK, May L, Hall A, Bullen T, Waldman S, Rodrigo J, et al. LBP rapid combined flu A/B and SARS-CoV-2 RNA polymerase chain reaction testing for emergency and ambulatory care settings. Accessed January 29, 2020., https://health.ucdavis.edu/blog/lab-best-practice/rapid-combined-flu-ab-and-sars-cov-2-rna-polymerase-chain-reaction-testing-for-emergency-and-ambulatory-care-settings/2020/11

Tsai CM, Lin CR, Zhang H, Chiu IM, Cheng CY, Yu HR, Huang YH. Using machine learning to predict bacteremia in febrile children presented to the emergency department. Diagnostics. 2020;10(5):307.

Tsao Y-T, Tsai Y-H, Liao W-T, Shen C-J, Shen C-F, Cheng C-M. Differential markers of bacterial and viral infections in children for point-of-care testing. Trends Mol Med. 2020;26:1118–32.

United States Preventive Services Task Force, Owens DK, Davidson KW, Krist AH, Barry MJ, Cabana M, et al. Screening for HIV infection: US preventive services task force recommendation statement. JAMA. 2019;321(23):2326.

Van Hecke O, Raymond M, Lee JJ, Turner P, Goyder CR, Verbakel JY, Van den Bruel A, Hayward G. In-vitro diagnostic point-of-care tests in paediatric ambulatory care: a systematic review and meta-analysis. PLoS One. 2020;15(7):e0235605.

Westlake P. Procise CRP Assay Receives CE Mark. 2020. Available at: https://clpmag.com/diagnostic-technologies/clinical-chemistry/procise-crp-assay-receives-ce-mark/.

White CB, Bass JW, Yamada SM. Rapid latex agglutination compared with the throat culture for the detection of group a streptococcal infection. Pediatr Infect Dis. 1986;5(2):208–12.

Whitley HP, Yong EV, Rasinen C. Selecting an A1C point-of-care instrument. Diabetes Spectr. 2015;28: 201–8.

Wilson E, Donovan CV, Campbell M, Chai T, Pittman K, Seña AC, et al. Multiple COVID-19 clusters on a University Campus—North Carolina, August 2020. MMWR Morb Mortal Wkly Rep. 2020;69: 1416–8.

Care of the Child with an Infectious Disease or Immunological Defect

Ashley N. Gyura and Emily R. Harrison

Learning Objectives

After completing the chapter, the learner should be able to:

1. Differentiate diagnostic lab tests used in pediatric infectious diseases.
2. Evaluate the clinical indications for diagnostic tests in a variety of pediatric infections.
3. Critique diagnostic tests with an understanding of their pitfalls.
4. Prioritize the best diagnostic tests to develop a diagnosis.
5. Discriminate different laboratory tests used in infectious diseases.

6.1 Introduction

The child who presents with a history of fever or symptoms that point to an infectious disease needs specific testing for a clinician to verify the diagnosis. It is important to understand the different types of tests and their limitations. There has been an explosion in the field of molecular testing. Rapid molecular testing allows for a depth of interrogation that cannot be obtained with conventional microbiology (Graf and Pancholi 2020;

Baird 2019). Due to the emergence of resistant strains and complex patient scenarios, new infectious disease tests provide rapid results with greater sensitivity than previously available. Diagnostic test stewardship asks clinicians to consider whether the right patient is receiving the right test at the right time (Messacar et al. 2017). The information in this chapter and the point of care chapter provides an overview of the available infectious disease testing.

6.2 Methods for Infectious Disease Testing

Laboratory detection of bacteria, fungi, and viruses is a fundamental and complex process that plays a critical role in therapeutic decision-making. Serology, antigen detection, molecular testing, culture, and direct tissue visualization are the foundation of infectious disease testing.

6.2.1 Serology

The immune system produces immunoglobulins (Ig) in response to immunogenic antigens. There are five Ig classes: IgA, IgD, IgE, IgG, and IgM. Infectious disease testing focuses primarily on the detection of IgG and IgM. Antibody testing is performed most commonly on serum or plasma, but other body fluids can be analyzed.

A. N. Gyura (✉) · E. R. Harrison
Department of Infectious Disease, Children's
Minnesota, St Paul, MN, USA

© The Author(s), under exclusive license to Springer Nature Switzerland AG 2022
R. M. John (ed.), *Pediatric Diagnostic Labs for Primary Care: An Evidence-based Approach*,
https://doi.org/10.1007/978-3-030-90642-9_6

Upon exposure to a new antigen, immature B lymphocytes differentiate into plasma cells, which, in turn, secrete soluble antibodies. The time course and amount of antibody produced depend on the infectious agent, the antigen's immunogenicity, and the host immune status. Typically, an initial antibody response with IgM is detectable 5–7 days after exposure; then, IgG becomes detectable 7–10 days after exposure (Theel 2019). IgM levels soon wane, while IgG levels increase, so that by 2–3 months after exposure, only IgG levels remain detectable. Often IgG can remain detectable for life, even without repeated exposure. With future exposure to the same antigen, resting memory B cells will rapidly stimulate antibody production—predominately IgG with some production of IgM. Detection of IgG may not indicate protection against reinfection.

Serologic tests can give qualitative or quantitative results. Quantitative results are reported with a titer, which is the greatest dilution of the sample with the detectable antibody activity. A higher titer indicates more antibodies present than a lower titer (e.g., 1:64 is higher than 1:4). Since there can be variability in measuring titers, a fourfold (or 2-dilution) difference is considered a significant change.

The presence of IgM antibodies may indicate acute infection. However, IgM can persist for months or years after exposure, so detection may not always indicate acute infection. False-positive IgM results may occur due to polyclonal B cell activation and cross-reactivity between closely related pathogens. It may take 1–2 weeks for IgM to become detectable; therefore, a negative result does not exclude early disease. The presence of IgG antibodies indicates past exposure either through infection or vaccination. A single IgG value cannot determine the stage of infection; high IgG titers do not necessarily indicate recent infection.

Change in antibody titers over time can provide more conclusive evidence of recent infection. Antibody titers from an acute sample collected soon after exposure are compared to titers from a convalescent sample collected 2–4 weeks later. Recent infection is confirmed when converting from negative to positive titers (seroconversion) or a fourfold rise in antibody titers.

Avidity testing can also help determine the time elapsed since exposure. Avidity is the antibody-antigen interaction's overall strength, strengthening with time since initial exposure and repeat exposures (Theel 2019). There is low avidity early in infection, followed by increased avidity later in infection. Timing of infection during pregnancy may be particularly important to assess the risk of congenital infection. Interpretation of avidity can be complicated by the persistence of low avidity IgG antibodies that can persist for months to years. Therefore, low avidity IgG does not always represent acute infection.

There are different serologic testing methods used to detect antibodies and antigens. Benefits and limitations are summarized in Table 6.1. Pathogens are tested with different assays standardized by laboratory protocol; the clinician typically does not select the type of immunoassay.

6.2.1.1 Agglutination Assay

Agglutination assays rely on antigen binding to its corresponding antibody to cause visible clumping, which is considered a positive reaction. IgM is a large molecule with multiple binding sites for antigens, making it more efficient at agglutination than IgG, which has few binding sites. Examples include the monospot test for detection of heterophile antibodies that are often present in Epstein-Barr virus (EBV) infection and rapid plasma reagin (RPR) and venereal disease research laboratory (VDRL) tests for detection of syphilis. The assay can also result in false negatives due to the prozone phenomenon when there is a lack of agglutination due to excessive antibodies in the sample (Theel 2019).

6.2.1.2 Complement Fixation

Complement fixation (CF) is a two-step process that uses complement to lyse indicator red blood cells (RBCs). In the first step, patient serum is mixed with lab-derived antigen plus standardized complement. If corresponding antibodies are present in the patient sample, they will form complexes with the antigen and bind ("fix") circulating complement. In step two, RBCs are added to the sample. If antibody-antigen complexes are

Table 6.1 Benefits and limitations of common immunoassays

Test	Benefits	Limitations
Agglutination assay	Inexpensive Easy to perform Semiquantitative	Limited sensitivity Possibility of prozone phenomenon False positives, particularly in the presence of rheumatoid factor
Complement fixation	Very sensitive Semiquantitative The only method for less commonly tested pathogens	Technically difficult Long turnaround time
Neutralization assay	Confirmatory assay	Technically difficult
Immunofluorescent assay	Easy to perform Semiquantitative	Requires special equipment Difficult to interpret
Chemiluminescent immunoassay	Very sensitive Inexpensive	Requires special equipment
Western blot and immunoblot	Confirmatory assay	Subjective interpretation by laboratory technicians
Enzyme immunoassays	Commonly used More objective Readily automated	False positives, particularly in the presence of rheumatoid factor

Adapted from Theel (2019)

present, complement is fixed, and RBCs are saved from lysis. However, if no antibodies are present, the complement remains active and will lyse RBCs. CF may be the only method available for less commonly tested pathogens. However, many CF assays have been replaced by enzyme immunoassays (EIAs).

6.2.1.3 Neutralization Assay

Neutralization assays detect the presence of neutralizing antibodies, which are antibodies that can reduce viral infectivity. The plaque reduction neutralization test (PRNT) is one method used in which a patient sample is incubated at serial dilutions with a live virus. If neutralizing antibody is present, it will inactivate the virus. The mixture is then inoculated into wells and assessed days later for plaque formation, indicating a live virus without neutralizing antibodies. This assay may be done as confirmatory testing by a reference laboratory. For example, PRNT for anti-Zika virus (ZIKV) IgM may be performed as a highly specific confirmatory test since other immunoassays are limited by cross-reactivity of ZIKV antibodies with other flaviviruses.

6.2.1.4 Immunofluorescent Assay

Immunofluorescent assays (IFAs) use fluorescently labeled antibodies to detect antigens or antibodies in serum. Direct IFAs use fluorescently labeled antibodies to detect an antigen in tissue or body fluid. Indirect IFAs incubate the antigen of interest with the patient sample for detection of patient antibodies. An antibody-antigen complex is formed, and secondary fluorescently labeled antibodies to human IgG or IgM are added to detect the complexes present.

6.2.1.5 Chemiluminescent Immunoassays

Chemiluminescent immunoassays (CIAs) use chemiluminescent labels tagged on an antigen, antibody, or enzyme reactant. The labels are detected during the oxidation of compounds that emit light.

6.2.1.6 Western Blot and Immunoblot

These assays demonstrate proteins that are recognized by patient antibodies. In Western blot, pathogen-specific proteins are separated into bands by electrophoresis according to molecular weight or charge and then transferred to a filter paper. Pre-blotted membranes can also be used. The immobilized proteins are incubated with patient serum; patient antibodies to specific separated proteins are visualized with enzymes conjugated to antihuman antibodies. Results are reported with the number of bands to which a sample has active antibodies and are interpreted based on a specific band pattern. These assays are used for confirmatory testing, as in the detection of antibodies to *Borrelia burgdorferi*.

6.2.1.7 Enzyme Immunoassay

EIAs are assays that use enzymes as labels. Enzyme-linked immunosorbent assay (ELISA) is often used interchangeably with EIA; however, it specifically refers to an assay in which the antibody-antigen complex adheres to a solid matrix and a second enzyme-labeled antibody is used for detection. The process can be referred to as "capture" or "sandwich" since the patient antibodies are "sandwiched" between the solid phase antigen and the labeling antibody. Enzyme labels can be fluorescent, luminescent, or chromogenic. Early assays had low sensitivity and specificity for IgM, although updated procedures have improved (Theel 2019). Table 6.1 reviews the benefits and limitations of common immunoassays.

6.2.2 Antigen Detection

Antigen testing identifies target proteins in a clinical specimen. Rapid immunoassays, specifically lateral flow immunoassays, are a commonly used format for antigen testing. While useful in infectious disease testing, this is also the format used at home or for rapid pregnancy tests. An antigen of interest in the patient sample is captured by dedicated antibodies, which, if present, appear as a visible line on the test strip. There is also a control band to confirm the test is working properly. Rapid antigen testing has many uses, including detecting HIV (especially in low-resource settings), malaria, *Streptococcus pneumoniae*, and group A streptococcus. Antigen testing is often inexpensive and easy to use, requires no specialized equipment, and has rapid turnaround time, making it ideal for point-of-care testing. However, these assays generally have lower sensitivity, cannot be automated, and require subjective test interpretation.

6.2.3 Molecular Diagnostics

Molecular tests detect the genetic material of a pathogen, either RNA, DNA, or nucleic acids.

Molecular testing can be point of care or laboratory-based. There are two main methods, non-amplified nucleic probes and nucleic acid amplification tests, which are described below. Box 6.1 provides examples of commonly used molecular diagnostic tests.

6.2.3.1 Non-amplified Nucleic Acid Probes

Nucleic acid probes are RNA or DNA segments with reporter molecules that bind to a complementary nucleic acid sequence in a clinical specimen. Often these probes cannot be used to test clinical specimens directly because too few organisms are present. However, non-amplified nucleic acid probes may be useful in clinical settings where a high number of organisms are present (e.g., group A streptococcus pharyngitis or genital infection with *Neisseria gonorrhoeae* or *Chlamydia trachomatis*). Probes also have utility in identifying organisms already isolated in cultures, such as mycobacteria or dimorphic fungi (Nolte and Wittwer 2016).

6.2.3.2 Nucleic Acid Amplification Tests

Nucleic acid amplification tests (NAATs) are widely used tests to amplify small amounts of genetic material for detection. NAATs can be performed on many different specimen types. Polymerase chain reaction (PCR) is a common technique; other NAAT techniques include transcription-based amplification methods, strand displacement amplification, and loop-mediated amplification.

PCR uses DNA polymerase to synthesize many copies of a nucleic acid target sequence. Conventional PCR techniques are used for DNA amplification. Reverse transcriptase PCR was developed to amplify RNA targets by first converting an RNA template to DNA and then proceeding through PCR amplification. Nested PCR refers to PCR amplification followed by a second round of PCR on the product of the first round. Nested PCR improves the sensitivity and specificity of testing but increases the risk of amplifying sample contaminants. Real-time PCR performs amplification and analysis simultaneously to provide results more quickly. Multiplex PCR panels are available that can amplify multiple targets simultaneously.

PCR results may be either qualitative or quantitative. Quantitative PCR testing can measure the initial number of copies present in the sample, which can be clinically useful in following response to therapy, such as monitoring HIV viral load.

NAATs generally have high sensitivity and specificity. However, they are susceptible to contamination, which may lead to false positives. Detection of genetic material does not confirm the presence of viable infectious material.

Box 6.1 Examples of Molecular Diagnostic Tests by Commonly Tested Source of Specimen

Respiratory
Respiratory multiplex panel (detects bacteria and viruses).
Group A streptococcus.
Mycoplasma pneumoniae.
Methicillin-resistant *Staphylococcus aureus.*
Mycobacterium tuberculosis.

Genitourinary
Chlamydia trachomatis.
Neisseria gonorrhoeae.
Trichomonas vaginalis.
Group B *streptococcus.*
Bacterial vaginosis.

Blood
HIV.
Hepatitis viruses (A, B, C).
Blood multiplex panel for positive blood culture (detects bacteria and yeast).
Carbapenem resistance in gram-negative bacteria.

Stool
Enteric multiplex panel (detects bacteria, viruses, and parasites).
Clostridium difficile.

Cerebrospinal fluid
Meningitis/encephalitis multiplex panel (detects bacteria and viruses).

Multiple specimen types
Varicella-zoster virus (specimen: superficial swabs, cerebrospinal fluid, blood).
Herpes simplex virus (specimen: superficial swabs, cerebrospinal fluid, blood).

Adapted from Murray et al. 2021

6.2.4   Culture

Conventional cultures remain a widely used method of detection for bacteria and fungi. However, the use of viral cultures to assist with clinical decision-making has diminished with the development of accurate and accessible molecular methods of viral detection. Importantly, culture-based methods rely on optimal environmental elements for growth; deviations from the optimal collection, storage, transport, and processing can decrease the likelihood of organism recovery.

6.2.4.1 Specimen Collection

The goal of microbial culture is to isolate and identify organisms that are causing infection. A key factor in specimen collection is avoiding introducing colonizing bacteria from the collection site through appropriate disinfecting techniques and optimized collection devices or obtaining samples during surgical procedures. Ideally, the sample should be collected soon after disease onset and before antimicrobial therapy initiation. Specimen collection type should be considered carefully based on anatomic site to optimize pathogen detection while preventing nonpathogenic or colonizing organism growth. For example, when collecting a sample for bacterial culture from the urinary tract, a midstream or catheterized urine may be considered appropriate, whereas "bagged" urine from infants is considered inappropriate (Thomson 2002). Specimen selection and collection guides are often made available to clinicians specific to their organization, and standardized guides can also be found online (Miller et al. 2018).

6.2.4.2 Specimen Storage and Transport

After collecting the specimen, the viability of the organism depends on proper storage and transport. The transport system should be chosen according to current guidelines. (Clinical and Laboratory Standards Institute [CLSI] 2019). The transport system is particularly important when specimens cannot be immediately taken to the laboratory after collection. Fastidious microbes are especially sensitive to environmental conditions and may have unusual transport and storage requirements to optimize detection (Wilson et al. 2015). Institutional laboratory test guides or manuals for specimen storage and transport should be followed closely to maintain the microorganism's viability.

6.2.4.3 Specimen Processing

Four primary elements promote the growth of an organism (Lagier et al. 2015). First, different organisms require different nutrients to promote optimal growth. Culture media contains the appropriate nutrients to sustain a microbe and can vary in different ingredients, allowing the medium to select for or against certain microbes. Second, different organisms utilize different methods of metabolizing compounds to create energy for growth, and the atmosphere should be adjusted for the specific organism that is being isolated. For example, aerobic bacteria require oxygen for growth, while anaerobic bacteria cannot grow in the presence of oxygen. Facultative organisms are the most versatile and can adapt to either aerobic or anaerobic conditions (Hentges 1996). Third, organisms have optimum temperatures for growth. Last, the incubation time needed to grow a pathogen differs dramatically based on the organism. Although many clinical pathogens will grow within 24–48 h, some pathogens may require a much longer incubation time (Wilson et al. 2015). When there is a high suspicion for an unusual or specific organism, the clinician should notify the laboratory to optimize culture techniques.

6.2.4.4 Antimicrobial Susceptibility Testing

The primary purpose of performing susceptibility testing is to guide decision-making for individual children. Selecting the appropriate antimicrobial medication to which a particular organism is susceptible can both optimize infection-related outcomes and reduce overall mortality (Kollef 2000). A secondary but important purpose for performing susceptibility testing is to amass data on the patient population of a particular facility or organization to create an antibiogram (Reller et al. 2009).

An antibiogram is a composite profile of antimicrobial susceptibility testing results of a specific organism to routinely tested and clinically useful antimicrobial drugs in a given population (Barlam et al. 2016). An antibiogram is useful for clinicians in making antibiotic choices when a pathogen is not isolated or susceptibilities are not yet available. For example, the choice of empiric therapy for a *Staphylococcus aureus* skin and soft tissue infection may differ significantly in geographical or organizational areas known to have elevated rates of methicillin-resistant *Staphylococcus aureus* (MRSA). Clinicians should be aware of the current antimicrobial susceptibility profiles in their area or facility to effectively treat patients.

Methods. A basic understanding of the methods utilized for susceptibility testing is useful when interpreting results. Susceptibility testing can be performed utilizing qualitative or quantitative methods. Qualitative susceptibility testing, primarily the disk diffusion or Kirby-Bauer method, utilizes small, antibiotic-impregnated disks placed onto an agar plate that has been inoculated with the organism. The antibiotic molecules diffuse out from the disk and inhibit the organism's growth in the area around the disk based on its susceptibility to the drug. This area, or zone diameter, in which the organism growth is inhibited is measured and compared to standardized measurements. Although this method is simple and inexpensive, it can also be prone to error depending on the antimicrobial, organism, and light source position. This method does not provide a minimum inhibitory concentration (MIC).

Quantitative methods are considered the reference methods for susceptibility testing as they have high reproducibility (Kuper et al. 2009). Examples of quantitative methods include agar dilution, the E test, and broth micro- and macrodilution. Importantly, quantitative methods of susceptibility testing can measure the MIC, defined as the lowest concentration of a specific antibiotic that inhibits an organism's visible growth (Andrews 2001). In the modern microbiology laboratory, there are now many different automated methods used to perform susceptibility testing and provide MICs. Importantly, these automated methods must be consistent with the quantitative reference methods.

Interpretation. Once complete, the results are compared to a set of standard interpretations, known as breakpoints, which define susceptibility and resistance to antimicrobials. Depending on the method used, these breakpoints are expressed either as a concentration or a zone diameter (Turnidge and Paterson 2007). Breakpoints are set by both the Food and Drug Administration (FDA) and the Clinical and Laboratory Standards Institute (CLSI), a non-profit, globally recognized standards development organization. The established breakpoints allow the organism to be classified into three interpretive categories for each antimicrobial tested: susceptible, intermediate, or resistant. The interpretive categories, laboratory findings, and clinical application of antimicrobial breakpoints are described in Table 6.2.

Although the interpretive categories are a practical necessity for most busy clinicians, there are considerations even within these interpretations. Routinely, the MICs of specific antimicrobials do not require comparison to choosing an effective treatment, as antimicrobials have different established breakpoints. The MIC can be important regardless of the interpretive category in some critical infections such as bacteremia or endocarditis. For example, in invasive MRSA infections, a vancomycin MIC of 1–2 ug/mL may be associated with treatment failure despite being considered susceptible per the established breakpoint (Soriano et al. 2008). In this scenario, a clinician may consider transitioning to a different medication despite a "susceptible" interpretation to vancomycin. Also, susceptibility in vitro does not always predict clinical success in vivo, nor does resistance in vitro always predict failure in vivo. The "90/60" rule was developed after observations that infections caused by susceptible isolates respond to appropriate therapy approximately 90% of the time. In contrast, infections caused by resistant isolates respond to inappropriate therapy about 60% of the time (Rex and Pfaller 2002).

There are also certain situations where a particular resistance factor may indicate clinical failure more than the MIC or the interpretative category (Doern and Brecher 2011). For example, extended-spectrum β-lactamases (ESBLs) can be produced by some members of the *Enterobacteriaceae* family, such as *Escherichia coli* and *Klebsiella pneumoniae*. Despite having low MICs to beta-lactam antimicrobials in vitro, a strain of *Escherichia coli* expressing an ESBL is likely to result in clinical treatment failure if treatment is attempted with a beta-lactam antibiotic (Yang et al. 2010).

6.2.4.5 Viral Cultures

Culture-based systems have been considered the gold standard for virus isolation for decades (Hodinka 2013). Traditional cell culture methods utilize different cell lines (e.g., primary rhesus monkey kidney cells or primary rabbit kidney cells) inoculated with a sample, incubated, and monitored daily for changes to the cells that indicate isolation of a virus. This method allows the detection of various viruses; however, it requires significant time for incubation, is labor-intensive, and is associated with high costs to purchase and maintain the various cell lines (Hematian et al. 2016). Novel methods of viral culture have decreased the necessary incubation time down to 1–2 days. For example, shell vial cultures modified the traditional cell culture to reduce virus detection time to 16–72 h. This method involves inoculation of the specimen into cells grown on coverslips, which are then centrifuged and incubated (Ginnocchio et al. 2015). Regardless of the method, viral cultures often require specialized facilities and technician expertise.

Table 6.2 Interpretation and clinical application of antimicrobial susceptibility breakpoints

Interpretive category	Laboratory finding		Clinical application
	Qualitative	Quantitative (MIC)	
Susceptible	Zone diameter ≥ established breakpoint	MIC ≤ established breakpoint	The organism is likely to respond to treatment with a standard antimicrobial dosage
Susceptible dose-dependent	N/A	N/A	Only reported for select antimicrobial/microbe combinations. Increased doses, dose frequency, or change in infusion times can predict susceptibility
Intermediate	Zone diameter between susceptible and resistant breakpoints	MIC close to achievable serum concentration for a standard dose of antimicrobial	"Buffer zone" between the susceptible and resistant categories to prevent serious interpretive errors. May consider the antimicrobial when it concentrates at the site of infection (such as in urine). May consider the antimicrobial if higher than standard dosages can be safely utilized
Resistant	Zone diameter ≤ established breakpoint	MIC ≥ established breakpoint	The organism is unlikely to respond to treatment with standard antimicrobial dosage. The dosage needed to treat will cause toxicity in humans

MIC minimum inhibitory concentration
Adapted from Turnidge and Paterson (2007), Nielsen et al. (2019)

6.2.5 Direct Visualization and Tissue Biopsy

When diagnosis remains unclear after less invasive testing, tissue and fluid samples from suspected infection sites can be tested. Specimens can be examined for histologic features of infection, incubated for culture growth, or submitted for molecular testing. Biopsy should be guided by the suspected organism or condition and pursued in collaboration with surgery or interventional radiology. For example, if there is suspicion for nontuberculous mycobacterium lymphadenitis, excisional biopsy is recommended rather than incision and drainage or fine needle aspirate (Griffith et al. 2007). Even a well-executed tissue biopsy may not collect a specimen with active infection. A negative biopsy cannot exclude infection.

6.3 Markers of Inflammation

Inflammatory markers can be very useful as ancillary tests in infectious disease testing, often providing clues for distinguishing viral from bacterial infection or determining the severity of illness. Table 6.3 compares commonly used inflammatory markers.

6.3.1 Erythrocyte Sedimentation Rate

Erythrocyte sedimentation rate (ESR) is a common and inexpensive laboratory test. ESR measures the distance that red blood cells (RBCs) separate from plasma and fall in a vertical column of anticoagulated whole blood over 1 h (International Committee for Standardization in Hematology 1973). However, automated methods are becoming more widely used in many laboratories (Jou et al. 2011). Sedimentation is affected by the RBCs' size and shape, the hemoglobin concentration, and the ratio of plasma proteins. RBCs normally have a negative charge that prevents them from clumping together; the presence of increased plasma proteins, such as fibrinogen and other acute phase reactants, can neutralize these charges. This allows the RBCs to form stacks, called rouleaux, which settle very quickly, increasing the ESR when inflammation is present (McPherson and Mcpherson 2011). The ESR generally rises 24–48 h after the onset of inflammation and declines slowly, which may align with the complete resolution of inflammation more closely than other acute phase reactants (Ramsay and Lerman 2015).

Table 6.3 Comparison of inflammatory markers

	Time to elevation	Relative elevation during infection			Elevation in non-infectious conditions
		Bacterial	Fungal	Viral	
Erythrocyte sedimentation rate	24–48 h	High	High	Normal or mildly elevated	Autoimmune/autoinflammatory conditions, malignancy, post-IVIG
C-reactive protein	4–12 h	High	High	Normal or mildly elevated It can be elevated in adenovirus, CMV, influenza	Autoimmune/autoinflammatory conditions, tissue necrosis, trauma, burns, inflammatory bowel disease, malignancy
Procalcitonin	3–6 h	High	High	Normal	Severe trauma, burns, extensive surgical procedures, T-lymphocyte antibody therapy, graft-versus-host disease
Ferritin	Days	High to very high	*	High	Macrophage activating syndrome or hemophagocytic lymphohistiocytosis, iron overload, hemolytic anemia, rheumatologic disease
Serum amyloid A	3–6 h	High	High	High	Acute pancreatitis, rejection in kidney transplant, liver disease, autoimmune disease, insulin resistance, obesity, amyloidosis, and some tumors

Adapted from Zhang et al. (2019). *Data on fungal illness impacting ferritin level is lacking
h hours, *IVIG* intravenous immunoglobulin, *CMV* cytomegalovirus

The clinical indications for an ESR are the result of a careful history and physical. It is indicated when there is clinical suspicion of systemic inflammation, as seen in infection, autoimmunity, autoinflammatory conditions, and malignancy. ESR is not sensitive or specific enough to be the sole indicator of most disease processes. Variations in ESR response prohibit its use in differentiating serious or invasive infections from milder infections (Batlivala 2009). ESR is used in the diagnostic algorithm of atypical Kawasaki disease to indicate that further laboratory testing and an echocardiogram should be performed (McCrindle et al. 2017). The Jones criteria for the diagnosis of acute rheumatic fever also use ESR elevation of >30 millimeters per hour (mm/h) and > 60 mm/h. in high-risk and low-risk populations, respectively (Gewitz et al. 2015).

The interpretation of the normal values for ESR depends on age and sex, and individual labs may vary in their reference ranges. Generally accepted normal ranges are listed in Table 6.4. Notably, the ESR also increases with age, with approximately a 0.85 mm/h. increase every 5 years beyond puberty (Miller et al. 1983). Any process that elevates fibrinogen may elevate the ESR. Interpretation should consider other factors that increase and decrease the ESR, as listed in Table 6.5.

ESR often does not differ significantly between viral and bacterial infections in children with febrile illnesses of short duration (Virkki et al. 2002). Bacterial and fungal infections of longer duration will often have elevated ESR values. ESR is usually <30 mm/h in viral infections (Putto et al. 1986). Some viral infections, such as adenovirus, influenza, and cytomegalovirus, can produce a much higher ESR (Cavallo et al. 2017; Barone et al. 2000). ESR values >40 mm/h can assist with differentiation between patients with septic arthritis and those with transient synovitis (Caird et al. 2006), and the ESR is elevated in 94% of patients with acute osteoarticular infections (Spruiell et al. 2017). Chronic or subacute osteomyelitis can present with normal or slightly elevated ESR values (Ceroni et al. 2014). An extreme elevation of ESR >100 mm/h warrants further investigation, with infection as the most common cause (Abbag and Al Qahtani 2007).

ESR is almost universally elevated in Kawasaki disease, and extreme elevations are associated with coronary artery involvement

Table 6.4 Normal erythrocyte sedimentation rate by age

Age	Normal range
One month to 12 years	≤20 mm/h
>12 years[a]	Males: ≤15 mm/h
	Female: ≤20 mm/h

Adapted from Miller et al. (1983), Long and Vodzak (2018)

mm/h millimeters per hour

[a]Every 5 years beyond puberty, the normal erythrocyte sedimentation rate increases by approximately 0.85 mm/h

Table 6.5 Possible influencing factors on erythrocyte sedimentation rate

Increased ESR	Decreased ESR
Infection	Polycythemia
Anemia	Extreme leukocytosis
IVIG	Sickle cell
Pregnancy	Spherocytosis
Obesity	Disseminated intravascular
Hypoalbuminemia	coagulation
(nephrotic syndrome)	Valproic acid
Macrocytosis	Congestive heart failure
Malignancy	Glucocorticoids
Autoimmune conditions	Technical factors (cold
Autoinflammatory	specimen, sample > 2 h
conditions	old)
Technical factors (tilted	Cachexia
tube, warm specimen)	
Advanced age	
Renal failure	
Hypercholesterolemia	

Adapted from Brigden (1999)

ESR erythrocyte sedimentation rate, *IVIG* intravenous immunoglobulin

(Ghelani et al. 2013). Periodic fever syndromes often also present with ESR elevations, with ESR resolution to normal ranges between flares (Dancey et al. 2012). An elevated ESR value has been shown to correlate well with flares in patients with systemic lupus erythematosus (Fernando and Isenberg 2005), and prolonged ESR elevation is considered a poor prognostic feature in juvenile idiopathic arthritis (Beukelman et al. 2011).

6.3.2 C-Reactive Protein

C-reactive protein (CRP) is an acute-phase protein that increases in response to both acute and chronic inflammatory conditions occurring somewhere in the body (Agrawal 2005). It was named after observations in the 1930s that it reacts with C-polysaccharides of pneumococcal cell walls (Tillett and Francis 1930). CRP is produced primarily by hepatocytes in response to interleukin (IL)-1β, IL-6, and tumor necrosis factor-alpha (TNF-α) as part of the innate immune response (Khalil and Al-Humadi 2020). CRP levels rapidly increase within 4–12 h of a stimulus and have a doubling time of 8 h. CRP peaks at 2–3 days at levels 100–1000 times normal, and once the resolution of the inflammatory process begins, the levels fall rapidly (Long and Vodzak 2018). The main pathophysiologic role of CRP is to recognize foreign pathogens, stimulate opsonization, and activate the classical pathway of the complement system (Marnell et al. 2005). Several different methods of measuring CRP provide rapid and reliable results, including EIAs, monoclonal-antibody-based methods that measure agglutination (Chiesa et al. 2004).

A CRP is indicated when there is a suspicion of acute or chronic inflammation or infection and can be elevated in rheumatologic disease, infection, necrosis, trauma, burns, and malignancy. CRP is frequently utilized in combination with other tests as part of a sepsis panel or fever of unknown origin workup (Downes et al. 2018; Downes et al. 2016). CRP has been studied extensively as a marker for bacterial infection in children. Many of these studies have attempted to identify a cutoff value for predicting serious bacterial infection (SBI) in children (Chiu et al. 2019; Sanders et al. 2008). Despite this, a single CRP cutoff value has not been identified to rule in or rule out bacterial illness in a febrile child (Andreola et al. 2007).

CRP is often trended in pediatric musculoskeletal infections to assess early response to therapy and assist with the timing of the transition from intravenous to oral antibiotic therapy (Wood and Johnson 2016). CRP is also useful in some inflammatory disorders such as Kawasaki disease, which utilizes an elevated CRP within the diagnostic algorithm to indicate that further laboratory testing and an echocardiogram should be performed ((McCrindle et al. 2017). CRP is used as a marker of disease activity in Crohn's disease and, in some studies, has been useful in the differential diagnosis of inflammatory bowel disease (Vermeire et al. 2004).

When interpreting CRP, clinicians should note that some laboratories report CRP in milligrams per deciliter (mg/dL) while others report the results in milligrams per liter (mg/L). Normal CRP ranges are variable by laboratory and method. A CRP level of <1 mg/dL (10 mg/L) is generally considered normal for clinical predictive purposes, and a CRP < 2 mg/dL can assist with ruling out an SBI when the duration of the disease is >12 h (Putto et al. 1986; Van den Bruel et al. 2011). Generally, CRP levels are higher in bacterial illness than in viral illness (Tsai et al. 2020), with a value >8–10 mg/dL more likely to be associated with a bacterial infection (Andreola et al. 2007; Lee et al. 2020). Notably, this is not consistent and should not be used as the sole indicator for initiation or discontinuation of antimicrobial therapy (Nohynek et al. 1995). Certain viruses such as adenovirus, cytomegalovirus, influenza, measles, and mumps can also increase CRP levels to >10 mg/dL (Appenzeller et al. 2002). In children with fever and leukocytosis >25,000, a high CRP concentration was strongly associated with the presence of an SBI. In contrast, for children in the same study, a CRP < 3.4 mg/dL had a low positive predictive value for SBI (Kim et al. 2019).

Some studies have shown that CRP levels >10–15 mg/dL are associated with greater treatment failure and development of coronary lesions in Kawasaki disease (Kim et al. 2016), but this has not been demonstrated consistently (Rahbarimanesh et al. 2005; Kim et al. 2015). Significant variations in CRP elevations exist among inflammatory disorders and should be interpreted accordingly. Crohn's disease and rheumatoid arthritis are often associated with elevated CRP values. In contrast, systemic lupus erythematosus, ulcerative colitis, and dermatomyositis may have normal to mildly elevated CRP values despite the presence of inflammation disease (Vermeire et al. 2004).

CRP should be carefully interpreted if done very early in the course of illness (Pratt and Attia 2007). The liver synthesizes CRP. Therefore, hepatic failure may impair CRP production and should not be relied upon as a marker of infection in individuals with overwhelming sepsis and fulminant hepatic failure (Silvestre et al. 2010).

6.3.3 Procalcitonin

Procalcitonin (PCT) is the precursor of calcitonin, a hormone produced in the thyroid to regulate serum calcium concentrations. PCT is primarily produced in the C cells of thyroid tissue in healthy individuals; when an infectious or inflammatory stimulus is introduced, essentially all parenchymal tissues and cell types in the body begin to produce PCT, resulting in a rapid increase in PCT levels (Standage and Wong 2011). Animal models have demonstrated that the introduction of an infection or endotoxin results in PCT elevation within 2–6 h and a peak at 12–48 h (Zannoni et al. 2012; Standage and Wong 2011). Compared to CRP, PCT elevations are observed earlier, peak earlier, and have more rapid normalization after the stimulus has resolved.

Although PCT has been studied extensively, the optimal clinical indication remains unclear. PCT has utility as a marker of infection, sepsis, and systemic inflammation. It has been identified as having a predictive value in neonatal sepsis (Chiesa et al. 2004; Vermeire et al. 2004), pyelonephritis (Xu et al. 2014), SBI in children presenting with fever without a source (Andreola et al. 2007; Luaces-Cubells et al. 2012), bacterial infection or coinfection in lower respiratory tract infections (Principi and Esposito 2017: Kotula 3rd et al. 2018), and SBI in febrile neutropenic pediatric oncology patients (Lin et al. 2012; Arif and Phillips 2019), among others. Meta-analyses conducted to standardize PCT use for therapeutic decision-making have produced conflicting evidence, and its utility for diagnosis and prognosis of the disease remains uncertain (Becker et al. 2008). Current PCT assays are FDA-approved to aid clinicians in the following scenarios: risk assessment of critically ill patients for progression to severe sepsis and septic shock, assessment of mortality in critically ill patients, decision-making regarding antibiotic therapy for a patient with suspected or confirmed lower respiratory tract infection, and decision-making regarding antibiotic discontinuation for patients with suspected or confirmed sepsis (Microbiology Devices Panel of the Medical Devices Advisory Committee 2016). Notably, this use of PCT is based primarily on adult data.

Consensus interpretation of normative values of PCT is difficult due to conflicting cutoff points for abnormal values and differences in assays in clinical studies. A normal PCT level in uninfected adults was found to be 0.033 ± 0.003 nanograms per milliliter (ng/mL) via a highly sensitive research assay (Lee 2013); currently available commercial assays are not as sensitive and therefore are unable to detect such low levels. The first commercial assay for procalcitonin measurement has a lower limit sensitivity of 0.5 ng/mL. The second-generation PCT assay has a lower limit of sensitivity 0.05 ng/mL, an important distinction for clinicians to make when interpreting results (Long and Vodzak 2018). PCT crosses the placenta, and levels can be high in neonates even after an uncomplicated delivery.

6.3.4 Ferritin

Ferritin is a protein involved in iron storage but is also an acute phase reactant. It is hypothesized to sequester iron from infectious agents that may use iron as a nutrient source (Taylor et al. 2020). In severe infections with sepsis, high levels of proinflammatory cytokines stimulate ferritin production (Garcia et al. 2007). Ferritin rises within days of illness onset and can remain elevated for weeks after the acute inflammatory process has resolved (Birgegard et al. 1978).

Ferritin can be elevated in both viral and bacterial infections. In EBV infection, ferritin can be moderately elevated (median level of 431 ng/mL) (van de Veerdonk et al. 2012). In severe bacterial sepsis and septic shock, elevated ferritin has been associated with increased mortality. Studies have evaluated different ferritin levels as markers of severe disease; ranges of >300 ng/mL to >3000 ng/mL are associated with worse outcomes in children with sepsis (Garcia et al. 2007; Bennett et al. 2011; Tonial et al. 2017). In children with severe sepsis, a ferritin level of >1980 ng/mL is associated with increased mortality when combined with an elevated CPR of >40.8 mg/L (Carcillo et al. 2017). In severely ill patients with elevated ferritin and CRP, extreme systemic hyperinflammation as in macrophage activating syndrome (MAS) or hemophagocytic lymphohistiocytosis (HLH) should be considered. Ferritin in these children should be >500 ng/mL but can be >10,000 ng/mL (Taylor et al. 2020). Elevated ferritin is also found in patients with iron overload and chronic hemolytic anemias and rheumatologic disease such as systemic juvenile idiopathic arthritis and refractory Kawasaki disease and is associated with lower survival before bone marrow transplant (Taylor et al. 2020).

6.3.5 Serum Amyloid A

Serum amyloid A (SAA) is an apolipoprotein mainly synthesized by the liver. It can be elevated during viral, bacterial, and fungal infections. During acute phase response, SAA rises within 3–6 h, peaks within 24–48 h, and returns to baseline quickly due to its short half-life (Todorov et al. 2019; Zhang et al. 2019).

During viral infections, SAA may peak around 10–100 μg/mL from a baseline of 1 μg/mL. During bacterial or fungal infection, SAA may reach 10–1000 μg/mL (Zhang et al. 2019). SAA can also be elevated in late-onset sepsis in preterm infants, acute pancreatitis, rejection in kidney transplant recipients, liver disease, autoimmune disease, insulin resistance, obesity, amyloidosis, and some tumors. Unlike CRP, which can be decreased by corticosteroids, SAA is not affected by corticosteroids (Zhang et al. 2019). SAA may help identify early viral disease as it may be elevated in the setting of normal CRP (Zhang et al. 2019).

6.3.6 Other Markers of Inflammation

Many other acute-phase proteins can increase or decrease with inflammation. Markers including ceruloplasmin, haptoglobin, hepcidin, fibrinogen, α_1-acid glycoprotein, and D-dimer can increase with inflammation (Bu et al. 2016; Gabay and Kushner 1999; Hedegaard et al. 2015; Lee et al. 2018). Others, such as albumin, decrease with inflammation (Gabay and Kushner 1999). Levels of cytokines, such as IL-1, IL-6, IL-8, and TNF-α, can be measured, with different cytokine response patterns seen in different disease states (Gabay and Kushner 1999; Hedegaard et al. 2015).

Key Learning about Methods of Testing for Pediatric Infectious Diseases

- Typically, IgM rises before the IgG, and the IgG will stay elevated for a longer period.
- Antigen testing is a common method used in point-of-care testing. This testing method does allow for rapid results but is less accurate than PCR testing.
- Molecular methods detect the genetic material of a pathogen, either RNA, DNA, or nucleic acids. PCR is a common method of nucleic acid amplification that can report both qualitative and quantitative results.
- NAATs generally have high sensitivity and specificity. However, they are susceptible to contamination, which may lead to false positives. Positivity may not represent the presence of a viable organism.
- For effective culture, optimal collection, storage, transport, and processing are key.
- Antibiograms can help guide empiric antimicrobial therapy.
- Inflammatory markers are nonspecific and must be interpreted with the patient's history and clinical presentation in mind.

6.4 Specific Viral Infections

6.4.1 Epstein-Barr Virus

EBV is a member of the *Herpesviridae* family of DNA viruses and is a known cause of many clinical syndromes, including infectious mononucleosis (IM), post-transplant lymphoproliferative disease, and malignancies. The clinical presentation of primary EBV infection ranges from asymptomatic to self-limited mononucleosis in healthy individuals to progressive infections in patients with immune system disorders (Cohen 2000). More than 90% of adults worldwide are seropositive for EBV, and the age of primary infection varies substantially according to socioeconomic factors (Dowd et al. 2013).

The clinical presentation of primary EBV infection in children varies with patient age. Young, healthy children are often asymptomatic or develop nonspecific symptoms. In contrast, approximately 50% of adolescents and adults develop symptomatic IM. IM is a clinical entity characterized by pharyngitis, cervical lymph node enlargement, fatigue, and fever; more than 10% of patients also develop splenomegaly, palatal petechiae, and hepatomegaly (Cohen 2000). Approximately 90% of IM is caused by EBV (Hurt and Tammaro 2007). A rash can occur, although this is more common in patients treated with amoxicillin or other penicillins (American Academy of Pediatrics [AAP] 2018). Although IM is a self-limiting illness, diagnosis may minimize complications as well as prevent unnecessary treatments.

There are several methods for EBV detection, including serology, molecular testing, and direct visualization. In addition to nonspecific heterophile antibodies, several methods can be utilized for serologic testing, such as IFAs, EIAs and ELISAs, immunoblot, and avidity testing. Molecular techniques are also important tools for the direct detection of EBV DNA, and a quantitative PCR is commonly used for measuring EBV viral load. In situations where direct visualization is necessary, in situ hybridization is the gold standard for detecting EBV-infected cells in tissues and tumors (Gartner and Preiksaitis 2015).

Several diagnostic tests are used to diagnose an EBV infection, and the common ones are listed below.

6.4.1.1 Heterophile Antibody Tests

Heterophile antibody tests, commonly called the monospot, are latex agglutination tests that identify heterophile antibodies. These antibodies are primarily IgM and develop during the first 2 weeks of illness (American Academy of Pediatrics 2018). Heterophile antibody tests can be useful in children ≥4 years when IM is suspected. A negative test should be supplemented by EBV-specific serology (Marshall-Andon and Heinz 2017). Although more expensive and less timely, EBV-specific serology is useful in diagnosing EBV in children <4 years, in patients with heterophile-negative IM, and in patients presenting with symptoms that are not classic for IM (American Academy of Pediatrics 2018).

Pitfalls. Heterophile antibody tests are qualitative tests; a positive test indicates that heterophile antibodies are present. In addition to EBV, heterophile antibodies can be found in acute HIV infection, lymphoma, or other infections, making this a nonspecific test for acute EBV infection. In adolescents, heterophile antibody tests' sensitivities range from 81% to 95% (Bruu et al. 2000). However, it has been demonstrated that only 5–50% of children <4 years develop heterophile antibodies following an acute EBV infection (Womack and Jimenez 2015: Sumaya and Ench 1985). One study found a sensitivity of 27% in children <2 years and 76% in children 25–48 months (Horwitz et al. 1981), while another identified the sensitivity to be 38% in children ≤12 years (Linderholm et al. 1994). Heterophile antibodies can be elevated up to 1 year after infection; therefore, positive heterophile antibodies can be considered diagnostic of acute EBV infection only when combined with a finding of >10% atypical lymphocytes on a complete blood count (CBC) (American Academy of Pediatrics 2018).

6.4.1.2 EBV-Specific Serology

EBV-specific serology includes EBV-specific antibodies, such as IgG and IgM antibodies to the viral capsid antigen (VCA), IgG antibody to the Epstein-Barr nuclear antigen (EBNA-1), and IgG antibody to EBV early antigen-diffuse (EA-D) (Luaces-Cubells et al. 2012). EBV-specific serology remains the method of choice for the exclusion or diagnosis of EBV infection, but challenges remain in interpreting these results. If VCA IgG, VCA IgM, EA-D, and EBNA-1 are performed in conjunction with the heterophile antibodies, 32 possible serological patterns could be generated, and disagreement remains on interpreting certain patterns (Klutts et al. 2009). Typically, VCA IgG and VCA IgM occur in high titers early in infection, whereas EBNA-1 is not present for weeks to months after infection onset. EA-D is not required for the routine assessment of EBV infection but could be helpful in some situations. For example, a highly positive EA-D in the presence of VCA IgG and EBNA-1 may indicate reactivation rather than past infection (Katz 2018). Table 6.6 describes possible interpretations of common serological patterns.

Importantly, other causes of IM should be considered if serologic markers are not consistent with acute EBV infection. These include acute HIV; CMV; toxoplasmosis; rubella; hepatitis A and B viruses; human herpesviruses 6, 7, and 8; and adenovirus (Katz 2018). Streptococcal pharyngitis also has significant overlap in presentation and often cannot be distinguished clinically from IM.

Table 6.6 Serologic markers in the diagnosis of Epstein-Barr virus infection

Possible interpretation	VCA IgM	VCA IgG	EA-D	EBNA IgG
EBV-naive	–	–	–	–
Early primary infection	+	+	+/–	–
Convalescent (3 months)	+/–	+	+/–	+/–
Past infection	–	+	+/–	+
Reactivation	–	+	+	+

Adapted from American Academy of Pediatrics (2018), Katz (2018)
VCA viral capsid antigen, *IgM* immunoglobulin M, *IgG* immunoglobulin G, *EA-D* early antigen-diffuse, *EBNA-1* Epstein-Barr nuclear antigen, *EBV* Epstein-Barr virus

6.4.1.3 Molecular Methods

Molecular methods, such as PCR, are useful in high-risk patients when a quantitative result is needed to monitor disease status and are especially helpful when evaluating EBV status in immunocompromised patients (AbuSalah et al. 2020). They are more expensive and are not needed in previously healthy children.

Key Learning about the Laboratory Diagnosis of Epstein–Barr Virus

- Serology is the method of choice for the diagnosis of EBV infection.
- Heterophile antibodies are nonspecific for EBV, but in combination with >10% atypical lymphocytes, they are considered diagnostic for acute EBV infection.
- Heterophile antibodies/monospot should only be tested in children ≥4 years due to high false-negative rates in younger children.
- Serological patterns can be difficult to interpret, and expert consensus has not occurred on all possible patterns.
- Molecular testing, including quantification of the virus, may be helpful for high-risk patients.

EBV Epstein-Barr virus.

6.4.2   Cytomegalovirus

Cytomegalovirus (CMV) is a member of the *Herpesviridae* family of DNA viruses. CMV infections manifest differently depending on the age and immune status of the host. The majority of immunocompetent children and adolescents who acquire CMV infection postnatally are asymptomatic, with only 1–10% of CMV-infected individuals developing symptoms (Adler and Marshall 2007). When symptoms are present, they may include symptoms similar to IM or mild influenza-like illness (Hodinka 2015). Other manifestations of CMV disease, such as CMV colitis, encephalitis, pneumonia, and migratory polyarthritis, have been described in immuno-

competent patients but are rare (Harrison 2014; Micallef and Galea 2018). In immunocompromised hosts, end-organ disease and severe, life-threatening complications of CMV disease are of significant concern. Symptoms may develop from primary infection, infection with a different CMV strain, or reactivation of the latent virus, leading to significant morbidity and mortality in this patient population (Kenneson and Cannon 2007). Congenital CMV is discussed in the newborn section.

In immunocompetent children or adolescents, CMV testing may be indicated in heterophile antibody-negative IM or as part of the clinical investigation for prolonged fevers (Pass 2018). Immunocompromised patients often present with fever, malaise, leukopenia, and CMV symptoms associated with the underlying disease process. Serology helps determine if a patient has ever been infected, which may be of particular importance in pregnant women, blood and organ donors, and organ transplant candidates (Pass 2018).

The laboratory diagnosis of CMV infection depends upon the specific CMV disease under consideration. Other methods, including PCR, antigenemia, and culture isolation, are also available (Hodinka 2015). Several diagnostic tests are used to diagnose a CMV infection, and the common ones are listed below.

6.4.2.1 Serological Assays for CMV

Various serologic assays are available to detect CMV IgG and IgM, including IFA, latex agglutination, and EIAs. ELISAs are the most commonly used serologic assay for identifying CMV IgM and have been found to have a positive predictive value of only 49% for primary CMV infection (De Paschale et al. 2010). The diagnosis of primary CMV infection is best accomplished by identifying CMV IgM presence in one sample while testing for CMV IgG in two patient samples at least 2 weeks apart to document seroconversion (American Academy of Pediatrics 2018). CMV IgG avidity testing may help some situations, as CMV IgG of low avidity is produced during the first few weeks to months after primary infection. CMV IgG of high avidity is produced with past or non-primary infections (Hodinka 2015). Therefore, demonstration of low-avidity CMV IgG antibody improves the specificity of a positive CMV IgM result for diagnosis of primary infection (Pass 2018).

Immunocompetent children or adolescents. Serologic detection may be utilized in a healthy child or adolescent to confirm primary CMV infection. Notably, CMV IgM has poor specificity for primary CMV infections; some individuals have persistent IgM for over 1 year after infection. IgM can also be produced during reinfection with a different CMV strain viral reactivation (Prince and Lapé-Nixon 2014).

Immunocompromised children or adolescents. Serology and viral cultures are not particularly useful in this population for diagnosing symptomatic disease because most patients are seropositive and may shed virus intermittently (Adler and Marshall 2007).

6.4.2.2 Cultures for CMV

Cultures of the urine, saliva, and blood for CMV may be positive during acute infection. However, this should be used as supporting evidence rather than confirmation of diagnosis (Adler and Marshall 2007).

6.4.2.3 PCR Testing for CMV

Immunocompromised children or adolescents. The diagnosis of CMV in immunocompromised children or adolescents can be highly complicated. Individuals at particularly high risk of CMV infection include solid organ transplant and hematopoietic stem cell transplant recipients if either the donor or the recipient is seropositive, as well as individuals with HIV and other primary or acquired immune disorders that affect T lymphocytes or natural killer cells (Pass 2018). Routine CMV quantitative PCR testing may be utilized as a screening tool for immunocompromised individuals during high-risk periods. In post-transplant patients, assays that quantify virus levels may be more useful, such as the quantitative PCR (American Academy of Pediatrics 2018). However, even detection of CMV by quantitative

PCR may represent shedding unrelated to clinical disease. The definitive diagnosis of CMV disease in the immunocompromised or post-transplant population often relies on detecting CMV in a specimen of the affected tissue to demonstrate end-organ disease (Kotton et al. 2018). The testing methods for different pediatric populations are summarized in Table 6.7.

6.4.3 Real-Life Example

An 11-year-old presented with a one-week history of sore throat, enlarged cervical adenopathy of 1.5 cm, fatigue, myalgia, and fever. A monospot was negative, and EBV serology was negative. The child's clinical presentation resembled mononucleosis, and on day 11, CMV serology was sent, which showed a positive CMV IgM and IgG. CMV was suspected as the cause of the mononucleosis, and the child recovered after 24 days of illness.

6.4.4 Varicella-Zoster Virus

Varicella-zoster virus (VZV) is a member of the *Herpesviridae* family of DNA viruses. Primary infection with VZV causes varicella, commonly called chickenpox. The virus develops latency in sensory ganglia and can reactivate to cause herpes zoster, commonly called shingles. Reactivation occurs with both wild-type VZV and vaccine-type VZV (Arvin 2018).

The classic presentation in unvaccinated individuals is a low-grade fever with a generalized, pruritic, maculopapular vesicular rash in varying stages of development and resolution, including papules, vesicles, and crusted lesions (American Academy of Pediatrics 2018). Breakthrough varicella cases, defined as chickenpox occurring >42 days after vaccination, can present with atypical clinical symptoms such as fewer and predominantly maculopapular lesions without vesicles (Weinmann et al. 2008). Varicella is more likely to cause severe disease in young infants, adolescents, and adults. Progressive and severe

Table 6.7 Overview of cytomegalovirus testing strategies in pediatric populations

Testing method		Testing strategies in various populations				Comments
		Immunocompetent	Immunocompromised	cCMV	Postnatal CMV	
PCR	Qualitative	X	X[a]	X	X	Sensitive, rapid
	DBS	–	–	X	X	Highly variable sensitivity Only performed at select research laboratories Not all infants with cCMV are viremic at birth
	Quantitative	–	X	X	X	Useful for monitoring therapy
Serology	IgM	X	–	–	–	Low specificity for primary CMV infection Very low sensitivity in newborns
	IgG	X	X	–	–	Detection of seroconversion in primary CMV infection Screening to determine serostatus (pregnant women, immunocompromised, transplant candidates, blood/organ donors) Not useful in newborns due to passive transfer of maternal antibody
Viral culture		X	X[a]	X	X	Standard tube culture: 2–4 weeks for results, not suitable for screening Shell vial assay: Rapid, expensive, variable sensitivity

Adapted from Britt (2016), Hodinka (2015), Pass (2018)

cCMV congenital cytomegalovirus, *CMV* cytomegalovirus, *PCR* polymerase chain reaction, *DBS* dried blood spot, *IgM* immunoglobulin M, *IgG* immunoglobulin G

[a] Positive qualitative PCR testing or viral culture in immunocompromised individuals may not indicate active disease

disseminated disease may occur in immunocompromised children and healthy children on high-dose steroids (Roderick and Finn 2012; Dowell and Bresee 1993). Complications of varicella in healthy and immunocompromised children may occur, including bacterial superinfection, central nervous system involvement, pneumonia, thrombocytopenia, Reye syndrome, myocarditis, hepatitis, and hemorrhagic complications (Ziebold et al. 2001). Clinical diagnosis of varicella is less reliable in the post-vaccine era. The classic maculopapular vesicular rash is seen less frequently, and the rash in vaccinated patients may lack vesicles or resemble other rashes. Therefore, laboratory testing or epidemiological linkage to a typical case or laboratory-confirmed case should be sought to confirm varicella infection (Centers for Disease Control and Prevention 2015a). Herpes zoster (shingles) typically manifests with acute neuralgia preceding the development of a unilateral vesicular eruption in the distribution of a sensory nerve and may disseminate in immunocompromised children (Centers for Disease Control and Prevention 2015a). For epidemiological purposes, primary care clinicians should confirm all suspected cases of herpes zoster in individuals <18 years.

The laboratory diagnosis of varicella can be made using direct fluorescent antibody (DFA) methods, PCR, viral culture, or a significant rise in varicella IgG.

6.4.4.1 Direct Fluorescent Antibody (DFA) Methods

A vesicular scraping for DFA staining can demonstrate VZV. This method is less sensitive than VZV PCR and cannot distinguish a wild-type from a vaccine-strain virus (American Academy of Pediatrics 2018).

6.4.4.2 Viral Culture

Viral culture for VZV, while specific, is less sensitive than PCR and can take up to 14 days to isolate (Miller et al. 2018).

6.4.4.3 PCR

The current diagnostic method of choice test for varicella is PCR of vesicular fluid, crusts, scabs, or maculopapular scraping (Centers for Disease

Control and Prevention 2015a). Laboratory techniques for PCR testing allow differentiation of wild-type and vaccine strains of VZV.

6.4.4.4 Serology

Serologic testing is rarely indicated in the diagnosis of acute infection. A fourfold increase in VZV IgG titers between acute and convalescent samples utilizing a standard serologic assay can retrospectively confirm a diagnosis, although this is unreliable in immunocompromised individuals (American Academy of Pediatrics 2018). IgG titers persist for life after primary infection. They may be useful as a screening tool to determine a person's immune status, guide decisions about the need for varicella vaccine, and evaluate the risk of infection or reactivation in individuals receiving immunosuppressive therapy (Arvin 2018). All currently available commercial assays for VZV IgM have poor sensitivity and specificity and should not be used to diagnose infection (Centers for Disease Control and Prevention 2015a). VZV laboratory testing is summarized in Table 6.8.

6.4.5   Herpes Simplex Virus

Herpes simplex virus (HSV) is a member of the *Herpesviridae* family of DNA viruses. There are two distinct HSV types, identified as HSV-1 and HSV-2. Traditionally, HSV-1 caused orolabial infections, and HSV-2 caused genital infections. However, both types can cause orolabial, genital, and neonatal disease. Due to increasing sexual preferences for oral sex, an increasing number of genital and neonatal herpes in the United States are HSV-1. However, HSV-2 is still predominant at this time (Pinniti and Kimberlin 2018; Alkhar et al., 2017). After primary infection, HSV-1 and HSV-2 remain latent in sensory neural ganglia and may reactivate periodically (Kimberlin and Prober 2018).

Common clinical syndromes in children and adolescents may include orolabial lesions or gingivostomatitis; genital herpes; keratoconjunctivitis; cutaneous infections such as a herpetic whitlow, herpes gladiatorum, or eczema herpeticum; and central nervous system disease such as

Table 6.8   Laboratory testing for varicella-zoster virus

Method	Specimen	Comments
PCR (recommended)	Vesicular fluid, crusts/scabs, maculopapular scraping, biopsy tissue, CSF	Rapid, sensitive, specific. Can distinguish wild-type from vaccine-type
DFA	Vesicular scraping	Rapid and specific Less sensitive than PCR
Viral culture	Vesicular fluid, maculopapular scraping, biopsy tissue, CSF	Specific Less sensitive than PCR and DFA Less timely than PCR and DFA
IgG	Serum	Acute and convalescent specimens may be used for retrospective diagnosis It may be useful for screening of immunity
IgM	Serum	Not recommended for use

Adapted from American Academy of Pediatrics (2018)
VZV varicella-zoster virus, *PCR* polymerase chain reaction, *CSF* cerebrospinal fluid, *DFA* direct fluorescent antibody, *IgG* immunoglobulin G, *IgM* immunoglobulin M

HSV encephalitis (American Academy of Pediatrics 2018).

Several diagnostic tests are used to diagnose an HSV infection, and the common ones are listed below.

6.4.5.1 Serology

Serology can help determine exposure status to HSV-1 and HSV-2 but should not be used as a primary diagnostic test and is not useful in neonates. Type-specific IgG antibodies indicate previous exposure to the corresponding viral serotype but do not differentiate past infection from active infection unless seroconversion is documented (Miller et al. 2018). Commonly used ELISAs for anti-HSV IgG have sensitivities between 80% and 98% (Liermann et al. 2014). Anti-HSV IgM assays have unacceptably high false-positive rates, and they cannot reliably differentiate HSV-1 and HSV-2. An elevated anti-HSV IgM can also occur with reactivation and, therefore, cannot distinguish

reactivation from primary infection (Kimberlin and Prober 2018).

6.4.5.2 Nucleic Acid Amplification Tests

HSV PCR is preferred over culture in detecting HSV from genital ulcers or vesicles and other mucocutaneous lesions due to improved sensitivity over culture (Strick and Wald 2006). PCR of CSF is the diagnostic method of choice for central nervous system disease, using an assay that distinguishes between HSV-1 and HSV-2 (Miller et al. 2018). The diagnosis of neonatal HSV infection should include testing of surface specimens (including the mouth, nasopharynx, conjunctivae, and anus), skin vesicles, CSF, and whole blood via PCR (or culture, if PCR is unavailable) for HSV-1 and HSV-2 (American Academy of Pediatrics 2018). Individual laboratories have developed many PCR assays, although there are now several FDA-approved HSV PCR tests with reported sensitivities and specificities >95% (Binnicker et al. 2014). Notably, performance characteristics of skin and mucous membrane specimens from neonates who are suspected of having HSV have not been studied. In HSV encephalitis, PCR assay can yield negative results early in the disease course (American Academy of Pediatrics 2018).

6.4.5.3 Viral Culture

Culture is the most specific method for diagnosing an active HSV infection, and HSV grows readily in traditional cell culture and shell vial culture. An enzyme-linked, virus-inducible system (ELVIS) is a commercially available rapid culture technique with a turnaround time of less than 1 day (Kowalski et al. 2002). Viral cultures may be performed on corneal scrapings, ocular swabs, neonatal surface swabs, and oral or genital lesion swabs. The sampling timing is important for viral cultures. HSV can be detected in >90% of genital lesions sampled during the vesicular stage instead of 25% from the crusted stage (Moseley et al. 1981). The specificity of viral culture for HSV is nearly 100%; however, the sensitivity can range anywhere from 30% to 95% depending on the clinical context, the sample obtained, and the timing of sample collection within the course of the disease. Also, sample collection methods, storage, and transport can negatively affect sensitivity (LeGoff et al. 2014).

6.4.6 HIV-1 Virus

HIV is an RNA virus classified into types 1 and 2. HIV-1 is more common than HIV-2 in the United States, but HIV-2 should be considered in patients with exposure from West Africa or exposure to an HIV-2-infected individual (Miller et al. 2018). For most populations, the recommended initial screening for HIV-1 and HIV-2 is a fourth-generation antigen/antibody combination immunoassay. DNA and RNA assays for HIV-1 are reviewed below; there are currently no molecular tests approved by the FDA for HIV-2, although specialized facilities may be able to perform this testing on individuals known to have HIV-2 (Branson et al. 2014).

HIV DNA or RNA assays are recommended in conjunction with an immunoassay (e.g., fourth-generation antigen/antibody combination assay) in children and adolescents outside the neonatal period to diagnose acute retroviral syndrome, commonly known as acute HIV. Acute retroviral syndrome is characterized by nonspecific mononucleosis-like symptoms, including fever, malaise, lymphadenopathy, and skin rash (American Academy of Pediatrics 2018). There are high levels of false-negative immunoassay results early after virus acquisition, so molecular tests are preferred in this time period. Molecular testing can also be used to confirm a new diagnosis of HIV and obtain information on viral load (Branson et al. 2014).

The timing of various diagnostic tests related to HIV exposure can dramatically affect the test's sensitivity and specificity. The sensitivity of molecular testing in patients with established HIV infection may also be lowered due to natural or therapeutic viral suppression (Miller et al. 2018).

6.4.6.1 HIV Immunoassays
Immunoassays are found in Chap. 5 under point-of-care tests.

6.4.6.2 Qualitative HIV-1 DNA and RNA PCR
These assays detect intracellular HIV-1 nucleic acids that are typically present 10–14 days after HIV exposure, in the form of either viral RNA in plasma or proviral DNA in peripheral blood mononuclear cells. It may be used to diagnose HIV-1 for children <24 months and individuals with acute or early HIV-1 infection. This test may also be utilized for early detection of HIV-1 infection in children and adolescents who may be receiving combination antiretroviral prophylaxis or preemptive treatment (Branson and Owen 2015). For diagnosis of acute HIV outside the neonatal period, qualitative HIV-1 DNA and RNA PCR tests have high specificity; false negatives may occur in the first 10 days after infection, but high sensitivity is achieved after day 10. In perinatally exposed infants, the specificity of qualitative PCR testing is high; the sensitivity is low at birth but is >90% at age 2–4 weeks and reaches 100% at ages 3 and 6 months (Lilian et al. 2012).

An "undetected" result indicates that the assay could not detect HIV-1 DNA and/or RNA within the specimen, while a "detected" result is consistent with HIV-1 infection. A first-time positive result should be repeated as soon as possible to confirm the diagnosis.

6.4.6.3 Quantitative HIV-1 RNA PCR
The quantitative HIV-1 RNA PCR, also known as a viral load, measures the quantity of HIV-1 nucleic acid RNA in plasma. HIV RNA is typically detectable in plasma 10–14 days after HIV exposure. It may be used to diagnose HIV-1 for children <24 months and individuals with acute or early HIV-1 infection. This test is primarily used to obtain a baseline viral load before therapy initiation and monitor disease progression or viral load changes during treatment (American Academy of Pediatrics 2018). HIV-1 RNA viral load assays have a high sensitivity and specificity when used to diagnose HIV infection in HIV-exposed infants and suspected acute HIV-infected patients (Lee et al. 2012).

An "undetected" result indicates that the assay was unable to detect HIV-1 RNA within the specimen. If RNA is detected, results are generally reported in copies/mL. The quantification result range varies by the test and the manufacturer. Assays known as "ultrasensitive" may provide a result that indicates HIV-1 RNA is detected but is below the lowest quantification limit of the assay. Possible causes may include false-positive results, very early HIV-1 infection, or a very low plasma HIV-1 viral load.

In children and adolescents outside the neonatal period with positive HIV DNA or RNA PCR results, a repeat sample should be sent as soon as possible to confirm the diagnosis. Positive PCR testing confirms the diagnosis of HIV.

6.4.7 Zika Virus

Zika virus (ZIKV) is an RNA virus of the *Flaviviridae* family. This virus is transmitted to humans primarily through the bite of an infected *Aedes* species mosquito. Perinatal, in utero, and presumed sexual and transfusion-related transmission events have been reported.

Testing for ZIKV infection may be considered in patients presenting with acute onset of fever, maculopapular rash, arthralgia, or conjunctivitis who live in or have traveled to an ongoing transmission area 2 weeks before the onset of symptoms (American Academy of Pediatrics 2018). The Centers for Disease Control and Prevention maintains information on countries or territories with current ZIKV outbreaks and provides travel recommendations. Dengue virus (DENV) and chikungunya virus (CHIKV) evaluations should also be initiated in patients with suspected ZIKV as these viruses have similar clinical manifestations and geographic distributions (Miller et al. 2018). Infants born to mothers with possible ZIKV exposure during pregnancy should be tested for ZIKV if they are (1) symptomatic or (2) asymptomatic with laboratory evidence of possible maternal ZIKV infection during pregnancy. Clinical findings consistent with congenital ZIKV syndrome include severe microcephaly, decreased brain tissue, ocular abnormalities, congenital contractures, and hypertonia (CDC 2019).

Testing for ZIKV depends on the presence of symptoms and a patient's pregnancy status. Dengue virus (DENV) and chikungunya virus (CHIKV) evaluations should also be initiated in patients with suspected ZIKV as these viruses have similar clinical manifestations and geographic distributions (Miller et al. 2018). The testing algorithm for symptomatic, non-pregnant patients with risk for both ZIKV and DENV is described in Fig. 6.1. Two diagnostic tests are used to diagnose a ZIKA infection and are listed below.

6.4.7.1 NAAT to Confirm the Presence of ZIKV RNA

ZIKV RNA may be detectable by NAAT several days before to several days after symptom onset and can be found in serum, whole blood, urine, and saliva. ZIKV RNA is only present transiently in body fluids; therefore, a negative PCR does not rule out infection (American Academy of Pediatrics 2018). ZIKV PCR is sensitive and specific, although the timing of sample collection is important (Jääskeläinen et al. 2019). ZIKV RNA in serum declines as antibody appears but can be shed in urine for a longer time and in higher titers than in serum (Landry and St. George 2016).

6.4.7.2 Serological Tests to Identify Antibodies Primarily Using IgM Assays and PRNT

ZIKV IgM appears 4–7 days after symptom onset and generally persists for 12 weeks, although prolonged positive ZIKV IgM has been noted years after primary infection (Mlakar et al. 2016). ZIKV IgM testing is performed utilizing an ELISA. False-positive results are common due to nonspecific reactivity and significant cross-reactivity with other flaviviruses, such as DENV. Neutralizing antibodies, consisting primarily of IgG antibodies, appear alongside IgM antibodies and can persist for years. PRNTs are quantitative assays that measure virus-specific neutralizing antibody titers for ZIKV and other flaviviruses. A titer value ≥ 10 in serum and ≥ 2 in CSF defines positive specimens and clarifies the interpretation of anti-ZIKV IgM antibody results (Sharp et al. 2019).

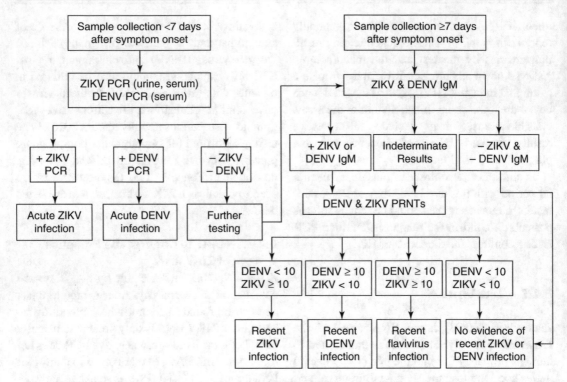

Fig. 6.1 Zika and dengue virus testing algorithm for symptomatic, non-pregnant patients with risk for both viruses. Adapted from Sharp et al. (2019). *ZIKV* Zika virus, *DENV* dengue virus, *PCR* polymerase chain reaction, *IgM* immunoglobulin M, *PRNTs* plaque reduction neutralization tests

6.4.8 Dengue Virus

DENV are RNA viruses and members of the *Flaviviridae* family. There are four types, designated DENV 1–4. A virus is transmitted to humans primarily through the bite of an infected *Aedes* species mosquito (Hills and Fischer 2018). Transmission in utero, perinatally, and, rarely, via breast milk, blood transfusions, or organ transplant has been reported (American Academy of Pediatrics 2018).

Testing for DENV may be considered in patients presenting with a clinically compatible illness (acute onset of fever plus ≥2 of the following: nausea, vomiting, rash, myalgias/arthralgias, leukopenia, or a positive tourniquet test) who live in or have traveled to an area with ongoing transmission within 2 weeks before the onset of symptoms. Approximately 75% of DENV infections are asymptomatic or cause a mild, self-limiting febrile illness (Hills and Fischer 2018). However, some patients may develop severe diseases, including pleural effusions, ascites, hypo-

volemic shock, and hemorrhage (Adebanjo et al. 2017). The Centers for Disease Control and Prevention maintains up-to-date information on countries or territories with current outbreaks of DENV and provides travel guidance. ZIKV and CHIKV evaluations should also be initiated in patients with suspected DENV, as these viruses have similar clinical manifestations and geographic distributions (Miller et al. 2018).

DENV diagnostic testing relies on molecular methods, detection of DENV nonstructural protein-1 (NS1) antigen, and serologic testing.

6.4.8.1 PCR Testing for DENV RNA

DENV RNA may be detectable via PCR testing several days before to 1 week after symptom onset. DENV PCR is highly sensitive and specific, although the timing of sample collection is important.

6.4.8.2 Antigen Testing

DENV NS1 antigens are present during the acute viremic phase and are detectable several days before to 1 week after symptom onset. Available assays for NS1 antigen include ELISA and rapid diagnostic tests, but these vary widely in sensitivity and specificity (Hills and Fischer 2018).

6.4.8.3 Serology for DENV Antibodies

DENV IgM is typically detectable 3–5 days after symptom onset. Similar to ZIKV testing, DENV IgM testing is performed with ELISA. False-positive results are more common with IgM antibody testing than with PCR due to nonspecific reactivity and significant cross-reactivity with other flaviviruses. Neutralizing antibodies, consisting primarily of IgG antibodies, appear alongside IgM antibodies and can persist for years. PRNTs are quantitative assays that measure virus-specific neutralizing antibody titers for DENV as well as other closely related flaviviruses, such as ZIKV. A value titer ≥ 10 in serum and ≥ 2 in cerebrospinal fluid defines positive specimens and clarifies the interpretation of anti-DENV IgM antibody results (Sharp et al. 2019).

Other tests, including DENV IgG and hemagglutination inhibition assays, are not specific for the diagnosis of DENV (American Academy of Pediatrics 2018).

The preferred testing for non-pregnant patients with clinical indications for DENV differs based on timing from symptom onset (see newborn chapter for Fig. 3.1). Although DENV may be tested independently from ZIKV, there is significant overlap in clinical presentation and geographical distribution, and ZIKV should be considered in the differential diagnosis. CHIKV may also be considered (Miller et al. 2018).

6.4.9 Chikungunya Virus

CHIKV is a small RNA virus of the family *Togaviridae*. CHIKV is primarily transmitted by infected *Aedes* species mosquitoes (Staples and Powers 2018). CHIKV infection should be considered in patients with acute onset of fever and polyarthralgia, especially travelers who recently returned from areas with known virus transmission. Other symptoms may include headache, myalgia, arthritis, conjunctivitis, nausea, vomiting, or rash. The majority of people infected with CHIKV become symptomatic (American Academy of Pediatrics 2018).

Routine diagnostic tests include detection of CHIKV RNA by PCR and serology.

6.4.9.1 PCR for CHIKV RNA

CHIKV RNA is detectable by PCR in serum samples up to 6–8 days after the onset of symptoms (Lanciotti et al. 2007, Lanciotti et al. 2008). CHIKV PCR tests are highly sensitive and specific when performed within this time frame. For patients with clinical indications for testing and symptom onset <6 days, initial testing should include CHIKV PCR assay on serum or CSF. A positive PCR result typically provides evidence of acute infection, and no additional antibody testing is indicated. If the PCR test is negative or serum is collected ≥ 6 days after symptom onset, CHIKV IgM antibody testing should be performed.

6.4.9.2 Serology for CHIKV Antibodies

CHIKV IgM antibodies are normally detectable in serum by day 5–7 after symptom onset and are highest 3–5 weeks after illness onset. CHIKV IgM antibodies typically persist between 30 and 90 days but have been detected up to 18 months post-infection (Grivard et al. 2007). Several methods of serologic testing are approved in the United States for CHIKV IgM antibody testing. The sensitivity of CHIKV serology improves with disease progression, with lower sensitivities at day 4 after symptom onset and higher sensitivity by day 8 (Yap et al. 2010). Neutralizing antibodies develop along with IgM antibodies and persist indefinitely and can be tested with PRNTs to discriminate false-positive tests due to cross-reacting IgM antibodies. If initial IgM antibody testing is positive, most laboratories and state health departments will perform confirmatory PRNTs. If IgM antibody testing is negative and clinical suspicion remains high, consider repeat CHIKV IgM antibody testing in 2 weeks (Johnson et al. 2016).

Blood precautions: It is important to note that CHIKV requires biosafety level 3 (BSL-3) precautions in the laboratory, and caution is recommended when handling infected blood samples. Testing for CHIKV RNA is limited by the number of facilities that can safely work with the virus. It is recommended that clinicians contact their state health department to facilitate testing.

6.4.10 COVID-19

Coronavirus disease 2019 (COVID-19) is caused by a novel coronavirus (CoV), designated SARS-CoV-2. Respiratory illness with this novel coronavirus was first reported in China at the end of 2019. By March 2020, the World Health Organization declared a global pandemic of COVID-19 due to a widespread disease outbreak. Other important coronaviruses include SARS-CoV, the cause of severe acute respiratory syndrome (SARS); MERS-CoV, the cause of the Middle East respiratory syndrome (MERS); and a group of less pathogenic CoV that cause community-acquired respiratory illness such as upper respiratory tract infection or the common cold (Tezer and Bedir Demirdağ 2020).

SARS-CoV-2 can result in asymptomatic to severe disease, including respiratory failure and death. SARS-CoV-2 can result in an excessive immune reaction due to a cytokine storm, leading to more inflammation, tissue damage, and an increased risk of clotting (Tezer and Bedir Demirdağ 2020). In general, children present with more mild or asymptomatic infections. Children can present with fever, headache, fatigue, myalgia, upper respiratory symptoms, pharyngitis, anosmia, cough, shortness of breath, tachypnea, pneumonia, bronchiolitis, and GI symptoms such as diarrhea and abdominal pain (Patel 2020). Neurological symptoms and signs include acute flaccid myelitis, Guillain-Barré syndrome, and febrile seizures (Christy 2020).

Multisystem inflammatory syndrome in children (MIS-C) is a rare complication of COVID-19 infection. The clinical signs and symptoms include cardiac dysfunction, shock, peripheral edema, fever, abdominal pain associated with diarrhea, conjunctivitis, rash, and peripheral edema. The laboratory findings included elevated inflammatory markers such as serum ferritin, CRP, D-dimer, and other inflammatory markers (Godfred-Cato et al. 2020). These markers were previously discussed (see Sect. 6.3). An elevated alanine aminotransferase, aspartate aminotransferase, creatine kinase, lactate dehydrogenase, blood urea nitrogen, and serum creatinine levels have also been reported (Nicola et al. 2020).

MIS-C can be similar in presentation to Kawasaki disease but has distinct features.

Testing for COVID-19 includes point-of-care testing, serological testing, and molecular testing. The point-of-care testing is discussed in Chap. 5.

6.4.10.1   Serological Testing

IgM and IgG antibodies increase nearly simultaneously by 2–3 weeks after the onset of COVID-19 symptoms. Still, some people develop antibodies within a week (CDC 2020d). A positive IgM indicates active or recent COVID-19 infection. Detection of IgG alone indicates past infection with COVID-19. Detection of both IgG and IgM together indicates that a patient may still be infectious. Duration of IgG and IgM detection is unknown, but in one study, antibody levels were shown to wane to undetectable levels on repeat testing (Self et al. 2020). Currently, the FDA has granted Emergency Use Authorization (EUA) to many commercial serologic assays. These detect either the spike or nucleocapsid proteins. The average sensitivity of currently available assays is 84%, and the specificity is 98% (Mathur and Mathur 2020), although individual test characteristics vary.

Serologic tests may be useful in evaluating a child who is recovering or has recovered from COVID-19 (Brooks and Das 2020). In particular, serology is helpful in the diagnosis of MIS-C to confirm recent exposure or infection to SARS-CoV-2. Documenting serologic conversion may also have utility in a child with persistently positive antigen or molecular testing, indicating an absence of acute infectious disease.

Point-of-care serologic tests use lateral flow devices to recognize IgG, IgG and IgM, or total antibodies in serum, plasma, whole blood, and/or saliva. The blood samples can be done by finger stick instead of venipuncture. ELISAs or CIAs are done in clinical laboratories.

6.4.10.2   Antigen Testing

Antigen tests detect certain SARS-CoV-2 proteins found on the viral surface as detected by swabbing the nose or nasopharynx (Brooks and Das 2020; CDC 2020e). The antigen tests are faster and cheaper than molecular tests. They are practical and quick, so they may be used when testing a large number of people. Currently, multiple commercial assays have been granted EUA by the FDA. The specificity of antigen tests is comparable to molecular-based tests. However, sensitivity is lower than molecular tests. Negative results should be interpreted in a clinical context and confirmed with molecular tests (CDC 2020e).

6.4.10.3 Molecular Testing

The molecular tests use PCR technology to detect virus while in the acute phase of a COVID-19 infection. The FDA has granted multiple assays EUA. Test characteristics vary between assays and are difficult to assess as there is no "gold standard" for COVID-19 diagnosis. Generally, these PCR assays have a high sensitivity and specificity (Hanson et al. 2020). It is preferred to collect samples for PCR testing from the nasopharynx, anterior nares, mid-turbinate ("deep nasal"), saliva, or combined anterior nares plus oropharyngeal swabs; oropharyngeal swab alone has lower sensitivity (Hanson et al. 2020). A limitation of currently available SARS-CoV-2 molecular tests is their inability to quantify viral load.

6.5 Viral Hepatitis (Hepatitis A, B, C, D, E)

While other viruses like EBV and CMV can cause a clinical hepatitis or inflammation of the liver, five well-known viruses are attributed to the majority of cases of hepatitis.

6.5.1 Hepatitis A Virus

Hepatitis A virus (HAV) is a cause of acute viral hepatitis that does not progress to chronic infection. Young children may be asymptomatic; older children often have nonspecific symptoms and may present with jaundice (American Academy of Pediatrics 2018). Hepatitis A is a vaccine-preventable illness, and vaccine recommendations are included in the childhood immunization schedule.

Antibody testing is commercially available and sufficient for HAV diagnosis (CDC 2020a). Anti-HAV IgM becomes detectable 5–10 days before symptom onset, peaks within 1 month of illness, and typically decreases to undetectable levels within 6 months of infection (CDC 2020a). IgM can persist for >1 year after infection. It is also detectable in up to 20% of HAV vaccine recipients for up to 2 weeks after vaccination. Anti-HAV IgM can be falsely positive (CDC 2020a). Positive IgM in the setting of a compatible clinical illness indicates current or recent HAV infection. Anti-HAV IgG appears shortly after detection of IgM and protects future HAV infection. Some assays test total anti-HAV antibodies, a total of both IgM and IgG against HAV. If positive, total anti-HAV indicates immunity to HAV but does not differentiate acute from past infection; further testing with anti-HAV IgM is needed to identify acute infection (CDC 2020a).

HAV RNA NAAT can detect the virus in stool and serum during the acute phase of HAV infection. However, NAATs are not routinely used to diagnose HAV as there are currently no FDA-approved assays (American Academy of Pediatrics 2018).

6.5.2 Hepatitis B Virus

Hepatitis B virus (HBV) often causes asymptomatic acute infection in children. However, HBV is an important pediatric illness as the risk of progression to chronic infection is related inversely to age at the time of exposure. The risk of progression from acute to chronic infection due to exposure in infancy (e.g., an infant born to a mother with active HBV infection or exposure in the first year of life) is 90%, whereas the risk in children exposed at 1–5 years is 25–35% and only 5–10% in older children and adults (American Academy of Pediatrics 2018; Terrault et al. 2018).

Box 6.2 reviews high-risk groups for whom HBV screening is indicated. Testing for HBV is based on the detection of HBV antigens and antibodies. It may include hepatitis B surface antigen

Table 6.9 Serologic tests recommended for testing of hepatitis B virus infection

Clinical indication for testing	Serologic testing recommended
Screening for chronic HBV infection	HBsAg, anti-HBs, anti-HBc
Suspicion for acute infection (possible recent exposure, increase in liver function tests)	HBsAg, anti-HBc IgM
Pregnancy screening	HBsAg
Children born to HBsAg-positive women who have received post-exposure immunoprophylaxis	HBsAg, anti-HBs
Post-vaccination titers	Anti-HBs

Adapted from American Academy of Pediatrics (2018), Davison and Strasser (2014)
HBV hepatitis B virus, *HBsAg* hepatitis B surface antigen, *Anti-HBs* hepatitis B surface antibody, *Anti-HBc* hepatitis B core antibody, *IgM* immunoglobulin M

(HBsAg), hepatitis B surface antibody (anti-HBs), and hepatitis B core antibody (anti-HBc). Anti-HBc IgM and IgG can be ordered separately to provide additional information on the timing of infection. Hepatitis B e antigen (HBeAg) and hepatitis B e antibody (anti-HBe) testing is also available. Initial screening tests requested depend on the clinical indication, as summarized in Table 6.9.

HBsAg is a marker of current infection. It appears in the serum 2–10 weeks after exposure to HBV (Trépo et al. 2014). Positivity may indicate acute or chronic infection. Chronic HBV carriers are defined by having HBsAg positivity for >6 months. Anti-HBc IgM and IgG begin to rise 1–2 weeks after the appearance of HBsAg. Anti-HBc IgG persists during chronic infection, while IgM typically wanes over time, although IgM can be detectable in some patients during periods of exacerbation of chronic HBV. Anti-HBs are a marker of immunity from previous vaccination or exposure. HBeAg is a marker of viral replication and infectivity. It has largely been replaced by HBV DNA testing, which directly measures viral load (Trépo et al. 2014). Most HBV DNA assays use PCR techniques. Interpretation of screening tests is summarized in Table 6.10.

6.5.2.1 Vaccination and Testing

The hepatitis B vaccine is a recombinant vaccine

Box 6.2 Groups at High Risk for Hepatitis B Virus Infection Needing Screening
- All persons born in countries with moderate to high HBV endemicity (HBsAg prevalence ≥2%).
- US-born persons not vaccinated in infancy whose parents were born in regions with high HBV endemicity (HBsAg prevalence ≥8%).
- Pregnant women.
- Children born to HBsAg positive mothers.
- Persons needing immunosuppressive therapy.
- Persons seeking treatment for sexually transmitted infections.
- Travelers to countries with moderate to a high prevalence of HBV.
- Persons with chronic liver disease or elevated ALT or AST of unclear etiology.
- Others with high-risk activities or exposures, including:
  - Males who have sex with males.
  - Persons who have had >1 sexual partner in the previous 6 months.
  - Persons who have ever injected drugs.
  - Persons at risk for occupational exposure to HBV.
  - Inmates of correctional facilities.

Adapted from Terrault et al. 2018
HBV hepatitis B virus, *HBsAg* hepatitis B surface antigen, *ALT* alanine aminotransferase, *AST* aspartate aminotransferase.

containing >95% HBsAg protein. After vaccination, serologic testing is not routinely indicated but can be considered in immunocompromised patients or sex partners of HBsAg-positive per-

Table 6.10 Interpretation of screening tests for hepatitis B virus infection

HBsAg	Anti-HBc	Anti-HBs	Interpretation	Management
–	–	–	Susceptible to infection	Vaccinate
–	–	+	Immune due to vaccination	No further testing
–	+	+	Immune due to natural infection	No further management unless immunosuppressed
+	+	–	Acute or chronic infection Anti-HBc IgM differentiates acute from chronic infection[a]: • Positive anti-HBc IgM indicates acute infection • Negative anti-HBc IgM indicates chronic infection	Acute and chronic infections require additional testing and management, potentially by a subspecialist
–	+	–	1. Recovery from acute infection 2. Distantly immune with low undetectable level anti-HBs 3. False-positive anti-HBc 4. Chronic, occult infection with undetectable HBsAg	HBV DNA testing if immunocompromised

Adapted from Terrault et al. (2018)
HBsAg hepatitis B surface antigen, *Anti-HBc* hepatitis B core antibody, *Anti-HBs* hepatitis B surface antibody, *HBV* hepatitis B virus, *IgM* immunoglobulin M
[a] Often anti-HBc IgM needs to be ordered separately

sons (CDC 2015b). Post-vaccination antibody levels to anti-HBs can be checked 1–2 months after the third vaccine dose (CDC 2015b). A robust immune response is demonstrated with an anti-HBs titer of >10 mIU/mL. After three doses, 90% of healthy adults and 95% of infants, children, and adolescents develop an adequate response to the vaccine. Titers decrease over time, although symptomatic infection is rare after immunization, suggesting immune memory (Trépo et al. 2014). Of note, transient HBsAg can be detected from 1 day to 3 weeks following vaccine administration (American Academy of Pediatrics 2018).

6.5.3   Hepatitis C Virus

Hepatitis C virus (HCV) screening is recommended for specific groups identified in Box 6.3. Screening should be performed with an HCV antibody test with reflex to HCV RNA (AASLD-IDSA 2020). Within 15 weeks of exposure and 5–6 weeks after onset of hepatitis, 80% of patients will have a positive HCV antibody. HCV antibody tests are available as laboratory-based and point-of-care assays with similar sensitivity and specificity (AASLD-IDSA 2020). Immunoassays are at least 97% sensitive and more than 99% specific (American Academy of Pediatrics 2018). A posi-

tive antibody test indicates active infection (acute or chronic), a past infection that has resolved, or, rarely, a false positive. An RNA test is used to detect active infection. Many laboratories offer HCV antibody tests with a reflex to HCV RNA PCR as a single orderable test.

> **Box 6.3 Groups for Whom Hepatitis C Screening Is Indicated**
> • As one-time routine testing in all adolescents and young adults over 18 years.
> • During routine prenatal care with each pregnancy.
> • In children less than 18 years with activities, exposures, conditions, or circumstances associated with increased risk of HCV infection, including:
> – Males who have sex with males.
> – Children born to HCV-infected women.
> – Persons with HIV infection.
> – Persons starting pre-exposure prophylaxis for HIV.
> – Persons with chronic liver disease or elevated ALT or AST of unclear etiology.
> – Persons who use injection drugs.
>
> Adapted from AASLD-IDSA 2020.
> *HCV* hepatitis C virus, *ALT* alanine aminotransferase, *AST* aspartate aminotransferase.

HCV RNA PCR becomes detectable within 1–2 weeks after exposure to HCV. HCV RNA PCR testing alone is indicated in immunocompromised patients, those with possible HCV exposure (e.g., needlestick) in the previous 6 months, and in neonates (American Academy of Pediatrics 2018). HCV RNA PCR is also monitored in HCV-infected patients receiving antiviral therapy.

6.5.4   Hepatitis D

Hepatitis D virus (HDV) causes infection only in those with hepatitis B infection since HDV requires HBsAg for replication. Testing should be considered in patients with severe or prolonged hepatitis or in patients who are HBsAg positive who have additional risk factors such as emigration from a region with endemic HDV, injection drug use, males who have sex with males, and high-risk sexual practices or have coinfection with HIV or HCV (American Academy of Pediatrics 2021). Screening for HDV is recommended with anti-HDV IgG followed by HDV RNA studies if antibody testing is positive (Terrault et al. 2018). Anti-HDV may not be detectable until several weeks after illness onset, so testing of acute and convalescent serum may be needed to make a diagnosis (American Academy of Pediatrics 2018).

6.5.5   Hepatitis E

Hepatitis E virus (HEV) is an important cause of acute hepatitis in resource-limited countries. Testing should be considered in symptomatic travelers from an endemic area with HEV or any symptomatic patients who have tested negative for serologic markers of hepatitis A, B, and C and other hepatotropic viruses (CDC 2020b). Diagnosis can be made by detecting anti-HEV IgM in serum. Detection of HEV RNA from serum or stool can confirm the diagnosis. Serologic and nucleic acid tests are commercially available, but none have been approved by the FDA (CDC 2020c).

> **Key Learning about Hepatitis Viruses**
> - Testing for viral hepatitis should be considered for specific groups or based on clinical presentation, including results of liver function testing.
> - Antibody testing for hepatitis A is sufficient for testing. Hepatitis A does not cause a prolonged carrier state.
> - Hepatitis B testing provides information about the acute and chronic state of the virus.
> - Hepatitis C screening should be performed with an HCV antibody test with reflex to HCV RNA.
> - Hepatitis D travels with hepatitis B since it requires HBsAg for replication.
> - Hepatitis E should be considered when a traveler returns with symptoms of hepatitis. Diagnosis can be made by detecting anti-HEV IgM in serum. Detection of HEV RNA from serum or stool can confirm the diagnosis.

6.5.6   Real-Life Example

A 9-year-old presented with mild abdominal pain, nausea, vomiting, and anorexia. His mother also reported similar symptoms, but she had icteric sclera. The child's liver enzymes were mildly elevated. A hepatitis panel showed a positive IgM for hepatitis A. The mother's icteric sclera helped the clinician consider hepatitis as the cause of their symptoms.

6.6   Bacterial and Parasitic Infections

6.6.1   Syphilis

Syphilis is a systemic disease caused by *Treponema pallidum* subspecies *pallidum*, a spirochete bacterium. Infection can be acquired during childhood or adulthood, usually during sexual activity or maternal-to-child transmission (congenital infection). Darkfield examinations and molecular tests can detect *T. pallidum* taken directly from lesion exudate or tissue and are considered definitive tests that can diagnose early syphilis and congenital syphilis (Workowski et al. 2021).

Infection acquired in childhood or adolescence can be divided into three stages—primary, secondary, and tertiary—with periods of latency between active stages. Primary syphilis is characterized by painless indurated ulcers on the skin or mucus membranes at the inoculation site; these chancres typically occur 3 weeks after initial exposure and spontaneously resolve within a few weeks. Secondary syphilis occurs 1–2 months after initial infection when *T. pallidum* invades organ systems throughout the body. Patients may present with nonspecific signs and symptoms, including fever, sore throat, muscle aches, rash, mucocutaneous lesions, and generalized lymphadenopathy. Tertiary syphilis occurs 15–30 years after infection, so it is not encountered frequently in the pediatric population. It can include gumma formation or cardiovascular involvement. There are periods of latency between times of active infection when a patient may be seroreactive but have no clinical manifestations of syphilis. Early latent syphilis is defined as an infection in the preceding year; late latent syphilis is an infection acquired more than 1 year prior or syphilis of unknown duration (American Academy of Pediatrics 2018; Larsen et al. 1995). Neurosyphilis can be seen in any stage of the acquired disease and congenital infection.

6.6.1.1 Serology for Syphilis

Serology is the cornerstone of syphilis diagnosis since there is a paucity of easy and widely avail-able tests for the direct detection of syphilis. Serology may be the only evidence of disease during latent, asymptomatic infection. There are two types of serologic tests, nontreponemal and treponemal, which must be considered together in the diagnosis of syphilis.

Nontreponemal tests. Nontreponemal tests include the rapid plasma reagin (RPR) test and the venereal disease research laboratory (VDRL) test. Nontreponemal tests measure IgM and IgG antibodies to antigens released from damaged host cell walls and antigens on the spirochete surface (Ratnam 2005). These antibodies can first be detected 1–4 weeks after the appearance of a primary syphilitic chancre and approximately 6 weeks after initial exposure (Peeling and Ye 2004). These tests utilize different antigen preparations resulting in varied reactivity levels (Larsen et al. 1995). The 2021 STI guidelines point to a fourfold change in titer (which is equivalent to a change of two dilutions: 1:16 to 1:4 or from 1:8 to 1:32), which is needed for clinically significant difference between two results from a nontreponemal test from the same type of serologic test and the same manufacturer to avoid any variation in results (Workowski et al. 2021).

Nontreponemal titers often correlate with disease activity, making them a useful tool for distinguishing active infection, untreated infection, or reinfection. After appropriate treatment of syphilis, titers decline and may become nonreactive over time (Workowski et al. 2021). Reinfection causes a rise in titers. Comparison of titers should be done between the same nontreponemal assays, ideally done at the same laboratory. Quantitative results between VDRL and RPR cannot be compared (Workowski et al. 2021).

Limitations of nontreponemal tests. Nontreponemal tests have low sensitivity in the early primary disease when there may be a slow rise in detectable titers and in late latent syphilis when there is a gradual decline in reactivity (Ratnam 2005). Specificity is generally high, although false positives occur with an incidence of 1–2%. False positives have been attributed to many factors, including infection with HIV, hepatitis, infectious mononucleosis, pneumococcal pneumonia, chickenpox, measles, and other viral infections; autoimmune conditions; pregnancy; injection drug use; older age; and malignancy (American Academy of Pediatrics 2018; Association of Public Health Laboratories 2018; Geusau et al. 2005; Larsen et al. 1995; Ratnam 2005). A quantitative titer is not useful for distinguishing true positive from false-positive results as false positives have been documented in patients with high titers (Larsen et al. 1995); however, 90% of false positives have a titer less than 1:8 (Ratnam 2005). False-negative results can occur due to the prozone phenomenon, in which a large amount of nontreponemal antibody interferes with the test assay. Diluting these samples results in increased reactivity. This reaction is seen in 1–2% of patients with secondary syphilis (Yap et al. 2010).

Nontreponemal tests have been utilized as screening tests for syphilis since they are widely available, inexpensive, convenient, and reflect treatment history (Larsen et al. 1995). Given the false-positive rate, positive tests should be followed up with a confirmatory test, especially in a low-risk population.

Treponemal tests. Treponemal tests detect IgM and IgG antibodies directed against specific *T. pallidum* antigens (Soreng et al. 2014). These antibodies are first detected approximately 3 weeks after initial exposure, often before nontreponemal antibodies (Peeling and Ye 2004). Currently available treponemal tests include treponemal antibody absorbed (FTA-ABS) test, *T. pallidum* passive particle agglutination (TP-PA) assay, *T. pallidum* EIA (TP-EIA), and *T. pallidum* CIA (TP-CIA).

Treponemal tests do not correlate with disease activity and remain positive regardless of appropriate treatment of syphilis. They should not be used to evaluate response to therapy or reinfection. The incidence of false-positive results is approximately 1% (Larsen et al. 1995). False positives can occur with autoimmune conditions, older age, and infection with antigenically similar spirochetes such as pinta, yaws, and Lyme disease (Larsen et al. 1995; Soreng et al. 2014; Ratnam 2005). The sensitivity and specificity of

commonly used treponemal and nontreponemal tests are reviewed in Table 6.11.

Traditionally, treponemal tests have been more costly and technically difficult to perform, so they have been used as confirmatory tests after positive nontreponemal tests (Larsen et al. 1995). Many treponemal assays, such as TP-EIA tests, have become available as high-throughput automated assays. This has given rise to the "reverse sequence screening approach," in which treponemal tests are used as screening tests.

Testing algorithms. Nontreponemal and treponemal tests should be used together to improve sensitivity and specificity. Typically, laboratories decide the testing approach used.

The conventional screening approach (Fig. 6.2) starts with a nontreponemal test and, if positive, reflexes to a treponemal test for confirmation. Up to 40% of untreated late latent cases are nonreactive on nontreponemal tests and would subsequently be undiagnosed using this screening scheme (Soreng et al. 2014).

The reverse sequence screen approach (Fig. 6.3) starts with a treponemal test to identify people who have previously had treated, incompletely treated, or untreated syphilis. A positive result is followed up with a nontreponemal test for confirmation. Discordant results (positive treponemal test and negative nontreponemal test) are further assessed with a different treponemal test, ideally based on a different antigen than the original test. This screening algorithm is gaining popularity as automated treponemal TP-EIA, and TP-CIA assays are fast and easy to perform, compared to nontreponemal tests, which generally need to be done manually. This approach is superior to the conventional approach in detecting early infection and late latent disease (Soreng et al. 2014). However, there is generally low specificity of first-line TP-EIA results. In one study, up to 56% of specimens with a positive TP-EIA had a negative RPR, of which 31% were ultimately negative on confirmatory treponemal test; this suggests the initial TP-EIA had many false positives (CDC 2011).

Post-treatment monitoring. After appropriate treatment, quantitative nontreponemal titers

Table 6.11 Sensitivity and specificity of nontreponemal and treponemal tests in the diagnosis of syphilis

| Test | | Sensitivity (%) by stage of untreated syphilis | | | | Specificity (%) |
		Primary	Secondary	Early latent	Late latent	
Nontreponemal	VDRL	78 (74–87)	100	95 (88–100)	71 (37–94)	98 (96–99)
	RPR	86 (77–100)	100	98 (85–100)	73	98 (93–99)
Treponemal	FTA-ABS	84 (70–100)	100 (95–100)	100	96	97 (94–100)
	TP-PA	88 (86–100)	100	100	86 (76–93)	96 (95–100)
	TP-EIA[a]	39–100	100 (96–100)	100 (90–100)	98 (92–99)	82 (78–86)
	TP-CIA[a]	98	100	100	91–100	98–100

Adapted from: Larsen et al. 1995; Association of Public Health Laboratories 2018; Park et al. 2019; Sena et al. 2010; Ratnam 2005

VDRL venereal disease research laboratory, *RPR* rapid plasma reagin, *FTA-ABS* treponemal antibody absorbed, *TP-PA* *T. pallidum* passive particle agglutination, *TP-EIA T. pallidum* enzyme immunoassays, *TP-CIA T. pallidum* chemiluminescent assay

[a]Limited data available for sensitivity and specificity of TP-EIA and TP-CIA

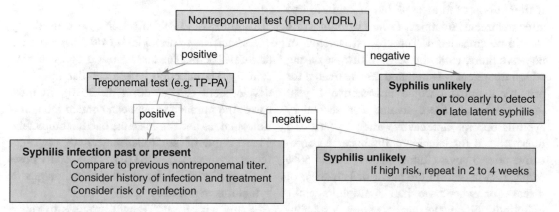

Fig. 6.2 Conventional screening approach for the diagnosis of syphilis. Adapted from Soreng et al. (2014), Workowski et al. (2021). *RPR* rapid plasma reagin, *VDRL* venereal disease research laboratory, *TP-PA T. pallidum* passive particle agglutination

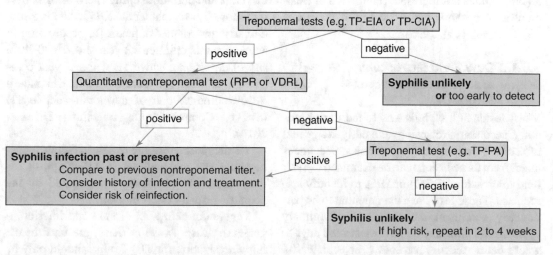

Fig. 6.3 Reverse sequence screening approach for the diagnosis of syphilis. Adapted from Soreng et al. (2014), Workowski et al. (2021). *TP-EIA T. pallidum* enzyme immunoassays, *TP-CIA T. pallidum* chemiluminescent assay, *VDRL* venereal disease research laboratory, *RPR* rapid plasma reagin, *TP-PA T. pallidum* passive particle agglutination

should be followed. The same nontreponemal test (RPR or VDRL) should be trended over time, ideally at the same laboratory. In children treated for congenital syphilis, nontreponemal titers should be obtained every 2–3 months until nonreactive. RPR or VDRL should decrease by 3 months and be nonreactive by 6 months (American Academy of Pediatrics 2018). In those treated for primary or secondary acquired syphilis, nontreponemal titers should be followed at 6 and 12 months after treatment. RPR or VDRL should decline fourfold by 3–4 months after treatment and decline eightfold by 6–8 months after treatment (Larsen et al. 1995). If titers do not fall as expected or begin to rise after treatment, treatment failure or reinfection should be considered. Time to retroversion, or negative titers, varies by stage of disease during which treatment was initiated. Those treated for primary syphilis become nonreactive 1 year after treatment, those treated for secondary syphilis become nonreactive after 2 years, and those treated for latent syphilis become nonreactive after 5 years (Ratnam 2005). About 50% of patients treated in the latent or late stage of disease or who have had multiple syphilis infections will develop persistent low-level nontreponemal titers (RPR 1:4 or less; VDRL 1:2 or less), known as a "serofast reaction." A "serofast reaction" does not represent reinfection or treatment failure (American Academy of Pediatrics 2018; Larsen et al. 1995).

6.6.1.2 Dark Field Microscopy and Direct Fluorescent Antibody

Moist lesions of syphilis—as found during primary, secondary, relapsing, and early congenital infection—contain many spirochetes. Specimens taken from these lesions can be examined by dark field microscopy (DFM) or DFA to identify spirochetes. These tests have the potential to be particularly useful in the diagnosis of primary syphilis, as DFM may be positive several days to weeks before reactive serology (Yap et al. 2010). However, these tests require specialized techniques and experienced personnel, making them largely obsolete (Larsen et al. 1995; Association of Public Health Laboratories 2018).

6.6.1.3 Nucleic Acid Amplification Tests

Nucleic acid amplification tests, such as PCR, are very sensitive for the detection of *T. pallidum*. PCR can detect as few as one to ten organisms per specimen (Peeling and Ye 2004: Ratnam 2005). Currently, there are no FDA-approved commercially available PCR tests for syphilis.

Diagnosis of infection acquired after birth relies primarily on serologic testing. Notes on testing by stage of infection are summarized in Table 6.12.

6.6.2 Tuberculosis

Tuberculosis (TB) infection is caused by *Mycobacterium tuberculosis* (*Mtb*) complex an, acid-fast bacilli. The disease can progress during primary TB infection before cellular immunity development (Fitzgerald et al. 2020). In most cases, the immune system can contain the infection but does not eliminate the bacilli completely. This period of controlled infection, or latent tuberculosis infection (LTBI), is defined by positive immune reactivity to *Mtb* with no signs or symptoms of infection.

Some with latent TB will progress to active TB infection. Risk factors for progression to the active disease include young age, diabetes mellitus, HIV, and high-dose corticosteroids or TNF-α inhibitors (Lewinsohn et al. 2017). Age is a particularly important risk factor for progression to active disease: children <2 years have a 30–40% risk of developing active TB within 1 year compared to children ≥5 years and adults who have a 5–10% lifetime risk of developing active TB (Starke, Committee On Infectious Diseases 2014).

TB diagnostic tests are reviewed below, focusing on LTBI and pulmonary TB diagnosis, as these are most commonly encountered by the pediatric primary care clinician.

Tuberculin skin tests (TSTs) and interferon-gamma release assays (IGRAs) are used in the initial evaluation for TB. Testing should only be pursued when there are risk factors for TB infection, a disease or condition that requires immunosuppression or suspected TB infection. In the primary care setting, children are often screened

Table 6.12 Recommended testing for postnatally acquired syphilis based on the infection stage

Stage of syphilis	Clinical presentation	Testing options	Comments and pitfalls
Primary syphilis	Painless ulcer, which may go unrecognized	Direct examination of spirochetes	DFM and DFA are not practical in most clinical settings. PCR is not widely available.
		Serology	Nontreponemal and treponemal antibodies are often not detected until 1–4 weeks after the chancre of primary syphilis has formed. Treponemal tests are positive before nontreponemal tests. If serology is negative, repeat testing in 2–12 weeks.
Secondary syphilis	1–2 months after initial infection when there is the dissemination of spirochetes	Serology	The sensitivity of nontreponemal and treponemal tests is nearly 100% during secondary syphilis. In people with a previous history of treated syphilis, a fourfold (or 2 dilutions) rise in nontreponemal titer is diagnostic of reinfection.
Latent syphilis	Asymptomatic period	Serology	Nontreponemal titers are reactive in early latent disease, but reactivity decreases with increasing latency.
Tertiary syphilis	15–30 years after infection; includes Gumma formation or cardiovascular involvement	Serology	Approximately 30% of patients with tertiary syphilis have a nonreactive nontreponemal test. The sensitivity of treponemal tests also declines with late-stage infection but is more likely to be reactive.

Adapted from Larsen et al. (1995), Ratnam (2005)
DFM dark field microscopy, *DFA* direct fluorescent antibody

after recent immigration from areas with high rates of tuberculosis (≥20 cases per 100,000), for employment or camp purposes, or when there is a concern for TB infection.

TSTs and IGRAs cannot distinguish LTBI from active TB disease, so positive screening TST or IGRA should be followed by evaluating signs and symptoms suggestive of TB disease and chest radiograph (Lewinsohn et al. 2017). If a chest radiograph shows findings of active TB, then respiratory samples are needed for testing. Isolation of *Mtb* confirms active TB disease. Even with optimal technique, *Mtb* is only isolated in fewer than 75% of infants and 50% of children with clinically diagnosed TB (American Academy of Pediatrics 2018). Therefore, a diagnosis of pulmonary TB in children can be made with high clinical suspicion and a lack of direct detection of *Mtb*.

6.6.2.1 Immunologic Tests

TST and IGRA detect cell-mediated immunity to *Mtb* and are used as screening tests for TB infection. TST or IGRA screening should be performed at least 2–10 weeks after presumed infection when reactivity can first be detected (American Academy of Pediatrics 2018). The

preferred test type is based on the child's age and test characteristics, as reviewed in Table 6.13 and discussed further in the text below.

Usually, either TST or IGRA is recommended, but both can be considered together in the following scenarios: (1) the initial and repeat IGRA are indeterminate/invalid; (2) the initial TST or IGRA is negative, but there remains high clinical suspicion for TB disease, or the child has a risk factor for TB and is at high risk for disease progression (e.g., on TNF-α inhibitors); (3) the initial TST is positive in patient ≥2 years with a history of bacille Calmette-Guerin (BCG) vaccine (Starke and Committee On Infectious Diseases 2014).

Tuberculin skin test. TST detects cell-mediated immunity to *Mtb*. Specifically, TST measures delayed-type hypersensitivity reaction to proteins shared by *Mtb*, nontuberculous mycobacteria, and the strain of *Mycobacterium bovis* (*M. bovis*) found in the BCG vaccine.

Purified protein derivative (PPD) is administered in a standardized volume intradermally on the volar surface of the arm (Mantoux method) (Lewinsohn et al. 2017). The test is interpreted after 48–72 h by measuring the area of induration, not the area of erythema. Measurement

Table 6.13 Suggested use of tuberculin skin test and interferon-gamma release assay by age

Age	Recommended initial screening test	Comments
<3 months	Unclear	TST and IGRA are both unreliable. Consult a specialist if concern for TB disease or exposure
3 months to <2 years	TST preferred	TST and IGRA with similar sensitivity. IGRA has higher rates of indeterminate/invalid results in this age group
≥2 years	IGRA preferred, TST acceptable	IGRA is preferred, especially in those who have received BCG vaccines or are unlikely to return for TST reading. In children 2–5 years, IGRA and TST have similar sensitivity. In children ≥5 years, IGRA has better sensitivity than TST

Adapted from Starke and Committee On Infectious Diseases 2014; Cruz and Reichman 2019; Kay et al. 2018
TST tuberculin skin test, *IGRA* interferon-gamma release assay, *TB* tuberculosis, *BCG* bacille Calmette-Guérin

Table 6.14 Positive tuberculin skin test related to size of induration and risk factors

Measurement of induration	Risk factors
≥5 mm	• Recent known or suspected exposure to a person with active/contagious TB • Children with immunosuppression, including those living with HIV, organ transplants, on prolonged therapy with corticosteroids, or receiving TNF-α inhibitors • Children with suspicion for TB based on clinical or radiographic evidence

≥10 mm	Children with increased risk of disseminated TB disease:
	• Children <5 years
	• Children with other medical conditions, including diabetes mellitus, severe kidney disease, malnutrition, lymphoma
	Children with increased risk of exposure to TB disease:
	• Children who were born in high-prevalence areas of the world or have traveled to high-prevalence areas of the world (within the last 5 years)
	• Children who are residents or employees of high-risk congregate settings, including prisons or jails, or homeless shelters
	• Children or adolescents who use injection drugs
	• Children who are exposed to adults who:
	  – Are at high risk for developing active TB (such as adults with HIV)
	  – Live in high-risk congregate settings such as homeless shelters, prisons, or jails or are residents of long-term care facilities
	  – Use injection drugs

≥ 15 mm	People with no known risk factors for TB

Adapted from Lewinsohn et al. 2017; CDC 2020f; Cruz and Reichman 2019
TST tuberculin skin test, *TB* tuberculosis

should be taken across the forearm or perpendicular to the long axis. In those with reactivity, the induration and erythema may persist for weeks. Interpretation is based on the size of induration and risk factors (see Table 6.14).

Without a gold standard for comparison, TST sensitivity and specificity are difficult to assess. Sensitivity is estimated to be 75–85% (Starke and Committee On Infectious Diseases 2014), and 10–40% of immunocompetent children with culture documented TB do not have a reactive TST initially (American Academy of Pediatrics 2018). False negatives may be due to anergy, which is the inability to react to the TST due to a weakened immune system. False negatives are more often seen with young age, malnutrition, those who have recently received live viral vaccines, those with immunosuppression (HIV infection, treatment with high-dose corticosteroids or TNF-α inhibitors), those with overwhelming illness including disseminated or extensive TB, and after recent viral or bacterial infection (Lewinsohn et al. 2017; American Academy of Pediatrics 2018). Testing in early infection, before TST reactivity develops, can cause false-negative results (Lewinsohn et al. 2017).

Table 6.15 Comparison of tuberculin skin test and interferon-gamma release assay test characteristics

		TST	IGRA
Technique		Intradermal injection with reading 48–72 h later	Single blood draw
Cross-reactivity	BCG vaccine	Yes	No
	NTM	Yes	Some
Boosting by previous TST		Yes	Possible
Estimated sensitivity[a]		75–85%	80–85%
Estimated[a] specificity	BCG unvaccinated	95–100%	90–95%
	BCG vaccinated	49–65%	89–100%

Adapted from Starke and Committee On Infectious Diseases 2014
TST tuberculin skin test, *IGRA* interferon-gamma release assay, *BCG* bacille Calmette-Guérin, *NTM* nontuberculous mycobacteria
[a] There is no reference standard for diagnosis of tuberculosis, making sensitivity and specificity ranges only estimates

BCG vaccine is an immunization against TB, prepared from an attenuated strain of *M. bovis*. Given the cross-reactivity between antigens in PPD and the BCG vaccine, the specificity of TST depends on previous vaccination with the BCG vaccine (see Table 6.15). Approximately half of the infants who received the BCG vaccine will have a TST with induration; by age 5, up to 90% of children who received the BCG vaccine in infancy will have a nonreactive (negative) TST (Starke, Committee On Infectious Diseases 2014). When there is a high risk for TB, the TST should be interpreted the same as children who have not received vaccination (American Academy of Pediatrics 2018). False-positive TST results can also occur with infection with nontuberculous mycobacteria (NTM).

TST reactivity can wane over time, especially when there is no ongoing exposure to *Mtb*. However, repeat TST testing can restore reactivity, which is called "boosting." Two negative tests 1–3 weeks apart can help distinguish waning reactivity from true negativity. BCG vaccine can also provide the basis for the boosting phenomenon. A child who previously received the BCG vaccine may have an initial negative TST, but repeat testing in 1–3 weeks may show induration

in the absence of a new TB infection. This repeated testing is important in those getting yearly TST, such as for employment, to differentiate waning reactivity with boosting from seroconversion due to new exposure (Lewinsohn et al. 2017).

Interferon-gamma release assay. Interferon-gamma release assays (IGRAs) are in vitro blood tests that measure interferon-gamma (IFN-γ) released by sensitized T cells in response to *Mtb* antigens. The antigen tested is not in the strain of *M. bovis* used in the BCG vaccine nor in most NTM (including *Mycobacterium avium* complex, the most commonly found pathogenic NTM); however, it is found in *M. kansasii*, *M. szulgai*, *M. marinum*, and wild-type *M. bovis* (Lewinsohn et al. 2017; Starke, Committee On Infectious Diseases 2014).

There are two commercially available IGRA assays: QuantiFERON-TB Gold In-Tube (QTF) test and T-Spot.*TB* test. The QTF test is an ELISA on whole blood. Two control tubes are drawn: one mitogen (positive) control with phytohemagglutinin stimulating T cells to ensure viable cells are present and one-nil (negative) control to examine background IFN-γ activity. A third tube reports IFN-γ activity in the presence of TB antigen (QuantiFERON®-TB Gold (QFT®) ELISA Package Insert 2016). T-SPOT.*TB* is an enzyme-linked immunosorbent spot (ELISPOT) assay on peripheral mononuclear cells. Peripheral blood mononuclear cells (lymphocytes) are separated, and IFN-γ activity is noted in wells with mitogen control, nil control, and TB antigens. The response is noted in "spot forming units." There are three possible results of IGRA assays:

- Positive: IFN-γ response of TB antigen minus nil activity is greater than the cutoff value. Background activity (from nil control) is subtracted from TB antigen test activity to determine activity specific to TB antigen.
- Indeterminate/invalid: Often due to lack of response to mitogen control or nil control with high background levels. Poor response to mitogen control may be due to technical errors in specimen collection or processing or related to host anergy (Lewinsohn et al. 2017).

Indeterminate values are associated with immunosuppression but can occur in immunocompetent patients (Lewinsohn et al. 2017). There are particularly high indeterminate results in children, with up to 35% of children with indeterminate results. Children <2 years have especially high rates of indeterminate results (Starke, Committee On Infectious Diseases 2014; Cruz and Reichman 2019: Kay et al. 2018).

- Negative: IFN-γ response of TB antigen minus nil activity is less than the cutoff value. No significant IFN-γ response to TB antigen.

The sensitivity of IGRAs is estimated to be 80–85% and specificity 89–100% (Starke, Committee On Infectious Diseases 2014). Given the use of antigens more specific to *Mtb* in IGRAs, specificity is higher than for TST. IGRA and TST are compared in Table 6.15.

Four to six weeks after administration of live viral vaccines, there can be false-negative tuberculin reactivity. Therefore, TST should be placed or blood drawn for IGRA on the same day as vaccines are given (American Academy of Pediatrics 2018). After effective treatment, TST reactivity can persist for years, while IGRA durability is less clearly defined. TST and IGRA should not be used to determine the efficacy of treatment or diagnosing reinfection (American Academy of Pediatrics 2018).

6.6.2.2 Direct Detection of *Mycobacterium Tuberculosis*

When there is suspicion for active pulmonary TB, respiratory samples should be collected to detect *Mtb*. Respiratory samples from children can be collected via spontaneous expectoration, induction, nasopharyngeal aspiration, gastric aspiration, or bronchoalveolar lavage. Spontaneous sputum production and expectoration are often successful in children ≥2 years. Induction with aerosolized hypertonic saline can help with sputum production and has been noted to be successful in infants, although sputum production requires special expertise in the very young (American Academy of Pediatrics 2018). Gastric aspiration is the collection of swallowed sputum from the stomach after an overnight fast and can be obtained from children unable to produce sputum. While any of these methods are acceptable, spontaneous or induced sputum is preferred, followed by gastric aspirates (American Academy of Pediatrics 2018). The highest yield for Mtb detection is achieved from the first-morning respiratory specimen (Lewinsohn et al. 2017). Three specimens (sputum or gastric aspirates) should be collected, ideally once each morning, to increase sensitivity.

Smear for acid-fast bacilli. In evaluating pulmonary TB, sputum specimens can be stained and examined by microscopy for acid-fast bacilli (AFB) of *Mtb*. A sputum AFB smear's sensitivity from a single specimen is 54% but increases to 70% with three specimens. Little increase in sensitivity is achieved by collecting more than three specimens. The specificity of sputum AFB smears is ≥90%. AFB smears cannot distinguish *Mtb* from NTM, accounting for some false-positive results. Gastric aspirates rarely are AFB smear-positive (Lewinsohn et al. 2017). AFB smears should not be used to definitively exclude or confirm pulmonary TB.

Nucleic acid amplification tests. NAATs can be used to detect Mtb in respiratory samples rapidly. It is recommended to perform NAAT on at least one respiratory sample when pulmonary TB is considered (CDC 2009). Results should be interpreted in relation to AFB smear results, as outlined in Table 6.16. All results should be confirmed with culture, which is also needed for drug susceptibility testing.

Molecular testing for drug susceptibility. If AFB smear or NAAT is positive for presumed *Mtb* on a respiratory sample, then rapid molecular drug susceptibility testing for rifampin and/or isoniazid resistance is recommended for children at high risk for drug resistance. Those at high risk include people who were treated for tuberculosis in the past, were born in or lived for at least 1 year in a foreign country with at least moderate tuberculosis incidence or a high primary multidrug-resistant TB prevalence, are contacts of patients with multidrug-resistant TB, or are HIV-infected (Lewinsohn et al. 2017).

Rapid molecular drug susceptibility testing for rifampin resistance has a sensitivity and specificity

Table 6.16 Interpretation of respiratory sample acid-fast bacilli smear and nucleic acid amplification test results in the diagnosis of pulmonary tuberculosis

		NAAT result	
		Positive	Negative
AFB smear results	Positive	TB is likely but confirm with culture.	TB is unlikely but confirm with culture. Consider testing for *Mtb* inhibitors to NAAT. May also consider NTM.
	Negative	TB is likely but confirm with culture.	TB is unlikely but confirm with culture. If intermediate to high suspicion of TB, the disease cannot be excluded.

Adapted from Lewinsohn et al. 2017; CDC 2009
AFB acid-fast bacilli, *NAAT* nucleic acid amplification test, *TB* tuberculosis, *NTM* nontuberculous mycobacteria, *NAAT* nucleic acid amplification test, *Mtb Mycobacterium tuberculosis*

of >97%, so results can be used to confirm or exclude rifampin resistance and guide initial treatment. Rapid molecular testing for isoniazid resistance has a sensitivity of 90% and a specificity of 99% (Lewinsohn et al. 2017); it can be used to confirm but not exclude isoniazid resistance. All molecular drug sensitivity testing should be confirmed with culture-based methods.

Culture. Culture is the gold standard for diagnosing TB disease; however, *Mtb* can take 2–6 weeks to grow in culture (CDC 2009). It is recommended to culture specimens on both liquid and solid media. The average time to detection is shorter with liquid culture methods (13.2–15.2 days) compared to solid culture methods (25.8 days) (Lewinsohn et al. 2017).

Drug susceptibility testing is performed on all *Mtb* culture isolates; given the slow rate of culture growth, these results may take weeks to become available. In a child with TB disease, the source case can provide likely drug susceptibilities. Culture and susceptibility should be pursued, especially when an isolated from the source case is not available; the presumed source case has drug-resistant TB; the child is immunocompromised or ill enough to require hospitalization; or in cases of extrapulmonary TB (American Academy of Pediatrics 2018).

Key Learning about Tuberculosis
- The specificity of an IGRA is higher than a TST.
- A TST is presently recommended for children between ages 3 months and 2 years since the IGRA has higher indeterminate/invalid results in this age group.
- An IGRA is a preferred test in children aged 2 years and over.
- NAATs can be used to detect Mtb in respiratory samples rapidly.
- Testing should only be pursued when there are risk factors for TB infection, a disease or condition that requires immunosuppression, or suspected TB infection.

6.6.3 Real-Life Example

A 10-year-old newly arrived immigrant came from Peru to the United States. He received BCG at birth. He was screened with an IGRA. The family history was positive for a 40-year-old uncle in Peru who recently died of an undiagnosed illness with a cough. The child's IGRA was positive, and a chest X-ray was obtained that was negative. Due to the history, the child was referred to the TB clinic for further management, which included routine treatment for latent tuberculosis infection (LTBI). All family members were screened with an IGRA.

6.6.4 Group A Streptococcus

Group A β-hemolytic *Streptococcus* (GAS), or *Streptococcus pyogenes*, can cause a range of clinical infections, including tonsillopharyngitis (colloquially known as "strep throat") and skin and soft tissue infections.

GAS causes an estimated 10% of cases of acute pharyngitis in children (Oliver et al. 2018). Untreated pharyngeal infection can lead to suppurative complications—including bacteremia and peritonsillar abscess—and nonsuppurative complications. The non-suppurative complications include acute rheumatic fever (ARF) and post-streptococcal glomerulone-phritis (PSGN), which occur 2–3 weeks after acute GAS infection. ARF is uncommon in children <3 years and in adults (Gerber et al. 2009). GAS pharyngitis can cause both ARF and PSGN. Prevention of ARF can be accomplished by treating GAS pharyngitis within 9 days of acute illness onset (Gerber et al. 2009). Given this time frame to initiate antibiotics, it may be reasonable in the appropriate clinical setting to defer treatment until a diagnostic evaluation is completed. GAS skin infections have not been proven to cause ARF but can cause PSGN (Shulman et al. 2012). Treatment of acute GAS pharyngitis or skin infection does not prevent PSGN (Shulman et al. 2012).

Testing should be guided by clinical suspicion for GAS pharyngitis, although there is significant overlap in the presentation of GAS pharyngitis and other causes of pharyngitis, such as viruses. GAS pharyngitis typically presents with a sore throat (usually sudden onset), pain with swallow-ing, and fever, although children may also pres-ent with headache, abdominal pain, nausea, and vomiting. On exam, there may be tonsillopharyn-geal erythema with or without exudate, anterior cervical lymphadenitis, soft palate petechiae, beefy swollen uvula, and scarlatiniform rash. Children <3 years may present more atypically with fever, mucopurulent rhinitis, excoriated nares, and diffuse adenopathy; exudative pharyn-gitis is rare in younger children. Features that may be more suggestive of a viral infection include the absence of fever, the presence of con-junctivitis, cough, hoarseness, coryza, anterior stomatitis, intraoral ulcerative lesions, viral exanthem, and diarrhea (Shulman et al. 2012). In temperate climates, cases of GAS pharyngitis are more common in the winter and spring.

Age may be considered when deciding to test for GAS pharyngitis. GAS pharyngitis is most common in children 5–15 years (Gerber et al. 2009). Children <3 years have a lower prevalence of GAS pharyngitis compared to children 5–15 years, with a prevalence of 10–14% and 15–20%, respectively (Shulman et al. 2012; Amir et al. 1994; Nussinovitch et al. 1999). Pairing this

lower prevalence with only rare reports of ARF in the younger age cohort, GAS testing is not rou-tinely indicated in children <3 years. Testing can be considered if there is a symptomatic house-hold contact or childcare outbreak of GAS pharyngitis.

Skin and soft tissue infections, including impetigo, erysipelas, and cellulitis, are com-monly caused by GAS. Perianal cellulitis due to GAS presents as sharply demarcated erythema. GAS can also cause more invasive diseases, including sepsis, toxic shock syndrome, osteo-myelitis, and necrotizing fasciitis.

Provider clinical judgment is not accurate in distinguishing GAS pharyngitis from viral phar-yngitis (Poses et al. 1985). Clinical scoring sys-tems, such as the Centor score, have been developed to help predict a positive GAS throat culture (Centor et al. 1981; McIsaac et al. 1998). However, scoring systems have proven unreliable in assessing the probability of GAS pharyngitis in children (Roggen et al. 2013). Clinical diagno-sis or scoring systems should not be used in place of other diagnostic testing for GAS pharyngitis.

Acute GAS infection can be diagnosed with the detection of the bacteria from an infected site. Three diagnostic tests—culture, rapid antigen detection test (RADT), and NAAT—are used to diagnose GAS as listed below.

6.6.4.1 Culture

A throat culture is a gold standard for the diag-nosis of GAS pharyngitis. A bacterial throat culture can be ordered as either a GAS-specific culture or general throat culture to detect all organisms. Bacterial throat culture has a sensi-tivity of 90–97% for detecting GAS pharyngitis (Shulman 1994). Swabs should be collected from both the surface of either tonsil plus the posterior pharyngeal wall to get a representa-tive sample for culture. Culture should be col-lected before antibiotics, as antibiotics administered before collection can inhibit bac-terial growth and cause false-negative results. The number of colonies grown on culture can-not differentiate colonization from active infec-tion (Shulman et al. 2012). Culture can also be performed on purulent fluid or swabs collected from skin or soft tissue infections. Culture is considered the diagnostic test of choice for skin or soft tissue infections.

Antibiotic susceptibilities are not routinely reported for GAS cultures since GAS is universally sensitive to penicillin (Shulman et al. 2012). In penicillin-allergic patients, susceptibility testing may be considered if there is a concern for antibiotic resistance to second-line therapies.

6.6.4.2 Rapid Antigen Detection Test

Since throat culture can take 1–2 days to grow, there is a role for rapid testing to help guide clinical treatment. Rapid antigen detection tests (RADTs) will be discussed in the point of care section.

RADTs for GAS can also be used for the detection of GAS from skin infections. Test characteristics depend on the assay used. For GAS detection in perineal infections, sensitivity ranges from 78 to 98% and specificity from 72% to 100% (Clegg et al. 2003; Cohen et al. 2015).

6.6.4.3 Nucleic Acid Amplification Tests

NAATs for the detection of GAS use PCR techniques. Current assays are only approved for the detection of GAS from throat swabs. They have high sensitivity and specificity compared to culture, with a sensitivity of 95–100% and a specificity of 97–100% (Parker et al. 2019). These tests are not true "point of care" as they require specialized equipment often unavailable in an ambulatory setting and can have a slightly longer turnaround time. They are also more costly compared to other methods of detection. Currently, no guidelines address whether these sensitive PCR-based tests can be used as a stand-alone diagnostic test without a follow-up culture of a negative test. Follow-up testing with throat culture may be considered, especially if symptoms persist or there is an ARF outbreak (Xpert Xpress Strep A Package Insert 2019; Cobas Strep A Package Insert 2017).

Pitfalls. Neither throat culture, RADT, nor NAAT can differentiate GAS pharyngitis from GAS colonization with a concurrent viral infection. Colonization, or GAS carriage, is characterized by the presence of GAS in the pharynx but no immunologic response. It can also be considered in an asymptomatic child with a persistently positive GAS throat culture after appropriate antibiotic treatment (Martin et al. 2004). 8–25% of asymptomatic children may be GAS carriers, with the higher rates noted in temperate climates in the winter and spring (Martin et al. 2004; Shaikh et al. 2010; Oliver et al. 2018). GAS carriers are unlikely to spread the organism to close contacts and are at very low risk, if any, of developing complications, including ARF. It is recommended to limit GAS testing to symptomatic children to avoid identifying carriers (Shulman et al. 2012).

Post-treatment GAS throat testing is not routinely recommended. Following appropriate treatment, up to 37% of children may continue to be positive on GAS throat culture. If these children are asymptomatic, they may be considered carriers (Shulman et al. 2012). Post-treatment repeat testing is indicated if there is a recurrence of classic GAS pharyngitis symptoms or there is a very high risk for ARF. Asymptomatic carriage of GAS has been noted in household contacts of individuals with GAS pharyngitis. Therefore, routine testing of asymptomatic household contacts is not indicated unless contacts develop symptoms (Shulman et al. 2012).

6.6.4.4 Serological Tests

Serology is important in diagnosing antecedent GAS infection when evaluating patients for post-GAS complications such as ARF and PSGN. These sequelae occur after acute GAS infection at a time when direct detection of bacteria is not always possible or may no longer be positive (Steer et al. 2015). Serology generally does not have a role in diagnosing acute GAS infection, as it is often negative at the time of acute infection.

Anti-streptolysin O. Streptolysin O is a toxin secreted by GAS that forms large pores in cell membranes. When GAS is cultured on blood agar plates, streptolysin O is responsible for the zone of β-hemolysis (complete clearing) due to lysis of RBC membranes (Steer et al. 2015; Parks et al. 2015). Streptolysin O is secreted by all β-hemolytic streptococcus, not just GAS, but expression varies between strains (Parks et al. 2015). Antibodies against streptolysin, or anti-streptolysin O (ASO), are clinically useful and commonly measured GAS antibodies.

ASO begins to increase 1 week after infection and peaks 3–5 weeks after infection (Wannamaker and Ayoub 1960). The decline is more variable but likely begins 6–8 weeks after infection and then returns to pre-infection levels by 6–12 months after acute infection, although it can persist beyond 1 year (Parks et al. 2015; Wannamaker and Ayoub 1960; Shet and Kaplan 2002; Johnson et al. 2010). Upper respiratory tract infections generally stimulate a robust ASO response compared to weak responses to skin infections. This may be due to free cholesterol in the skin binding to streptolysin O and reducing its immunogenicity (Shet and Kaplan 2002). Only about 80% of patients with a documented GAS infection will develop measurable ASO titers (Wannamaker and Ayoub 1960; Johnson et al. 2010). This may be due to the variable expression of streptolysin O by different strains of GAS.

False-positive ASO may occur due to the presence of non-group A streptococcal species that also produce streptolysin O, such as group C and G streptococcus (Parks et al. 2015). An old serum sample or specimen contaminated with bacteria may cause a falsely elevated titer (Shet and Kaplan 2002). False positives may occur in patients with myeloma, hypergammaglobulinemia, liver disease, and autoimmune disease with increased rheumatoid factor (Parks et al. 2015). Host hyperlipidemia may cause false-negative ASO (Wannamaker and Ayoub 1960).

Anti-deoxyribonuclease B. Deoxyribonuclease B (DNAse B or streptodornase) is an enzyme secreted by GAS that degrades extracellular DNA. It has an important role in allowing GAS to spread in the skin and soft tissue infections (Steer et al. 2015). DNAse B is more specific to GAS and less commonly found in other streptococci, such as group C and group G streptococci (Steer et al. 2015). Antibodies against DNAse B, or anti-DNAse B (ADB), are

commonly used to diagnose recent GAS infection.

ADB peaks 6–8 weeks after infection, decreases at 12 weeks after infection, and may return to pre-existing levels by 12 months, although it can persist longer than 1 year (Johnson et al. 2010; Ayoub and Wannamaker 1962). Both upper respiratory tract infections and skin infections can stimulate a strong ADB response. This rise in ADB after either respiratory or skin infection makes it particularly useful in diagnosing PSGN (Parks et al. 2015). False-negative ADB may occur due to acute hemorrhagic pancreatitis or infection with a GAS strain with no or minimal DNAse B production (Steer et al. 2015; Shet and Kaplan 2002).

Other GAS serologic tests. Other available GAS antibody tests, such as anti-streptokinase, anti-streptococcal hyaluronidase, anti-nicotinamide adenine dinucleotidase (NADase), type-specific M antibody, and anti-A carbohydrate, are not ordered routinely and are primarily used in research or reference laboratories.

The streptozyme test is a hemagglutination test that detects antibodies to five streptococcal antigens. While it historically gained some popularity, it suffered from variability and false-positive results, so it is no longer recommended (Parks et al. 2015; Shet and Kaplan 2002).

Serologic interpretation. As with other serology, GAS antibody levels can be interpreted by either comparing a single value to a reference value or examining a change in titer over time.

The 80th percentile defines the upper limit of normal for GAS serology. However, the upper limit of normal varies by age, season, and geography, with increased GAS prevalence increasing the upper limit of normal. Children ages 5–15 years have more frequent GAS exposure, so higher titers are seen in this age group (Kaplan et al. 1998). In temperate climates where GAS is more common in the winter and spring, GAS titers are higher during those seasons (Shet and Kaplan 2002). GAS titers are also generally higher in warmer climates, where GAS impetigo is more common (Steer et al. 2015). It is important to interpret ASO and ADB results based on age-stratified and geographic-specific data when possible. Age-stratified data for children in the United States is presented in Table 6.17. Commercially available tests often report the upper limit of normal ranges from adults or an inadequately defined population, so they should not be relied upon when interpreting results. Antibiotic use likely does not affect the subsequent development of ASO or ADB (Johnson et al. 2010).

Interpretation of a single GAS titer may have utility, especially when it is not feasible to obtain a second specimen in 2–4 weeks to evaluate trends. The rise in ASO occurs 1 week after GAS infection and may correspond to the development of ARF or PSGN, which typically occurs 2–3 weeks after acute infection (Wannamaker and Ayoub 1960). ASO or ADB above the upper limit of normal may be diagnostic for a recent GAS infection. Only 80% of patients with ARF develop ASO, but additional evaluation of other GAS antibodies increases detection of antecedent GAS infections to 92–98% (Ayoub and Wannamaker 1962). Therefore, if ASO is negative, ADB should be measured.

It is often preferable to document a trend in titer over 2–4 weeks. Reference values can be difficult to interpret, with some people having a peak value less than the upper limit of normal (Johnson et al. 2010; Ayoub and Wannamaker 1962). A rise in ASO or ADB over time, even if the value never exceeds the upper limit of normal for age and location, may be diagnostic of a recent GAS infection. A fourfold increase in ASO is typically considered a significant rise; a clinically significant rise in ADB is less well defined. In some, titers may be elevated for many months, so elevated titers over time (with possible slow decline) may represent old infection (Johnson et al. 2010). In another scenario, serum drawn at initial presentation for ARF or PSNG may already have peak antibody levels, which may decline with time. As noted above, in this case, an initial value above the upper limit of normal may help diagnose a recent GAS infection.

The utility of GAS serology is not well studied in other conditions, including post-streptococcal reactive arthritis, pediatric autoimmune neuropsychiatric disorder associated with streptococcal infection, and acute demyelinating encephalomyelitis.

Key Learning about the Diagnosis of Group A Streptococcus

- GAS pharyngitis prevalence varies by age, with the highest prevalence in children ages 5–15 years.
- It is important to diagnose and treat GAS infection to prevent acute rheumatic fever.
- Throat culture, RADT, and NAAT cannot differentiate GAS pharyngitis from GAS colonization with a concurrent viral infection.
- ASO and ADB titers should be interpreted according to age-stratified and geographic-specific normal values.

  GAS group A streptococcus, *RADT* rapid antigen detection test, *NAAT* nucleic acid amplification test, *ASO* anti-streptolysin O, *ABD* anti-deoxyribonuclease B.

Table 6.17 Age-based upper limit of normal (80th percentile) values for serum streptococcal antibody in US children

Age (years)	ASO titer upper limit normal (IU/mL)	ADB titer upper limit normal (IU/mL)
2	160	240
3	120	60
4	120	240
5	160	320
6	240	480
7	240	640
8	240	640
9	240	640
10	320	640
11	320	800
12	320	480

Adapted from Kaplan et al. 1998
ASO anti-streptolysin O, *ADB* anti-deoxyribonuclease B, *IU/mL* international units per milliliter

6.6.5 Mycoplasma

Mycoplasma pneumonia is a pleomorphic bacteria that lack a cell wall. It can cause infections of both the upper and lower respiratory tract, including pharyngitis, bronchitis, pneumonia, and otitis media, with severity ranging from mild to severe. Pharyngitis due to *M. pneumoniae* typically lacks exudate or associated lymphadenopathy. Otitis media related to mycoplasma is uncommon but can present with bullous myringitis; this finding was thought to be pathognomonic for mycoplasma, but other organisms can cause this as well (Waites et al. 2017). Children >5 years are most commonly affected with mycoplasma pneumonia, and the disease is often mild (Waites et al. 2017; Jain et al. 2015).

Mycoplasma can less commonly cause extrapulmonary manifestations, which may be attributed to direct effects of the organism or immune-mediated phenomena. Concurrent pulmonary symptoms may be absent. Extrapulmonary manifestations can include central nervous system disease (e.g., encephalitis, aseptic meningitis, Guillain-Barré syndrome, and transverse myelitis), dermatologic disorders (e.g., urticaria, erythema multiforme, erythema nodosum, and Stevens-Johnson syndrome), cardiac disease (e.g., pericarditis and myocarditis), arthritis, and hematologic abnormalities (e.g., hemolytic anemia and thrombocytopenic purpura) (American Academy of Pediatrics 2018; Waites et al. 2017). Hemolytic anemia is due to the development of cold-sensitive IgM autoantibodies to an antigen on RBCs, which at sufficient levels can cause hemolysis. These autoantibodies, called "cold agglutinins," can be found in 50% of people with *M. pneumoniae* but may be life-threatening in those with underlying hematologic disorders (Waites et al. 2017).

Diagnosis of *M. pneumoniae* is primarily accomplished with NAAT and/or serologic testing. Acute respiratory tract infection due to mycoplasma can be diagnosed with NAAT testing, as this is often positive early in the disease course before the development of antibodies. Serology with IgM can supplement the diagnosis of acute disease, especially in those treated with antibiotics who may have a negative PCR. IgM antibody plus NAAT together provides the most reliable early diagnosis of *M. pneumoniae,* especially in children.

Extrapulmonary mycoplasma infection can be difficult to diagnose, but paired acute and convalescent serology should be compared for seroconversion, as there is often an immunologic basis for disease. Detection of the organism can be attempted with molecular testing of extrapulmonary specimens such as blood, CSF, pericardial fluid, or skin biopsy tissue (Waites et al. 2017). Further information about the tests used in diagnosing *M. pneumoniae* is seen below.

6.6.5.1 Nucleic Acid Amplification Tests

Direct detection of *M. pneumoniae* DNA can be accomplished by NAATs, which replace culture as the "new gold standard" for diagnosing acute *M. pneumoniae*. Most commonly, PCR-based testing is used. Both monoplex and multiplex commercial assays are available for *M. pneumoniae* detection from respiratory specimens. Few studies compare the two types of assays directly; multiplex assays are slightly less sensitive but have the advantage of screening multiple pathogens (Loens and Ieven 2016).

Various respiratory specimens can be sent for PCR testing, including nasopharyngeal or oropharyngeal swabs, tracheal aspirates, lung tissue obtained from biopsy, pleural fluid, sputum, and bronchoalveolar lavage fluid. Sputum is the best specimen for detection of *M. pneumoniae* by PCR in the respiratory tract, which may be explained by a greater number of the organism in the pulmonary alveoli compared to the epithelium of the upper respiratory tract as demonstrated in nonhuman animal models (Loens et al. 2009). However, good-quality sputum samples are often difficult for young children to produce, so oropharyngeal or nasopharyngeal swabs are commonly collected as readily available and easy-to-obtain alternatives. There is no significant difference in PCR detection of *M. pneumoniae* from oropharyngeal compared to nasopharyngeal swabs. However, children can be positive in one site and not the other, so combining both sites' results provides the highest yield. Nasopharyngeal swabs may be more likely to be rejected for testing compared to oropharyngeal swabs due to the presence of PCR inhibitors or lack of respiratory epithelium (Loens et al. 2009).

PCR detection of *M. pneumoniae* from the respiratory tract is not able to distinguish colonization from infection. It is unclear if there is an asymptomatic carriage of *M. pneumoniae* in adults and children. Several studies have examined the presence of *M. pneumoniae* by PCR in the upper respiratory tract of healthy asymptomatic children and found carriage rates of <3% up to 56% (Jain et al. 2015; Spuesens et al. 2013; Wood et al. 2013).

6.6.5.2 *M. Pneumoniae* Serology

There are many commercial *M. pneumoniae* antibody assays. Historically, CF assays have been used; however, CF has been replaced by testing methods with improved sensitivity and specificity quantifying IgM and IgG. ELISA is the most widely used. Detection of antibodies does not indicate immunity to future reinfection (Waites et al. 2017).

IgM. Detection of IgM may represent acute *M. pneumoniae* infection. IgM is produced during the first week of infection, peaks during the third week of illness, and declines to low levels within a few months (Jacobs et al. 1986). In some people, IgM can persist for months. The highest sensitivity for IgM detection is achieved when a specimen is collected 7–10 days into illness (Waites et al. 2017).

There are limitations to IgM testing. IgM may not be produced in some primary infections. In particular, children less than 12 months of age seem to mount a less vigorous IgM response to *M. pneumoniae* infection (He et al. 2013). IgM may not be produced in reinfection; however, children are more likely than adults to be experiencing primary infection, making IgM a potentially useful test in the pediatric population. The prolonged persistence of IgM in some patients can make this an unreliable marker of acute disease. Generally, there is a low sensitivity of IgM for the diagnosis of acute infection. Estimates of sensitivity range from 32 to 35% compared to IgG seroconversion and 35–77% compared to PCR (Waites et al. 2017).

IgA. IgA is produced early in the course of *M. pneumoniae* infection and returns to low levels before the decline of IgM and IgG (Waites et al. 2017; Daxboeck et al. 2003). Studies have shown no advantage in children of selective IgA testing compared to IgM and IgG testing (Waites et al. 2017; Lee et al. 2017). There are few commercially available assays for IgA.

IgG. IgG levels rise more slowly throughout infection, usually reaching detectable levels 2 weeks after IgM has been detected. IgG peaks 4–5 weeks after illness onset with detectable levels that can persist for up to 4 years (Jacobs et al. 1986; Daxboeck et al. 2003). Acute and convalescent sera drawn at least 2 weeks apart and showing at least a fourfold rise in IgG are convincing evidence of recent *M. pneumoniae* infection (Daxboeck et al. 2003; Loens et al. 2010). A single IgG titer is not diagnostic for acute infection as the timing of seroconversion is not known.

6.6.6 Cat-Scratch Disease

Cat-scratch disease is a bacterial infection caused by *Bartonella henselae* that predominantly manifests as regional lymphadenopathy or lymphadenitis in immunocompetent children. *B. henselae* is a fastidious gram-negative bacillus with a low yield on routine cultures; molecular methods can be used in some laboratories to test tissues or body fluids when these specimens are available (Hansmann et al. 2005). Diagnosis of cat-scratch disease is routinely made with the presence of antibodies to *B. henselae* in the appropriate clinical setting. A combination of both serologic and molecular methods can increase detection accuracy (Allizond et al. 2019).

Cat-scratch disease should be considered in children with known exposure to cats who present with lymphadenopathy or lymphadenitis. Typically, a skin papule or pustule is found at the site of inoculation 3–10 days after the inoculating event, with subsequent development of lymphadenopathy proximal to the inoculation site. The lymphadenopathy is typically unilateral and solitary. It may be tender, warm, or erythematous and may suppurate spontaneously in up to 25% of cases (Carithers 1985). Testing for cat-scratch disease can also be considered in children with fever of unknown origin with or without lymphadenopathy (Murakami et al. 2002). Additionally, atypical disease or disseminated disease may occur, and *Bartonella* species are a known cause of culture-negative endocarditis (Edouard et al. 2015).

6.6.6.1 Serological Testing

Serologic testing for *B. henselae* commonly utilizes indirect IFAs or EIAs. Elevation in IgM may be brief. Therefore, a positive IgM may support the diagnosis, but a negative IgM should not exclude acute infection (Abarca et al. 2013). Diagnosis primarily relies on IgG titers for confirmation of diagnosis. Although the best evidence for acute infection is the demonstration of rising IgG titers, many patients already have high titers at the time of presentation, and titers can persist for up to 1 year (Dalton et al. 1995). Generally, an IgG titer <1:64 indicates a negative test, whereas a titer >1:256 is consistent with acute infection. IgG titers between 1:64 and 1:256 may indicate past or acute infection and may be repeated in 2 weeks to assess the trend (American Academy of Pediatrics 2018).

IFA assays for *B. henselae* IgG have been found to have sensitivities ranging from 93% to 100%, while specificity may be lower, from 70% to 98% (Murakami et al. 2002; Dalton et al. 1995; Sander et al. 1998). EIA tests are more specific, with a specificity of IgG assays up to 98% (Metzkor-Cotter et al. 2003; Giladi et al. 2001; Otsuyama et al. 2016; Tsuruoka et al. 2012). Cross-reactivity among the different *Bartonella* species on the serologic assays is common, and the available tests do not accurately differentiate the species (Stevens et al. 2014). Also, there is no standard timeline of anti-*B. henselae* IgG and IgM production in individuals with cat-scratch disease, making the diagnosis challenging (Bergmans et al. 1997).

6.6.7   Toxoplasmosis

Toxoplasmosis is caused by infection with the parasite *Toxoplasma gondii* and is one of the most common parasitic infections in humans. Although most individuals infected with *T. gon-*

dii are asymptomatic, clinical manifestations of acute infection or reactivation of chronic infection may occur in both immunocompetent and immunocompromised patients. Serologic testing is the primary method of diagnosis. Molecular methods may also be used and are commonly utilized when congenital toxoplasmosis is suspected (Contopoulos-Ioannidis and Montoya 2018).

Toxoplasmosis may be considered in patients who present with an infectious mononucleosis-like syndrome without evidence of an alternate diagnosis, such as EBV. Symptoms may be non-specific, such as malaise, fever, headache, sore throat, arthralgia, and myalgia. Both localized (solitary occipital) and generalized lymphadenopathy may be seen, often nonsuppurative and nontender (Contopoulos-Ioannidis and Montoya 2018). *T. gondii* is the most common infectious cause of retinitis and should be considered in any patient presenting with chorioretinitis (Miller et al. 2018).

Although *T. gondii* is found worldwide, the seroprevalence of *T. gondii* varies by geographic location and socioeconomic status. Toxoplasmosis should be considered in ill travelers of an endemic area with persistent fevers, myocarditis, myositis, hepatitis, pericarditis, encephalitis, and life-threatening pneumonia (American Academy of Pediatrics 2018).

6.6.7.1 Serological Testing

IgG-specific antibodies to *T. gondii* typically appear within 1–2 weeks after acute infection, peak within 1–5 months, and remain positive indefinitely. There are various commercial kits to measure IgG, including agglutination tests, IFAs, and EIAs (McAuley et al. 2015), and each test has varying sensitivity and specificity. IgM-specific antibodies can typically be detected 2 weeks after infection, with a peak at approximately 1 month. Most patients will have decreasing IgM titers that become undetectable within 6–9 months, although some patients can have persistent IgM for years.

Initial testing for *T. gondii* IgG and IgM antibodies in immunocompetent children and adolescents may be performed by non-reference or commercial laboratories; however, there are high

IgM false-positive rates. Confirmatory testing for *T. gondii* for all sera with positive IgM test results should be submitted to a reference laboratory with expertise in *T. gondii* assays and their interpretation, such as the Dr. Jack S. Remington Laboratory for Specialty Diagnostics, previously the Palo Alto Medication Foundation Toxoplasma Serology Laboratory (American Academy of Pediatrics 2018). Dr. Jack S. Remington Laboratory for Specialty Diagnostics helps clinicians identify the appropriate IgG and IgM assays based on patient age and exposure. Serologic tests performed at this laboratory have improved sensitivity and specificity compared to commercial assays (Montoya 2002; Pomares and Montoya 2016).

Additional testing may be useful in determining the timing of infection in patients with a positive IgM test, as well as for infants with concern for congenital toxoplasmosis. These tests, which are available at toxoplasma reference labs, include an IgG avidity test, the differential agglutination test, and IgA- and IgE-specific antibody tests (Goldstein et al. 2008).

6.7   Tick-Borne Infections

Ticks are the vector for various pathogens. The epidemiology of tick-borne diseases depends on the geographic distribution of the primary tick vector and human behaviors that put a child at risk for tick exposure. These infections should be considered in children with known or possible tick exposure in an area with endemic tick-borne disease.

6.7.1   Lyme Disease

Lyme disease is caused by *Borrelia burgdorferi*, which is transmitted by a bite from the ticks *Ixodes scapularis* or *Ixodes pacificus*. Serologic testing is the basis for Lyme disease diagnosis, although molecular testing may be sent on select specimens (CSF or synovial fluid).

Infection with *B. burgdorferi* can cause three distinct stages: early localized, early disseminated, and late disease. The diagnostic approach and expected serologic results vary based on the stage of disease clinically suspected (as summarized in Table 6.18).

Early localized disease is characterized by a primary erythema migrans rash, which develops at the site of an infected tick bite. Diagnosis of primary erythema migrans is based on the appearance of the rash. The lesion becomes apparent 7–14 days (range 3–30 days) after an infected tick is detached or removed (Wormser et al. 2006). The lesion can be somewhat variable with homogenous erythema, an area of central clearing, or a distinct target-like appearance. Untreated lesions may persist for weeks to months (Wormser et al. 2006).

Table 6.18 Diagnostic tests recommended for stages of Lyme disease

Lyme disease manifestation		Recommended diagnostic test	Comments
Early localized		N/A	Clinical diagnosis of rash Serology not recommended
Early disseminated	Multiple erythema migrans	Serology	Symptoms <4 weeks, Western blot IgM only may be positive; symptoms >4 weeks IgG should also be positive If IgG is negative, can repeat serology in 2–4 weeks to confirm the development of IgG
	Early neurologic (e.g., CN palsies, lymphocytic meningitis)	Serology Meningitis: CSF for *B. burgdorferi* antibodies and PCR	
	Carditis	Serology	
Late disseminated	Arthritis	Serology Synovial fluid for *B. burgdorferi* PCR	Western blot IgG should be positive. Western blot only positive for IgM is nondiagnostic
	Late neurologic	Serology	

Adapted from American Academy of Pediatrics 2018; Steere 2020
There is no clinical role for *B. burgdorferi* PCR or culture from the blood
CN cranial nerve, *CSF* cerebrospinal fluid, *PCR* polymerase chain reaction, *IgM* immunoglobulin M, *IgG* immunoglobulin G

When a child presents with a primary erythema migrans rash, serology is <40% sensitive for the diagnosis of Lyme disease, making this an unreliable test (Sanchez et al. 2016). If there is diagnostic uncertainty, Lyme antibodies tested on acute and convalescent serum can be compared to look for seroconversion. There is no clinical role for *B. burgdorferi* PCR or culture from the blood.

Early disseminated Lyme disease is characterized by multiple erythema migrans lesions, early neurologic manifestations, and carditis. Disseminated erythema migrans occur several days to weeks after untreated primary erythema due to the hematogenous spread of *B. burgdorferi* beyond the primary tick bite site (Steere 2020). Early neurologic involvement, including cranial neuropathies and lymphocytic meningitis, can begin after several weeks to months of untreated infection. Cranial nerve 7 palsy (Bell's palsy) is the most common cranial neuropathy and can be bilateral (Wormser et al. 2006). In children with cranial nerve 7 palsy and no clinical concern for meningitis, there are no clear recommendations on whether or not to perform a lumbar puncture. If performed, CSF may show lymphocytic pleocytosis, antibodies to *B. burgdorferi*, or positive *B. burgdorferi* PCR. Lumbar puncture is always indicated if there are associated signs or symptoms of meningitis (Wormser et al. 2006). For the diagnosis of central nervous system disease, especially meningitis, *B. burgdorferi* antibodies and PCR can be sent from CSF; however, they have low sensitivity (Sanchez et al. 2016). Cardiac manifestations of Lyme Disease may arise within several weeks after exposure (Steere 2020). Typically, there is acute onset of varying degrees of intermittent atrioventricular heart block, sometimes with associated myopericarditis (Wormser et al. 2006).

Over 80% of people with early neurologic and cardiac manifestations of Lyme disease are seropositive (Wormser et al. 2006). For the seronegative child at initial presentation, the convalescent serum should be tested for seroconversion 2 weeks later. For those with symptoms for <4 weeks, IgM only may be positive; however, if symptoms have persisted for >4 weeks, IgG should also be positive.

Late Lyme disease can manifest as joint or neurological complications. Monoarticular or oligoarticular arthritis due to *B. burgdorferi* can occur 3–6 months after untreated infection (Kullberg et al. 2020). The knee is most commonly involved, but other joints can be affected (Wormser et al. 2006). In Lyme arthritis, synovial fluid can show mild to moderate leukocytes, and *B. burgdorferi* PCR is often positive. *B. burgdorferi* PCR from the synovial fluid is >75% sensitive in patients with Lyme arthritis (Sanchez et al. 2016). Late neurologic disease with encephalomyelitis, peripheral neuropathy, and encephalopathy is a rare complication of untreated Lyme disease. In Lyme encephalomyelitis and some cases of encephalopathy, CSF can be positive for *B. burgdorferi* antibodies. PCR testing from CSF has very low sensitivity (Wormser et al. 2006). By the time of presentation with late Lyme disease, serology is positive for IgG antibodies.

6.7.1.1 Serologic Testing

Two-tiered serologic testing is recommended in the diagnosis of Lyme disease. This testing algorithm increases specificity as similar antibodies can be produced to other spirochetal infections, spirochetes in normal oral flora, other acute infections, and autoimmune diseases (American Academy of Pediatrics 2018).

The first tier of testing is an EIA or IFA. If this test is positive or equivocal, then the same serum sample is sent for second-tier testing, consisting of IgM and IgG Western blots. Alternatively, second-tier testing can be accomplished with an FDA-approved EIA confirmatory test (American Academy of Pediatrics 2021). Western blots for each IgM and IgG are interpreted as positive or negative based on the number of bands present (Table 6.19). A single EIA or IFA result should not be interpreted alone. A second-tier EIA confirmatory test or Western blot with sufficient bands confirm a positive result.

C6 EIA. Serologic testing with C6 EIA can detect antibodies to a peptide on *B. burgdorferi*. C6 EIA seems to have improved sensitivity in adults for detecting early Lyme disease and Lyme disease acquired in Europe. When used

Table 6.19 Criteria for positive Western blot in diagnosis of Lyme disease

IgM is considered positive when….	2 out of 3 of the following bands are present[a]: 23/24, 39, 41 kDa
IgG is considered positive when…	5 out of 10 of the following bands are present: 18, 23/24, 28, 30, 39, 41, 45, 60, 66, 93 kDa

Adapted from American Academy of Pediatrics 2018; Steere 2020

IgM immunoglobulin M, *IgG* immunoglobulin G, *kDa* kilodaltons

[a] 23 and 41 kDa bands together may represent a false-positive result

alone, its specificity is lower than the traditional two-tier testing (American Academy of Pediatrics 2018).

Pitfalls. In endemic areas, Lyme seropositivity population rates are 5%, with rates up to 50% in hunters (Kullberg et al. 2020). Therefore, it is important to correlate results with clinical findings. Some people treated with appropriate antibiotics for early localized Lyme disease may never develop antibodies (American Academy of Pediatrics 2018). For those who develop antibodies, serum Lyme IgG may persist for decades following appropriate treatment (Kullberg et al. 2020).

Lyme IgM should be interpreted with particular caution. IgM Western blot can be falsely positive, and it is only useful in a disease of <4 weeks' duration (American Academy of Pediatrics 2018). Positive IgM can be confirmed by evaluating for seroconversion of positive IgG in convalescent serum collected 2–4 weeks later.

Key Learning about Lyme Disease Serology

- Lyme disease testing should only be done when there are symptoms that are consistent with Lyme disease.
- Serologic testing for Lyme disease is recommended with two-tiered testing. If the first-tier EIA or IFA is positive or equivocal, a second tier of testing is completed.
- IgG bands should be present in patients who have had symptoms for >4 weeks.

6.7.2 Real-Life Example

A 17-year-old male presented to the office with a classic erythema migrans rash over his shoulder. His history was remarkable for hiking in the woods in northern Minnesota for 6 h 1 week ago. He admitted to seeing several ticks on his clothing but did not check himself for ticks after the hike. Based on the history and the physical exam, he was diagnosed with early localized Lyme disease. No serologic testing was ordered since the testing may be negative early in the course of Lyme disease. The child's lesion resolved after a ten-day course of doxycycline.

6.7.3 Human Granulocytic Anaplasmosis

Human granulocytic anaplasmosis (HGA) is caused by *Anaplasma phagocytophilum*, a rickettsial bacteria transmitted by the ticks *Ixodes scapularis* or *Ixodes pacificus*. *A. phagocytophilum* causes intracellular infection predominately of granulocytes (Biggs et al. 2016). In the United States, it is found primarily in the Northeastern states, upper Midwestern states, and Northern California; it can also be found in Europe and Asia (American Academy of Pediatrics 2018).

HGA may present as an acute febrile illness, headache, chills, malaise, myalgia, and nausea. General laboratory findings include leukopenia with neutropenia, thrombocytopenia, mild anemia, and mild elevations in liver transaminases (Biggs et al. 2016).

6.7.3.1 Diagnostic Testing for HGA

A specific diagnosis can be made with blood smear, PCR, or serology (see Table 6.20). A blood smear can show characteristic inclusions within neutrophils; however, a smear is very insensitive and should not be relied upon for diagnosis (Tickborne Diseases of the United States 2018). PCR of whole blood for detecting *A. phagocytophilum* is most sensitive during the first week of illness when the pathogen circulates in blood cells. The sensitivity of PCR may decrease after starting ther-

Table 6.20 Diagnostic tests for detection of common tick-borne diseases

Disease	Primary cell type infected	Diagnosis		
		Blood smear	PCR	Serology
Human granulocytic anaplasmosis	Granulocytes	Inclusions may be seen in granulocytes during the first week of illness	Yes – During the first week of illness	IgG often reaches ≥1:640 during acute infection; a single IgG titer ≥1:64 supports but does not confirm a recent disease diagnosis Compare acute and convalescent serum
Human monocytic ehrlichiosis	Monocytes and tissue macrophages	Inclusions may be seen in monocytes during the first week of illness	Yes – During the first week of illness	A single IgG titer ≥1:64 supports but does not confirm a diagnosis of recent disease Compare acute and convalescent serum
Babesiosis	Erythrocytes	Parasites may be seen in erythrocytes	Yes – During acute illness	IgG often reaches ≥1:1024 during acute infection; a single IgG titer ≥1:64 supports but does not confirm a recent disease diagnosis Compare acute and convalescent serum
Rocky Mountain spotted fever	Endothelial cells	N/A	No – Not sensitive	A single IgG titer ≥1:64 supports but does not confirm a diagnosis of recent disease Compare acute and convalescent serum

Adapted from Wormser et al. 2006; Sanchez et al. 2016; Biggs et al. 2016: MDPH et al., 2018; Ruebush et al. 1981
IgG immunoglobulin G

apy with tetracycline-class antibiotics (Biggs et al. 2016). Antibody titers often reach ≥1:640 during acute infection, but a single IgG titer ≥1:64 can suggest disease (Sanchez et al. 2016; Biggs et al. 2016). Serology can show a rise in IgG between acute and convalescent samples.

6.7.4 Human Monocytic Ehrlichiosis

Human monocytic ehrlichiosis (HME) is caused by infection with *Ehrlichia chaffeensis*, *E. ewingii*, or *E. muris eauclairensis*, which are transmitted by the ticks *Amblyomma americanum* or *Ixodes scapularis* (Biggs et al. 2016; MDPH et al., 2018). *Ehrlichia* species are intracellular bacteria that infect monocytes and tissue macrophages. In the United States, *E. chaffeensis* is predominantly found in the Southeast, South-central, and East coast states; *E. ewingii* is predominantly in the Southeast, South-central, and Midwestern states. Both *E. chaffeensis* and *E. ewingii* have been reported outside of the United States. *E. muris eauclairensis* has only been identified in Minnesota and Wisconsin.

HME may present as an acute febrile illness with headache, chills, malaise, myalgia, rash, and nausea. In the first week of illness, general labo-

ratory findings include leukopenia with lymphopenia, thrombocytopenia, and mild elevation in liver transaminases. Later in infection, anemia and mild to moderate hyponatremia may be apparent (Biggs et al. 2016).

6.7.4.1 Diagnostic Testing for HME
A specific diagnosis can be made with blood smear, PCR, or serology (see Table 6.20). A peripheral blood smear may show morulae in monocytes during the first week of illness; however, this is highly insensitive. Blood PCR is useful during the acute phase of infection since the pathogen is found in circulating blood cells. A single IgG titer ≥1:64 supports but does not confirm the diagnosis of recent disease (Biggs et al. 2016). Paired serology can show the development of IgG between acute and convalescent samples.

6.7.5 Babesiosis

Babesiosis is most often caused by infection with *Babesia microti*, transmitted by the tick *Ixodes scapularis.* Like malaria, it is a protozoal infection of RBCs. It is primarily found in the United States in the Northeastern and upper Midwestern states (MDPH et al., 2018).

Babesiosis is often asymptomatic but may present with fever and mild, nonspecific symptoms such as chills, myalgia, headache, or nausea. Notably, the infection can be severe in immunocompromised and asplenic children (American Academy of Pediatrics 2018). General laboratory findings include hemolytic anemia with elevated reticulocyte count, thrombocytopenia, proteinuria, elevated liver transaminases, and elevated blood urea nitrogen and creatinine (Wormser et al. 2006).

6.7.5.1 Diagnostic Testing for Babesiosis

A specific diagnosis can be made with blood smear, PCR, or serology (see Table 6.20). Microscopic identification of parasites can be made on Giemsa- or Wright-stained thin blood smears. Only a few RBCs may be infected, so multiple blood smears should be examined, although a negative smear does not exclude disease. *Babesia* species can be difficult to distinguish from malaria species (*Plasmodium falciparum*) on blood smears (American Academy of Pediatrics 2018). Blood PCR for the detection of *Babesia* species is more sensitive than blood smear during acute illness (Sanchez et al. 2016). A single IgG titer ≥1:64 supports the diagnosis of recent disease, but often, during acute infection, the IgG titer will be ≥1:1024 (Sanchez et al. 2016). Serology can demonstrate seroconversion of IgG between acute and convalescent samples (Wormser et al. 2006).

6.7.6 Rocky Mountain Spotted Fever

Rocky Mountain spotted fever (RMSF) is caused by infection with *Rickettsia rickettsii*, transmitted by the ticks *Dermacentor variabilis*, *D. andersoni*, or *Rhipicephalus sanguineus*. *R. rickettsii* is an intracellular bacterium that primarily infects endothelial cells and causes systemic, small-vessel vasculitis with high morbidity and mortality in untreated patients. RMSF is widespread in the United States, although most cases are reported in the South Atlantic, Southeast, and South-central states (MDPH et al., 2018).

Common symptoms of RMSF include fever, severe headache, myalgia, edema around the eyes and on the back of the hands, and gastrointestinal symptoms. A characteristic erythematous macular or maculopapular rash may appear within 2–4 days of symptom onset, first on the wrists and ankles and then spreading to the trunk, palms, and soles. Many patients seek care before rash onset, and approximately 10% of patients never develop a rash (Biggs et al. 2016; MDPH et al., 2018). General laboratory tests may be normal early in the disease course, but abnormalities may arise, including slightly increased leukocyte count, thrombocytopenia, slightly elevated liver transaminases, and hyponatremia (Biggs et al. 2016).

6.7.6.1 Diagnostic Testing for Rocky Mountain Spotted Fever

Blood PCR for *R. rickettsii* is not sensitive since there are low numbers of rickettsia in the bloodstream without advanced disease (Biggs et al. 2016). IgM and IgG begin to rise in the first week of infection. IgM is less specific, and IgG testing is preferred; an IgG titer ≥1:64 can suggest recent disease if positive. IgG may be negative in the first week of infection, although a titer ≥1:64 can suggest recent disease if positive. Serum samples taken 2–4 weeks after disease onset can show a rise in IgG. Very early therapy with tetracycline-class antibiotics may diminish or delay the development of antibodies to RMSF.

6.7.7 Pitfalls of Tick-Borne Infection Testing

Given the potential severity of illness, treatment should not be delayed for RMSF, HGA, or HME while awaiting diagnostic studies (Biggs et al. 2016).

Ixodes scapularis can transmit *B. burgdorferi*, *A. phagocytophilum*, *E. muris eauclairensis*, and *B. microti*. In endemic areas, coinfection with these organisms can occur. Coinfection can be considered in patients with early Lyme disease (erythema migrans) who present with more severe symptoms than typically seen in patients with Lyme disease alone or who have continued or worsening viral-like symptoms despite appropriate treatment for Lyme disease.

When considering serologic testing, IgG is often negative in the first week of infection when patients first present for care. It is recommended to test paired acute and convalescent serum for IgG 2–4 weeks apart (Biggs et al. 2016). Confirmation of infection can be made with ≥ fourfold rise in IgG titers in the setting of a compatible clinical illness. IgM is less specific and should not be used independently for diagnosis. Antibodies can persist for many years after acute infection (Biggs et al. 2016).

Many commercial laboratories offer tick-borne disease PCR and antibody panels. The PCR panels often include *A. phagocytophilum*, *Ehrlichia* species, and *Babesia* species. Lyme and RMSF are absent from these panels as routine blood PCR is not recommended in their diagnosis. Antibody panels often include serology to *A. phagocytophilum*, *E. chaffeensis*, *B. microti*, and *B. burgdorferi*. *R. rickettsii* antibodies need to be ordered separately. Table 6.20 reviews diagnostic tests for common tick-borne diseases.

6.8 Evaluation of the Child with Recurrent Infections

Recurrent infections in children can be concerning and frustrating for both the family and the primary care clinician. Young children may routinely have 6–12 acute respiratory tract illnesses per year, with similar numbers of acute otitis media episodes (Monto and Ullman 1974). Daycare attendance and secondhand smoke exposure may further increase the number of infections in children (Schuez-Havupalo et al. 2017; Kuehni and Barben 2015).

6.8.1 Immunodeficiency Warning Signs

The Jeffrey Modell Foundation developed a list of ten warning signs (Box 6.4) to assist clinicians in identifying patients at risk for primary immunodeficiency (PID) and suggested that patients with greater than or equal to two warning signs should be evaluated (The Jeffrey Modell Foundation [JMF] 2020). Clinicians should recognize that

this list will not detect all cases of PID (Arkwright and Gennery 2011). Although a large number of infections may prompt parents or clinicians to question the child's immune status, the number alone is unlikely to be predictive of PID. Important and more predictive factors may include severe, complicated, or deep-seated infections at multiple sites; a family history of immunodeficiency; failure to thrive; infections caused by atypical organisms; and the need for parenteral antibiotics to treat infections (Reda et al. 2013).

Concern for immunodeficiency should prompt a thorough history, physical exam, height, and weight records review. Anatomic and physiologic abnormalities and underlying conditions can predispose children to recurrent infections; initial abnormal findings may be supplemented with directed imaging and laboratory evaluation (Buescher 2018). Testing should generally be guided by the type of deficiency for which there is clinical concern. There are over 400 immunodeficiencies; examples of various immunodeficiencies are provided in Box 6.5 (JMF 2020).

Box 6.4 Jeffrey Modell Foundation Warning Signs for Patients at Risk for Primary Immunodeficiency

1. Four or more new ear infections within 1 year.
2. Two or more serious sinus infections within 1 year.
3. Two or more months on antibiotics with little effect.
4. Two or more pneumonias within 1 year.
5. Failure of an infant to gain weight or grow normally.
6. Recurrent, deep skin or organ abscesses.
7. Persistent thrush in mouth or fungal infection on skin.
8. Need for intravenous antibiotics to clear infections.
9. Two or more deep-seated infections including septicemia.
10. A family history of primary immunodeficiency.

Adapted from JMF 2020

Box 6.5 Examples of Specific Immunodeficiencies

Predominantly antibody deficiencies

Hyper-immunoglobulin M syndromes.
Immunoglobulin G subclass deficiency.
Selective immunoglobulin M deficiency.
Selective immunoglobulin A deficiency.
Common variable immunodeficiency.
Transient hypogammaglobulinemia of infancy.
X-linked agammaglobulinemia (Bruton).
Autosomal recessive agammaglobulinemia.

Combined immunodeficiencies

Severe combined immunodeficiency.
CD8 deficiency.

Other cellular immunodeficiencies

Wiskott-Aldrich syndrome.
Ataxia-telangiectasia.
DiGeorge anomaly.
Multiple cytokine deficiency.

Defects of phagocytic function

Chronic granulomatous disease.
Leukocyte adhesion defects.
Neutrophil G6PD deficiency.
Severe congenital neutropenia (Kostmann).
Cyclic neutropenia (elastase defect).

Secondary immunodeficiencies

Splenic deficiency.
Immunosuppression (corticosteroids, chemotherapy).
Chronic lung disease.
HIV infection.
Drug-induced hypogammaglobulinemia.

This list is not all-inclusive.
Adapted from Ochs et al. 2004

6.8.2 Diagnostic Testing for Immunodeficiency

If there are no history and physical findings to guide a directed investigation, an initial laboratory evaluation may be initiated (Table 6.21). The Jeffrey Modell Foundation has recommended a four-stage approach to the child with suspected immunodeficiency, which may be a useful strategy for the primary care clinician. Stage 1 testing includes a CBC with differential and total immunoglobulins. A chemistry panel, urinalysis, and inflammatory markers are recommended to rule out causes of secondary immunodeficiency if not previously performed. Stage 2 testing includes a specific antibody response to tetanus toxoid and diphtheria toxoid, pneumococcal antigen, and IgG subclass analysis (JMF 2020). The primary care clinician may also include a total hemolytic complement (CH50) in the early stages of testing to evaluate the classic complement pathway's functional integrity. Further laboratory examinations for PID often require specialized laboratory expertise and facilities, and consultation with an immunologist is recommended even during the early diagnostic process (Alkhater 2009).

6.8.2.1 Assessment of Antibody Levels

Predominant antibody deficiencies are the most common type of immunodeficiency, accounting for approximately 50–70% of all PID (Bonilla et al. 2015). Children with antibody deficiencies or defects of antibody function are predisposed to recurrent sinopulmonary infections, including recurrent otitis media, pneumonia, or rhinosinusitis, as well as recurrent gastroenteritis and sepsis (Bousfiha et al. 2013). They are particularly susceptible to infection with polysaccharide-encapsulated organisms, including *Streptococcus pneumoniae* and *Haemophilus influenzae*. Quantitative testing of serum IgG, IgM, and IgA should be performed as part of the initial laboratory screening for primary immunodeficiency. IgE may be performed; IgD levels are not part of the initial screening.

There is significant variation in normal values with different age groups, testing methods, and laboratories. For this reason, the results must be compared to age-matched controls for the specific method being used (McCusker et al. 2018). Quantitative antibody levels assist in the diagnosis of profound antibody deficiencies, such as X-linked agammaglobulinemia, as well as less severe antibody deficiencies, such as transient hypogammaglobulinemia of infancy. Antibody deficiencies may also be present in genetic

Table 6.21 Initial laboratory evaluation for immunodeficiency

	Test	Purpose
Stage 1	CBC with differential	• Assess numbers and morphology: Leukopenia or leukocytosis, anemia, thrombocytopenia, cell inclusions – Lymphopenia for age is cause for concern (ALC < 2500 cells/μL in infants: <1500 cell/μL in children) – Neutropenia could indicate cyclic or congenital neutropenia – Persistent leukocytosis may be seen with infection or leukocyte adhesion deficiency – Anemia could indicate malnutrition, red blood cell disorder (thalassemia, sickle cell), or aplastic anemia – Thrombocytopenia can be seen in Wiskott-Aldrich syndrome or autoimmune cytopenias
	Chemistry panel	• Assists with identification of liver or renal disease, diabetes, and malnutrition as etiologies of secondary immunodeficiency
	Urinalysis	• Proteinuria may suggest protein loss via kidneys
	Inflammatory markers	• Elevations may be seen with infection and other inflammatory disorders
	Total IgG, IgM, IgA[a]	• Assists with identification of antibody deficiencies • Quantification identifies increased or decreased levels for age
Stage 2	Antibody titers to diphtheria and tetanus toxoid, HIB	• Assess antibody production in response to specific protein antigens (e.g., antibody function)
	Antibody titers to pneumococcal antigen	• Assess antibody production in response to specific polysaccharide antigens (e.g., antibody function)
	IgG subclass analysis	• Assess for specific IgG subclass deficiencies
Consider	CH50[b]	• Evaluation of the classic complement pathway (C1-C9)

CBC complete blood count, *ALC* absolute lymphocyte count, *BUN* blood urea nitrogen, *IgG* immunoglobulin G, *IgM* immunoglobulin M, *IgA* immunoglobulin A, *HIB Haemophilus influenzae* B, *CH50* total hemolytic complement
Adapted from Buescher 2018; Ochs et al. 2004; Sullivan and Winkelstein 2004
[a] Immunoglobulin E and D testing is not routinely performed during the initial evaluation
[b] May consider CH50 as part of a broader initial evaluation; referral to an immunologist should be sought early in this process, when possible

syndromes and secondary immunodeficiencies (Ochs et al. 2004). Notably, antibody levels may be difficult to interpret during active infection episodes; testing during wellness periods is preferred.

6.8.2.2 Assessment of Antibody Function

Bacterial antigens are predominantly either complex polysaccharides or proteins. Children may have impaired response to polysaccharide antigens or have impaired response to both polysaccharide and protein antigens; it is atypical for a patient to have a poor response to only protein antigens. IgG titers to vaccines that contain protein or polysaccharide antigens can be used to determine specific antibody responses to each type of antigen (Perez et al. 2017).

Evaluation of response to polysaccharide antigens in children. Typically, the 23-valent pneumococcal polysaccharide vaccine (PPV-23) is used to assess an individual's response to polysaccharide antigens. The conjugate pneumococcal vaccine that is routinely administered to young children, previously Prevnar 7 (PCV 7) and currently Prevnar 13 (PCV 13), is not useful in assessing the response to polysaccharide antigens. The PPV-23 should only be utilized in children >2 years old for assessing responsiveness to polysaccharide antigens. Children <2 years old often do not have a robust response to polysaccharide vaccines, and routine conjugate vaccines may be less effective if administered after polysaccharide vaccines. Children should receive at least three doses of conjugate vaccine before receiving PPV-23. Commercially available pneumococcal titer panels vary—the primary care clinician should request a panel of at least 14 and ideally 23 serotypes.

Interpretation. When assessing pneumococcal serotype titers in children who have received conjugate vaccines previously, only non-conjugate serotypes should be evaluated for response. Table 6.22 is a list of the serotypes in commonly administered pneumococcal vaccines in the United States. The initial measurement of serum titers should be obtained before immunization with PPV-23 to assess the magnitude of increased response caused by vaccination. After administering PPV-23, post-vaccination titers should be measured ≥4 weeks after administering the vaccine but no more than 12 weeks post-vaccination. A serotype-specific IgG concentration ≥ 1.3 mcg/mL, or an increase in the titer of at least two-fold, is considered a normal response to polysaccharide antigens (Orange et al. 2012). This level should be used instead of the laboratory-provided reference range when assessing titers. Table 6.23 reviews the acceptable percentage of positive PPV-23 serotypes post-vaccination by age. An insufficient response to PPV-23 indicates a poor response to polysaccharide antigens.

Pitfalls. Assessing responses to vaccine serotypes <4 weeks after vaccination with PPV-23

Table 6.22   Serotypes in pneumococcal vaccines

Prevnar 7[a]	Prevnar 13	Pneumovax 23	
4	4	4	Serotypes limited to PPV-23[b]
6B	6B	6B	2
9 V	9 V	9 V	8
14	14	14	9 N
18C	18C	18C	10A
19F	19F	19F	11A
23F	23F	23F	12F
–	1	1	15B
–	5	5	17F
–	3	3	20
–	7F	7F	22F
–	19A	19A	33F
–	6A	6A	

Adapted from Centers for Disease Control and Prevention (2015a)

PPV-23 Pneumovax 23

[a] Children vaccinated before the widespread use of Prevnar 13 may have received Prevnar 7

[b] There is a Prevnar 15 vaccine product in development that includes 22F and 33F in addition to the serotypes included in Prevnar 13

Table 6.23 Acceptable percentage of Pneumovax 23-specific serotypes post-vaccination by age

Age	Percent positive (≥ 1.3 mg/dL or twofold increase)
<6 years	50%
≥6 years	70%

Adapted from Orange et al. 2012

may result in low titers. The response to vaccination cannot reliably be evaluated in patients who have received immune globulin in the past 4–6 months or who have received specific immunoglobulins to prevent infections in the past 3–5 months. Pre- and post-vaccination titers should be performed at the same laboratory using the same assay as differences in methodology may affect interpretation.

6.8.2.3 Evaluating Response to Protein Antigens

Diphtheria, tetanus, and *Haemophilus influenzae* B (HIB) vaccines may be used to evaluate an individual's response to protein antigens. Tetanus and diphtheria vaccines are both toxoid vaccines. The HIB vaccine is a conjugate vaccine composed of polysaccharide polyribosylribitol phosphate (PRP) as the primary antigen, which is conjugated to immunogenic proteins of either diphtheria toxoid or the outer membrane protein complex of meningococcus. Antibodies are produced to the protein component so that the HIB conjugate vaccine can measure protein response. Anti-diphtheria toxin, anti-tetanus toxin, and anti-PRP antibodies should be measured after a series of three immunizations has been completed, generally after 6 months of age.

Interpretation. The levels of anti-diphtheria, anti-tetanus, and anti-PRP IgG titers that are suggestive of a vaccine response are noted in Table 6.24. Antibody titers that suggest vaccine response but remain relatively low may not confer long-term protection; accepted antibody titers that suggest a long-term protective level are also noted in Table 6.24. Timing of the immunization to the titer assessment should be considered in the interpretation of values. For example, detectable but relatively low titers in a patient who was recently immunized may not be sufficient to

Table 6.24 Interpretation of antibody titers to protein antigens

Antibody	Peak antibody levels	Suggestive of vaccine response	Suggestive of long-term protection
Anti-diphtheria	2–3 weeks	>0.01 IU/mL	>0.1 IU/mL
Anti-tetanus	2–3 weeks	>0.01 IU/mL	>0.15 IU/mL
Anti-PRP (HIB)	3–4 weeks	>0.15 mcg/mL	≥1 mcg/mL

Adapted from Orange et al. (2012), Hammarlund et al. (2016), WHO (2017), Gergen et al. (1995), Peltola et al. (1977), Käyhty et al. (1983), Käyhty et al. (1983)
PRP polysaccharide polyribosylribitol phosphate, *HIB Haemophilus influenzae* B

interpret as an appropriate response, as a more robust response would be anticipated; conversely, low titers in a patient who was vaccinated several years prior may not be indicative of immune dysfunction, as the exact timing of waning antibody after vaccination has not been established. In this case, it is reasonable to administer a booster dose of vaccine and reassess titers post-vaccination. After receiving the conjugated HIB vaccine, PRP antibodies do not rule out a defect in response to polysaccharide antigens.

6.8.2.4 Immunoglobulin G Subclasses

Measurement of IgG subclasses may be useful as part of the immune evaluation, particularly in patients with a clinically concerning history of infections and normal total immunoglobulin concentrations. An IgG subclass deficiency refers to a decrease in the serum concentration of one or more IgG subclass, despite a normal level of total IgG. Children with a symptomatic IgG subclass deficiency may present with recurrent otitis media, rhinosinusitis, pneumonia, allergic asthma, allergic rhinitis, or autoimmune conditions. More serious infections, such as septicemia, meningitis, and osteomyelitis, may also occur (Parker et al. 2017).

The normal ranges for IgG subclasses vary with the method of analysis and the child's age. The primary care clinician should ensure that the laboratory provides age-matched reference ranges for the method being used. Notably, an IgG subclass deficiency may not be clinically relevant, particularly in the setting of normal total immunoglobulins and normal response to vaccines (Buckley 2002). A clinically significant IgG subclass deficiency may be diagnosed in the setting of recurrent infections and evidence of inadequate vaccine response. Abnormal IgG subclass concentrations should be confirmed with at least one additional measurement 1 month after the initial test (Parker et al. 2017).

6.8.2.5 Total Serum Hemolytic Complement

Measurement of CH50 activity is a useful screening tool for detecting deficiencies of the classical complement pathway. All nine classical pathway components (C1 through C9) are required for a normal CH50; deficiency of any complement protein within this pathway leads to decreased or absent activity (Buescher 2018). The clinical presentation of complement deficiencies includes increased susceptibility to infection, rheumatic disease, and angioedema. The particular presentation and the kind of bacteria that most commonly causes infection relate to the deficient component's normal physiologic role (Sullivan and Winkelstein 2004).

An undetectable or extremely low CH50 result suggests a specific complement deficiency and requires further testing to determine the abnormal complement component. Recurrent infections like meningococcemia may be a sign of a complement deficiency (Lewis and Ram 2014). Both decreased and elevated levels of CH50 may be found during an active infection, and decreased levels may also be found in rheumatologic and immune complex diseases. Neonates have reduced CH50, as there is little to no maternal complement transfer to the fetus in utero. Neonates generally reach adult values of complement proteins by 6–18 months of age (Hong and Lewis 2016). A common cause of a low CH50 is improper specimen handling, as several complement proteins are unstable. A very low CH50 should be confirmed with a new sample.

6.8.3 Real-Life Example

A one-year-old male had a history of four episodes of otitis media and one episode of sinusitis and most recently had a second episode of pneumonia requiring hospitalizations. The child was growing on the fifth to the tenth percentile. There was no family history of immune deficiency. A B cell deficiency was suspected, and the child was referred for evaluation of possible X-linked agammaglobulinemia due to recurrent sinopulmonary infection (Smith and Cunningham-Rundles 2019). The diagnosis was confirmed by infectious disease. The clinician was made aware of the increased risk of leukemia and lymphoma (Hoshino et al. 2015).

Key Learning Points about Immunodeficiencies in Pediatrics

- The number of infections alone is not predictive of immunodeficiency.
- Type and location of the infection, family history, growth history, organisms involved, and treatment course may be predictive factors for immunodeficiency.
- The initial screening for immunodeficiency may include CBC with differential and total immunoglobulins, as well as additional testing to rule out possible causes of secondary immunodeficiency.
- When possible, consultation with an immunologist is recommended even during the early diagnostic process to help guide testing.

Questions

1. A child has a negative hepatitis B surface antigen, negative anti-HBc, and positive anti-HBs. What does this indicate?
   - (a) The child has hepatitis B.
   - (b) The child had hepatitis B in the past and is immune.
   - (c) The child has been vaccinated.
   - (d) The child needs to be revaccinated.

2. A child has a negative hepatitis B surface antigen but positive anti-HBs and anti-HBc. What does this indicate?
   - (a) The child has not been vaccinated.
   - (b) The child has hepatitis B in the past and is immune.
   - (c) The child has active hepatitis B.
   - (d) The child needs to be revaccinated.

3. A 5-year-old has his second case of meningococcemia. What should you suspect?
   - (a) A T cell defect.
   - (b) A B cell defect.
   - (c) A complement defect.
   - (d) A neutrophil defect.

4. A 16-year-old female presents with 12 days of fever, pharyngitis, fatigue, and cervical lymphadenopathy. She reports four sexual partners in the past year. A throat culture for group A streptococcus, a monospot, and a VCA IgG, VCA IgM, and EBNA for EBV are all negative. What is the next step?
   - (a) Send a QuantiFERON test.
   - (b) Send an HIV fourth-generation antigen/antibody test.
   - (c) Send initial PCR for Zika virus.
   - (d) Send an HIV NAAT.

5. A child has EBV serology as follows: VCA IgM negative, VCA IgG positive, EA-D negative, and EBNA IgG positive. What is an appropriate interpretation of this pattern?
   - (a) EBV-naïve.
   - (b) Past infection.
   - (c) Convalescent infection.
   - (d) Early primary infection.

6. A healthy six-year-old child with no known risk factors for mycobacterium tuberculosis and no history of BCG vaccine. The child requires a tuberculin skin test for summer camp paperwork. The induration is measured at 7 mm, although there is erythema that measures at 18 mm. What is the interpretation of this result?
   - (a) The results are considered a positive test. The child should have a chest X-ray.
   - (b) The test was administered incorrectly and should be performed again.
   - (c) The child has active tuberculosis.
   - (d) The results are considered a negative test. No further examination is required.

7. A patient's serology for Zika virus and dengue virus is as follows: Zika virus IgM positive, dengue virus IgM positive, Zika virus plaque reduction neutralization test is ≥10, and dengue virus plaque neutralization test is <10. How is this interpreted?
   (a) Recent Zika virus infection.
   (b) Recent dengue virus infection.
   (c) Recent flavivirus infection – unable to determine the specific virus.
   (d) No evidence of recent Zika or dengue virus infection.

8. A child presents in February with swelling and redness of the right knee. He reports tick exposure the previous summer. Before being referred to the emergency department, Lyme serology is obtained. The result shows first-tier EIA positive and second-tier Western blot with 2 IgM and 2 IgG bands positive. How is this result interpreted?
   (a) Suggestive of early localized Lyme disease.
   (b) Suggestive of early disseminated Lyme disease.
   (c) Suggestive of Lyme arthritis.
   (d) The child has a disease not related to Lyme.

9. A 5-year-old previously healthy boy presents with pharyngitis and fever. He is positive for group A streptococcus (GAS) using a molecular test for strep. He is started on a 10-day course of amoxicillin. He completes 8 days of a ten-day course of Amoxil but returns with rhinorrhea, cough, and sore throat. On exam, he has pharyngeal erythema without exudate and a macular rash on his trunk. What is the next step?
   (a) Provide reassurance.
   (b) Obtain a throat culture for GAS and order susceptibilities.
   (c) Provide a prescription for azithromycin.
   (d) Send anti-streptolysin O and anti-deoxyribonuclease levels.

10. A 17-year-old girl presents to get screened for sexually transmitted infections. She is currently asymptomatic. She has had multiple partners in the past and comes in for routine screening every 6 months. She is found to have positive testing for syphilis with TP-PA positive and RPR 1:64. She is treated for early latent syphilis with one dose of benzathine penicillin G IM. Six months later, she returns and is found to have TP-PA positive and RPR 1:1. What is the next step?
    (a) Retreat with benzathine penicillin G.
    (b) Re-test in 2–4 weeks.
    (c) Re-test in 6 months.
    (d) Get a lumbar puncture to look for neurosyphilis.

11. For which patient would you begin a workup for immunodeficiency?
    (a) A 7-month-old girl with recurrent oral thrush despite treatment. She is growing well.
    (b) A 5-year-old boy with recurrent ear infections between 1 and 3 years that resolved with tympanostomy tubes. He now presents with multiple viral illnesses since starting kindergarten.
    (c) An 8-year-old girl with two admissions for bacteremia and severe pneumonia in the last 2 years, now presenting for a third sinus infection this year.
    (d) A 10-year-old boy with asthma receiving antibiotics once or twice a year for asthma exacerbation with concurrent pneumonia.

Rationale

1. Answer: C
   The child has been vaccinated. In this case scenario, the child only has a positive anti-HBs. If the child had the disease and recovered, he would have positive anti-HBs and anti-Hbs. If he had a positive HbsAg, and a positive anti-HBc IgM but a negative anti-HBs, he would have an acute infection.

2. Answer: B
   See rationale above.

3. Answer: C
   Patients with a complement defect may present with recurrent meningococcemia.

4. Answer: D

Acute HIV is included in the differential diagnosis in patients with a presentation similar to infectious mononucleosis without evidence of EBV infection or streptococcal pharyngitis. A fourth-generation HIV antigen/antibody test is unlikely to capture acute HIV as antibodies do not develop for 2–4 weeks after HIV exposure. An HIV NAAT, such as a quantitative HIV-1 RNA PCR, becomes positive within 10–14 days. Adolescents may or may not report sexual activity to their providers. Therefore, presenting this testing as a common component of this workup in children of all ages may be beneficial. This clinical presentation is not consistent with pulmonary tuberculosis. Testing for ZIKV infection may be considered in patients presenting with acute onset of fever, maculopapular rash, arthralgia, or conjunctivitis who live in or have traveled to an ongoing transmission area 2 weeks before the onset of symptoms.

5. Answer: B

Past infection is consistent with a positive VCA IgG and positive EBNA IgG, +/− EA-D. Convalescent infection may be difficult to determine as this typically presents with a positive VCA IgG, with or without VCA IgM, EA-D, or EBNA IgG. EBV-naïve patients would have negative results for all EBV antibodies. Early primary infection typically presents with a positive VCA IgM and positive VCA IgG, +/− EA-D.

6. Answer: D

When reading tuberculin skin tests, measurements should be performed of the induration rather than erythema. Children with no risk factors for tuberculosis require induration measured ≥15 mm to be considered a positive test. Induration <15 mm in children with no risk factors is considered a negative test.

7. Answer: A

There is significant cross-reaction among IgM testing for flaviviruses. Although this patient had positive Zika and dengue serology, the plaque neutralization test revealed a positive result only for Zika virus, indicating a recent Zika virus infection.

8. Answer: D

This patient presents with clinical concern for Lyme arthritis. This manifestation of Lyme occurs 3–6 months after a bite from an infected tick. By this time, IgG will be positive. This patient had a positive first-tier screen, but only IgM is considered positive, with two out of three bands positive. Less than five out of ten IgG bands are positive, so IgG is interpreted as a negative result. Since Lyme IgG is negative, this patient's arthritis is not due to Lyme disease. In early localized disease, serology is often negative. In early disseminated disease, if symptoms have occurred for <4 weeks, Western blot IgM only may be positive, and IgG may be negative. This patient's results could be consistent with early disease Lyme disease, but the clinical picture does not support this diagnosis.

9. Answer: A

This child is getting appropriate treatment for GAS pharyngitis and now presents with symptoms more consistent with a viral infection, including rhinorrhea, cough, and absence of fever. Reassurance and supportive care can be provided. Repeat culture is not indicated since he may continue to be GAS positive on throat culture despite appropriate treatment. Susceptibility testing is not indicated as GAS is universally sensitive to penicillin (and amoxicillin). Azithromycin can be used to treat GAS in children with true penicillin and cephalosporin allergy; however, this child's rash and symptoms are more consistent with a viral infection and not an allergy. There is no role for serologic testing in the diagnosis of acute GAS infection.

10. Answer: C.

After appropriate treatment for syphilis, nontreponemal titers will decline over time, while treponemal titers will remain positive regardless of treatment. This patient declined in RPR from 1:64 to 1:1 (titer of 1:64 indicates more antibody is present compared to the lower titer of 1:1), which indicates successful treatment. Repeat nontreponemal testing is recommended 12 months after treatment, which should be repeated in another 6 months.

11. Answer: C.

A child with two deep-seated infections plus two or more sinus infections in a year concerns an immunodeficiency. With recurrent sinopulmonary infections, there is a concern for antibody deficiency or defects in function.

References

AASLD-IDSA. HCV in children. Recommendations for testing, managing, and treating hepatitis C. https://www.hcvguidelines.org/unique-populations/children. Accessed November 20, 2020.

Abarca K, Winter M, Marsac D, Palma C, Contreras AM, Ferrés M. Accuracy and diagnostic utility of IgM in Bartonella henselae infections. Rev Chil Infectol. 2013;30(2):125–8.

Abbag F, Al Qahtani J. Extreme elevation of the erythrocyte sedimentation rate in children. Ann Saudi Med. 2007;27(3):175–8.

AbuSalah MAH, Gan SH, Al-Hatamleh MAI, Irekeola AA, Shueb RH, Yean C. Recent advances in diagnostic approaches for Epstein-Barr virus. Pathogens. 2020;9(3):226.

Adebanjo T, Godfred-Cato S, Viens L, et al. Update: interim guidance for the diagnosis, evaluation, and management of infants with possible congenital zika virus infection—United States, October 2017.

Adler SP, Marshall B. Cytomegalovirus infections. Pediatr Rev. 2007;28(3):92–100.

Agrawal A. CRP after 2004. Mol Immunol. 2005;42(8):927–30.

Alkhater SA. Approach to the child with recurrent infections. J Family Community Med. 2009;16(3):77–82. PMID: 23012196; PMCID: PMC3377046.

Allizond V, Costa C, Sidoti F, et al. Serological and molecular detection of Bartonella henselae in specimens from patients with suspected cat-scratch disease in Italy: a comparative study. PLoS One. 2019;14(2):e0211945.

American Academy of Pediatrics. Summaries of infectious diseases. In: Kimberlin DW, Brady MT, Jackson MA, Long SS, editors. Red book: 2018 report of the committee on infectious diseases. American Academy of Pediatrics; 2018. p. 235–901.

American Academy of Pediatrics. Summaries of infectious diseases. In: Kimberlin DW, Brady MT, Jackson MA, Long SS, editors. Red book: 2021 report of the committee on infectious diseases. American Academy of Pediatrics; 2021. Section 3.

Amir J, Shechter Y, Eilam N, Varsano I. Group a beta-hemolytic streptococcal pharyngitis in children younger than 5 years. Israel J Med Sci. 1994; 30(8):619.

Andreola B, Bressan S, Callegaro S, Liverani A, Plebani M, Da Dalt L. Procalcitonin and C-reactive protein as diagnostic markers of severe bacterial infections in febrile infants and children in the emergency department. Pediatr Infect Dis J. 2007;26(8): 672–7.

Andrews JM. Determination of minimum inhibitory concentrations. J Antimicrob Chemother. 2001;48(Suppl 1):5–16.

Appenzeller C, Ammann RA, Duppenthaler A, Gorgievski-Hrisoho M, Aebi C. Serum C-reactive protein in children with adenovirus infection. Swiss Med Wkly. 2002;132(25–26):345–50.

Arif T, Phillips RS. Updated systematic review and meta-analysis of the predictive value of serum biomarkers in the assessment and management of fever during neutropenia in children with cancer. Pediatr Blood Cancer. 2019;66(10):e27887.

Arkwright PD, Gennery AR. Ten warning signs of primary immunodeficiency: a new paradigm is needed for the 21st century. Ann N Y Acad Sci. 2011;1238:7–14.

Arvin AM. Varicella-Zoster virus. In: Long SS, editor. Principles and practice of pediatric infectious diseases. 5th ed. Philadelphia, PA: Elsevier; 2018. p. 1065–72.

Association of Public Health Laboratories. Consultation on laboratory diagnosis of syphilis, meeting summary report. 2018.

Ayoub EM, Wannamaker LW. Evaluation of the streptococcal desoxyribo-nuclease b and diphosphopyridine nucleotidase antibody tests in acute rheumatic fever and acute glomerulonephritis. Pediatrics. 1962;29(4):527–38.

Baird GS. The choosing wisely initiative and laboratory test stewardship. Diagnosi. 2019;6(1):15–23.

Barlam TF, Cosgrove SE, Abbo LM, et al. Implementing an antibiotic stewardship program: guidelines by the Infectious Diseases Society of America and the Society for Healthcare Epidemiology of America. Clin Infect Dis. 2016;62(10):e51–77.

Barone SR, Pontrelli LR, Krilov LR. The differentiation of classic Kawasaki disease, atypical Kawasaki disease, and acute adenoviral infection: use of clinical features and a rapid direct fluorescent antigen test. Arch Pediatr Adolesc Med. 2000;154(5):453–6.

Batlivala SP. Focus on diagnosis: the erythrocyte sedimentation rate and the C-reactive protein test. Pediatr Rev. 2009;30(2):72–4.

Becker KL, Snider R, Nylen ES. Procalcitonin assay in systemic inflammation, infection, and sepsis: clinical utility and limitations. Crit Care Med. 2008;36(3):941–52.

Bennett TD, Hayward KN, Farris RW, Ringold S, Wallace CA, Brogan TV. Very high serum ferritin levels are associated with increased mortality and critical care in pediatric patients. Pediatr Crit Care Med. 2011;12(6):e233–6.

Bergmans AM, Peeters MF, Schellekens JF, et al. Pitfalls and fallacies of cat scratch disease serology: evaluation of Bartonella henselae-based indirect fluorescence assay and enzyme-linked immunoassay. J Clin Microbiol. 1997;35(8):1931–7.

Beukelman T, Patkar NM, Saag KG, et al. 2011 American College of Rheumatology recommendations for the treatment of juvenile idiopathic arthritis: initiation and safety monitoring of therapeutic agents for the treatment of arthritis and systemic features. Arthritis Care Res (Hoboken). 2011;63(4):465–82.

Biggs HM, Behravesh CB, Bradley KK, et al. Diagnosis and management of tickborne rickettsial diseases: Rocky Mountain spotted fever and other spotted fever group rickettsioses, ehrlichiosis, and anaplasmosis—United States: a practical guide for health care and public health professionals. MMWR: Recomm Rep. 2016;65(2):1–44.

Binnicker MJ, Espy MJ, Irish CL. Rapid and direct detection of herpes simplex virus in cerebrospinal fluid by use of a commercial real-time PCR assay. J Clin Microbiol. 2014;52(12):4361–2.

Birgegard G, Hallgren R, Killander A, Stromberg A, Venge P, Wide L. Serum ferritin during infection. A longitudinal study. Scand J Haematol. 1978;21(4):333–40.

Bonilla FA, Khan DA, Ballas ZK, et al. Practice parameter for the diagnosis and management of primary immunodeficiency. J Allergy Clin Immunol. 2015;136(5):1186–205. e1178

Bousfiha AA, Jeddane L, Ailal F, et al. A phenotypic approach for IUIS PID classification and diagnosis: guidelines for clinicians at the bedside. J Clin Immunol. 2013;33(6):1078–87.

Branson BM, Owen SM. Human immunodeficiency viruses. In: Jorgenson JH, Pfaller MA, Carroll KC, et al., editors. Manual of clinical microbiology. 11th ed. Washington, DC: ASM Press; 2015. p. 1436–57.

Branson BM, Owen SM, Wesolowski LG, et al. Laboratory testing for the diagnosis of HIV infection : updated recommendations. In: T. B. Prevention, Division of HIV/AIDS Prevention, editor. Centers for disease control & prevention, association of Public Health Laboratories, National Center for HIV/Aids VH. Atlanta, GA; 2014. https://doi.org/10.15620/cdc.23447.

Brigden ML. Clinical utility of the erythrocyte sedimentation rate. Am Fam Physician. 1999;60(5):1443–50.

Britt W. Cytomegalovirus. In: Wilson CB, Nizet V, Maldonado YA, Remington JS, Klein JO, editors. Remington and Klein's infectious diseases of the fetus and newborn infant. 8th ed. Philadelphia, PA: Elsevier Saunders; 2016. p. 724–65.

Brooks ZC, Das S. COVID-19 testing. Am J Clin Pathol. 2020;154(5):575–84.

Bruu AL, Hjetland R, Holter E, et al. Evaluation of 12 commercial tests for detection of Epstein-Barr virus-specific and heterophile antibodies. Clin Diagn Lab Immunol. 2000;7(3):451–6.

Bu X, Chen J, Wan Y, Xu L. Diagnostic value of D-dimer combined with WBC count, neutrophil percentage and CRP in differentiating between simple and. Clin Lab. 2016;62(9):1675–81.

Buckley RH. Immunoglobulin G subclass deficiency: fact or fancy? Curr Allergy Asthma Rep. 2002;2(5):356–60.

Buescher ES. Evaluation of the child with suspected immunodeficiency. In: Long SS, editor. Principles and practice of pediatric infectious diseases. 5th ed. Philadelphia, PA: Elsevier; 2018. p. 1128–31.

Caird MS, Flynn JM, Leung YL, Millman JE, D'Italia JG, Dormans JP. Factors distinguishing septic arthritis from transient synovitis of the hip in children. A prospective study. J Bone Joint Surg. 2006;88(6):1251–7.

Carcillo JA, Sward K, Halstead ES, et al. A systemic inflammation mortality risk assessment contingency table for severe sepsis. Pediatr Crit Care Med. 2017;18(2):143–50.

Carithers HA. Cat-scratch disease. An overview based on a study of 1,200 patients. Am J Dis Child. 1985;139(11):1124–33.

Cavallo ML, Castrovilli A, D'Introno A, et al. A systemic and severe infection via cytomegalovirus and other herpesviruses in a young apparently immunocompetent patient: a case report. J Med Cases. 2017;8(9):265–8.

Centers for Disease Control and Prevention. Discordant results from reverse sequence syphilis screening- five laboratories, United States, 2006–2010. MMWR. 2011;60:5.

Centers for Disease Control and Prevention. Epidemiology and prevention of vaccine-preventable diseases. Washington D.C.: Public Health Foundation; 2015a.

Centers for Disease Control and Prevention. Hepatitis a. In: Hamborsky J, Kroger A, Wolfe S, editors. Epidemiology and prevention of vaccine-preventable diseases. 13th ed. Washington D.C.: Public Health Foundation; 2015b.

Centers for Disease Control and Prevention. Hepatitis B. In: Hamborsky J, Kroger A, Wolfe S, editors. Epidemiology and prevention of vaccine-preventable diseases. 13th ed. Washington D.C.: Public Health Foundation; 2015c.

Centers for Disease Control and Prevention. NEW Zika and dengue testing guidance. 2019. https://www.cdc.gov/zika/hc-providers/testing-guidance.html. Assessed December 1, 2020.

Centers for Disease Control and Prevention. Prevention of hepatitis a virus infection in the United States: recommendation of the advisory committee on immunization practices, 2020. MMWR. 2020a;69:5.

Centers for Disease Control and Prevention. Hepatitis E questions and answers for health professionals. 2020b. https://www.cdc.gov/hepatitis/hev/hevfaq.htm#section4. Accessed December 1, 2020.

Centers for Disease Control and Prevention. Hepatitis E. In: CDC yellow book 2020: health information for international travel. New York: Oxford University Press; 2020c.

Centers for Disease Control and Prevention. (2020d). How COVID-19 spreads. Retrieved from https://www.cdc.gov/coronavirus/2019-ncov/prevent-getting-sick/how-covid-spreads.html

Centers for Disease Control and Prevention. Interim guidance for antigen testing for SARS-CoV-2. https://www.cdc.gov/coronavirus/2019-ncov/lab/resources/antigen-tests-guidelines.html. 2020e Accessed February 11, 2021.

Centers for Disease Control and Prevention. Tuberculin skin testing fact sheet. https://www.cdc.gov/tb/publications/factsheets/testing/skintesting.htm Accessed December 20, 2020. 2020f.

Centers for Disease Control and Prevention (CDC). Updated guidelines for the use of nucleic acid amplification tests in the diagnosis of tuberculosis. MMWR Morb Mortal Wkly Rep. 2009;58(1):7–10.

Centor RM, Witherspoon JM, Dalton HP, Brody CE, Link K. The diagnosis of strep throat in adults in the emergency room. Med Decis Mak. 1981;1(3):239–46.

Ceroni D, Belaieff W, Cherkaoui A, Lascombes P, Schrenzel J, de Coulon G, et al. Primary epiphyseal or apophyseal subacute osteomyelitis in the pediatric population: a report of fourteen cases and a systematic review of the literature. J Bone Joint Surg Am. 2014;96(18):1570–5.

Chiesa C, Panero A, Osborn JF, Simonetti AF, Pacifico L. Diagnosis of neonatal sepsis: a clinical and laboratory challenge. Clin Chem. 2004;50(2):279–87. https://doi.org/10.1373/clinchem.2003.025171. PMID: 14752012.

Chiu IM, Huang L-C, Chen IL, Tang K-S, Huang Y-H. Diagnostic values of C-reactive protein and complete blood cell to identify invasive bacterial infection in young febrile infants. Pediatr Neonatol. 2019;60(2):197–200.

Christy A. COVID-19: a review for the pediatric neurologist. J Child Neurol. 2020;35(13):934–9.

Clegg HW, Dallas SD, Roddey OF, et al. Extrapharyngeal group a streptococcus infection: diagnostic accuracy and utility of rapid antigen testing. Pediatr Infect Dis J. 2003;22(8):726–31.

Clinical and Laboratory Standards Institute. Quality control of microbiological transport systems; approved standard—second edition. Wayne, PA: Clinical and Laboratory Standards Institute; 2019.

Cobas Strep A Package Insert. In: Liat c, ed 2017.

Cohen JI. Epstein–Barr virus infection. N Engl J Med. 2000;343(7):481–92.

Cohen R, Levy C, Bonacorsi S, Wollner A, Koskas M, Junget C, al. Diagnostic accuracy of clinical symptoms and rapid diagnostic test in group a streptococcal perianal infections in children. Clin Infect Dis. 2015;60(2):267–70.

Contopoulos-Ioannidis D, Montoya JG. Toxoplasma gondii (Toxoplasmosis). In: Long SS, editor. Principles and practice of pediatric infectious diseases. 5th ed. Philadelphia, PA: Elsevier; 2018. p. 1352–63.

Cruz AT, Reichman LB. The case for retiring the tuberculin skin test. Pediatrics. 2019;143:6.

Dalton MJ, Robinson LE, Cooper J, Regnery RL, Olson JG, Childs JE. Use of Bartonella antigens for serologic diagnosis of cat-scratch disease at a national referral center. Arch Intern Med. 1995;155(15):1670–6.

Dancey P, Benseler S, Junker AK, et al. The challenge of periodic fevers in children. Paediatr Child Health. 2012;17(3):123.

Davison SA, Strasser SI. Ordering and interpreting hepatitis B serology. BMJ. 2014;348:g2522.

Daxboeck F, Krause R, Wenisch C. Laboratory diagnosis of mycoplasma pneumoniae infection. Clin Microbiol Infect. 2003;9(4):263–73.

De Paschale M, Agrappi C, Manco MT, Clerici P. Positive predictive value of anti-HCMV IgM as an index of primary infection. J Virol Methods. 2010;168(1–2):121–5.

Doern GV, Brecher SM. The clinical predictive value (or lack thereof) of the results of antimicrobial susceptibility tests. J Clin Microbiol. 2011;49(9 Supplement):S11–4.

Dowd JB, Palermo T, Brite J, McDade TW, Aiello A. Seroprevalence of Epstein-Barr virus infection in U.S. children ages 6-19, 2003-2010. PLoS One. 2013;8(5):e64921.

Dowell SF, Bresee JS. Severe varicella associated with steroid use. Pediatrics. 1993;92(2):223–8.

Downes KJ, Fitzgerald JC, Schriver E, et al. Implementation of a pragmatic biomarker-driven algorithm to guide antibiotic use in the pediatric intensive care unit: the optimizing antibiotic strategies in sepsis (OASIS) II study. J Pediatr Infect Dis Soc. 2018;9(1):36–43.

Downes KJ, Weiss SL, Gerber JS, et al. A pragmatic biomarker-driven algorithm to guide antibiotic use in the pediatric intensive care unit: the optimizing antibiotic strategies in sepsis (OASIS) study. J Pediatr Infect Dis Soc. 2016;6(2):134–41.

Edouard S, Nabet C, Lepidi H, Fournier P-E, Raoult D. Bartonella, a common cause of endocarditis: a report on 106 cases and review. J Clin Microbiol. 2015;53(3):824–9.

Fernando MMA, Isenberg DA. How to monitor SLE in routine clinical practice. Ann Rheum Dis. 2005;64(4):524–7.

Fitzgerald DW, Sterling TR, Hass DW. Mycobacterium tuberculosis. In: Bennett JE, Dolin R, Blaser MJ, editors. Mandell, Douglas, and Bennett's principles and practice of infectious diseases. 9th ed. Philadelphia: Elsevier; 2020.

Gabay C, Kushner I. Acute-phase proteins and other systemic responses to inflammation. N Engl J Med. 1999;340(6):448–54.

Garcia PC, Longhi F, Branco RG, Piva JP, Lacks D, Tasker RC. Ferritin levels in children with severe sepsis and septic shock. Acta Paediatr. 2007;96(12):1829–31.

Gartner BC, Preiksaitis JK. Epstein-Barr virus. In: Jorgenson JH, Pfaller MA, Carroll KC, et al., editors.

Manual of clinical microbiology. 11th ed. Washington, DC: ASM Press; 2015. p. 1728–53.

Gerber MA, Baltimore RS, Eaton CB, et al. Prevention of rheumatic fever and diagnosis and treatment of acute streptococcal pharyngitis: a scientific statement from the American Heart Association Rheumatic Fever, Endocarditis, and Kawasaki Disease Committee of the Council on Cardiovascular Disease in the Young, the Interdisciplinary Council on Functional Genomics and Translational Biology, and the Interdisciplinary Council on Quality of Care and Outcomes Research: endorsed by the American Academy of Pediatr. Circulation. 2009;119(11):1541–51.

Gergen PJ, McQuillan GM, Kiely M, Ezzati-Rice TM, Sutter RW, Virella G. A population-based serologic survey of immunity to tetanus in the United States. N Engl J Med. 1995;332(12):761–6.

Geusau A, Kittler H, Hein U, Dangl-Erlach E, Stingl G, Tschachler E. Biological false-positive tests comprise a high proportion of venereal disease research laboratory reactions in an analysis of 300,000 sera. Int J STD AIDS. 2005;16(11):722–6.

Gewitz MH, Baltimore RS, Tani LY, et al. Revision of the Jones criteria for the diagnosis of acute rheumatic fever in the era of Doppler echocardiography. Circulation. 2015;131(20):1806–18.

Ghelani SJ, Kwatra NS, Spurney CF. Can coronary artery involvement in Kawasaki disease be predicted? Diagnostics. 2013;3(2):232–43.

Giladi M, Kletter Y, Avidor B, Metzkor-Cotter E, Varon M, Golan Y, et al. Enzyme immunoassay for the diagnosis of cat-scratch disease defined by polymerase chain reaction. Clin Infect Dis. 2001;33(11):1852–8.

Ginnocchio CC, Van Horn G, Harris P. Reagents, stains, media, and cell cultures: virology. In: Jorgenson JH, Pfaller MA, Carroll KC, et al., editors. Manual of clinical microbiology. 11th ed. Washington, DC: ASM Press; 2015. p. 1422–31.

Godfred-Cato S, Bryant B, Leung J, Oster ME, Conklin L, Abramset J, et al. COVID-19–associated multisystem inflammatory syndrome in children—United States., March–July 2020. MMWR. 2020;69:1074–80.

Goldstein EJC, Montoya JG, Remington JS. Management of toxoplasma gondii infection during pregnancy. Clin Infect Dis. 2008;47(4):554–66.

Graf EH, Pancholi P. Appropraite use and future direction of molecular diagnostic testing. Curr Infect Dis Rep. 2020;22:5.

Griffith DE, Aksamit T, Brown-Elliott BA, Catanzaro A, Daley C, Gordin F, et al. An official ATS/IDSA statement: diagnosis, treatment, and prevention of nontuberculous mycobacterial diseases. Am J Respir Crit Care Med. 2007;175(4):367–416.

Grivard P, Le Roux K, Laurent P, Fianu A, Perrau J, Gigan J, et al. Molecular and serological diagnosis of chikungunya virus infection. Pathol Biol (Paris). 2007;55(10):490–4.

Hammarlund E, Thomas A, Poore EA, et al. Durability of vaccine-induced immunity against tetanus and diphtheria toxins: a cross-sectional analysis. Clin Infect Dis. 2016;62(9):1111–8.

Hansmann Y, DeMartino S, Piémont Y, Meyer N, Mariet P, Heller R, et al. Diagnosis of cat scratch disease with detection of Bartonella henselae by PCR: a study of patients with lymph node enlargement. J Clin Microbiol. 2005;43(8):3800–6.

Hanson K, Caliendo A, Arias C, et al. The Infectious Disease Society of America Guidelines on the Diagnosis of COVID-10: Molecular Diagnostic Testing. 2020. Accessed February 11, 2021. www.idsociety.org/COVID19guidelines/dx.

Harrison GJ. Cytomegalovirus. In: Cherry JD, Harrison GJ, Kaplan SL, editors. Feigin and Cherry's textbook of pediatric infectious diseases. 7th ed. Philadelphia, PA: Elsevier Saunders; 2014.

He XY, Wang XB, Zhang R, et al. Investigation of mycoplasma pneumoniae infection in pediatric population from 12,025 cases with respiratory infection. Diagn Microbiol Infect Dis. 2013;75(1):22–7.

Hedegaard SS, Wisborg K, Hvas AM. Diagnostic utility of biomarkers for neonatal sepsis—a systematic review. Infect Dis (Lond). 2015;47(3):117–24.

Hematian A, Sadeghifard N, Mohebi R, Taherikalani M, Nasrolahi A, Amraei M, Ghafourian S, et al. Traditional and modern cell culture in virus diagnosis. Osong Public Health Res Perspect. 2016;7(2):77–82.

Hentges DJ. Anaerobes: general characteristics. In: Baron S, editor. Medical microbiology. Galveston, TX: University of Texas Medical Branch at Galveston; 1996.

Hills SL, Fischer M. Flaviviruses. In: Long SS, editor. Principles and practice of pediatric infectious diseases. 5th ed. Philadelphia, PA: Elsevier; 2018. p. 1128–31.

Hodinka RL. Point: is the era of viral culture over in the clinical microbiology laboratory? J Clin Microbiol. 2013;51(1):2–4.

Hodinka RL. Human cytomegalovirus. In: Jorgenson JH, Pfaller MA, Carroll KC, et al., editors. Manual of clinical microbiology. 11th ed. Washington, DC: ASM Press; 2015. p. 1718–38.

Hong DK, Lewis DB. Developmental immunology and role of host defenses in fetal and neonatal susceptibility to infection. In: Wilson CB, Nizet V, Maldonado YA, Remington JS, Klein JO, editors. Remington and Klein's infectious diseases of the fetus and newborn infant. 8th ed. Philadelphia, PA: Elsevier Saunders; 2016. p. 81–188.

Horwitz CA, Henle W, Henle G, et al. Clinical and laboratory evaluation of infants and children with Epstein-Barr virus-induced infectious mononucleosis: report of 32 patients (aged 10-48 months). Blood. 1981;57(5):933–8.

Hoshino A, Okuno Y, Migita M, Ban H, Yang X, Kiyokawa N, et al. X-linked agammaglobulinemia associated with B-precursor acute lymphoblastic leukemia. J Clin Immunol. 2015;35(2):108–11.

Hurt C, Tammaro D. Diagnostic evaluation of mononucleosis-like illnesses. Am J Med. 2007;120(10):911.e911–8.

International Committee for Standardization in Hematology. Reference method for the erythrocyte sedimentation rate (ESR) test on human blood. Br J Haematol. 1973;24(5):671–3.

Jääskeläinen AJ, Korhonen EM, Huhtamo E, Lappalainen M, Vapalahti O, Kallio-Kokko H. Validation of serological and molecular methods for diagnosis of zika virus infections. J Virol Methods. 2019;263: 68–74.

Jacobs E, Bennewitz A, Bredt W. Reaction pattern of human anti-mycoplasma pneumoniae antibodies in enzyme-linked immunosorbent assays and immunoblotting. J Clin Microbiol. 1986;23(3):517–22.

Jain S, Williams DJ, Arnold SR, et al. Community-acquired pneumonia requiring hospitalization among U.S. children. N Engl J Med. 2015;372(9):835–45.

Jeffrey Modell Foundation. Four stages of primary immunodeficiency testing. Assessed January 25, 2020., http://www.cipo.ca/wp-content/uploads/2019/01/The-Four-Stages-of-PI-Testing.pdf

Johnson BW, Russell BJ, Goodman CH. Laboratory diagnosis of chikungunya virus infections and commercial sources for diagnostic assays. J Infect Dis. 2016;214(suppl 5):S471–4.

Johnson DR, Kurlan R, Leckman J, Kaplan EL. The human immune response to streptococcal extracellular antigens: clinical, diagnostic, and potential pathogenetic implications. Clin Infect Dis. 2010;50(4):481–90.

Jou JM, Lewis SM, Briggs C, Lee SH, De La Salle B, et al. ICSH review of the measurement of the erythrocyte sedimentation rate. Int J Lab Hematol. 2011;33(2):125–32.

Kaplan EL, Rothermel CD, Johnson DR. Antistreptolysin O and anti-deoxyribonuclease B titers: normal values for children ages 2 to 12 in the United States. Pediatrics. 1998;101(1):86–8.

Katz BZ. Epstein-Barr virus (mononucleosis and lymphoproliferative disorders). In: Long SS, editor. Principles and practice of pediatric infectious diseases. 5th ed. Philadelphia, PA: Elsevier; 2018. p. 1088–94.

Kay AW, Islam SM, Wendorf K, Westenhouse J, Barry PM. Interferon-γ release assay performance for tuberculosis in childhood. Pediatrics. 2018;141(6):e20173918.

Käyhty R, Peltola H, Karanko V, Mäkelä PH. The protective level of serum antibodies to the capsular polysaccharide of haemophilus influenzae type b. J Infect Dis. 1983;147(6):1100.

Kenneson A, Cannon MJ. Review and meta-analysis of the epidemiology of congenital cytomegalovirus (CMV) infection. Rev Med Virol. 2007;17(4): 253–76.

Khalil RH, Al-Humadi N. Types of acute phase reactants and their importance in vaccination (review). Biomed Rep. 2020;12(4):143–52.

Kim BY, Kim D, Kim YH, Ryoo E, Sun YH, Jeon IS, et al. Non-responders to intravenous immunoglobulin and coronary artery dilatation in Kawasaki disease: predictive parameters in Korean children. Korean Circ J. 2016;46(4):542–9.

Kim JH, Lee JY, Cho HR, Lee JS, Ryu JM, Lee J. High concentration of C-reactive protein is associated with serious bacterial infection in previously healthy children aged 3 to 36 months with fever and extreme leukocytosis. Pediatr Emerg Care. 2019;35(5): 347–52.

Kim JJ, Yun SW, Yu JJ, Yoon KL, Lee KY, Kil HR, et al. Common variants in the CRP promoter are associated with a high C-reactive protein level in Kawasaki disease. Pediatr Cardiol. 2015;36(2):438–44.

Kimberlin DW, Prober CG. Herpes simplex virus. In: Long SS, editor. Principles and practice of pediatric infectious diseases. 5th ed. Philadelphia, PA: Elsevier; 2018. p. 1056–64.

Klutts JS, Ford BA, Perez NR, Gronowski AM. Evidence-based approach for interpretation of Epstein-Barr virus serological patterns. J Clin Microbiol. 2009;47(10):3204–10.

Kollef MH. Inadequate antimicrobial treatment: an important determinant of outcome for hospitalized patients. Clin Infect Dis. 2000;31(Suppl 4):S131–8.

Kotton CN, Kumar D, Caliendo AM, et al. The third international consensus guidelines on the management of cytomegalovirus in solid-organ transplantation. Transplantation. 2018;102(6):900–31.

Kotula JJ 3rd, Moore WS 2nd, Chopra A, Cies JJ. Association of procalcitonin value and bacterial coinfections in pediatric patients with viral lower respiratory tract infections admitted to the pediatric intensive care unit. J Pediatr Pharmacol Ther. 2018;23(6):466–72.

Kowalski RP, Karenchak LM, Shah C, Gordon JS. ELVIS: a new 24-hour culture test for detecting herpes simplex virus from ocular samples. Arch Ophthalmol. 2002;120(7):960–2.

Kuehni CE, Barben J. Protecting children from second-hand smoke. 2015;46(3):601–603.

Kullberg BJ, Vrijmoeth HD, van de Schoor F, Hovius JW. Lyme borreliosis: diagnosis and management. BMJ. 2020;369:m1041.

Kuper KM, Boles DM, Mohr JF, Wanger A. Antimicrobial susceptibility testing: a primer for clinicians. Pharmacotherapy. 2009;29(11):1326–43.

Lagier J-C, Edouard S, Pagnier I, Mediannikov O, Drancourt M, Raoult D. Current and past strategies for bacterial culture in clinical microbiology. Clin Microbiol Rev. 2015;28(1):208–36.

Lanciotti RS, Kosoy OL, Laven JJ, et al. Chikungunya virus in US travelers returning from India, 2006. Emerg Infect Dis. 2007;13(5):764–7.

Lanciotti RS, Kosoy OL, Laven JJ, et al. Genetic and serologic properties of Zika virus associated with an epidemic, Yap State, Micronesia, 2007. Emerging Infect Dis J. 2008;14(8):1232.

Landry ML, St. George K. Laboratory diagnosis of Zika virus infection. Arch Pathol Lab Med. 2016;141(1):60–7.

Larsen SA, Steiner BM, Rudolph AH. Laboratory diagnosis and interpretation of tests for syphilis. Clin Microbiol Rev. 1995;8(1):1–21.

Lee BE, Plitt SS, Jayaraman GC, Chui L, Singh AE, Preiksaitis JK. Use of quantitative HIV RNA detection for early diagnosis of HIV infection in infants and acute HIV infections in Alberta, Canada. J Clin Microbiol. 2012;50(2):502–5.

Lee H. Procalcitonin as a biomarker of infectious diseases. Korean J Intern Med. 2013;28(3): 285–91.

Lee JW, Her SM, Kim JH, et al. D-dimer as a marker of acute pyelonephritis in infants younger than 24 months with urinary tract infection. Pediatr Nephrol. 2018;33(4):631–7.

Lee TG, Yu ST, So CH. Predictive value of C-reactive protein for the diagnosis of meningitis in febrile infants under 3 months of age in the emergency department. Yeungnam U J Med. 2020;37(2):106–11.

Lee WJ, Huang EY, Tsai CM, et al. Role of serum mycoplasma pneumoniae IgA, IgM, and IgG in the diagnosis of mycoplasma pneumoniae-related pneumonia in school-age children and adolescents. Clin Vaccine Immunol. 2017;24:1.

LeGoff J, Péré H, Bélec L. Diagnosis of genital herpes simplex virus infection in the clinical laboratory. Virol J. 2014;11:83.

Lewinsohn DM, Leonard MK, LoBue PA, et al. Official American Thoracic Society/Infectious Diseases Society of America/Centers for Disease Control and Prevention Clinical Practice Guidelines: diagnosis of tuberculosis in adults and children. Clin Infect Dis. 2017;64(2):e1–e33.

Lewis LA, Ram S. Meningococcal disease and the complement system. Virulence. 2014;5(1):98–126.

Liermann K, Schäfler A, Henke A, Sauerbrei A. Evaluation of commercial herpes simplex virus IgG and IgM enzyme immunoassays. J Virol Methods. 2014;199:29–34.

Lilian RR, Kalk E, Bhowan K, et al. Early diagnosis of in utero and intrapartum HIV infection in infants prior to 6 weeks of age. J Clin Microbiol. 2012;50(7): 2373–7.

Lin SG, Hou TY, Huang DH, et al. Role of procalcitonin in the diagnosis of severe infection in pediatric patients with fever and neutropenia—a systemic review and meta-analysis. Pediatr Infect Dis J. 2012;31(10):e182–8.

Linderholm M, Boman J, Juto P, Linde A. Comparative evaluation of nine kits for rapid diagnosis of infectious mononucleosis and Epstein-Barr virus-specific serology. J Clin Microbiol. 1994;32(1): 259–61.

Loens K, Goossens H, Ieven M. Acute respiratory infection due to mycoplasma pneumoniae: current status of diagnostic methods. Eur J Clin Microbiol Infect Dis. 2010;29(9):1055–69.

Loens K, Ieven M. Mycoplasma pneumoniae: current knowledge on nucleic acid amplification techniques and serological diagnostics. Front Microbiol. 2016;7:448.

Loens K, Van Heirstraeten L, Malhotra-Kumar S, Goossens H, Ieven M. Optimal sampling sites and methods for detection of pathogens possibly causing community-acquired lower respiratory tract infections. J Clin Microbiol. 2009;47(1):21–31.

Long SS, Vodzak J. Laboratory manifestations of infectious diseases. In: Long SS, editor. Principles and practice of pediatric infectious diseases. 5th ed. Philadelphia, PA: Elsevier; 2018. p. 1447–59.

Luaces-Cubells C, Mintegi S, García-García JJ, Astobiza E, Garrido-Romero R, Velasco-Rodríguez J, Benito J, et al. Procalcitonin to detect invasive bacterial infection in non-toxic-appearing infants with fever without apparent source in the emergency department. Pediatr Infect Dis J. 2012;31(6):645–7.

Marnell L, Mold C, Du Clos TW. C-reactive protein: ligands, receptors and role in inflammation. Clin Immunol. 2005;117(2):104–11.

Marshall-Andon T, Heinz P. How to use … the Monospot and other heterophile antibody tests. Arch Dis Child Educ Pract Ed. 2017;102(4):188–93.

Martin JM, Green M, Barbadora KA, Wald ER. Group A streptococci among school-aged children: clinical characteristics and the carrier state. Pediatrics. 2004;114(5):1212–9.

Mathur G, Mathur S. Antibody testing for COVID-19. Am J Clin Pathol. 2020;154(1):1–3.

McAuley JB, Jones JL, Singh K. Toxoplasma. In: Jorgenson JH, Pfaller MA, Carroll KC, et al., editors. Manual of clinical microbiology. 11th ed. Washington, DC: ASM Press; 2015. p. 2373–86.

McCrindle BW, Rowley AH, Newburger JW, Burns JC, Bolger AF, Gewitz M, et al. Diagnosis, treatment, and long-term management of Kawasaki disease: a scientific statement for health professionals from the American Heart Association. Circ. 2017;135(17):e927–99.

McCusker C, Upton J, Warrington R. Primary immunodeficiency. Allergy Asthma Clin Immunol. 2018;14(Suppl 2):61.

McIsaac WJ, White D, Tannenbaum D, Low DE. A clinical score to reduce unnecessary antibiotic use in patients with sore throat. Can Med Assoc J. 1998;158(1):75–83.

McPherson RA, Mcpherson. Henry's clinical diagnosis and management by laboratory methods. New York: NY Elsevier; 2011.

Messacar K, Parkder SK, Todd JK, Dominquez SR. Implementation of rapid molecular infectious disease diagnostic: the role of diagnostic and antimicrobial stewardship. J Clin Microbiol. 2017;55(3): 715–23.

Metzkor-Cotter E, Kletter Y, Avidor B, et al. Long-term serological analysis and clinical follow-up of patients with cat-scratch disease. Clin Infect Dis. 2003;37(9):1149–54.

Micallef S, Galea R. CMV encephalitis in an immune-competent patient. BMJ Case Rep. 2018;2018:bcr-2018-224740.

Microbiology Devices Panel of the Medical Devices Advisory Committee. FDA executive summary: over-the-counter diagnostic tests for the detection of pathogens causing. Infect Dis. 2016; https://www.fda.gov/media/99873/download

Miller A, Green M, Robinson D. Simple rule for calculating normal erythrocyte sedimentation rate. Br Med J (Clin Res Ed). 1983;286(6361):266.

Miller JM, Binnicker MJ, Campbell S, Carroll KC, Chapin KC, Gilligan PH, et al. A guide to utilization of the microbiology laboratory for diagnosis of infectious diseases: 2018 update by the Infectious Diseases Society of America and the American Society for Microbiologya. Clin Infect Dis. 2018;67(6):e1–e94.

Mlakar J, Korva M, Tul N, et al. Zika virus associated with microcephaly. N Engl J Med. 2016;374(10):951–8.

Monto AS, Ullman BM. Acute respiratory illness in an American Community: the Tecumseh study. JAMA. 1974;227(2):164–9.

Montoya JG. Laboratory diagnosis of toxoplasma gondii infection and toxoplasmosis. J Infect Dis. 2002;185(Supplement_1):S73–82.

Moseley RC, Corey L, Benjamin D, Winter C, Remington ML. Comparison of viral isolation, direct immunofluorescence, and indirect immunoperoxidase techniques for detection of genital herpes simplex virus infection. J Clin Microbiol. 1981;13(5):913–8.

Murakami K, Tsukahara M, Tsuneoka H, et al. Cat scratch disease: analysis of 130 seropositive cases. J Infect Chemother. 2002;8(4):349–52.

Murray PR, Rosenthal KS, Pfaller MA. Molecular diagnosis. In: Medical microbiology. 9th ed. Elsevier; 2021. p. 24–9.

Nicola M, O'Neill N, Sohrabi C, Agha KM, M, Aghae R. Evidence-based management guideline for the COVID-19 pandemic—review article. Int J Surg. 2020;77:206–16.

Nielsen LE, Forrester JB, Girotto JE, Dassner AM, Humphries R. One-size fits all? Application of susceptible-dose dependent breakpoints to pediatric patients and laboratory reporting. J Clin Microbiol. 2019; JCM.01446-01419

Nohynek H, Valkeila E, Leinonen M, Eskola J. Erythrocyte sedimentation rate, white blood cell count and serum C-reactive protein in assessing etiologic diagnosis of acute lower respiratory infections in children. Pediatr Infect Dis J. 1995;14(6):484–90.

Nolte FS, Wittwer CT. Nucleic acid amplification methods overview. In: Persing DH, Tenover FC, Hayden RT, et al., editors. Molecular microbiology: diagnostic principles and practice. 3rd ed. Washington, DC: ASM Press; 2016. p. 3–18.

Nussinovitch M, Finkelstein Y, Amir J, Varsano I. Group A Beta-Hemolytic streptococcal pharyngitis in preschool children aged 3 months to 5 years. Clin Pediatr. 1999;38(6):357–60.

Ochs HD, Stiehm ER, Winkelstein JA. Antibody deficiencies. In: Ochs HD, Stiehm ER, Winkelstein JA, editors. Immunologic disorders in infants & children. Philadelphia, PA: Elsevier Saunders; 2004. p. 357–426.

Oliver J, Malliya Wadu E, Pierse N, Moreland NJ, Williamson DA, Baker MG. Group A streptococcus pharyngitis and pharyngeal carriage: a meta-analysis. PLoS Negl Trop Dis. 2018;12(3):e0006335.

Orange JS, Ballow M, Stiehm ER, Ballas ZK, Chinen J, De La Morena M, et al. Use and interpretation of diagnostic vaccination in primary immunodeficiency: a working group report of the basic and clinical immunology interest section of the American Academy of Allergy, Asthma & Immunology. J Allergy Clin Immunol. 2012;130(3, Supplement):S1–S24.

Otsuyama K, Tsuneoka H, Kondou K, et al. Development of a highly specific IgM enzyme-linked immunosorbent assay for Bartonella henselae using refined N-lauryl-sarcosine-insoluble proteins for serodiagnosis of cat scratch disease. J Clin Microbiol. 2016;54(4):1058–64.

Park IU, Fakile YF, Chow JM, et al. Performance of treponemal tests for the diagnosis of syphilis. Clin Infect Dis. 2019;68(6):913–8.

Parker AR, Skold M, Ramsden DB, Ocejo-Vinyals JG, López-Hoyos M, Harding S. The clinical utility of measuring IgG subclass immunoglobulins during immunological investigation for suspected primary antibody deficiencies. Lab Med. 2017;48(4): 314–25.

Parker KG, Gandra S, Matushek S, Beavis KG, Tesic V, Charnot-Katsikas A. Comparison of 3 nucleic acid amplification tests and a rapid antigen test with culture for the detection of group a streptococci from throat swabs. J Appl Lab Med. 2019;4(2):164–9.

Parks T, Smeesters PR, Curtis N, Steer AC. ASO titer or not? When to use streptococcal serology: a guide for clinicians. Eur J Clin Microbiol Infect Dis. 2015;34(5):845–9.

Pass RF. Cytomegalovirus. In: Long SS, editor. Principles and practice of pediatric infectious diseases. 5th ed. Philadelphia, PA: Elsevier; 2018. p. 1073–81.

Patel NA. Pediatric COVID-19: systematic review of the literature. Am J Otolaryngol. 2020;41(5):102573.

Peeling RW, Ye H. Diagnostic tools for preventing and managing maternal and congenital syphilis: an overview. Bull World Health Organ. 2004;82: 439–46.

Peltola H, Käyhty H, Sivonen A, Mäkelä H. Haemophilus influenzae type b capsular polysaccharide vaccine in children: a double-blind field study of 100,000 vaccinees 3 months to 5 years of age in Finland. Pediatrics. 1977;60(5):730–7.

Perez EE, Orange JS, Bonilla F, et al. Update on the use of immunoglobulin in human disease: a review of evidence. J Allergy Clin Immunol. 2017;139(3, Supplement):S1–S46.

Pinniti SG, Kimberlin DW. Neonatal herpes simplex virus infections. Sem Perinatol. 2018;42(3):168–75.

Pomares C, Montoya JG. Laboratory diagnosis of congenital toxoplasmosis. J Clin Microbiol. 2016;54(10):2448–54.

Poses RM, Cebul RD, Collins M, Fager SS. The accuracy of experienced physicians' probability estimates for patients with sore throats: implications for decision making. JAMA. 1985;254(7):925–9.

Pratt A, Attia MW. Duration of fever and markers of serious bacterial infection in young febrile children. Pediatr Int. 2007;49(1):31–5.

Prince HE, Lapé-Nixon M. Role of cytomegalovirus (CMV) IgG avidity testing in diagnosing primary CMV infection during pregnancy. Clin Vaccine Immunol. 2014;21(10):1377–84.

Principi N, Esposito S. Biomarkers in Pediatric community-acquired pneumonia. Int J Mol Sci. 2017;18(2):447.

Putto A, Ruuskanen O, Meurman O, Ekblad H, Korvenranta H, Mertsola J, et al. C reactive protein in the evaluation of febrile illness. Arch Dis Child. 1986;61(1):24–9.

QuantiFERON®-TB Gold (QFT®) ELISA Package Insert. In: QIAGEN, ed 2016.

Rahbarimanesh AA, Salamati P, Ghafourian S, Zekavat M. Relationship between ESR, CRP, platelet count and coronary artery disease in Kawasaki disease. Iran J of Pediatr. 2005;15(2):139–44.

Ramsay ES, Lerman MA. How to use the erythrocyte sedimentation rate in paediatrics. Arch Dis Child. 2015;100(1):30–6.

Ratnam S. The laboratory diagnosis of syphilis. Can J Infect Dis Med Microbiol. 2005;16:45.

Reda SM, El-Ghoneimy DH, Afifi HM. Clinical predictors of primary immunodeficiency diseases in children. Allergy Asthma Immunol Res. 2013;5(2):88–95.

Reller LB, Weinstein M, Jorgensen JH, Ferraro MJ. Antimicrobial susceptibility testing: a review of general principles and contemporary practices. Clin Infect Dis. 2009;49(11):1749–55.

Rex JH, Pfaller MA. Has antifungal susceptibility testing come of age? Clin Infect Dis. 2002;35(8):982–9.

Roderick M, Finn AAVR. Chickenpox in the immuno-compromised child. Arch Dis Child. 2012;97(7):587–9.

Roggen I, van Berlaer G, Gordts F, Pierard D, Hubloue I. Centor criteria in children in a paediatric emergency department: for what it is worth. BMJ Open. 2013;3:4.

Ruebush TK, Chisholm ES, Sulzer AJ, Healy GR. Development and persistence of antibody in persons infected with Babesia Microti. Am J Trop Med Hyg. 1981;30(1):291–2.

Sanchez E, Vannier E, Wormser GP, Hu LT. Diagnosis, treatment, and prevention of Lyme disease, human granulocytic Anaplasmosis, and Babesiosis: a review. JAMA. 2016;315(16):1767–77.

Sander A, Posselt M, Oberle K, Bredt W. Seroprevalence of antibodies to Bartonella henselae in patients with cat scratch disease and in healthy controls: evaluation and comparison of two commercial serological tests. Clin Diagn Lab Immunol. 1998;5(4):486–90.

Sanders S, Barnett A, Correa-Velez I, Coulthard M, Doust J. Systematic review of the diagnostic accuracy of C-reactive protein to detect bacterial infection in non-hospitalized infants and children with fever. J Pediatr. 2008;153(4):570–574.e573.

Schuez-Havupalo L, Toivonen L, Karppinen S, Kaljonen A, Peltola V. Daycare attendance and respiratory tract infections: a prospective birth cohort study. BMJ Open. 2017;7(9):e014635.

Self WH, Tenforde MW, Stubblefield WB, et al. Decline in SARS-CoV-2 antibodies after mild infection among frontline health care personnel in a multistate hospital network—12 states, April–August 2020. MMWR Morb Mortal Wkly Rep. 2020;69:1762–6. https://doi.org/10.15585/mmwr.mm6947a2.

Sena AC, White BL, Sparling PF. Novel Treponema pallidum serologic tests: a paradigm shift in syphilis screening for the 21st century. Clin Infect Dis. 2010;51(6):700–8.

Shaikh N, Leonard E, Martin JM. Prevalence of streptococcal pharyngitis and streptococcal carriage in children: a meta-analysis. Pediatrics. 2010;126(3):e557–64.

Sharp TM, Fischer M, Muñoz-Jordán JL, et al. Dengue and Zika virus diagnostic testing for patients with a clinically compatible illness and risk for infection with both viruses. Morb Mortal Wkly Rep. 2019;68(1):1–10.

Shet A, Kaplan EL. Clinical use and interpretation of group a streptococcal antibody tests: a practical approach for the pediatrician or primary care physician. Pediatr Infect Dis J. 2002;21(5)

Shulman ST. Streptococcal pharyngitis: diagnostic considerations. Pediatr Infect Dis J. 1994;13(6):567–71.

Shulman ST, Bisno AL, Clegg HW, et al. Clinical practice guideline for the diagnosis and management of group a streptococcal pharyngitis: 2012 update by the Infectious Diseases Society of America. Clin Infect Dis. 2012;55(10):e86–102.

Silvestre JP, Coelho LM, Póvoa PM. Impact of fulminant hepatic failure in C-reactive protein? J Crit Care. 2010;25(4):657.e657–12.

Smith T, Cunningham-Rundles C. Primary B-cell immunodeficiencies. Hum Immunol. 2019;80(6):351–62.

Soreng K, Levy R, Fakile Y. Serologic testing for syphilis: benefits and challenges of a reverse algorithm. Clin Microbiol Newsl. 2014;36(24):195–202.

Soriano A, Marco F, Martínez JA, et al. Influence of vancomycin minimum inhibitory concentration on the treatment of methicillin-resistant Staphylococcus aureus Bacteremia. Clin Infect Dis. 2008;46(2):193–200.

Spruiell MD, Searns JB, Heare TC, Roberts JL, Wylie E, Pyle L, et al. Clinical care guideline for improving pediatric acute musculoskeletal infection outcomes. J Pediatr Infect Dis Soc. 2017;6(3):e86–93.

Spuesens EB, Fraaij PL, Visser EG, Hoogenboezem T, Hop WC, van Adrichem LN, et al. Carriage of mycoplasma pneumoniae in the upper respiratory tract of symptomatic and asymptomatic children: an observational study. PLoS Med. 2013;10(5):e1001444.

Standage SW, Wong HR. Biomarkers for pediatric sepsis and septic shock. Expert Rev Anti-Infect Ther. 2011;9(1):71–9.

Staples JE, Powers AM. Togaviridae (Alphaviruses). In: Long SS, editor. Principles and practice of pediatric infectious diseases. 5th ed. Philadelphia, PA: Elsevier; 2018. p. 1126–31.

Starke JR, Committee On Infectious Diseases. Interferon-γ release assays for diagnosis of tuberculosis infection and disease in children. Pediatrics. 2014;134(6):e1763–73.

Steer AC, Smeesters PR, Curtis N. Streptococcal serology: secrets for the specialist. Pediatr Infect Dis J. 2015;34(11):1250–2.

Steere AC. Lyme disease (Lyme Borreliosis) due to Borrelia burgdorferi. In: Bennett JE, Dolin R, Blaser MJ, editors. Mandell, Douglas, and Bennett's principles and practice of infectious diseases. 9th ed. Philadelphia: Elsevier; 2020. p. 2911–22.

Stevens DL, Bisno AL, Chambers HF, et al. Practice guidelines for the diagnosis and management of skin and soft tissue infections: 2014 Update by the Infectious Diseases Society of America. Clin Infect Dis. 2014;59(2):e10–52.

Strick LB, Wald A. Diagnostics for herpes simplex virus: is PCR the new gold standard? Mol Diagn Ther. 2006;10(1):17–28.

Sullivan KE, Winkelstein JA. Deficiencies of the complement system. In: Ochs HD, Stiehm ER, Winkelstein JA, editors. Immunologic disorders in infants & children. Philadelphia, PA: Elsevier Saunders; 2004. p. 357–426.

Sumaya CV, Ench Y. Epstein-Barr virus infectious mononucleosis in children. II. Heterophil antibody and viral-specific responses. Pediatrics. 1985;75(6):1011–9.

Taylor MD, Allada V, Moritz ML, et al. Use of C-reactive protein and ferritin biomarkers in daily pediatric practice. Pediatr Rev. 2020;41(4):172–83.

Terrault NA, Lok ASF, McMahon BJ, et al. Update on prevention, diagnosis, and treatment of chronic hepatitis B: AASLD 2018 hepatitis B guidance. Hepatology. 2018;67(4):1560–99.

Tezer H, Bedir Demirdağ T. Novel coronavirus disease (COVID-19) in children. Turkish J Med Sci. 2020;50(SI-1):592–603.

The Jeffrey Modell Foundation. 10 warning signs of primary immunodeficiency Accessed 12, 2020.

Theel ES. Immunoassays for the diagnosis of infectious diseases. In: Carroll KC, Pfaller MA, Landry ML, et al., editors. Manual of clinical microbiology. 12th ed. Washington, DC: ASM Press; 2019. p. 124–38.

Tickborne Diseases of the United States, A Reference Manual for Healthcare Providers. In: Centers for Disease Control and Prevention, editor. 5th ed 2018.

Thomson JRJ. Use of microbiology laboratory tests in the diagnosis of infectious disease. In: Tan JS, editor. Expert guide of infectious disease. Philadelphia, PA: American College of Physician; 2002. p. 1–41.

Tillett WS, Francis T. Serological reactions in pneumonia with a non-protein somatic fraction of pneumococcus. J Exp Med. 1930;52(4):561–71.

Todorov I, Gospodinova M, Bocheva Y, Popcheva G. Serum amyloid a protein in the course of infectious mononucleosis. Ther Adv Infect Dis. 2019;6:2049936118811208.

Tonial CT, Garcia PCR, Schweitzer LC, et al. Cardiac dysfunction and ferritin as early markers of severity in pediatric sepsis. J Pediatr. 2017;93(3):301–7.

Trépo C, Chan HLY, Lok A. Hepatitis B virus infection. Lancet. 2014;384(9959):2053–63.

Tsai C-M, Lin C-HR, Zhang H, et al. Using machine learning to predict Bacteremia in febrile children presented to the emergency department. Diagnostics. 2020;10(5):307.

Tsuruoka K, Tsuneoka H, Kawano M, et al. Evaluation of IgG ELISA using N-lauroyl-sarcosine-soluble proteins of Bartonella henselae for highly specific serodiagnosis of cat scratch disease. Diagn Microbiol Infect Dis. 2012;74(3):230–5.

Turnidge J, Paterson DL. Setting and revising antibacterial susceptibility breakpoints. Clin Microbiol Rev. 2007;20(3):391–408.

van de Veerdonk FL, Wever PC, Hermans MH, et al. IL-18 serum concentration is markedly elevated in acute EBV infection and can serve as a marker for disease severity. J Infect Dis. 2012;206(2):197–201.

Van den Bruel A, Thompson MJ, Haj-Hassan T, et al. Diagnostic value of laboratory tests in identifying serious infections in febrile children: systematic review. BMJ. 2011;342:d3082.

Vermeire S, Van Assche G, Rutgeerts P. C-reactive protein as a marker for inflammatory bowel disease. Inflamm Bowel Dis. 2004;10(5):661–5.

Virkki R, Juven T, Rikalainen H, Svedström E, Mertsola J, Ruuskanen O. Differentiation of bacterial and viral pneumonia in children. Thorax. 2002;57(5):438–41.

Waites KB, Xiao L, Liu Y, Balish MF, Atkinson TP. Mycoplasma pneumoniae from the respiratory tract and beyond. Clin Microbiol Rev. 2017;30(3): 747–809.

Wannamaker LW, Ayoub EM. Antibody titers in acute rheumatic fever. Circulation. 1960;21(4):598–614.

Weinmann S, Chun C, Mullooly JP, et al. Laboratory diagnosis and characteristics of breakthrough varicella in children. J Infect Dis. 2008;197(Supplement _2):S132–8.

Wilson ML, Weinstein MP, Reller LB. Laboratory detection of bacteremia and fungemia. In: Jorgenson JH, Pfaller MA, Carroll KC, et al., editors. Manual of clinical microbiology. 11th ed. Washington, DC: ASM Press; 2015. p. 15–28.

Womack J, Jimenez M. Common questions about infectious mononucleosis. Am Fam Physician. 2015;91(6):372–6.

Wood JB, Johnson DP. Prolonged intravenous instead of oral antibiotics for acute hematogenous osteomyelitis in children. J Hosp Med. 2016;11(7):505–8.

Wood PR, Hill VL, Burks ML, et al. Mycoplasma pneumoniae in children with acute and refractory asthma. Ann Allergy Asthma Immunol. 2013;110(5):328–334 e321.

Workowski KA, Bachmann LH, Chan PA, Johnston CM, Muzny CA, Park I, et al. Sexually transmitted infections treatment guidelines, 2021. MMWR Recomm Rep. 2021;70(4):1–187.

World Health Organization. Diphtheria vaccine: review of evidence on vaccine effectiveness and immunogenicity to assess the duration of protection ≥10 years after the last booster dose. 2017.

Wormser GP, Dattwyler RJ, Shapiro ED, et al. The clinical assessment, treatment, and prevention of Lyme disease, human granulocytic anaplasmosis, and babesiosis: clinical practice guidelines by the Infectious Diseases Society of America. Clin Infect Dis. 2006;43(9):1089–134.

Xpert Xpress Strep A Package Insert. In: Cepheid; 2019.

Xu R-Y, Liu H-W, Liu J-L, Dong J-H. Procalcitonin and C-reactive protein in urinary tract infection diagnosis. BMC Urol. 2014;14(1):45.

Yang YS, Ku CH, Lin JC, et al. Impact of extended-spectrum β-lactamase-producing Escherichia coli and Klebsiella pneumoniae on the outcome of community-onset bacteremic urinary tract infections. J Microbiol Immunol Infect. 2010;43(3):194–9.

Yap G, Pok K-Y, Lai Y-L, et al. Evaluation of chikungunya diagnostic assays: differences in sensitivity of serology assays in two independent outbreaks. PLoS Negl Trop Dis. 2010;4(7):e753.

Zannoni A, Giunti M, Bernardini C, Gentilini F, Zaniboni A, Bacci ML, Forni M, et al. Procalcitonin gene expression after LPS stimulation in the porcine animal model. Res Vet Sci. 2012;93(2):921–7.

Zhang Y, Zhang J, Sheng H, Li H, Wang R. Acute phase reactant serum amyloid A in inflammation and other diseases. Adv Clin Chem. 2019;90:25–80.

Ziebold C, von Kries R, Lang R, Weigl J, Schmitt HJ. Severe complications of varicella in previously healthy children in Germany: a 1-year survey. Pediatrics. 2001;108(5):e79.

Genetics and Pediatric Patient

Rita Marie John and Angela Kenny

Learning Objectives

After completing the chapter, the learner should be able to:

1. Understand the importance of family history in evaluating a child with a possible genetic disorder.
2. Apply the understanding of the red flags of the family and medical history that put a child at higher risk for cancer.
3. Understand the pros and cons of genetic testing.
4. Evaluate the different genetic tests and when they are used in clinical practice.
5. Accurately describe the differences between different genetic tests.
6. Apply their knowledge of different genetic tests in clinical practice.
7. Continue to enhance their understanding of genetic testing by reading and continuing education.

R. M. John (✉)
School of Nursing, Columbia University,
New York, NY, USA
e-mail: rmj4@cumc.columbia.edu

A. Kenny
Developmental-Behavioral Pediatrics, Mary Bridge
Children's Hospital, Tacoma, WA, USA

7.1 Introduction

The genetic causes for a child's disease have dramatically increased due to the availability of newer genetic tests. Clinicians need to understand that genetic testing can change decisions about treatments. Clinicians must identify at-risk individuals, offer education about genetic testing, and refer to genetic specialists to enhance the family's understanding of genetic information. Ideally, all clinicians should have ready availability to a geneticist, genetic counselor, and host of subspecialists. Ordering and interpreting genetic tests are complicated. Direct-to-consumer websites are growing, and patients can now order testing on themselves without the benefit of genetic counseling, leading to unnecessary stress or worry. The number of gene panel tests has grown. An accurate genetic diagnosis requires a complete patient medical history, including family history, a knowledge of dysmorphology, and careful test selection (Farmer et al. 2019). It is impossible to do this within a 20-minute primary care visit. Once the genetic testing is back, medical management should include family education and counseling and ensure that the family understands penetrance and residual risk. Errors in genetic testing carry with it the risk of missed or delayed diagnosis, improper medical management, inefficient utilization of healthcare dollars, false reassurance, psychosocial stress, and increased morbidity or mortality (Farmer et al.

© The Author(s), under exclusive license to Springer Nature Switzerland AG 2022
R. M. John (ed.), *Pediatric Diagnostic Labs for Primary Care: An Evidence-based Approach*,
https://doi.org/10.1007/978-3-030-90642-9_7

2019). The chapter hopes to inform clinicians about the expanding field of genetics. It should be kept in mind that the field of genetics is exploding, so continuing education is very important.

7.2 Family History

The importance of accurate three-generation family history cannot be stressed enough. For various cultural and religious reasons, families may hesitate to give an accurate history to clinicians, or within families, possible genetic diseases are a family secret. This lack of knowledge can affect pediatric patients and cause significant distress for parents. Clinicians can help families identify genetic risks by keeping track of their family history through the My Family Health Portrait tool designed by the CDC which is available at https://phgkb.cdc.gov/FHH/html/index. html. The link can be shared with other family members to add to it and clinicians to plan care.

Clinicians need to recognize recurrent diseases within a family and understand what red flags put patients at increased risk of a particular disease. Chen and Saul (2012) developed a rule of two/too. A family history with two or more affected family members, two or more generations that are affected, too many clinical findings, or too early an age of onset is a significant or positive family history for a particular disease. Family history may not reveal a problem if the trait is autosomal recessive, atypical female-predominant X-linked, or matrilineal mitochondrial patterns (Kim and Bodurtha 2019). Table 7.1 reviews the red flags in the family history that put an individual patient at increased risk for genetic cancers. Table 7.2 reviews the increased risk for cancer in patients with certain genetic syndromes.

7.2.1 Clinical Responsibilities Regarding Genetics

Once a family has seen a genetic counselor and/ or a geneticist, the family may have unanswered questions. Clinicians need to be able to answer

Table 7.1 Red flags and genetic cancer risk

History	Physical assessment
Cancer genetic risk factors	
The same kind or related kinds of cancer in the same side of the family affecting multiple members	Presence of Spitzoid melanoma or the giant congenital nevi (can have somatic mutation involving NRAS and NRAS (Merkel et al. 2019)
A family history of adenomatous colon polyps and colon cancer at a young age or having ten or more adenomatous polyps (The Jackson Laboratory 2021)	Multiple café au lait spots or hypopigmented macules can indicate a neurocutaneous disorder
Moderately increased risk of cancer • A single first-degree relative with common cancer at average age only • One first- and one second-degree relative or two second-degree relatives with common cancer at average ages (The Jackson Laboratory 2021)	Hemihypertrophy syndromes will have enlargement of one side of the body
High risk for cancer • Three or more relatives with cancers that are either similar or related • Two generations of cancer cases with one relative diagnosed earlier than expected • Known hereditary mutation for cancer	Eczematoid rashes that do not respond to usual care and large platelets may indicate Wiskott-Aldrich syndrome
Early-onset cancer or adenomatous polyps <50 years suggest an underlying susceptibility	Multiple atypical nevi (Soura et al. 2016)
Ionizing radiation and benzene can predispose to childhood leukemia (Jin et al. 2016)	Pallor of skin and mucus membranes, tachycardia due to anemia, recurrent infections

Adapted from The Jackson Laboratory (2021), Jin et al. (2016), Merkel et al. (2019), Soura et al. (2016)

Table 7.2 Genetic diseases and risk of cancers

Genetic diseases and risk of cancers	
Down syndrome	AML, ALL
WAGR, Denys-Drash syndrome	Wilms' tumor
Hemihypertrophy syndromes (Beckwith-Wiedemann)	Hepatoblastoma, Wilms' tumor
Neurocutaneous syndromes (NF, TSC, von Hippel-Lindau disease)	Optic glioma, CNS tumor Neurofibrosarcoma Peripheral nerve sheath tumor Leukemia Wilms' tumor
Immunodeficiency disorders (Wiskott-Aldrich, common/severe combined immunodeficiency)	Leukemia, non-Hodgkin lymphoma
Lynch syndrome (formerly hereditary nonpolyposis colorectal cancer [HNPCC])	Colorectal cancers, as well as other cancers depending on which of the five genes are affected. Screening for colon cancer five years younger than the youngest person in the family who had cancer
Multiple endocrine neoplasia, type 1	Cancers of the parathyroid gland, islet cells of the pancreas, adrenal cortical tumors, neuroendocrine tumors, pituitary tumors, and rare pheochromocytomas
Multiple endocrine neoplasia, type 2a (95% of all cases of MENS 2)	100% prevalence of medullary thyroid carcinoma (MTC) in association with pheochromocytoma (PHEO) or primary hyperthyroidism (PHPT) or both in some patient
Multiple endocrine neoplasia, type 2b (5.0% of all cases of MENS 2)	Early-onset 100% prevalence of an earlier onset and more severe MTC, PHEO, but not PHPT
Li-Fraumeni syndrome	Germline mutation of the TP53 gene on chromosome 17p13.1. A patient with a sarcoma before age 45, a first-degree relative with cancer before 45 years, and a first- or second-degree relative with cancer before 45 years or a sarcoma at any age. Cancer types include sarcomas, carcinomas, brain tumors, and leukemia (Correa 2016)
Peutz-Jeghers syndrome (PJS)	The child presents with mucocutaneous pigmentation that can fade over time, but the intraoral pigmentation does not fade. The child with PJS tends to develop gastrointestinal polyps early and has characteristic mucocutaneous freckling. They are at increased risk for cancers of the esophagus, stomach, rectum, colon, ovary, testis, and pancreas, with a 93% risk of developing cancer as an adult. The STK11 (tumor suppressor gene) is the defective gene, which is either autosomal dominant or a de novo mutation (Latchford et al. 2019)
Familial atypical mole/multiple melanomas (FAMMM)	FAMMM is fairly rare with most familial melanoma due to family sun exposure in families with susceptible skin types. FAMMM presents with multiple nevi, with some with marked atypia and a family history of melanoma. Hereditary melanoma is autosomal dominant. Screening for melanoma should begin in late adolescence. There is a proven association between CDKN2A melanoma, multiple nevi, pancreatic cancer (Soura et al. 2016)
PTEN hamartoma tumor syndrome (Cowden syndrome, Bannayan-Riley-Ruvalcaba syndrome, adult Lhermitte-Duclos disease, and autism spectrum disorders associated with macrocephaly)	The child will present at birth or in early childhood with genital lentigines, macrocephaly, intestinal hamartoma, polyposis, lipomas, developmental delay, or developmental disability if not identified until after age 5. Cancer risk includes thyroid, breast, endometrial, and renal cancers. The PTEN variant gene has cancer risk, and the disease is autosomal dominant (Pilarski 2019)
Familial adenomatous polyposis (Gardner syndrome, Turcot syndrome)	FAP is an autosomal dominant, rare genetic disorder associated with hundreds to thousands of gastrointestinal polyps and early colon cancer (usually by 40 years). By 15 years, at least 50% have colorectal adenomas. Other cancer complications include hepatoblastomas and thyroid, brain, biliary, and pancreatic cancers. Other noncancer complications include nasal angiofibroma, multiple osteomas (frontal bone is the most common location), and dental abnormalities. Congenital hypertrophy of retinal pigment epithelium is found in 90% of patients and may be seen in the retina at birth (Dinarvand et al. 2019)

Adapted from Correa (2016), Dinarvand et al. (2019), Latchford et al. (2019), Pilarski (2019), Roades and Steuber (2020), Soura et al. (2016)

questions and/or to contact the genetic team for clarification. Having subspecialists available to the practicing clinician can help facilitate the best care for the patient. It is important to keep up with current changes in genetic testing so that when a child requires additional testing, the clinician can further explain the need for testing. The primary care clinician needs to receive any communications sent to the family and receive a follow-up letter after a consult is requested. When the clinician needs to order the test themselves, they should review the genetic testing and obtain consent after in-depth education with the family. Types of errors that can occur are seen in Table 7.3.

Clinicians need to keep current about genetic testing to provide the best care to their patients. Table 7.4 is a list of resources for clinicians to keep current.

7.2.2 Direct-to-Consumer Testing

In the past genetic testing occurred at specialist genetic centers. These centers provided a diagnosis, risk to future offspring, extensive counseling with a genetic counselor, surveillance for complications of the genetic disease, and support as families with rare genetic conditions may have significant anxiety (Payne et al. 2018). Several companies do

Table 7.3 Types of errors by clinician when ordering genetic tests

Reason for ordering the wrong test	
Lack of knowledge	
Problem	Implications
Failure to recognize a rare genetic syndrome	The wrong test was ordered since the type of genetic variation was not identified
Clinician's lack of knowledge of the genetic etiology of the suspected disease	No testing was ordered since a genetic etiology was not suspected
The clinician's lack of knowledge led to a misinterpretation of the results of the genetic test	The clinician told the patient that the risk of the disease was lower or higher than expected since the clinician did not understand how to determine the risk of the disease for the next child
The clinician ordered the wrong genetic test	When the wrong genetic test is ordered, it can lead to a delay in diagnosis. For example, a patient can have a rare genetic variant of a disease that is not picked up when common genetic panels are ordered
Inadequate communication	
Failure to get a complete family history either due to clinician's error or patient not being fully informed of the family history or want to share it with the clinician	At times, families do not fully disclose important information. At other times, the clinician fails to probe more into the family history to develop the family history fully
The patient received inadequate communication about the test results	The explanation given to the family did not follow health literacy guidelines. Patients need to make sure they ask three specific questions to their clinicians: • What is my main problem? • What do I need to do? • Why is it important for me to do this? (Institute for Healthcare Improvement 2021)
The patient failed to receive any information about the results of the genetic testing	The family can fail to follow up with the provider that ordered the testing
Inadequate follow-up	
Additional testing was needed, and the clinician did not order it	
Laboratory reporting error	
The result interpretation or documentation by the testing laboratories was erroneous	The report by the laboratory was based on old data, or the lab reported the test as negative despite the fact the test was positive for the specific variant that ran in the family

Adapted from Farmer et al. (2019); Institute for Healthcare Improvement (2021); Lalonde et al. (2020)

Table 7.4   Resources for clinicians

Name of organization/website	Potential information
The Jackson Laboratory (JAX) www.jax.org/ccep	Online courses and case studies
Genetic science learning Center at the University of Utah https://learn. genetics.utah.edu/content/disorders/)	Information about genetics and health
GRACE by JAX www.jax.org/grace	Information about cancer risk assessment
Genomics education programme for health education England https://www. genomicseducation.hee. Nhs.Uk/	Online education for clinicians Resources
GEC-KO http://geneticseducation.ca	Evidence-based resources for clinicians
Genereviews	This website will give you resources for evidence for genomic/precision medicine
Radygenomics.Org	Free grand rounds about genomic medicine. Clinicians can sign up for grand rounds
TOXNET and Reprotox	Databases that can be used when there is a history of in utero exposure to a chemical
Online Mendelian inheritance in man (OMIM)	Can highlight a genetic problem based on one or more clinical findings and is free
Face2Gene application for smartphone	This smart application uses the pictures of standard syndromes and undiagnosed malformation and the London Dysmorphology database to generate a list of diagnoses based on the picture the clinician takes of the patient
Findingzebras.com	This website allows you to enter history and physical exam findings, and the search engine generates a list of possible diagnoses. It is a free decision support tool
Isabel.com	Another decision support website to help clinicians identify rare syndromes by using information gathered from history and physical examination

genetic analyses of ethnicity that may include medical data such as BRCA genes. DTC testing companies often specify that raw data files should not be used to inform medical care. In some cases, families are reassured even though they have a genetic problem. Recently DTC whole-genome sequencing testing was offered for 400 hundred dollars. This decrease in cost will make it increasingly likely that families will seek genetic testing without the benefit of clinician involvement.

7.2.3   Real-Life Example

A 26-year-old mother gave birth to her first child without any prenatal testing. The baby was a full-term infant born to a para 1001 mother. The child had anencephaly at birth and subsequently died four days later. The parents were referred to a genetic counselor who requested a three-generation family tree. While completing the tree, the mother learned that her maternal aunt had had two infants who died at birth, one from anencephaly and the other from spina bifida and anencephaly. As a result, the mother's seven siblings learned that they were at increased risk of having a child with a neural tube defect.

A 19-year-old male was seen by a primary provider requesting testing for multiple endocrine neoplasia type 2 (MEN2). The testing was ordered and was negative. However, the adolescent was worried, and he sought a second opinion since he felt he had the symptoms of MEN2. The clinician reviewed the testing and realized that a RET analysis had not been done, but rather a gene testing for MEN1 was ordered. The clinician ordered the right test and confirmed that the adolescent had the molecular diagnosis of MEN2.

Key Learning from Genetics Overview
- Family history is key to understanding a family's genetic risk. Families may have secrets that prevent clinicians from obtaining a complete history.
- There are red flags in history that require the clinician to probe further.
- The rule of two/too can help understand the significance of family history.
- Several genetic diseases have an increased risk of cancer.
- There are several resources that clinicians can use to continue education and to develop a differential diagnosis.

7.3　Types of Genetic Tests

There are different kinds of genetic tests that are used to identify different kinds of genetic problems. The clinician ordering the test must know the right test to evaluate the patient's problem. Before discussing any genetic tests, Table 7.5 will help define genetic terms used in the chapter.

Table 7.6 reviews the pros and cons of genetic testing.

7.3.1　Traditional Approaches to Diagnosis

Before ordering any genetic tests, it is important to ask families what genetic testing has been

Table 7.5 Definition of terms for facilitating understanding of genetic testing

Term	Definition
Aneuploidy	Loss of gain of an entire chromosome
Bionano Genomics	It is a new technique that can give a direct, high-resolution exam of long, intact DNA molecules (Pauly and Schwartz 2020)
Chain termination sequencing or sanger sequencing	Used in the human genome project
Chromosomal rearrangement	A change in the usual location of a piece of a chromosome
Chromosomal microarray	Chromosomal microarray analysis (CMA) is performed either by array comparative genomic hybridization (aCGH) or by using a single nucleotide polymorphism (SNP) array. CMA can detect imbalances in DNA copy numbers. The imbalances are called copy number variants (CNV). The presence of CNV does not mean that this points to an abnormal or pathogenic phenotype. Many CNVs are insignificant clinically, and very small CNVs are likely to be benign (Levy and Wapner 2018)
Comparative genomic hybridization microarray (aCGH)	aCGH compares the patient's DNA to the normal control DNA sample and can note over- or underrepresented areas in the patient's DNA. An aCGH diagnostic capability depends on the number and types of probes that are used to evaluate the entire genome. Most labs report when there are imbalances ranging from 50 to 100 Kb. Triploidy cannot be evaluated by this method (Levy and Wapner 2018)
Single nucleotide polymorphism (SNP) microarray analysis (SOMA)	SOMA involves using high-density oligonucleotide-based arrays where the target probes involve DNA locations that vary between individuals by a single base pair (Levy and Wapner 2018). The labs will report CNVs that are of known clinical significance, ranging from 50 to 100 Kb and higher. Uniparental disomy (UPD), mosaicism, zygosity, parent of origin, triploidy, and consanguinity can be evaluated using SNP microarray
Copy number variant (CNV)	Changes in the amount of DNA. There are five kinds of copy number variants (CNVs): (1) pathogenic, (2) likely pathogenic variants, (3) variants of unknown significance, (4) likely benign variants, (5) benign variants (Stoler 2017)
Epigenome	Altered genetic information without any change in DNA sequence (Zoghbi and Beaudel 2016)

Table 7.5 (continued)

Term	Definition
Epigenetic modification	Control gene expression patterns in a cell but do not modify the genes themselves. DNA methylation and histone modification can occur through DNA methylation that affects the gene expression without altering the somatic cells' nucleotide DNA structure (Pauly and Schwartz 2020). Some diseases are a result of genetic mutations that disrupt a gene's function. On the other hand, epigenetic defects usually misregulate gene expression by altering the chromatin context of the locus
Genomic imprinting (GI)	GI is a type of epigenetic regulation where the expression of a gene is dependent on whether the gene is from the mother or father (Zoghbi and Beaudel 2016)
Insertions	In smaller regions of DNA that change in the structure of the chromosome
Isochromosome	An unbalanced structural abnormality occurs when the arms of the chromosome are mirror images. The chromosome has two copies of the long arm or the short arm due to isochromosome formation. It is equivalent to a simultaneous duplication and deletion of genetic material
Methylation	Inactivation of a missing or extra methyl group modification
Mitochondrial genomic variant	A change in a gene within a mitochondrial genome
Monogenic diseases	Conditions related to genomic changes within a single gene (Petrikin et al. 2015)
Mosaicism	The cells within the same person have two or more types of genetic makeup within cells that result in a change in the person's phenotype. While each person has a few different cells with genetic differences, the disease is expressed when the number of cells with abnormal genetic material exceeds the cells with normal genetic material. So, the degree of mosaicism determines the severity of the disease along with the severity of the mistake in the genetic makeup
Mutation	Causes changes in the DNA structure
Partial chromosomal structural variant	A missing or extra piece of a chromosome
Precision/genomic medicine	The ability to tailor the therapeutic plan to the underlying mechanism caused by the mutation (Myers et al. 2019)
RNA-seq	A complementary tool to genomic sequencing that can detect transcript level changes and detect pathogenic coding variants. RNA-seq increases diagnostic yield by about 35% (Pauly and Schwartz 2020)
Single gene variant	A change in the gene that is within the nuclear genome, such as found in repeat expansions, missing pieces, extra pieces, or nucleotide sequence change
Single nucleotide variants Short insertions/ deletions	Change the sequence of the chromosome
Transcriptomics	Transcriptomics studies the transcriptome or the complete set of RNA transcripts produced by the genome. This technique is done under specific circumstances or within a specific cell. The method uses high-throughput techniques like microarray analysis
Translocations	In smaller regions of DNA that change in the structure of the chromosome
Uniparental disomy	Occurs when a person inherits both homologous chromosomes or a segment of a chromosome from the same parent. As a result, there is a lack of gene expression from the other parent, and all genetic material is expressed on one parental allele
Whole-chromosome aneuploidy	An extra or missing chromosome

Adapted from Kim and Bodurtha (2019); Lalonde et al. (2020); Levy and Wapner (2018); Myers et al. (2019); Pauly and Schwartz (2020); Petrikin et al. (2015); Stoler (2017); Zoghbi and Beaudel (2016)

Table 7.6 Pros and cons of genetic testing

Pros	Cons
It may help explain the reason for the child's problem	May not identify the reason for the child's problem
It may help soothe a parent's guilt	May lead to the identification of a new genetic problem and give additional guilt
It may help provide access to life-saving treatment	Results for this testing may be confusing to parents
It may help with identifying sources of support for the family, including support groups	The wait for the results may cause additional stress and confuse the causes for the child's problem
It may be helpful in future family planning	It may have a finding without any genetic significance
The results may be added to a data bank to identify a new genetic problem	It may have negative effects on future insurance coverage
May help identify associated health problems and screen appropriately for them	Pain and stress associated with venipuncture

done previously and its results. The traditional genetic tests identify a causative single genetic variant that has a recognizable clinical presentation.

7.3.1.1 Karyotype

Traditional karyotyping or G-banded karyotype examines large structural changes in the chromosome. It can identify aneuploidies, structural rearrangements, and mosaicism. It is the first-line test when patients are suspected of having an aneuploidy such as trisomy or sex chromosome aneuploidy. Examples include Down syndrome, triple X, or Klinefelter syndrome (Lalonde et al. 2020). It will also pick up balanced changes such as rings, translocations, inversions, and insertions. It will also show isochromosomes and CNV of >5–10 MB. The test is used in mothers who have a history of recurrent miscarriages or infertility. Karyotype analysis, FISH, and whole-genome sequencing (WES) can detect structural changes, especially when they are balanced. Still, the latter is more expensive [WES is generally only ordered by a geneticist and may have insurance limitations] (Lalonde et al. 2020).

7.3.1.2 Single Gene Testing

Single gene testing can be used as a primary test when a specific disease is suspected or a secondary test when the pathogenic or likely pathogenic variant is detected in a disease gene known to have an autosomal recessive mode of inheritance. For example, a pathogenic variant within the gene, SCN1A, causes Dravet syndrome in 80% of children. Single gene testing can evaluate expansion mutations (DRPLA and EPM1) or can assess the methylation at a specific locus, such as seen in Angelman syndrome (Myers et al. 2019). The reporting for a single gene testing is based on detecting all pathogenic variants, variants of uncertain clinical significance, and benign variants (Fogel et al. 2016).

7.3.1.3 Fluorescence in Situ Hybridization (FISH Testing)

FISH testing emerged in the 1980s and helped determine whether discrete segments of DNA are present or absent. The FISH probe uses targeted probes to identify microdeletions and microduplications (Stoler 2017). It allows for deletions and duplications to be identified. It is useful to confirm the clinical diagnosis of known disorders such as Wolf-Hirschhorn syndrome and cri du chat syndrome. It also helps to define the translocations or chromosomes that are identified as abnormal in a karyotype. FISH testing will identify aneuploids, CNV, translocation, inversions, and insertions. The probes are designed for specific aberration. The most common resolution is from 200 to 400 kilobase pair (kb), but some labs will do 5–10 megabase (Mb). There are one million base pairs in an Mb and one thousand base pairs in a kb (Corfield 2021). FISH testing is used when there is identified prenatal aneuploidy, follow-up for abnormal karyotype, and in parental studies for proband with some identified structural rearrangements whether balanced or unbalanced or CNV (Lalonde et al. 2020). FISH is used in cytogenetic follow-up studies or tests for recurrent changes found in Williams syndrome. If a patient is found to have mosaic gain in CMA testing, then FISH studies help to determine the exact numbers of deletions.

7.3.1.4 Multiplex Ligation-Dependent Probe Amplification (MLPA, Real-Time PCR)

Multiplex ligation-dependent probe amplification (MLPA) is a technique that assesses copy numbers. It is used to detect smaller CNV involved in single gene deletion or recurrent microdeletion or duplication syndrome (Lalonde et al. 2020). Sixty to eighty-five percent of patients with Duchenne's muscular dystrophy (DMD) have either a deletion or a duplication of the DMD gene in the X chromosome (Lalonde et al. 2020). High resolution of the CNVs is critical as patients with out-of-frame CNV will have the aggressive form of DMD, whereas patients with inframe CNV will have Becker's MD. CMA done SNO may not detect the differences, but aCGH may have the resolution to detect single exon changes (Lalonde et al. 2020).

7.3.1.5 Sanger Sequencing

Sanger sequencing (SS) or chain termination sequencing was the first and the most common DNA sequencing method used for decades (Fogel et al. 2016). SS is a genotyping test used to evaluate the patient for a known disease or treatment-associated variant. SS is best used when a single shorter gene causes the disease. It does not capture mosaicism that is less than 15–20% (Lalonde et al. 2020). SS does not pick up deletion, structural genetic rearrangements, and duplications. Today, genomic tests rely on next-generation sequencing (NGS) technologies, and there has been a decline in the use of Sanger sequencing (Payne et al. 2018).

For example, in common disorders related to the HBB gene, SS can be reliably used. In thalassemia, loss-of-function variants or β^0 results in no production of the protein, whereas other variants cause reduced production of the HBB protein or β^+. The HBB gene is small and has three exons which can be sequenced with two amplicons. Therefore, Sanger sequencing can detect sequence variants, and MLPA can detect deletions (Lalonde et al. 2020).

7.3.2 Newer Genetic Tests

Advances in genomics enable clinicians to assess the submicroscopic of chromosome structure using CMA and the ability to detect pathogenic variants to the resolution of a single base pair using NGS (Mone et al. 2018). While NGS gives more detailed information, CMA is less expensive. Chromosomal microarray (CMA) has greater sensitivity than karyotype and is an older test than NGS. It can be used for microdeletions and microduplications (Stoler 2017). It is preferred for patients with a developmental delay, autism spectrum disorder (ASD), intellectual disability (ID), and multiple congenital anomalies of unknown clinical significance (Lalonde et al. 2020). It has a diagnostic yield of 12–15% (Levy and Wapner 2018). Approximately 6% of people with intellectual disability and 10% of those with dysmorphic features will have an abnormal CMA (Stoler 2017). The clinician should realize that patients in their teens may not have previously received this kind of testing, and the testing should be offered to parents.

CMA has a high sensitivity for submicroscopic aberrations, as tiny as 5–10 Kb. This resolution is as much as 1000 times more sensitive than conventional karyotyping (Mone et al. 2018). There are two types of chromosomal microarray analysis (CMA) to detect copy number variants: genome-wide single nucleotide polymorphism (SNP) and array comparative genomic hybridization (aCGH). CMA is a DNA test done by a single nucleotide polymorphism array (SNP) or oligoarray. The oligoarray uses a small segment of DNA as a problem, but the SNP uses a single nucleotide. SNP array problems are restricted to a specific position within the genome that is known polymorphic. The probe density determines the resolution of both kinds of arrays. The SNP is in the range of 10–100 kb for a clinical platform. SNP greatly increases the resolution compared to karyotype. Unfortunately, balanced changes, including insertions, inversion, or translocations, will not be detected since there is no loss in the material. When duplication is detected, the placement in the genome cannot be determined. SNP is best in identifying multi-gene or larger CNV and can better detect low-level mosaicism. SNP focuses on identifying moderate to high allele frequencies (Petersen et al. 2017). aCGH is useful for gene-level CNV. Some aCGH platforms can identify CNV down to one exon.

NGS was developed in 2005 and initially was very expensive (Fogel et al. 2016). The entire human genome can be sequenced in less than 2 days at the cost of under 1000 dollars (https://www.genome.gov/about-genomics/fact-sheets/). When parents do not have answers to what is wrong with their children, they are likely to have increased distress. These newer technologies can identify if there is a genetic problem (Pauly and Schwartz 2020). NGS includes targeted panels, whole-exome sequencing (WES), and whole-genome sequencing (WGS). NGS is a relatively new method for evaluating inherited (germline) and acquired mutations (somatic) genetic mutations (Yohe and Thyagarajan 2017). While targeted panels for genes are used when a clinical phenotype is identified, whole-exome sequencing is used when the targeted testing has not been helpful (Yohe and Thyagarajan 2017) or when the child is critically ill, and information about the diagnosis must be obtained quickly. However, the genome-based diagnostic test may report incidental findings not related to the clinical presentation, and different labs will handle the reporting of incidental findings differently (Payne et al. 2018). These new tests may offer an increased chance of diagnosis by moving the gene-based diagnostic test to whole-genome sequencing. By avoiding the sequential single gene tests or gene panel tests, time to diagnosis can shorten the time to appropriate, effective clinical intervention (Smith et al. 2019).

Next-generation sequencing was very expensive in 2007 but has steadily decreased to under 1000 dollars over the past five years. Information regarding current costs can be found at: https://www.genome.gov/about-genomics/fact-sheets/Sequencing-Human-Genome-cost. However, introducing these tests into clinical practice comes with additional costs as the cost of the test does not account for the time spent in developing

clinical guidelines and the time clinicians spent in counseling families. In truth, the actual cost of providing services to deliver genomic tests is not well documented (Payne et al. 2018). More research is needed to understand the impact of next-generation sequencing testing to demonstrate these tests' cost-effectiveness and clinical utility (Smith et al. 2019). It is critical to consider diagnostic stewardship and choose the right test on the right patient at the right time, especially as more costly tests become available (Smith et al. 2019).

7.3.2.1 Chromosomal Microarray (CMA)

CMA is valuable since it can show submicroscopic imbalances (also known as microdeletions or microduplications) or copy number changes (CNVs) that are not seen on a standard karyotype (Levy and Wapner 2018). Genetic tests like a chromosomal microarray (CMA) screen individuals by locating specific alleles of a gene by using specific probes. Since CMA uses comparison of the patient's DNA to normal controls, it can only report differences in the patient's DNA to the controls. As a result, balanced rearrangements cannot be detected (Levy and Wapner 2018). The test procedure is outlined as followed:

- DNA probes are small sections of DNA that are complementary to a known DNA sequence. The probes are labeled to facilitate their identification using fluorescence, an enzyme, or radioactivity.
- DNA probes locate the mutant, disease-causing allele using the following steps.
- First, the sequencing of the mutant allele is calculated by sequencing the DNA or by retrieving the desired DNA sequence in a genetic database.
- Then a probe is developed by synthesizing a fragment of DNA with a complementary base sequence to the disease-causing allele.
- A probe is a labeled molecule that binds specifically to a molecule of interest.
- The DNA probe is then labeled with a fluorescent marker.
- The DNA probe is amplified using PCR to produce many copies of the probe. The copies of

the DNA from the specimen are then heated until they are denatured and separated into single strands using a process called denaturation.

- The separated strands of DNA are mixed with DNA probes, followed by temperature reduction.
- If the specimen contains the mutant allele, the probe then binds to the complementary DNA fragments. When two single-stranded nucleic molecules of complementary basis form a double-stranded hybrid, the process is called hybridization. Nucleic acid hybridization is used in PCR, DNA microarray, and in situ hybridization.
- The DNA is then washed clean of any unattached probes, and the hybrid DNA can be detected due to the presence and intensity of the fluorescence.

Hundreds of diseases can be screened using different DNA probes on an array arranged on a glass slide. DNA probes are complementary to the sequences of DNA known to disease. The DNA probes will fluoresce only when bound to a fragment of DNA via hybridization (Govindarajan et al. 2012; Khan Academy 2021).

7.3.2.2 Targeted Panels

Single gene testing and targeted gene panels rely on PCR technology and can identify various targeted disorders (Stoler 2017). The revolution in PCR technology enables targeted CNV detection in even smaller regions, allowing for the detection of CNV. Single gene testing is used when a particular condition is considered as the most likely by the clinician. For example, the FGFR3 gene codes for achondroplasia, and single gene testing would be the best one to use. Targeted gene panels are used when there are multiple genes known to cause a problem. For example, targeted epilepsy gene panels will look for anywhere between 100 and 300 known genes for epilepsy (Myers et al. 2019). These panels are equal in cost to Sanger gene sequencing tests.

The problems with multi-gene panels include those variants of uncertain significance and pathogenic variants of moderate risk in 20–30% of the tests. The data regarding newer genes may

be restricted, and unexpected pathogenic variants may not align with the patient's history. In addition, testing technique differences include different technologies and the difference in interpretation or reporting by the genetic laboratories (Farmer et al. 2019). Some labs may elect not to report benign variants or variants of unknown clinical significance.

7.3.2.3 Whole-Exome Sequencing (WES)

Next-generation sequencing includes WGS and WES. Both WGS and WES can increase diagnostic yield compared to multi-gene panels (MGP). WES targets around 1–2% of the genome versus WGS, covering 95–98% of the genome (Pauly and Schwartz 2020). WES can identify various nontargeted disorders. Exome sequencing is unbiased and therefore reduces the impact of disease variability on the strategies for genetic testing. This method weighs all disease genes the same, and therefore all variants can be assessed simultaneously in terms of the clinical presentation (Fogel et al. 2016). Therefore, the true phenotypic variation of a disease can be assessed that is not dependent on previously published single gene phenotypes. This allows for better medical management, preventive care, reproductive counseling, and genetic counseling and increases the likelihood of the patient being identified for a clinical trial (Fogel et al. 2016).

Patients need to understand that WES assesses all exons that encode 20,00 genes. It can detect a genetic problem to the precision of a single base pair. Some of the changes are of uncertain significance, and therefore parental blood may be needed to assess the inheritance pattern. The use of WES may reveal incidental findings, posing ethical considerations (Mone et al. 2018). Ethical considerations include that non-paternity or consanguinity being discovered as a result of testing. Another ethical consideration is who owns the genetic information results and should other relatives have access to the result (Mone et al. 2018). These ethical considerations should be discussed in the pre-counseling and consent discussion.

WES also improves the detection of de novo genetic disorders such as achondroplasia and

Kabuki syndrome. Secondary findings detected during exome sequencing may be reported by the lab, or as suggested by recent guidelines, the patient may opt not to receive these secondary results. Cystic fibrosis has over 1000 mutations, and today WES can detect a variety of mutations.

7.3.2.4 Whole-Genome Sequencing (WGS)

Whole-genome sequencing (WGS) can identify nontargeted disorders. The advantages of WGS include the detection of CNVs, a uniform evaluation across the genome, and in-depth coverage to detect mosaicism (Pauly and Schwartz 2020).

WES has been shown to have a higher yield in identifying the causes of the person's clinical problem. Lionel et al. (2018) evaluated the differences between targeted gene panels and CMA as compared to WGS. The WGS identified a diagnostic variant in 41% versus 24% using the conventional testing of CMA or targeted gene panels. A recent scoping review suggested that more research is needed to determine the economic effectiveness and the outcome of testing (Smith et al. 2019).

7.3.2.5 Rapid Whole-Genome Sequencing

This technique has been used to evaluate the sick neonate to identify the genetic nature of the problem and develop an appropriate treatment plan. Rapid WGS can treat and understand that the patient's prognosis cannot be improved, and supportive care can be initiated (Char 2015). Rapid WGS is useful in the NICU when used in critically ill neonates; the cause of the neonatal illness is discovered in 57% (Petrikin et al. 2015). The impact of genetic diseases on the family is significant, with noted increases in maternal depression, anxiety, and an increase in divorce (Petrikin et al. 2015). The diagnosis generated using rapid WGS may not have been considered since the classical disease presentation may not have developed, or the presentation was rarer. In some cases, WGS enabled life-saving treatment and shorter NICU stays (Petrikin et al. 2015).

Rapid WGS cannot be used for triplet repeats expansion disorders or diseases with nonfunctional but highly homologous areas called pseudogenes. False-positive and false-negative results can occur with underreporting of de novo variants (Petrikin et al. 2015). False-negative and false-positive results occur due to technical errors related to assay design, instrumentation, and target coverage (Lalonde et al. 2020). False negative may result from laboratories restricting the analysis to variants that are more likely to impact protein sequence, noncoding, and intronic and synonymous variants, which can impact the transcription of genes. There is also disagreement among good laboratories about what is considered pathogenic, uncertain or likely benign, or benign.

7.3.2.6 Multi-Omic Analysis

This technique is part of a comprehensive variant assessment program to determine the significance of variants of unknown significance, particularly in complex patients with significant developmental delay, ID, and ASD. This technique involves doing WGS, genome-wide methylation profiling, and a CNV array analysis as a first-tier and as a second-tier and doing bionano genomic, structural variant analysis, RNA-seq analysis, and transcriptomics to develop a comprehensive genomic analysis leading to a functional assay (i.e., clustered regularly interspaced short palindromic repeats [CRISPR]) (Pauly and Schwartz 2020). This kind of testing is reserved for complex patients. The future use of these tests means that scientists need to work together to move genomic data into clinical use so patients can benefit from their use (Petersen et al. 2017).

Companion diagnostic tests. These diagnostic tests (typically an in vitro diagnostic) can further clarify NGS applications' results in more complex patients. Other NGS applications detect modulation of gene activity by using RNA-seq, which can direct the transcript sequence and detect differently methylated sites. A metagenomic sequence of the host-associated microbiome can determine microbiota diversity (Petersen et al. 2017). The application of multi-omics data can give a better overall picture of the disease and the molecular underpinnings. Other newer diagnostic tests include circulating tumor DNA testing, human leukocyte antigen (HLA) typing done by sequencing, and microbial analysis.

RNA-seq. Messenger RNA sequencing provides different information than DNA sequencing. It detects allele-specific expression, examines mRNA abundance, interrogates the results of splicing, and identifies germline variants in coding regions. It is a hybrid test to assess the abnormal expression and is capable of detecting pathogenic coding variants. The RNA-seq could detect abnormal splicing in DNA when other NGS are negative (Gonorazky et al. 2019).

7.3.3 Real-Life Example

A five-day-old presented with the classic features of Turner's syndrome, including a webbed neck and coarctation of the aorta. You explain to the mother that you are ordering a karyotype to confirm your clinical suspicions. She asks about whole-genome sequencing as she just read an article in the newspaper. She wants the latest testing. After explaining that a karyotype is done in patients with suspected sex chromosome aneuploidy, she accepts your opinion. The testing confirms Turner's syndrome.

> **Key Learning about Genetic Test**
> - A karyotype is an appropriate test for a child with the clinical features of a syndrome. It is a first-tier test for patients suspected of having an aneuploidy such as trisomy or sex chromosome aneuploidy.
> - A single gene test is a primary test when a specific disease is suspected or a secondary test when the pathogenic or likely pathogenic variant is detected in a disease gene known to have an autosomal recessive mode of inheritance.

- The FISH probe uses targeted probes to identify microdeletions and microduplications.
- Multiplex ligation-dependent probe amplification (MLPA) is a technique that assesses copy numbers. It is used to detect smaller CNV involved in single gene deletion or recurrent microdeletion or duplication syndrome.
- Advances in genomics enable clinicians to assess the submicroscopic of chromosome structure using CMA and the ability to detect pathogenic variants to the resolution of a single base pair using next-generation sequencing.
- Single gene testing and targeted gene panels rely on PCR technology and can identify various targeted disorders.
- Rapid WGS is useful in the NICU since when used in critically ill neonates.
- Next-generation sequencing includes WGS and WES. Both WGS and WES have the potential to increase diagnostic yield when compared to multi-gene panels.
- Other NGS applications detect modulation of gene activity by using RNA-seq, metagenomic sequence of the host-associated microbiome, and can improve the understanding of the clinical picture by combining first-line NGS with RNA-based testing.

7.4 Specific Conditions and Genetic Testing

7.4.1 Neurological Disorders

Almost all neurological disorders can have some degree of heritability (Fogel et al. 2016). NGS has vastly improved the diagnosis of neurological diseases.

Epilepsy is a common neurological disorder with a lifetime risk of 3% and a prevalence of 5–8 people per 1000. The estimates of epilepsy heritability range from 8% to 69% (Myers et al. 2019). Monozygotic twins have a greater risk of epilepsy, reflecting the heritability of the disease. The risk of epilepsy in first-generation relatives to the proband is five to ten times higher. Current evidence suggests that genetic abnormalities account for a major proportion of children with epilepsy. Knowing the genetic variation can promote early treatment. It is important to note that certain generalized epilepsy syndromes with pathogenic variants in SLC2A1 that encode the GLUT1 transporter will be more responsive to a ketogenic diet (Hebbar and Mefford 2020).

In neonates with early-onset, infantile epileptic encephalopathies (EIEE), the molecular tests add to the diagnostic process and allow for timely and accurate diagnosis. An example is a neonate with EIEE with a vitamin B6 deficiency resulting from a genetic defect. With early identification of the genetic problem, vitamin B6 supplementation can treat EIEE. While NGS testing can provide valuable information for treatment, it is not without drawbacks. NGS tests for neonates with EIEE take up to 6 weeks depending on the hospital, and some institutions use rapid WES with 48 hours turnaround. With WES or WGS, there may be additional information about adult-onset diseases included in the report. How the results are reported will depend on the laboratory, with some labs only reporting information pertinent to the clinical condition. The risk of additional information must be explained to the parent when the consent for testing is reviewed. A more detailed chart of neonatal EIEE diseases and the possible benefits of identifying the genetic defect can be found in the article by Myers et al. (2019). Still, it is not needed for the objectives of this chapter.

NGS is unnecessary when there is a specific clinical presentation, and EIEE is part of the recognizable syndrome. Diseases like Rett and Rett-like syndromes can be tested with a single gene or a restricted panel made up of a few genes. Other recognizable syndromes such as Miller-Dieker syndrome or Wolf-Hirschhorn syndrome can be identified using FISH, karyotype, or genomic hybridization instead of NGS testing (Myers et al. 2019). Testing by panel testing provides diagnosis in 15%–25% of cases (Myers

et al. 2019). While the primary care provider will not be ordering these tests, the clinician must be aware that the epileptologist and geneticist may order testing and, depending on the lab, discover a risk for other diseases. A referral to a neurologist specializing in metabolic disease should be considered if developmental regression and laboratory findings are consistent with a metabolic disorder. A dysmorphic examination should be done to evaluate for any recognizable syndromes associated with seizures.

Another example of the early identification of the genetic problem can be seen in tuberous sclerosis (TS), which results from a mutation in TSC1 or TSC2. The TSC1 gene normally makes a protein called hamartin, and the TSC2 gene makes a protein called tuberin. These proteins normally will bind and form a protein complex involved in mTOR (mammalian target of rapamycin). The abnormality of TSC function increases Rheb activity, leading to hyperactivity in mTOR. This hyperactivity in mTOR leads to disinhibition of protein synthesis and cell growth (Lee et al. 2015). Clinically, the patients will have the early onset of seizures, cortical tubers, ID, brain malformation, and a higher incidence of ASD. The physical exam in TS may be suspected by the skin findings (hypopigmented, ash leaf macules, or orange peel lesion) or the discovery of a cardiac rhabdomyoma. The early control of seizures with vigabatrin in TS can improve the neurodevelopmental outcome. Targeted medication is an example where a specific drug is effective against a specific gene mutation and can tailor therapy – a precision medicine concept. WES and WGS can increase diagnostic yield when seeking the genetic reasons for a child's epilepsy and developmental delay (Fogel et al. 2016).

Several genetic syndromes have a single gene variation. Table 7.7 reviews the various syndromes associated with epilepsy and a developmental delay and intellectual disability.

Neuromuscular diseases in pediatrics challenge diverse genetic etiological, overlapping clinical presentation, and phenotypic heterogeneity (Herman et al. 2021). Due to recent advances in treatment, identifying the molecular diagnosis

Table 7.7 Common syndromes associated with epilepsy and ASD

Syndrome	Clinical presentation
Down syndrome	Distinctive facies, intellectual disability, congenital anomalies, higher rate of ASD and epilepsy in 8–13%. The problem involves chromosome 21
Fragile X syndrome	ID, large ears, long face, macroorchidism. Problem in FMR1 region
Tuberous sclerosis complex	Hamartomas in the brain, lung, heart, kidney, skin. The problem is in TCS 1/2 region
PTEN-related disorders	Hamartomas, genetic cancer risk, ASD-associated syndrome. Problem in PTEN region
MECP2-related disorder (includes Rett syndrome, ASD, PPMX syndrome, duplications of MECP2, MECP2-related severe neonatal encephalopathy)	A severe neurodevelopmental disorder, arrested development by 6–18 months with regression of skills, microcephaly, loss of speech, seizures, ID, and stereotypical hand movements. Problem with MECP2 gene is on the long (q) arm of the X chromosome, band 28 MECP2
Phelan-McDermid syndrome/ SHANK3 deletion	The child will have hypotonia in early life, developmental delay including speech, autism-like behaviors, kidney problems, lymphedema, gastroesophageal reflux The problem is due to a deletion of 22q13.3 containing the SHANK3 gene
CDKL5-related disorders	X-linked condition with early onset of epilepsy, usually infantile spasms. A patient will have microcephaly, severe neurodevelopmental delay including lack of speech, dysmorphic features, hand stereotypies that resemble MECP2 disorders, and absent spoken language
FOXG1-related disorders	Presents with infantile spasms and will have a developmental disability that includes autistic-like features. The problem is in duplications of FOXG1 on chromosome 14q12
CASK-related disorders	Presents with postnatal microcephaly accompanied by pontine/cerebellar hypoplasia, intellectual disability, growth retardation abnormalities of the eye, and facial dysmorphisms. Epilepsy is as high as 50% in females. Located on the short arm of the X chromosome
SCN2A-related disorders	Presents with ASD; epilepsy with a developmental delay SCN2A is responsible for the neuronal sodium channel, which is one of several neuronal sodium channel genes that help the action potential of nerves. It is located on chromosome 2

Adapted from Lee et al. (2015); Sanders et al. (2018)

can facilitate treatment, allow for genetic counseling, increase participation in clinical trials, decrease psychosocial burden, and identify the risk of reoccurrence (Ravi et al. 2019). The use of NGS has a higher diagnostic yield than other genetic tests and, given the newer genetic treatments for a neuromuscular disease, should be considered (Herman et al. 2021).

7.4.2 Neurodevelopmental Delays

Chromosomal microarray (CMA), including single nucleotide polymorphism (SNP) array and array-based comparative genomic hybridization (aCGH), is commonly ordered for children with a developmental delay. The common clinical cutoff is 50Kb. Gene-disrupting and protein-damaging

rare variants or ultra-rare variants can play a role in neurodevelopmental disorders, including ASD, as well as in children with epilepsy. Rare CNVs are responsible for some neurodevelopmental disorders such as global developmental delay, ID, and ASD (Lowther et al. 2017).

Attention deficit hyperactivity disorder (ADHD) and ASD are neurodevelopmental disorders with onset in childhood. Both disorders are highly heritable, and genetics account for 70–80% of the phenotypes (Antshel and Russo 2019; Grimm et al. 2020). No specific genes have accounted for the two diseases, but rare copy number variants in similar loci have been identified (Antshel and Russo 2019). Rare variants likely account for some of the inheritability of ADHD (Grimm et al. 2020). Single nucleotide variants (SNPs) account for approximately 22% of the inheritability of ADHD (Grimm et al. 2020). Children with ADHD can have a higher rate of comorbidity with autism, bipolar disorder, anxiety, depression, and substance use disorder. Children with ASD are known to have ADHD symptoms, and this occurs around 40–70%. Twenty to sixty percent of children diagnosed with ADHD also demonstrate social impairment similar to ASD. Inattention, hyperactivity/impulsivity, and poor social functioning occur at a higher rate in children in these two diagnoses. Polygenic risk scores (PRS) may prove increasingly helpful in predicting which group of children will go on to develop adult ADHD. PRS utilizes the summary statistics of SNP results from large GWAS to predict the risk of a specific trait (Grimm et al. 2020).

In patients with ASD, approximately 0.5–3% have reciprocal duplications of the maternally inherited copy of chromosome 15q11-q13 region. Prader-Willi and Angelman syndromes also have deletions in this region (Lee et al. 2015). ADHD has a higher frequency in a child with several genetic syndromes, including fragile X syndrome, neurofibromatosis, tuberous sclerosis complex, Turner's syndrome, Klinefelter syndrome, velo-cardio-facial/DiGeorge syndrome, and Williams-Beuren syndrome.

7.4.3 Imprinting Disorders

A child inherits a set of chromosomes from the father and a set of chromosomes from the mother. Most of the autosomal genes are expressed from both the paternal and maternal alleles. Only one member of allele or gene pair is expressed in patients with an imprint disorder and X-inactivation. There can be transcriptional silencing of one parental gene allele, which causes major changes in fetal growth and placental development (Butler 2020). In imprinting, the expression of a few genes is expressed on one parental allele. When the child has paternal UPD, the expression of maternal alleles is absent, and there is a greater level for paternally expressed genes (Zoghbi and Beaudel 2016). The parent determines this expression during the gamete production due to an epigenetic process resulting from DNA methylation (Butler 2020).

Genomic imprinting occurs when there is methylation or inactivation of cytosine bases in the CpG dinucleotides of the DNA molecule. The bases of the dinucleotides are important in regulating the elements of genes (Butler 2009, 2020). It is important to understand that a methylated gene can be reactivated in the gamete in the next generation.

Prader-Willi syndrome, Silver-Russell syndrome, Angelman syndrome, Beckwith-Wiedemann syndrome, and Albright hereditary osteodystrophy are other examples of imprinting disorders. Prader-Willi syndrome is an example of an imprinting disorder resulting from a paternal deletion of chromosome 15q11-q13 or when both pairs of chromosome 15 s are from one parent (uniparental disomy). However, the allele expression may not be complete, and the imprinted gene expression is not absolute. It is believed that an event early in the pregnancy causes imprinting. Angelman syndrome is also an imprinting disorder with a typical 15q11-q13 as seen in PWS and maternal origin. Uniparental paternal disomy 15 causes Angelman syndrome in about 5–7% (Butler 2020). Over one dozen genes within the 15q11 -13q region play a role in PWS and Angelman syndrome. Several epigenetic tests are performed at the clinical laboratory to evaluate Prader-Willi syndrome, Angelman syndrome, Beckwith-Wiedemann syndrome, and others (García-Giménez et al. 2017).

The risk of imprinting disorders increases with assisted reproductive technology (ART) (Butler 2020; Kim and Bodurtha 2019). ART may affect the development and expression of imprinted genes due to pre- and periconception environmental factors. Babies born using ART contribute to 5% of all infants with low birth weight (Marjonen et al. 2018).

Imprinting disorder can cause a variety of oncological problems. In these patients, inappropriate methylation may result in tumor formation. This process either is the result of tumor-suppressing genes being silenced or growth-stimulating genes being activated. Imprinting disorders may be responsible for various psychiatric disorders, including schizophrenia, alcohol dependency, and possibly bipolar disorder (Butler 2009).

7.4.4   Repeat Expansion Disorders

Repeat expansion disorders in pediatric patients include fragile X syndrome, myotonic dystrophy, oculopharyngeal muscular dystrophy, spinal and bulbar muscular atrophy, Friedrich's ataxia, and spinocerebellar ataxia. Short tandem repeats, also known as microsatellites, vary in length, and the length of the pathogenic repeats varies from disorder to disorder. The longer the length of the repeats, the worse the disease and the earlier the onset of the disease. The testing for this is specific. Repeated primed PCR is more efficient in the identification of expanded repeats. For example, in fragile x, the FMR1 gene contains 5–44 CGG repeats in healthy people. The CGG repeats are between 55 and 200 repeats in the premutation range, and the premutation alleles can expand to full mutation, which is considered >200 repeats to over 1000 repeats (Lalonde et al. 2020).

NGS is not as accurate in identifying the problem, but emerging technology like long-read sequencing has been developed and may be helpful (Lalonde et al. 2020).

7.4.5   Hypertrophic Cardiomyopathy

Hypertrophic cardiomyopathy (HCM) is a genetically varied cardiac muscle disorder. In HCM, there is unexplained left ventricular hypertrophy (LVH) due to myocyte enlargement and disarray along with myocardial fibrosis. The disease is characterized by varying sarcomere dysfunction. HCM is autosomal dominant and incomplete and has variable penetrance. In adults, the prevalence is 1 in 500 people. Genetic testing has allowed for the identification of children with HCM before the onset of disease symptoms, including fatigue, exertional dyspnea, syncope, lightheadedness, atypical chest pain, and sudden cardiac death (Teekakirikul et al. 2019). HCM is the most common cause of sudden death in young adults. Arrhythmias such as atrial fibrillation (AF) and ventricular tachycardia can occur before the development of heart failure. The risk of thromboembolic stroke occurs as a result of AF. Myosin

heavy chain (MYH7) and myosin binding protein C (MYBPC3) cause most disease-causing variants with 5–10% of HCM involving mutations in non-sarcomere genes associated with neuromuscular diseases such as Friedreich ataxia, Noonan's syndrome, or Barth syndrome (Teekakirikul et al. 2019).

The phenotypic diversity is due to environmental factors, modifying gene variants, epigenetics, and other regulatory mechanisms of gene expression (Teekakirikul et al. 2019). Genetic testing used to rely on polymerase chain reaction (PCR) amplification and Sanger sequencing of amplicons of HCM genes. Due to advances in NGS, families previously offered genetic counseling should receive information about new advances in testing to identify risks in their offspring. Recent evidence demonstrated that a certain sarcomere mutation could predict early disease onset and adverse clinical outcomes, including ventricular arrhythmia and heart failure. Therefore, identifying the genotype can direct the clinical management of patients with HCM (Teekakirikul et al. 2019).

7.4.6   Psychiatric Disorders

Today, an understanding of the genetics of psychiatric disorders is rapidly expanding. Disorders such as Tourette's syndrome, once thought to be inherited as an autosomal dominant disorder, are now recognized as a combination of various genetic and environmental factors (Qi et al. 2019). NGS methods have vastly improved the understanding of the genetics of psychiatric disorders. The molecular etiology of any disease with a genetic basis will help develop drugs that target the defective genetic material. The development of CRISPR can allow the affected genes to be permanently modified with the body's cells, helping to identify novel therapeutic targets and synergistic drugs that can target multiple molecular pathways at a time, which is critical to drug discovery (Foley et al. 2017).

A meta-analysis of the Psychiatric Genomics Consortium (PGC) has documented that some copy number variants, while rare, can play a moderate to a large role in developing schizophrenia. While schizophrenia is largely heritable, social and environmental factors such as adversity and migration contribute to the risk of developing the disorder (Foley et al. 2017). Genome-wide association studies (GWAS) contribute to the understanding of psychiatric genetics. The studies use array-based methods to assay the common SNPs, and the results have been put into a database that the PGC analyzes. GWAS provide an unbiased approach to test associations of common genetic variants across the whole genome. GWAS evaluate hundreds of thousands to several million variants. GWAS require a large sample size. It is hoped that identifying the specific genetic difference allows drug therapy to be developed targeting the genetic problem. Understanding genetics may help develop a more effective treatment for psychiatric disease. For example, only 60% of patients with a depressive disorder (MDD) are responsive to antidepressant medications. The lack of response to medications points to the need for a greater understanding of the molecular etiology of MD.

In addition, the polygenetic risk scores (PRS) of patients can help target prevention methods. PRS are calculated using the weighted sum of the risk alleles divided by the weighted risk allele effect sizes derived from genome-wide association study data. It is used to develop the person's risk of developing a particular disease after genetic testing is done. PRS is used in precision medicine. High-throughput screening of molecular targets is developing using CRISPR technology (Foley et al. 2017). Whole-genome sequencing is likely to provide a better picture of genomic risk in the future.

Anxiety disorders are common, with approximately 20% lifetime incidence. However, they are very complex and polygenic. There are only a few risk loci identified in these disorders (Meier and Deckert 2019). First-degree relatives of patients with an anxiety disorder have a four to six times higher rate of developing anxiety (Meier and Deckert 2019). Similarly, depression has a 37% heritability based on twin studies. The GWAS have failed to identify risk genes. Depression is another complex, polygenic disorder that arises from many genetic variants with individual small effect sizes (Mullin and Lewis 2017).

Anorexia nervosa (AN) may also have a genetic basis as gene meta-analyses implicate serotonin genes in the genetic etiology. One genome-wide significant locus was identified in three GWA studies. A shared genetic risk seems likely between AN and many psychiatric and medical phenotypes (Baker et al. 2017).

7.4.7 Deafness

Hearing loss involves hundreds of associated genes that may be autosomal recessive, X-linked, and autosomal dominant or involves mitochondrial patterns of inheritance (Abou Tayoun et al. 2016). Hearing loss genetics is complex, and therefore multiple tests may be needed to determine the reason for hearing loss. Most nonsyndromic hearing loss involves two genes: (1) gap junction protein β-2 (GJB2) and stereocilin (STRC) gene. GJB2 causes severe to profound autosomal hearing loss, and STRC is the most common cause of mild to moderate hearing loss (Sloan-Heggen et al. 2016). Nonsyndromic hearing loss accounts for 70% of congenital hereditary deafness. The other 30% are syndromic hearing loss. Examples of syndromic hearing loss include Usher syndrome and Jervell Lange Nielsen syndrome. Usher syndrome causes blindness and hearing loss and vestibular dysfunction. Jervell Lange Nielsen syndrome causes long QT syndrome and hearing loss.

Molecular genetic testing should be done to evaluate the patient for hereditary syndromic hearing loss. Sanger sequencing was the standard DNA sequencing done before the advent of next-generation sequencing in 2005.

It is important to remember that parents with hearing loss may not have had a genetic workup for syndromic and nonsyndromic hearing loss. In addition to family history, temporal bone MRI to evaluate for an enlarged vestibular aqueduct, urinalysis, thyroid function studies, and ECG were usually done as part of the evaluation. Today, a complete history, physical examination, and audiogram are done initially, but genetic testing is likely to be done (Shearer and Smith 2012).

However, to capture all possible genetic causes of hearing loss, a comprehensive testing strategy is needed that includes sequencing (Sanger or next-generation sequencing followed) by an SNP array to detect large CNVs upstream of the gene. The most common mutation of non-syndromic hearing loss is mutations in the STRC gene. Clinicians should remember that older adolescents with congenital deafness likely would not have had newer genetic testing done when they were initially evaluated for their deafness.

7.4.8   Real-Life Example

A mother reported a family history of fragile X syndrome (FXS) in two cousins on the mother's side and a sibling. She was concerned that her three-year-old son had FXS. The clinician ordered a karyotype rather than an FMR1 expansion testing for CGG, the right test. The laboratory technician called the clinician as she knew this was the wrong test. The testing confirmed that the child had >200 repeats, and the clinician confirmed that the child had FXS.

A clinician evaluated a 9-year-old female with ASD, ID, and seizures. The clinician ordered MECP2 testing, which was positive. The family failed to follow up with the clinician, and the family was not called to follow up. The family was known to another clinician who had ordered a CMA and karyotype, which was negative. A two-year delay before the clinician ordered the MECP2 testing called the patient back for a follow-up visit. The results of the tests were reviewed. The lack of diagnosis caused the family significant psychosocial distress.

> **Key Learning about Specific Conditions and Genetic Testing**
> - Genetic testing has improved the diagnosis of neurological diseases, and there are genetic treatments for some neurological diseases such as spinal muscular atrophy, type 1.

- Current evidence suggests that genetic abnormalities account for a major proportion of children with epilepsy. Knowing the genetic variation can promote early treatment. Certain generalized epilepsy syndromes with pathogenic variants in SLC2A1 that encode the GLUT1 transporter will be more responsive to a ketogenic diet.
- Chromosomal microarray (CMA), including single nucleotide polymorphism (SNP) array and array-based comparative genomic hybridization (aCGH), is commonly ordered for children with a developmental delay. NGS may be considered in patients for whom CMA generates no diagnosis.
- Hypertrophic cardiomyopathy (HCM) is a genetically varied cardiac muscle disorder, which can present as sudden cardiac death as the first sign of the disease. The advances in next-generation sequencing have improved the identification of children at risk for the disorder.
- Repeat expansion disorders include fragile X, myotonic dystrophy, and bulbar and spinal muscular atrophy. Repeated primed PCR are efficient in the identification of expanded repeats, and therefore, specific testing can be done for these disorders.
- The genetics of psychiatric disorders have improved our understanding of these diseases. Most psychiatric diseases are a combination of a variety of genetic and environmental factors.
- The evaluation for the child with congenital deafness should include genetic testing. NGS followed by an SNP array to detect large CNVs upstream of the gene can help understand the genetic contribution in congenital deafness.

Questions

1. You see a 19-year-old for the first time. The child has an intellectual impairment and has autistic-like qualities. The 37-year-old mother reports that she recently married a 33-year-old male and wants to have a second child. She is worried that the child may be at risk of having similar problems. What is the best next step?
   (a) Take a three-generation family history, probing for developmental problems.
   (b) Order a chromosome microarray.
   (c) Order a single gene test.
   (d) Order a whole-exome sequencing test.

2. You suspect a newborn has Down syndrome. What is the best genetic test to order?
   (a) Order a karyotype.
   (b) Order a chromosome microarray.
   (c) Order a single gene test.
   (d) Order a whole-exome sequencing test.

3. You are practicing in rural Alaska. Which of the following is the best genetic test to evaluate a 3-year-old female for Angelman syndrome?
   (a) Whole genomic sequencing.
   (b) Chromosomal microarray.
   (c) Single gene testing.
   (d) Karyotype.

4. A two-year-old has physical symptoms of Wolf-Hirschhorn syndrome. What would be the best test to order to evaluate this child?
   (a) FISH study.
   (b) Chromosomal microarray.
   (c) Single gene testing.
   (d) Karyotype.

5. A 5-year-old is seen for the first time in the office. During the history, the mother reports that her 20-year-old son died suddenly while playing basketball. Her husband also died at age 39 after mowing the lawn. What is the best approach in evaluating this child?
   (a) Do a review of systems, including any signs of hypertrophic cardiomyopathy.
   (b) Evaluate the child for signs of heart failure.
   (c) Do a complete cardiac examination.
   (d) Refer to genetics for further testing.

6. A 15-month-old male presents with a long face, large ears, macrocephaly, developmental delay, poor social reciprocity, and mild hypermobility. What is the best genetic test to order?
   (a) Whole-genome sequencing.
   (b) Whole-exome sequencing.
   (c) A karyotype.
   (d) FMR expansion testing.

7. A mother brings her 7-year-old to the office for her first well visit. Family history reveals that the father had ADHD as a child but outgrew the disease. She wonders what the risk is that her child will have ADHD. Which of the following is the best response?
   (a) There is a 25% risk of ADHD.
   (b) There is a 40% risk of ADHD.
   (c) There is a 50% risk of ADHD.
   (d) There is a 70–80% risk of ADHD.

8. What is the most likely genetic test that a child with a neurodevelopmental delay would have had in the past ten years?
   (a) Chromosomal microarray.
   (b) Whole-exome sequencing.
   (c) Whole-genome sequencing.
   (d) Karyotype.

9. Which of the following is true about the genetics of depression and anxiety?
   (a) There are clear genes involved in depression and anxiety.
   (b) The genes involved in depression and anxiety are similar to Tourette's syndrome.
   (c) Both depression and anxiety are complex polygenic disorders.
   (d) There is a similar gene locus to ADHD, depression, and anxiety.

10. A child has congenital sensorineural deafness in the range of 80–100 dB across all frequencies. After a history and physical, what is the next step in evaluating this child?
    (a) Urinalysis and ECG.
    (b) MRI of the temporal bone and urinalysis.
    (c) Whole-genome sequencing (WGS).
    (d) Karyotype.

Rationale

1. Answer: a

   The next step is to take a family history. A complete family history is always the first step in evaluating a patient and should be done before testing is ordered.

2. Answer: a

   A karyotype is the first-line test when patients are suspected of having an aneuploidy such as trisomy or sex chromosome aneuploidy.

3. Answer: c

   Angelman syndrome is an imprinting disorder and involves a single gene on chromosome 15. Single gene testing would be the most cost-effective test to order.

4. Answer: a

   The FISH probe uses targeted probes to identify microdeletions and microduplications (Stoler 2017). It allows for deletions and duplications to be identified. It is useful to confirm the clinical diagnosis of known disorders such as Wolf-Hirschhorn syndrome.

5. Answer: d

   This child is likely asymptomatic, and genetic testing would be the best way to evaluate this child for hypertrophic cardiomyopathy.

6. Answer: d

   In this patient, you should consider fragile X syndrome. As a result, testing for repeat primed PCR for FMR looking for repeats of CCG would be the best available test. A karyotype would be better for aneuploidy or sex chromosome aneuploidy. Next-generation sequencing is not the best test for repeat expansion diseases.

7. Answer: d

   The risk of ADHD is approximately 70–80% in offspring of a parent with ADHD.

8. Answer: a

   Children with a neurodevelopmental delay are more likely to have had a chromosomal microarray done as part of their initial workup for the neurodevelopmental delay.

9. Answer: c

   Both depression and anxiety are complex polygenic psychiatric diseases without clear genetic loci.

10. Answer: c

    After a history and physical, the best test to order is a next-generation sequencing test such as whole-genome sequencing with the advent of next-generation sequencing.

References

Abou Tayoun AN, Al Turki SH, Oza AM, Bowser MJ, Hernandez AL, Funke BH, et al. Improving hearing loss gene testing: a systematic review of gene evidence toward more efficient next-generation sequencing-based diagnostic testing and interpretation. Genet Med. 2016;18(6):545–53.

Antshel KM, Russo N. Autism spectrum disorders and ADHD: overlapping phenomenology, diagnostic issues, and treatment considerations. Curr Psychiatry Rep. 2019;21(5):34.

Baker, Schaumburg, Munn-Chernoff. Genetics of anorexia nervosa. Curr Psychiatry Rep. 2017;19:84.

Butler MG. Imprinting disorders: a mini-review. Assist Reprod Genet. 2009;26:477–86.

Butler MG. Imprinting disorders in humans: a review. Curr Opin Pediatr. 2020;32(6):719–29.

Char DS. Whole-genome sequencing in critically ill infants and emerging ethical challenges. Semin Perinatol. 2015;39(8):573–5.

Chen E, Saul RA. Building an accurate family history, constructing a pedigree: an overview for primary care. Time out genetics webinar series presented by the genetics in primary care institute. April 26, 2012.

Corfield J. Base pairs. Retrieved from https://www.britannica.com/science/base-pair on July 31, 2021.

Correa H. Li-Fraumeni syndrome. J Pediatr Genet. 2016;5(2):84–8.

Dinarvand P, Davaro EP, Doan JV, Ising ME, Evans NR, Phillips NJ, et al. Familial adenomatous polyposis syndrome: An update and review of extraintestinal manifestations. Arch Pathol Lab Med. 2019;143(11):1382–98.

Farmer MB, Bonadies DC, Mahon SM, Baker MJ, Ghate SM, Munro C, et al. Adverse events in genetic testing: the fourth case series. Cancer J. 2019;25(4):231–6.

Fogel BL, Lee H, Strom SP, Deignan JL, Nelson SF. Clinical exome sequencing in neurogenetic and neuropsychiatric disorders. Ann N Y Acad Sci. 2016;1366(1):49–60.

Foley C, Corvin A, Nakagome S. Genetics of schizophrenia: ready to translate? Curr Psychiatry Rep. 2017;19(9):61.

García-Giménez JL, Seco-Cervera M, Tollefsbol TO, Romá-Mateo C, Peiró-Chova L, Lapunzina P, Pallardó FV. Epigenetic biomarkers: current strategies and future challenges for their use in the clinical laboratory. Crit Rev Clin Lab Sci. 2017;54(7–8):529–50.

Gonorazky HD, Naumenko S, Ramani AK, Nelakuditi V, Mashouri P, Wang P, et al. Expanding the boundaries of RNA sequencing as a diagnostic tool for rare Mendelian disease. Am J Hum Genet. 2019;104(3):466–83.

Govindarajan R, Duraiyan J, Palanisamy M. Microarray and its application. J Pharm Bioallied Sci. 2012;4(2):S310–2.

Grimm O, Krantz TM, Reif A. Genetics of ADHD: what should the clinician know? Curr Psychiatry Rep. 2020;22:18.

Hebbar M, Mefford HC. Recent advances in epilepsy genomics and genetic testing. F1000Res. 2020;9.:F1000 Faculty Rev:185.

Herman I, Lopez MA, Marafi D, Pehlivan D, Calame DG, Abid F, Lotze TE. Clinical exome sequencing in the diagnosis of pediatric neuromuscular disease. Muscle Nerve. 2021;63(3):304–10.

Institute for Healthcare Improvement. Retrieved from http://www.ihi.org/resources/Pages/Tools/Ask-Me-3-Good-Questions-for-Your-Good-Health.aspx on July 1, 2021.

Jin MW, Xu SM, An Q, Wang P. A review of risk factors for childhood leukemia. Eur Rev Med Pharmacol Sci. 2016;20(18):3760–4.

Khan Academy. Microarray. Retrieved from https://www.khanacademy.org/test-prep/mcat/biomolecules/dna-technology/v/hybridization-microarray, 2021.

Kim AY, Bodurtha JN. Dysmorphology. Pediatr Rev. 2019;40(12):609–18.

Lalonde E, Rentas S, Lin F, Dulik MC, Skraban CM, Spinner NB. Genomic diagnosis for pediatric disorders: revolution and evolution. Front Pediatr. 2020;8:373.

Latchford A, Cohen S, Auth M, Scaillon M, Viala J, Daniels R, et al. Management of Peutz-Jeghers Syndrome in children and adolescents: a position paper from the ESPGHAN Polyposis Working Group. J Pediatr Gastroenterol Nutr. 2019;68(3):442–52.

Lee BH, Smith T, Paciorkowski AR. Autism spectrum disorder and epilepsy: disorders with a shared biology. Epilepsy Behav. 2015;47:191–201.

Levy B, Wapner R. Prenatal diagnosis by chromosomal microarray analysis. Fertil Steril. 2018;109(2):201–12.

Lionel AC, Costain G, Monfared N, Walker S, Reuter MS, Hosseini SM, Thiruvahindrapuram B, et al. Improved diagnostic yield compared with targeted gene sequencing panels suggests a role for whole-genome sequencing as a first-tier genetic test. Genet Med. 2018;20(4):435–43.

Lowther C, Costain G, Baribeau DA, Bassett AS. Genomic disorders in psychiatry-what does the clinician need to know? Curr Psychiatry Rep. 2017;19(11):82.

Marjonen H, Auvinen P, Kahila H, Tšuiko O, Kõks S, Tiirats A, et al. rs10732516 polymorphism at the *IGF2/H19* locus associates with genotype-specific effects on placental DNA methylation and birth weight of newborns conceived by assisted reproductive technology. Clin Epigenetics. 2018;10:80.

Meier SM, Deckert J. Genetics of anxiety disorder. Curr Psychiatry Rep. 2019;21:16.

Merkel EA, Mohan LS, Shi K, Panah E, Zhang B, Gerami P. Paediatric melanoma: clinical update, genetic basis, and advances in diagnosis. Lancet Child Adolesc Health. 2019;3(9):646–54.

Mone F, Quinlan-Jones E, Kilby MD. Clinical utility of exome sequencing in the prenatal diagnosis of congenital anomalies: a review. Eur J Obstet Gynecol Reprod Biol. 2018;231:19–24.

Mullin N, Lewis CM. Genetics of depression: Progress at last. Curr Psychiatry Rep. 2017;19:43.

Myers KA, Johnstone DL, Dyment DA. Epilepsy genetics: current knowledge, applications, and future directions. Clin Genet. 2019;95(1):95–111.

Pauly R, Schwartz CE. The future of clinical diagnosis: moving functional genomics approaches to the bedside. Clin Lab Med. 2020;40(2):221–30.

Payne K, Gavan SP, Wright SJ, Thompson AJ. Cost-effectiveness analyses of genetic and genomic diagnostic tests. Nat Rev Genet. 2018;19(4):235–46.

Petersen BS, Fredrich B, Hoeppner MP, Ellinghaus D, Franke A. Opportunities and challenges of whole-genome and -exome sequencing. BMC Genet. 2017;18(1):14.

Petrikin JE, Willig LK, Smith LD, Kingsmore SF. Rapid whole-genome sequencing and precision neonatology. Semin Perinatol. 2015;39(8):623–31.

Pilarski R. *PTEN* hamartoma tumor syndrome: a clinical overview. Cancers (Basel). 2019;11(6):844.

Qi Y, Zheng Y, Li Z, Liu Z, Xiong L. Genetic studies of tic disorders and Tourette syndrome. Methods Mol Biol. 2019;2011:547–71.

Ravi B, Antonellis A, Sumner CJ, Lieberman A. Genetic approaches to the treatment of neuromuscular diseases-evaluation of current practice and literature review. Neuromuscul Disord. 2019;29(1):14–20.

Roades WA, Steuber CP. Clinical assessment and differential diagnosis of the child with suspected cancer. In: Blaney SN, Helman LL, Adamson PC, editors. Pizzo and Poplack's principles and practice of Pediatric oncology. 8th ed. Philadelphia: Lippincott; 2020. p. 106–13.

Sanders SJ, Campbell AJ, Cottrell JR, Moller RS, Wagner FF, Auldridge AL, et al. Progress in understanding and treating SCN2A-mediated disorders. Trends Neurosci. 2018;41(7):442–56.

Shearer AE, Smith RJ. Genetics: advances in genetic testing for deafness. Curr Opin Pediatr. 2012;24(6):679–86.

Sloan-Heggen CM, Bierer AO, Shearer AE, Kolbe DL, Nishimura CJ, Frees KL, et al. Comprehensive genetic testing in the clinical evaluation of 1119 patients with hearing loss. Hum Genet. 2016;135(4):441–50.

Smith HS, Swint JM, Lalani SR, Yamal JM, de Oliveira Otto MC, et al. Clinical application of genome and exome sequencing as a diagnostic tool for Pediatric patients: a scoping review of the literature. Genet Med. 2019;21(1):3–16.

Soura E, Eliades PJ, Shannon K, Stratigos AJ, Tsao H. Hereditary melanoma: update on syndromes and management: genetics of familial atypical multiple mole melanoma syndromes. J Am Acad Dermatol. 2016;74(3):395–407.

Stoler JM. Prenatal and postnatal genetic testing: why, how, and when? Pediatr Ann. 2017;46(11):e423–7.

Teekakirikul P, Zhu W, Huang HC, Fung E. Hypertrophic cardiomyopathy: An overview of genetics and management. Biomol Ther. 2019;9(12):878.

The Jackson Laboratory. Retrieved from www.jax.org/ccep, on July 1, 2021.

Yohe S, Thyagarajan B. Review of clinical next-generation sequencing. Arch Pathol Lab Med. 2017;141(11):1544–57.

Zoghbi HY, Beaudel AL. Epigenetics and human disease, 2018. Cold Spring Harb Perspect Biol. 2016;8(2):a019497.

Hematology

8

Rita Marie John and Caroline Anne Bell

Learning Objectives

After completing the chapter, the learner should be able to:

1. Describe common uses of complete blood count (CBC), and develop an organized approach to interpreting every CBC.
2. Discuss red blood cells (RBCs) disorders, white blood cells (WBCs), and platelets.
3. Interpret the common morphology of the blood's cellular components.
4. Describe key history points in a child with a hematological disorder.
5. Describe the pathophysiology and appropriate workup of a child with possible hemolytic anemia.
6. Develop a method to further work up a child with a microcytic versus macrocytic anemia.
7. List the initial workup for a child with possible immunodeficiency.

8. Discuss the features of bleeding disorders due to factor deficiency versus platelet disorder.
9. Discuss the clinical features that might be present in a patient with a bleeding disorder.
10. Discuss the initial workup of a child with a suspected bleeding disorder in primary care.

8.1 Introduction

Hematological problems in pediatrics are common. The clinician orders hematological tests based on the patient's history, the family history, and the physical exam. The child with pallor or bleeding may require testing to evaluate renal, gastrointestinal, infectious, or rheumatological diseases. The chapter focuses on hematological tests and their interpretation.

8.2 The CBC

The CBC with differential is one of the commonly requested tests in clinical practice (Buoro et al. 2017). A CBC is drawn in a purple top tube that contains ethylenediaminetetraacetic acid (EDTA) to prevent coagulation of the blood. It examines the WBC, RBC, and platelets using a

R. M. John
School of Nursing, Columbia University,
New York, NY, USA

C. A. Bell (✉)
Division of Pediatric Hematology, Oncology and Cellular Therapy, Children's Hospital at Montefiore, Bronx, NY, USA
e-mail: ccanty@montefiore.org

© The Author(s), under exclusive license to Springer Nature Switzerland AG 2022
R. M. John (ed.), *Pediatric Diagnostic Labs for Primary Care: An Evidence-based Approach*,
https://doi.org/10.1007/978-3-030-90642-9_8

modern hematology analyzer, enabling the clinician to receive high-resolution measurements of the blood's cellular components (Higgins 2015). The CBC's cellular components are primarily the result of activity in the bone marrow, and the normal RBC span is from 100 to 120 days (Higgins 2015).

The WBC or leukocyte components include information about WBC's different types and percentages, including the neutrophils, lymphocytes, monocytes, eosinophils, and basophils. The basic technology used includes electric impedance and light scatter. The automated analyzer directly measures the RBC or erythrocyte count, hemoglobin, MCV, leukocyte, and platelet count (Walters, Abelson, 2002; Cascio and De Loughery 2017). The MCH and the MCHC are calculated using the formulas seen in Table 8.1.

Both RBC and WBC are measured as they pass through large apertures and use flow cytometry to measure the forward and side light as they pass through the aperture. Measures critical to the RBC picture include the RBC count, the hemoglobin (HB), the hematocrit (Hct), the mean corpuscle volume (MCV), the mean corpuscle HB (MCH), the mean corpuscular HB concentration (MCHC), and the red cell distribution width (RDW). The CHr/Ret-He is a new index that the newer automated analyzers are now reporting. The reticulocyte MCV and the reticulocyte MCHC are needed to derive the MCH (CHr/Ret-He). CHr/Ret-He's value will fall at the onset

of iron deficiency and will be the first index to increase after therapeutic iron is started.

An automated reticulocyte count (RC) measures the rate of RBC production (Higgins 2015). It can help the clinician determine whether the anemia is due to production deficits, another destructive process, or hemolysis. An RC is generally a separate test and is not included in a CBC. It must be adjusted for anemia.

The platelet count includes the mean platelet volume (MPV) and is one component of the patient's coagulation profile. They are counted as they pass through the smallest aperture of the automated hematology analyzer.

8.2.1 CBC Specimen Evaluation Pitfalls

Timing of the Specimen: Delayed sample analysis is not uncommon in modern practice due to weekend closure and distance from where the sample is drawn to the lab. Also, poor storage conditions could lead to unreliable and inaccurate results, leading to poor clinical decisions (Briggs et al. 2014; Lippi and Simundic 2012). A recent systematic review and meta-analysis pointed out that most lab errors occur in the pre-analytical phase, with reliable specimen storage being key to high-quality results. When blood storage is prolonged, time and temperature changes can occur with acceptable stability after 24 h for RBC parameters, WBC count, and platelet count. Some measurements, including WBC differential, can be stable for up to 72 h if the collection is stored at 4C refrigerated (Ashenden et al. 2013; Robinson et al. 2011). The WBC differential may not be stable over time (Hill et al. 2009). The MPV does change over time, making it more inaccurate than the actual count (Wu and Fen Wang 2017). Values are less stable when the specimen is stored for longer than 24 h without refrigeration. Refrigeration at 4° centigrade (C) is a better choice for specimen accuracy (Wu and Fen Wang 2017).

Failure to use appropriate pediatric normal as well as technical artifact is a laboratory pitfall.

Table 8.1 Formula for calculating the MCH and MCHC

Measure	Formula calculation
Hemoglobin content	
MCH	MCH = Hb(g/L)/RBC ($10^{6\wedge}$/μL) Tends to go in the same direction as the MCV
MCHC	HB (g/dL)/Hct (%) Increased in spherocytosis
CHr/Ret-He	Decreased in iron deficiency Reduced in thalassemia and hemoglobinopathies must be excluded if the clinician uses CHr/Ret-He to assess iron status

Adapted from Walter and Abelson (1996): Cascio and De Loughery 2017 with Laboratory pitfalls include failure to use age adjusted pediatric values as well as technical artifact.

RBC agglutination or cold agglutinins may increase the MCV, leading to inaccurate hematocrit and elevated MCV (Walter and Abelson 1996). Hyperleukocytosis can elevate the Hb, Hct, RBC, and MCV. Hyperosmolar plasma can cause the Hct and the MCV to be falsely elevated. The rule of threes can help the clinician determine if the artifact is the cause of the problem since the HB is three times the RBC and the Hct is three times the HB values (Walter and Abelson 1996).

It is also common for transient viral illnesses to cause mild normocytic anemia and WBC alterations such as leukopenia, neutropenia, or leukocytosis. Measles vaccination can cause a mild decline in hemoglobin, returning to normal by days 21–30 (Olivares et al. 1989).

8.2.2 Statistical Problems

As stated in Chap. 1, a normal reference range for the results is two standard deviations from the mean, meaning the normal range reported is from the third to the 97th percentile. One in 20 tests can be below or above two standard deviations from the mean. When those results are reported, they are prominently highlighted, leading parents and clinicians to worry.

The clinician must carefully evaluate the history and physical in the face of relatively mild anemia associated with leukocytosis, neutropenia, thrombocytosis, or thrombocytopenia. The measurement may indicate something more serious.

8.2.3 Clinical Indications for a CBC

According to the AAP periodicity table, there are no specific indications for a CBC (American Academy of Pediatrics [AAP] 2019). A CBC is ordered when a child has symptoms or signs of anemia, unexplained pallor, is suspected of having an oncological problem, a genetic disease

affecting the elements of a CBC, having recurrent infections, or prolonged and unexplained fever. A yearly routine CBC is not indicated in a well-child exam without physical exam findings.

8.2.4 Real-Life Example

A child is seen for a 1-year-old visit. The mother reports that the child had 3 days of mild vomiting and diarrhea, which ended 4 days ago. The history is unremarkable, and the child is getting a daily vitamin with iron as she is a picky eater. The child looks slightly pale, but the rest of the exam is normal. You order a finger stick lead and Hct. The Hct is 10.1. You decide to order a CBC. You emphasize that viruses can cause transient anemia and ask that the mother to for wait 10 days. The worried mother decides to go immediately to the lab for the CBC. The results come back with normocytic anemia with a Hct of 9.8 and an MCV of 83 and elevated monocytes. Mild anemia is not uncommon in a child recovering from a viral illness. However, the mother reviews the CBC and sees the bolded area in the Hct and monocytes. She calls and wanting to know what your plan is regarding the anemia. Due to the mother's failure to wait until her child recovered from the viral infection, a repeat CBC was done after 10 days. As expected, the child's CBC returned to normal.

8.3 Red Blood Cells

The components of the RBC determine if anemia or polycythemia is present. The RBC is a biconcave disc of lipid material with a protein "skeleton." Hemoglobin makes up 99% of the protein content, and the cell has a diameter of 7.5 μm (Diez-Silva, et al. 2010). RBCs are used for oxygen exchange, so they must have an easily transformed shape and adequate hemoglobin (Haley 2017). The RBC does not have nuclei, ribosomes, or mitochondria (Grace and Glader 2018). The bone marrow is constantly producing the RBC, and as new RBCs are produced, old RBCs are cleared, and their components recycled.

The characteristics of the RBC change during the lifespan with a decrease in volume of 20% and a 15% decrease in hemoglobin over the lifecycle. The RBC's initial changes occur faster, and later changes in the RBC occur slower (Franco et al. 2013; Willekens et al. 2003). To prevent oxidative damage and maintain RBC shape, the RBC relies on anaerobic metabolism. When an acquired problem with hemoglobin synthesis occurs, problems with the protein that forms the RBC membrane or a deficiency of enzymes responsible for the membrane will have a shortened lifespan, and erythrocytosis

will occur. The RBC mass is mostly the result of the HB mass, and the HB concentration determines the density. After the first week, the RBC density and HB concentration tend not to change (Franco et al. 2013; Willekens et al. 2003). After the RBC dies, the HB is transported to the liver and spleen for recycling.

With acute anemia, the patient will experience shortness of breath, a higher heart rate, or pallor. If the anemia is due to hemolysis of the RBC, jaundice will likely occur. Severe acute anemia can lead to heart failure, particularly in younger children, as their ability to increase stroke volume

Table 8.2 RBC indices

RBC indices	What it means
RBC count	
Hemoglobin (HB)	• Assesses the oxygen-carrying capacity of the RBC • Unit: gm/dl • Directly measured by the modern hematology analyzer • Can be affected by age, gender, race, and degree of sexual maturation altitude • Nadir of hemoglobin occurs at 12 weeks for a full-term infant and 6 to 8 weeks for a preterm infant • The lower limit of normal is 11 + 0.1 X (age in years)
Hematocrit (Hct)	• Unit of a percentage of whole blood by centrifugation of the RBC • Estimated by the electronic cell counter • Are three times the HB
Mean corpuscular volume (MCV)	• The lower limit of normal is 70 + 1 X (age in years). Use this formula to age 10 and after age 1 • Directly measured (Hermiston and Mentzer 2002; Cascio and De Loughery 2017) • A spurious increase in the MCV can occur in the presence of cold agglutinins due to RBC clumping measures as RBC size by an automated hematology analyzer. Rewarming the specimen can result in the correct MCV (Kujovich 2016)
Mean corpuscular hemoglobin (MCH)	• The measure of the size or volume of the average red blood cell • Measured indirectly
Mean corpuscle hemoglobin concentration (MCHC)	• Measures the amount of hemoglobin in the average red cell to its size • Increased in spherocytosis • Measured indirectly
Red cell distribution width (RDW)	• Variability of the RBC size with the difference in RBC cell volume (anisocytosis) is reflected in RDW • A small RDW means there is little variation in the size, but you do not know whether they are small or large • A large RDW means mixed RBC and reticulocytes • An increase in RDW can precede an abnormality of hemoglobin • Abnormal production of erythropoietin or decreased responsiveness to erythropoietin due to chronic inflammation • A significant relationship between RDW increase in iron deficiency, vitamin B_{12}, and folate deficiency as well as proinflammatory cytokines (Litao and Kamat 2018)
CHr/ret-he	• Falls with the onset of iron deficiency and will be the first to rise once iron is initiated • It may be reduced in thalassemia (Cascio and De Loughery 2017)

Adapted from Cascio and De Loughery (2017), Hermiston and Mentzer (2002); Kujovich (2016), Litao and Kamat (2018), Walter and Abelson (1996)

is limited. The patient with chronic anemia will be less symptomatic and may tolerate mild anemia without any complaints.

The clinician needs to be aware of each of the RBC components to evaluate the child's anemia. Table 8.2 describes the components of the RBC in more detail.

8.3.1 Red Blood Cell Smear

Certain types of RBC can offer an insight into the child's diagnosis. A pathologist or technologist's formal blood smear review can help evaluate all three cell lines found in the blood. There is also the availability of digital technology that can capture images of a smear. The smear can confirm red cell size as a normocytic RBC when it is the same size as the lymphocyte nucleus, whereas a macrocytic RBC is larger than the lymphocyte nucleus. It is important to evaluate color (hypochromic or normochromic) and variations in size and shape. Hypochromia presents with central pallor in the RBC nucleus as the hemoglobin goes below 10 g/dl. Anisocytosis is a variation in the RBC size, whereas poikilocytosis presents a variation in RBC shape (Cascio and De Loughery 2017). The smear can also provide the arrangement or rouleaux formation and whether there are inclusions such as nucleated RBC, Howell-Jolly bodies, or

Table 8.3 Different RBC findings

Type of RBC	Reason for abnormality	Clinical significance
Acanthocytes (or spur cells)	Spiked RBC cell membranes with irregularly distributed projections that are thorn-like due to an increase in cholesterol in the RBC membrane (Cascio and De Loughery 2017)	Acanthocytes are commonly found in blood smears Abetalipoproteinemia Liver disease McLeod syndrome Pyruvate kinase deficiency
Anisopoikilocytosis	A variation in size and shape of an RBC	Iron deficiency
Bite cells (degmacytes)	A by-product of degradation of Heinz body Due to stress, hemoglobin denaturation, and removal of denatured hemoglobin by macrophages in the spleen removal	Glucose-6-phosphate dehydrogenase deficiency Drug-induced oxidant hemolysis
Coarse basophilic stippling	Ribosomal remnants (Cascio and De Loughery 2017)	Lead poisoning Marrow stress Thalassemia
Dacrocyte (teardrop cells)	A tail-like projection caused by RBC cytoplasmic projection	Marrow myelophthisis (found in metastatic carcinoma) Marrow fibrosis Extramedullary hematopoiesis Severe iron deficiency
Drepanocytes (sickle cells)	Bipolar red cells with points at each end of the RBC	Sickle cell disease (SCD)
Echinocytes (burr cells)	Artifact due to prolonged storage before smear is done	Reported more often in blood smears Found pathologically in end-stage renal disease Obstructive liver disease Hyperlipidemia
Elliptocytes	The hemoglobin is at either end of the RBC, and the RBC has the central pallor The ends of the RBC are elongated	Hereditary elliptocytosis Iron deficiency may be more pencil shaped
Heinz bodies	Denatured hemoglobin in round inclusions within the RBC. To be seen, supravital stains must be used	Hemolysis Hyposplenism-spleen does not function, and Heinz bodies are not removed Alpha (α) thalassemia

(continued)

Table 8.3 (continued)

Type of RBC	Reason for abnormality	Clinical significance
Howell-jolly bodies	Single small, dense basophilic inclusions at the periphery of the RBC that are RNA remnants (Cascio and De Loughery 2017)	Indicates hyposplenism state either from functional or anatomic removal of the spleen
Nucleated red blood cell (NRBC)	RBC with a nucleus In the marrow, the nucleus is only present for a short period, and the nucleus is eliminated before release into the bloodstream	Not normal in the peripheral smear Severe hemolysis Hemoglobinopathy Myelophthisic process Severe physiologic stress
Ovalocytes	Oval-shaped RBC with a lack of central pallor	Reported more frequently in blood smears
Polychromatophilic cells	Macrocytic with blue-gray color due to the presence of residual polyribosomes	Marrow stress or hemolysis Raised RC Beta (β) thalassemia/hemoglobin E disease
Rouleaux	Stack of greater than three RBCs	
Schistocytes (helmet cells)	RBC fragment, irregular shape, jagged with pointed ends	Intravascular coagulation hemolytic anemia Thrombotic thrombocytopenia purpura Hypertension Preeclampsia Mechanical heart valves Ventricular assist device Toxin- or stress-related hemolysis
Spherocytes	Mutation in proteins that maintain the vertical interaction between the spectrin-based cytoskeleton and the lipid layer	Hereditary spherocytosis (HS) Immune hemolytic anemia Microangiopathy hemolytic anemia
Stomatocyte	Linear areas of pallor rather than a circular central zone of pallor	Obstructive liver disease Hereditary stomatocytosis Rh null syndrome Ovalocytosis in Asian patients
Target cells	Bull's-eye appearance due to the congregation of Hb in the center of the cell Target cells in liver disease are due to lipid metabolism alterations In thalassemia, there is a lack of hemoglobin production	Excess red cell membrane to the amount of hemoglobin Thalassemia Hemoglobin C and E disease Obstructive liver disease

Adapted from Cascio and De Loughery (2017)

malaria. Rounded aggregates of RBC due to the presence of an antibody are called autoagglutination and are usually from IgM autoantibodies, also called cold agglutinins. If the clinical findings are not clear cut or nonspecific, a pathologist review of the smear can help determine the diagnosis (Chabot-Richards and Foucar 2017). Table 8.3 reviews the types of RBC morphology that could be reported with the CBC.

8.3.2 Red Cell Precursors

8.3.2.1 Reticulocytes

The reticulocyte is a precursor of the RBC produced in the bone marrow and is released at a steady state into the bone marrow in a healthy child. The RBC has six stages to maturity—pronormoblast, basophilic normoblast, polychromatophilic normoblast, orthochromic normoblast, reticulocyte, and finally mature RBC. If the reticulocyte in the bone marrow is shifted to the circulation earlier than the usual 2–3 days for maturity, it is called a shift or stress reticulocyte. The stress or shift reticulocyte has more filamentous reticulum than the mature

Table 8.4 Formulas for the reticulocyte production index, reticulocyte index, and absolute reticulocyte count

Reticulocyte production index	Formula 1 RPI = RC × hemoglobin/normal hemoglobin × 0.5
	Formula 2 RPI = (Hct/45) * retic/maturation Maturation = 1.0 for Hct ≥ 40% Maturation = 1.5 for Hct 30–39.9% Maturation = 2.0 for Hct 20–29.9% Maturation = 2.5 for Hct < 20% Maturation = 1.0 for Hct ≥ 40% Maturation = 1.5 for Hct 30–39.9% Maturation = 2.0 for Hct 20–29.9% Maturation = 2.5 for Hct < 20% An RPI >3 indicates a normal marrow response to anemia. An RPI <2 indicates an inadequate response to anemia. With a normal Hb and Hct, an RPI of 1 is normal From: https://www.merckmanuals.com/medical-calculators/ReticProdIndex.htm
Reticulocyte index (RI) or corrected reticulocyte count (CRC)	RI or CRC = RC × hematocrit/normal hematocrit RI ≥2 indicates an adequate response RI < 2% with anemia shows a decrease in the production of reticulocytes (i.e., an inadequate response to correct the anemia)
Absolute reticulocyte count (ARC)	Is the actual number of reticulocytes in 1 l of blood ARC = RC in percentage/RBC count * 100 The normal ARC is 50–100 × 10^9/L In aplastic anemia, ARC of <25 × 10^9/L With nutritional disease, the ARC 25–50 × 10^9/L In infiltrative disorders, infections, anemia, or hemolysis, the ARC is >100 × 10^9/L (Priya and Subhashree 2014)

Adapted from Priya and Subhashree (2014)

reticulocyte, which has more granular dots. The automated RC measures RBCs' production, and flow cytometry is the most accurate way of measuring it (Higgins 2015).

The RC is not a routine part of a CBC and must be ordered separately. An RC is higher in newborns when it ranges from 2% to 6%, dropping after 1–2 weeks. The size of the reticulocyte is about twice as large as a mature RBC. When the RC is high, the MCV goes up. For each 1% increase in reticulocytes, there is 1 fl increase in the MCV (Green and Dwyre 2015). The RC helps distinguish between different kinds of anemia, such as RBC destruction versus lack of RBC production. When someone develops mild anemia, there is a compensatory increase in the RC to make more RBC. If someone has severe anemia, there would be a greater increase in the RC. However, to determine whether the reticulocyte production magnitude is sufficient, the RC must be corrected to the degree of anemia (Higgins 2015). If the RC is elevated, it would likely indicate blood loss or hemolysis. If the RC is decreased to <0.1%, it indicates red cell aplasia or aplastic anemia (Cascio and De Loughery 2017).

However, in anemia, the reticulocyte production index (RPI) or corrected RC should be calculated. The RPI is the rate of effective erythropoiesis in pediatric patients with anemia (Ishii and Young 2015). During times of stress, the bone marrow's reticulocyte time is shortened from 3 days to 1 day. Table 8.4 shows formulas to determine if the results are normal.

8.3.2.2 Pitfalls of the RC

The automated RC is imprecise. Repeating measurements on the same blood sample can show a variation of more than 10%, and repeat measures in the same healthy person can vary by as much as 30%. Flow cytometry with fluorescent staining increases the accuracy of the RC. However, even given this variation, the RC's measure helps evaluate anemia (Higgins 2015). The blood and stain must be well mixed before the sample is analyzed

Table 8.5 The common causes of reticulocytosis and reticulocytopenia

Reticulocyte result	Possible causes
Reticulocytopenia	• Disordered RBC maturation due to nutritional deficiencies (iron, B_{12}, folate), hypothyroidism, anemia of chronic illness, rarely sideroblastic anemia • Bone marrow suppression due to chemotherapy, aplastic anemia, or bone marrow failure • Certain viral illnesses such as parvovirus 19, sepsis • Liver disease • Bone marrow infiltrate due to metabolic disorder or oncological process • Blood transfusion (Noronha 2016)
Reticulocytosis	• Post-iron deficiency anemia treatment or rarer in children folate or B_{12} supplementation • Hemoglobinopathy such as SCD or thalassemia major • Acute hemolysis causing anemia • Acute blood loss, most commonly from trauma or GI tract loss • Post-splenectomy

Adapted from Noronha (2016)

due to the reticulocyte's higher specific gravity. The stain must be allowed to sit for 10 min before it is examined. High glucose also can inhibit staining. Certain cells, such as Howell-Jolly bodies, Heinz bodies, and Pappenheimer bodies, can be confused with reticulocytes and leads to a higher RC. Table 8.5 reviews the common causes of reticulocytosis and reticulocytopenia.

8.3.3 Real-Life Example

A child is noted to be pale following a viral illness. You do an office-based Hct, and it is 29.4. You decide to order a CBC with reticulocytes. The indices are normal except for mild normocytic anemia with a Hct of 29.4 and an RC of 10. Using an online calculator from Google Search for the RPI calculator, you note the RPI is 3.3. Based on this result, the bone marrow response is normal. The child had a viral suppression of

bone marrow during the illness and is on the way to recovery.

8.4 White Blood Cells

The WBC includes five common cells—lymphocytes, neutrophils, monocytes, eosinophils, and basophils. The clinician needs to compare the results of the WBC differential with age-adjusted normal. The clinician must ensure all five WBC types are identified in the results and be aware of any premature WBC in the WBC count. The granulocyte count is broken down into neutrophils and bands in some labs. The WBC portion of a CBC can be affected by infections and inflammatory disorders, hematopoietic malignancies, and drugs, including cytotoxic agents. Leukopenia can be a normal variation in African-American males and can also occur in a child with a viral illness.

Reactive changes in the WBC count are usually in the neutrophil and lymphocyte count. Reactive neutrophils generally have prominent azurophilic granules, Dohle bodies, and cytoplasmic vacuoles. Dohle bodies are found in the cells' periphery and make the endoplasmic reticulum rough (Wahed et al. 2020). In lymphocytes, reactive lymphocytes are known as Downey cells. When the WBC is remarkably high, distorted white cells or smudge cells may be seen. Smudge cells can be seen in chronic lymphocytic leukemia (CLL).

Historically, an elevated WBC would be used to evaluate for a serious bacterial infection in children. Current data suggests that the WBC has a sensitivity of 58% and a specificity of less than 73% (Yo et al. 2012). It should be kept in mind that leukocytosis may not occur in 25% of children with an acute bacterial infection. However, a total neutrophil count should be part of the evaluation. In a patient recovering from a viral illness, it is not uncommon to see a transient increase in the monocyte count, eosinophil count, and lymphocytes with a decrease in the granulocyte count. During childhood, the values shift from a predominance of lymphocytes to a slightly greater

Table 8.6 Significant ANC values

ANC is less than 1500 and greater than 1000 (1.0 to 1.5 × 10³)	Mild neutropenia It may be normal in the African-American population
ANC is less than 1000 and greater than 500 (0.5–1.0 × 10³)	Moderate neutropenia
ANC is less than 500 (less than 0.5 × 10³)	Severe neutropenia

Adapted from Schwartz and Fulkerson (2018)

neutrophil count after age 10. The next part of the section will review several types of WBCs.

8.4.1 Neutrophils

The absolute neutrophil count or ANC is an important part of the evaluation of a CBC evaluation. Neutrophils predominate in the newborn CBC but rapidly decreases to a level of 20–30% in infancy. By the age of 5 years, the neutrophil and lymphocyte counts are equal. However, by 8 years of age, the neutrophils are the dominant WBC comprising 70% of the WBC count (Boxer 2003).

The absolute neutrophil count (ANC) is calculated by multiplying the entire WBC count by the total neutrophil count (segmented and band forms). Among children, infectious diseases, particularly viral infections, can cause neutropenia. Viral infections will drop the neutrophil count in the first 24 to 48 following infections and cause persistent neutropenia for 3–8 days. Newborns are at greater risk of depleting their neutrophils' supply, leading to death in sepsis (Boxer 2003). Other factors that cause neutropenia include drugs, autoimmune diseases, and a genetic disease known as Kostmann disease that causes an arrest in bone marrow production.

Clinical signs and symptoms of neutropenia include recurrent infections, mouth ulcers, gingivitis, and growth failure. Table 8.6 shows the significance of the ANC as it falls below 1500. If a child has neutropenia when the CBC is done, it should be repeated in 3–4 weeks (Boxer 2003). When the CBC shows an increase in the number of segmented neutrophils or bands or both, a shift to the left is present. Pseudoneutrophilia results

from trauma, pain, exercise, stress, hypoxia, smoking, and seizures.

8.4.2 Lymphocytes

Lymphocytes are predominant in the first 5 years of life. A lymphocytosis generally follows a viral infection and is called a shift to the left. It is not as common in bacterial infection except for *Bordetella pertussis* infection. Reactive lymphocytes can be seen during infection, known as Downey cells (Wahed et al. 2020). With the Epstein-Barr virus, there is a lymphocytosis with large, atypical lymphocytes, with at least 10% of the lymphocytes being reactive (Wahed et al. 2020).

Atypical lymphocytes vary in shape and size. They have a deep blue cytoplasm, with cytoplasmic borders that are irregular (skirting). The nuclei have an irregular shape, unlike typical lymphocytes that have a smooth border.

Lymphopenia is a count of less than 3000 in children. Immunodeficiencies like severe combined immunodeficiency can present with a marked lymphopenia of <3000 (Wahed et al. 2020).

8.4.3 Eosinophils

Eosinophils are part of the WBC count and the innate immune system. They typically represent less than 5–6% of the circulating WBC (Schwartz and Fulkerson 2018). The eosinophil will leave the circulation and live in specific tissue for several weeks. The GI tract has the largest tissue reserve (Schwartz and Fulkerson 2018). They are toxic to parasitic worms and are elevated in pediatric patients with this infection. In well children, they are found in much smaller quantities. They contain eosinophilic granules and have a bilobate nucleus. When activated by interleukin factor V, IgE, IgM, and complements, they release major basic protein (MBP), damaging normal cells, leading to allergy and autoimmune disease. Table 8.7 presents the three mnemonics for remembering the differential diagnosis of eosinophilia.

Table 8.7 Mnemonics for eosinophilia

N: Neoplasms (Hodgkin's lymphoma, chronic myelocytic leukemia (CML))

A: Allergy/atopy/asthma

A: Addison's disease (adrenal insufficiency)

C: Collagen vascular disease (systemic lupus erythematosus (SLE), Churg-Strauss syndrome)

P: Parasitic infection

A: Addison's disease

L: Lymphoma (Hodgkin's lymphoma and other lymphomas)

L: L-tryptophan deficiency (eosinophilia-myalgia syndrome)

E: Eczema, pemphigus, dermatitis herpetiformis

R: Respiratory (asthma, Hay fever, allergic aspergillosis)

G: Gastroenteritis (eosinophilic gastroenteritis)

I: Infections (parasitic, fungi-like *Coccidioides*, idiopathic)

C: Collagen vascular disease (SLE, Churg-Strauss syndrome)

C: Collagen vascular disease (SLE, Churg-Strauss syndrome)

H: Helminth infections

I: Infections (parasitic, fungi-like *Coccidioides*, idiopathic)

N: Neoplasms (Hodgkin's lymphoma, CML)

A: Allergic diseases

Adapted from Schwartz and Fulkerson (2018), Dewaswala (2020), Barone (2020)

8.4.3.1 Lab Workup for a Patient with Hypereosinophilia

In patients with hypereosinophilia, a diagnostic evaluation should include a CBC with a peripheral smear, comprehensive metabolic panel, urinalysis, serum troponin, vitamin B_{12} level, stool for ova and parasites (O&P), and an ESR/CRP (Schwartz and Fulkerson 2018). Further testing may be needed depending on the results. Children with an extremely high eosinophil count of $\geq 20,000$ should be hospitalized to determine the cause of the hypereosinophilic syndrome. Hypereosinophilic syndrome can lead to end-organ damage to the heart and kidney (Schwartz and Fulkerson 2018). The following example helps illustrate this.

8.4.4 Monocytes

Monocytes are a type of WBC that can convert to macrophages and dendritic cells within the immune system. The count is usually under 5,

Key Learning about WBCs

- Make sure that you confirm that the lab has reported all five types of white cells. Some labs may only report four types when one type is absent.
- Calculating the ANC is part of the interpretation of the CBC.
- Reticulocyte counts are not a part of the CBC and can be helpful in the evaluation of the CBC as well as the response to iron deficiency.

but monocytosis occurs in infections such as tuberculosis brucellosis, malaria, Rocky Mountain spotted fever, and typhus. Monocytosis also occurs in autoimmune diseases as well as oncological processes such as CML, HL, and AML (Wahed et al. 2020).

8.4.5 Basophils

Basophil counts are generally under 5, and they increase due to inflammatory mediators such as histamine. Basophils, like mast cells, have receptors for IgE. Basophilia is uncommon but may occur in viral infections such as varicella, inflammatory conditions such as ulcerative colitis, CML or other myeloproliferative disorders, and hypothyroid patients (Wahed et al. 2020).

8.4.6 Real-Life Example

A 17-year-old male presents for follow-up after treatment with Keflex for a 2.5-cm hard, firm, immobile neck mass. He denies any night sweats or fatigue. There is no history of recent illness, and the child reports that the mass does not hurt him when he palpates it. He denies any exposure to kittens or cats. There is no travel history. The physical exam is normal except for a matted, hard, firm neck mass in the posterior triangle. The result of a recent CBC shows a total WBC of 11,000 with an eosinophil count of 25% and a sedimentation rate of 60.

On follow-up, further testing was done that included the labs above. The CRP was 25, and the ESR was elevated to 90, while the lactate dehydrogenase (LDH) was elevated to 980, and uric acid was also elevated at 5.6. The B_{12} level was significantly decreased. An ultrasound was consistent with possible Hodgkin's lymphoma, and the child was referred to hematology and surgery. A biopsy confirmed HL.

8.5   Platelets

Platelets are small, ranging from 2 to 5 μm in size, and play an important role in angiogenesis, immunity, hemostasis, and inflammation. The precursors of platelets are formed in the bone marrow and are called megakaryocytes. Megakaryopoiesis is supported by a growth factor called thrombopoietin. The megakaryocyte is responsible for making platelets by thousands. The platelet's lifespan is 7 to 10 days, with 2/3 of the platelets in the blood and 1/3 in the spleen. Platelets play an important role in both primary and secondary hemostasis. Platelet cytoskeletal proteins play a role in changing the shape of the platelet. Each platelet contains alpha granules containing von Willebrand factor (VWF), fibrinogen, and factor V, XI, XII, and GPIIb/GPIIIa (Haley 2020). The dense granules in platelets contain magnesium, serotonin, adenosine diphosphate, adenosine triphosphate, and serotonin. These substances play a role in platelet activation when there is a disruption in the vasculature's endothelium. While the normal platelet count across the lifespan is usually 150–450 × 10^3/μL, the platelets needed for hemostasis are less than 150 μL. A lower than average platelet count may not be clinically apparent. Disorders of platelets will be discussed later in the chapter.

8.6   Evaluation of the CBC

Having reviewed the CBC components, the next section will review the importance of a systematic evaluation of the CBC. History is extremely important in evaluating the CBC. A

neonatal history of prolonged jaundice or maternal pregnancy history of anemia or pica should be obtained. A family history of anemia, cancer, bleeding disorders, transfusions, splenectomy, jaundice, or gallstones is important. A history of recent infections, mucocutaneous bleeding, prolonged menstrual bleeding, easy bruisability, petechiae, purpura, liver disease, or endocrinopathy should be explored. Also, when available, prior CBC results should be reviewed. The dietary history should include specifics about milk and fluid intake along with the ingestions of nonfood items. A complete history of pallor, shortness of breath, or complaints of the rapid heart rate should be obtained (Hermiston and Mentzer 2002). Yet, patients who have been gradually become anemic may be asymptomatic as they can tolerate a chronic hemoglobin concentration of 7 g/dl (Cascio and De Loughery 2017).

Evaluation of a CBC's Components: When evaluating the CBC, it is important to be organized and look at all three components reported. Table 8.8 reviews the method that the clinician should look at the CBC. The details within each cell line will be discussed separately and in greater detail in the following sections. It is important to remember that the CBC values need to be age-adjusted (Green and Dwyre 2015). For example, while the MCV

Table 8.8 Stepwise evaluation of the CBC

Evaluation of the CBC	
Evaluate RBC line first	1. First, determine whether there is anemia by looking at the Hct/Hb
	2. Then look at the MCV to determine the type of anemia—Microcytic, normocytic, macrocytic
	3. If the child has microcytic anemia, do Mentzer's index (or alternatives listed below)
	4. If the child has normocytic anemia, look at the MCHC. If it is elevated, think about spherocytosis
Evaluate the WBC line next	1. Look to make sure that all five types of WBCs are listed in the differential
	2. Calculate the ANC
Evaluate the platelet count next	1. Look at the platelet line—Is there thrombocytosis or thrombocytopenia?
	2. Look at the size of the platelet by evaluating the MPV

John (2018)

Table 8.9 Microcytosis: Formulas to discriminate between iron deficiency anemia (IDA) and β-thalassemia trait (β-TT)

Name of indices/formula	Mathematical formula	Likely diagnosis from result		Sensitivity (Sn) and specificity (Sp) (%)		PPV and NPV	
				IDA	β-TT	IDA	β-TT
Red blood cell (RBC) count	Part of CBC	<5 IDA	>5 (β-TT)	Sn 100–85.7 Sp 86.0–74.4	Sn 74–94.8 Sp 100–70.5	PPV 96.6–84.2 NPV 90.5–77.4	PPV 90.5–77.4 NPV 92.3–84.2
RBC distribution width (RDW)	Part of CBC	>14 IDA	<14 β-TT	Sn 99.0–83.9 Sp 6.0–74.73	Sn 6.0–83.1 Sp 99.0–76.4	PPV 51.2–80 NPV 97.29–75	PPV 80–97.29 NPV 51.1–80
Mentzer's index	MCV/RBC	>13	<13	Sn 93–78 Sp 82–69.47	Sn 98.7–69.47 Sp 98.7–78	PPV 98.2 NPV 86.3	PPV 86.3–75 NPV 98.2–51
Shine and Lal index	MCV [2]*MCH/100	>1530	<1530	Sn 100–1.7 Sp 97–100	Sn 100–91 Sp 100–1.7	PPV 100–76.23 NPV 50–100	PPV 100–50 NPV 100–76.23
Srivastava index	MCH/RBC	>3.8	<3.8	Sn 81–69.6 Sp 85.7–61	Sn 85.7–61 Sp 81–69.6	PPV 81.6–68.64 NPV 77.6–75.32	PPV 75.32–77 NPV 81.6–68.64
Green and king index	MCV2 X RDW/100Hb	>65	<65	Sn 99.3–73.2 Sp 76.7–55.78	Sn 83.1–74.4 Sp 96–73.2	PPV 84.9–70.21 NPV 98.14–77.6	PPV 95.4–77.6 NPV 84.9–79.3
Ricerca index (R)	RDW/RBC	<4.4	>4.4	Sn 85.7–4.7 Sp 100–65.5	Sn 100–65.7 Sp 85.7–14.7	PPV 92.2–100 NPV 57–92.63	PPV 57 NPV 100
England and Fraser's index	MCV-RBC-5Hb-3.4	Result is +	Result is -	Sn 100–14 Sp 100–45.26-	Sn 100–66.2 Sp 98.2–14	PPV 87.5–65.36 NPV 100–53.2	PPV 96.3–53.2 NPV 87.5–69

Adapted from AlFadhli et al. (2006), Okan et al. (2009), Vehapoglu et al. (2014), Valiya et al. (2019)

is generally smaller in children than in adults during the first 6 months of life, the MCV is larger (Green and Dwyre 2015). During pregnancy, the MCV is large by about 4 fl (Green and Dwyre 2015).

To evaluate the CBC, the clinician must look at the RBC line and all the components outlined above. As noted, the MCH and MCHC are derived values and are not directly measured by the automated system (Cascio and De Loughery 2017). Table 8.8 is a stepwise method to evaluate every CBC that the clinician interprets, followed by Table 8.9, which shows the various formulas to help discriminate a microcytosis. You can see the range of specificity

Key Learning about the CBC

- Taking a good nutrition history is important in evaluating the child with pallor.
- It is important to have an organized approach to the CBC to avoid errors in interpretation.
- Only use formulas like Mentzer's index in interpreting microcytic anemia.
- Acute-phase reactants such as ferritin can be normal in the face of iron deficiency if the patient has inflammation or an infection.

(SP), sensitivity (SN), positive predictive value (PPV), and negative predictive value (NPV) as no one formula is perfect.

When evaluating a patient with microcytic anemia, the Mentzer's index is the best-known formula and considered the best by Vehapoglu et al. (2014). Still, some authors suggest that England and Fraser's index is the best formula (Amal-Zaghloui et al. 2016). Some clinicians feel that Shine and Lai's formula has the best data (Okan et al. 2009). In contrast, Valiya et al. (2019) feel that Ricerca is the best formula (Valiya et al. 2019). Matos et al. (2016) suggested that close patient follow-up is important since no formula can completely differentiate between IDA and thalassemia trait. Based on the conflicting data in Table 8.9, the text authors suggest that if you are in doubt about the diagnosis, use at least two formulas to confirm iron deficiency, and closely follow the response to iron.

8.7 Disorders of Erythrocyte

Anemia is classified by two mechanisms—the size of the RBC and the pathophysiology of the anemia. Table 8.10 reviews the two ways to think about the cause of anemia. Depending on the type of anemia, the clinician can determine which tests to order in an organized fashion.

8.8 Microcytosis

In children, the clinician must make sure that they look at the MCV on the CBC. The two most common causes of microcytosis are iron deficiency and thalassemia. Very mild anemia with a small MCV may point to thalassemia.

8.8.1 Iron Deficiency

Iron deficiency is a common nutrient deficiency worldwide, found in industrial and

Table 8.10 Anemia classification and differential diagnosis

Classification of anemia	Possible causes
Size of the red cell	*Possible cause*
Microcytic anemia	• Iron deficiency due to menstrual loss, pregnancy, GI loss, bariatric surgery, celiac disease, and hematuria • Thalassemia • Anemia of chronic illness/inflammation • Sideroblastic anemia • Copper deficiency[a]
Normocytic anemia	• Blood loss • Hemolysis • Renal disease • Oncological disorder
Macrocytic anemia	• Marked reticulocytosis can elevate the MCV • Thyroid disease, including hypothyroidism • Aplastic anemia • Liver disease • B_{12} and folate deficiency • Chemotherapy • Myelodysplastic systemic • Copper deficiency[a]
Pathophysiology of the anemia	*Possible cause*
Increased loss	Hemorrhage–GI bleeding, menorrhagia, or much less common renal disease Trauma Hemolysis due to intrinsic red cell defects such as enzymopathy or red cell shape disorder, immune-mediated hemolysis, or a hemoglobinopathy
Decreased production	Bone marrow disorder causing stem cell dysfunction Nutritional disorder—Iron, B_{12}, folate deficiency, and copper deficiency Toxin/drug Lack of erythropoietin due to renal disease or anemia of chronic illness Interference with iron metabolism by a decrease in hepcidin Myelophthisic process from infection, cancer, and fibrosis

Adapted from Daugherty and De Loughery (2017), De Loughery (2017), Witmer (2013)
[a]Copper deficiency most commonly causes macrocytosis but can also cause microcytosis

nonindustrialized countries (Witmer 2013). Iron is distributed into three pools in the body, including transport, functional, and storage. Gastrointestinal absorption occurs in the proximal duodenum with hepcidin as the main regulator. Absorbed iron is bound in the plasma by transferrin and accounts for 0.1% of total body iron. Functional iron is used in hemoglobin production and accounts for 75% of the body's total iron. Finally, excess iron is stored in the liver (primarily), spleen, and bone marrow (Witmer 2013). At the time of birth, infants have high total body stores of iron, but iron-enriched cereals should be added at 6 months. Preterm infants should receive iron supplements due to the rapid postnatal growth, which can exhaust the iron stores by 2–3 months (Witmer 2013).

There are two risk periods for iron deficiency in normal children, toddlerhood and adolescence, especially for menstruating females and athletes. Toddlers are most often iron deficient when they switch to cows' milk around 12 months. Cows' milk contains no iron and interferes with iron absorption. Picky eaters will often drink large quantities of milk, leading to a decrease in iron-rich food content, and this combination will lead to IDA. Approximately 11% of adolescent females develop iron deficiency, whereas 15% of toddlers develop iron deficiency (Powers and Buchanan 2019).

Athletes develop iron deficiency due to exercise-induced hemolysis and urinary iron loss. The hemolysis in athletes results from a foot strike, intense muscle contraction, and higher hepcidin levels, resulting in decreased GI absorption (De Loughery 2017). Pregnancy is also associated with increased iron demands. Excessive blood loss can cause iron deficiency, and gastrointestinal bleeding is far more common than hematuria as a reason for this (De Loughery 2017). Inadequate iron absorption due to loss of or dysfunction of absorptive enterocytes occurs in celiac disease, infections with *Helicobacter pylori*, bariatric surgery, inflammatory bowel disease, or bowel resection (De Loughery 2017; Witmer 2013). Antacid therapy, a high gastric pH, and genetic defects of intestinal iron uptake also decrease iron absorption (Witmer 2013).

Symptoms of anemia include fatigue, lack of endurance, cold intolerance, and tachycardia. Fatigue is the most profound symptom that occurs early in the process. Iron deficiency causes systemic symptoms, including neurocognitive defects, angular stomatitis, glossitis, koilonychia, or nail spooning, pica and pallor of the mucous membranes can be seen.

While iron deficiency is usually classified as microcytic anemia, it may be normocytic early in the course. A thrombocytosis in the range of 500,000 to 700,000 is common. In terms of laboratory findings, the serum ferritin is the first test to decrease in iron deficiency, followed by decreased transferrin, decreased Hb, and elevated RDW, with a decreased MCV being the last test to show iron depletion (Witmer 2013).

Table 8.11 shows the tests that can be used to confirm an iron deficiency. Serum ferritin is the most cost-effective test (De Loughery 2017); however, it is an acute-phase reactant and can be elevated or normal in the face of inflammation or infection. Table 8.11 reviews the different types of tests used to confirm iron deficiency; however, it is perfectly acceptable to diagnose iron deficiency based on anemia. Microcytosis on the CBC indices confirms iron deficiency. Starting iron therapy results in an increase in reticulocyte within 2–3 days and an increase in hemoglobin in 1 week with normalization of the hemoglobin by 4–6 weeks (Witmer 2013). A follow-up visit at 1 week is needed to confirm a reticulocyte and Hb response to iron. It is also helpful to confirm that the child is getting the correct iron dose in 1 week.

8.8.2 Thalassemia

Understanding Hemoglobin. A basic understanding of hemoglobin helps with an understanding of thalassemia. Hemoglobin molecules are formed by two pairs of globin chains forming a tetramer with a heme compound joined to each chain. In the newborn, fetal hemoglobin consists of two α-globins and two gamma (γ)-globins. Fetal hemoglobin has a higher affinity for oxygen. Usually, by 12 months of life, the γ-globin is replaced by β-globin to form hemoglobin A, the predominant hemoglobin of most children (Noronha 2016).

Table 8.11 Tests in iron deficiency

Test	Measures	Results are influenced by
Total iron-binding capacity (TIBC)	TIBC is an indirect measure of transferrin. It measures the availability of iron-binding sites on the transferrin molecule	Normal in thalassemia Elevated in IDA, infection, inflammation, recent oral iron intake, and diurnal variation Decreased in anemia of inflammation, malnutrition, and cancer
Serum iron	Amount of iron in the blood	Decreased in IDA and normal in thalassemia (Witmer 2013) Normally low in anemia of inflammation but can be elevated if the patient is taking oral iron
Transferrin saturation	This is a calculated number = (serum iron/TIBC) X 100	Elevated in infection, inflammation, and recent oral iron intake
Serum ferritin	Regulated by cellular iron content. It is a storage compound for iron. Correlates with body iron stores in healthy patients	Low in IDA Normal in thalassemia Normal to elevated in infection and inflammation First-line test if there is confusion about the cause of the microcytic anemia
Soluble transferrin receptor (sTfR)	Iron is transferred into cells by iron transferrin complexes. The iron transferrin complexes bind to transferrin receptors outside the cells and where the iron is released into the cell's cytoplasm. Proteolytic cleavage occurs, and the soluble transferrin receptor is released into the plasma. Iron deficiency results in a high sTfR, whereas iron depletion results in low sTfR	Elevated in iron deficiency, thalassemia, and SCD It can also be increased by hemolytic anemia or blood loss Not affected by inflammation
Free erythrocyte protoporphyria (FEP)	Decreased iron supply to the RBC causes the generation of free zinc protoporphyria resulting in the release of FEP	Normal in thalassemia Elevated in lead poisoning, in IDA, and in anemia of inflammation
Mean corpuscle volume (MCV)	MCV is directly measured and is indicative of RBC size	Decreased in MCV in IDA and thalassemia Normal to decreased MCV in anemia of inflammation
Red blood cell distribution width (RDW)	Variation in RBC size or how much the RBC look like each other	Normal in thalassemia but will be low if the patient has thalassemia and IDA Increased RDW in IDA but can be normal in early iron deficiency

Adapted from Bruno et al. (2015), Cascio and De Loughery 2017, Hermiston and Mentzer (2002), Witmer (2013)

Hemoglobin A has two α-globin chains and two β-globin chains and makes up 97% of hemoglobin in the normal person. The remaining hemoglobin comprises hemoglobin A_2 and F. Hemoglobin A_2 is composed of a pair of α-globin chains and a pair of delta globin chains. Two genes on chromosome 16 each code for two α-globins, and one gene on chromosome 11 codes for each of the two β-globins. Two abnormal hemoglobins are Bart's hemoglobin and hemoglobin H. Hemoglobin E is a β-globin variant common in Asian populations (Noronha 2016). Bart's hemoglobin is composed of γ-globins and hemoglobin H. While this text is focusing on the most common variants of hemoglobin, it should be noted that there are over 1000 naturally occurring hemoglobin variants due to a single amino acid substitution in the hemoglobin molecule (Thom et al. 2013).

Thalassemia is prevalent in as much as 5% of the world's population, having a deficient production of either α- or β-globin chains (Piel and Weatherall 2014). Hemoglobin E is a common β-thalassemia variant among Asian populations and produces a thalassemia-like picture (Noronha 2016).

Thalassemia is an inherited genetic disorder that can vary from very mild to very severe anemia. Patients who have defective α-globin genes have α-thalassemia, while patients with defective β-globin genes have β-thalassemia (Martin and Thompson 2013). The genes for the α-chains and the γ-chains are duplicated (α α/α α, γ γ/γ γ). The genes for the β-chains are encoded by a single gene locus (β/β), but the β-chains can be completely deficient β^0 or partially deficient β^-. The clinical presentation varies with the number of defective globin chains. Several studies confirm that patients that carry thalassemia are less susceptible to infection with *Plasmodium Falciparum*. β-Thalassemias are the most common types. While thalassemia's prevalence is about 5% worldwide (Piel and Weatherall 2014), it is highest in Cambodian and Laotian people. It is also present among Vietnamese, Thai, African, Chinese, Filipino, Mediterranean, Middle Eastern, and Thai persons (Piel and Weatherall 2014). The most common test to diagnose thalassemia is hemoglobin electrophoresis.

8.8.2.1 Alpha (α) Thalassemia

The symptoms of α-thalassemia are based on the production of α-globin genes. Since there are four α-chains, a deficiency of one of the chains tends to be asymptomatic. These children are considered silent carriers and may have microcytosis and normal iron stores with normal hemoglobin electrophoresis. DNA sequencing determines the presence or absence of α-chain deletions (Cascio and De Loughery 2017).

Children with a two-gene deletion have α-thalassemia traits and are considered to have α-thalassemia or thalassemia minor. The child will have mild microcytic anemia that does not cause growth impairment (Cascio and De Loughery 2017).

Hemoglobin H disease has a three-gene deletion and will have decreased α-globin production plus insoluble tetramer of γ-globins. It is identified in the newborn screen as Bart's hemoglobin. As the switch from γ-globins occurs during the first year of life, hemoglobin electrophoresis identifies it as hemoglobin H. Hemoglobin H causes chronic hemolysis. During the second decade of life, the child may need RBC transfusions leading to iron overload. It is mild, but severe phenotypes have been reported (Piel and Weatherall 2014).

A recent MMWR indicated that 41 of 44 newborn screening programs (93%) report Bart's hemoglobin as part of the hemoglobin screening for SCD, but there is little guidance on what to do with these results. The higher Bart's hemoglobin result is, the more severe the degree of α-thalassemia (Bender et al. 2020). However, some programs only report that Bart's hemoglobin is present and advise follow-up in 6 months, but other programs report the percentage of Bart's hemoglobin. Only 80% reported that they advised follow-up for patient retesting based on the percentage of Bart's Hb. The recommendations varied and included confirmatory testing, CBC, RC, and referral to genetic counseling and a pediatric hematologist. Only a few programs reported the abnormal results to parents, so the clinician needs to follow up on this testing result (Bender et al. 2020).

In patients with a four-gene deletion, hydrops fetalis and intrauterine heart failure mean certain deaths. However, today, intrauterine transfusions enable the fetus to survive, but they will need chronic transfusions and a bone marrow transplant.

8.8.2.2 Beta (β) Thalassemia

β-Globin genes control the production of β-globin. Some β-globin gene produces no β-globins and is described as β^0, whereas other β-genes produce some β-globins that are noted as

---

Key Learning about Thalassemia

- Bart's hemoglobin on a newborn's screen needs to be followed up by age 6 months.
- A patient can have a hemoglobinopathy, but it cannot be detected by the particular method used as different hemoglobins may be better seen in different mediums.
- Thalassemia trait is not uncommon and should be considered in the face of microcytosis and lack of response to iron therapy.

β^-. Over 200-point mutations cause β-thalassemia that have a variable clinical presentation depending on how much β-globin is produced. β-Thalassemia trait occurs when one of the genes produce no β-globin or the two β-genes produce a mild to moderate amount of β-globins. The mutation occurs more commonly in the Middle East, Central Asia, the Far East, and the Mediterranean. In β-thalassemia, the level of hemoglobin A2 is increased. Hemoglobin A2 is composed of two α- and two delta chains. There is a decreased production of β-chains, and A2 increases as a compensatory mechanism. The expected results of an A2 elevation are found in the hemoglobin electrophoresis. The CBC will show a microcytosis with a decreased MCV, the Mentzer's index will be below 13, and the iron studies are normal. A study of Indonesian patients showed that the Shine and Lai index could predict all carriers of β-thalassemia with mutations at c92 + 5G > C and c.79G > A (Okan et al. 2009). The hemoglobin electrophoresis is discussed under tests used in microcytosis.

8.8.3 Anemia of Inflammation

Anemia of inflammation or anemia of chronic disease (ACD) can be seen in acute or chronic illness due to abnormal iron homeostasis, impaired response to erythropoietin, and suboptimal erythropoiesis. The diseases that cause this include infections, cancer, autoimmune diseases, chronic kidney disease transplant patients, and congestive heart failure patients. During infection, limiting iron available for microbes to multiply is protective and positively affects the innate immune system (Weiss 2015). Limiting iron availability also inhibits malignant cells from proliferating (Weiss 2015). ACD with IDA is possible, but the underlying etiology of the ACD must be determined as the administration of iron might result in increased bacterial growth. Many of the tests used to determine IDA may not be appropriate in the face of ACD and IDA. For example, ferritin is an acute-phase reactant that may be normal in the face of ACD and IDA (Weiss 2015).

The pathophysiology centers around hepcidin, a central regulatory hormone of iron metabolism. Hepatocytes primarily produce hepcidin, but there are areas in the brain that produce hepcidin (Yazici et al. 2019). Hepcidin produces ferroportin, causing it to block iron exportation to the circulation. Certain cytokines, particularly IL-6, are responsible for the upregulating hepcidin expression, resulting in iron sequestration by macrophages and hypoferremia (D'Angelo 2013). An increase in hepcidin occurs in iron deficiency, hypoxia, increased erythropoiesis, and anemia. Inflammation decreases hepcidin, leading to decreased iron availability and causing microcytosis (Ilkovska et al. 2016). There is a significant positive correlation between hepcidin levels and serum ferritin (Kumar et al. 2019), except in hemochromatosis where the ferritin is high and the hepcidin level is low (D'Angelo 2013). The kidneys play a role in hepcidin clearance; thus, with decreased hepcidin, anemia develops (D'Angelo 2013).

Hepcidin levels are not available from the major laboratories in the United States, and the availability of these levels is found in specialty labs. However, hepcidin levels have diurnal changes and are lowers in the a.m. and increase in the afternoon. The levels are affected by dietary iron intake, and there are considerable laboratory problems with this measure (D'Angelo 2013). Normal levels for hepcidin in pediatric patients have been determined on small samples of patients (Cangemi et al. 2013; Sdogou et al. 2015), but ethnicity does affect the results (Kumar et al. 2019). Thus, hepcidin's pathophysiology does explain the anemia of inflammation, but hepcidin measures are not readily available.

8.8.4 Copper Deficiency

This anemia is severe, with macrocytosis being more common than microcytosis, and is often associated with severe neutropenia. Thrombocytopenia rarely occurs, and a normal platelet count is usually seen. The most common reason for this deficiency is bariatric surgery, but excessive zinc intake can also cause copper deficiency since both zinc and copper use the same transporter. Patients with a developmental delay or autism may develop extremely limited diets due to self-selection causing copper and zinc deficiency. Symptoms of Wilson's disease center around the eye, the brain, and the liver. A Kayser-Fleischer ring is an annular area of copper with a golden to brown appearance located in the limbus of the eye. The patient may have liver disease with an enlarged liver causing abdominal pain, nausea, and vomiting. The patient may also have myelopathy presenting as weakness, pain, sensory abnormalities, gait abnormalities, and limb paresthesia. Pica for pennies results in copper deficiency since pennies are 97.5% zinc. Low ceruloplasmin levels can detect the deficiency of copper (Bandmann et al. 2015).

8.8.5 Rare Microcytic Anemias

Several rare microcytic anemias involve a defect in iron metabolism or heme metabolism. They include sideroblastic anemia, hereditary hypotransferrinemia, hereditary aceruloplasminemia, congenital erythropoietic porphyrias, and erythropoietic protoporphyria. There are several kinds of sideroblastic anemia, but they are all characterized by ringed sideroblasts within the bone marrow. The retention of iron in the mitochondria results in a hypochromic anemia. High serum ferritin with a high serum iron and normal transferrin is typical of sideroblastic and nonsideroblastic anemia (Bruno et al. 2015). Sideroblastic anemia is rare and may not be seen until midlife. It is not a common type of anemia, but one type is associated with ataxia, whereas another type is associated with splenomegaly and dark skin (Bruno et al. 2015).

8.8.6 Tests Commonly Used in Microcytosis

When microcytosis is present, iron deficiency and thalassemia are the most common causes. The table above reviews the common lab tests used in microcytosis when iron deficiency is suspected. However, in primary care, the CBC and the use of one of the indices to determine the cause of the microcytosis are all that are usually done. Therapeutic iron is usually started, and the clinical response to iron is sufficient to establish the diagnosis. When there is doubt, serum ferritin is the cheapest way to establish iron deficiency, but it is prone to error due to its role as an acute-phase reactant. When the CBC evaluation and the indices point to thalassemia, hemoglobin electrophoresis is done.

8.8.6.1 Hemoglobin (Hb) Electrophoresis

Hb variants can be suspected through physical examination, particularly skin color variations with blue or ruddy tones, and confirmed by simple testing via hemoglobin electrophoresis. In this test, RBCs are placed on gels, then an electric field is applied, and the proteins separate based on charge. A heme stain enables the identification, depending on where the RBC migrated on the gel (Siddon, Torney 2019). The test is carried out on a medium such as cellulose acetate, filter paper, starch gel, citrate agar gel, or an agarose gel (Wahed et al. 2020; Kumar and Derbigny 2019). The separation of different Hbs is largely, but not solely, dependent on the charge of the Hb molecule (Wahed et al. 2020). Hemoglobin electrophoresis is conducted using alkaline and acidic HB electrophoresis methods to separate the different hemoglobin fractions. Cellulose acetate electrophoresis at alkaline pH as a supporting medium for zone electrophoresis was first introduced by Kohn (1957). It should be kept in mind that different hemoglobins may be better seen in a different medium. For example, citrate agar electrophoresis at an acidic pH can help detect hemoglobin S and F (Thom et al. 2013). A more expensive method, called isoelectric focusing, can separate the hemoglobins (Siddon, Torney 2019).

Since some abnormal Hbs do not separate well from hemoglobin A on either agar or acetate gel, DNA sequencing of the globin genes can help identify the amino acid and nucleotide alterations and confirm a rarer Hb (Thom et al.

2013; Siddon, Torney 2019). Chapter 7 discusses the various genetic techniques in further detail.

8.8.6.2 Ceruloplasmin (CP) Test

If the symptoms or physical exam findings, particularly a Kayser-Fleischer ring and neurological or liver disease, is present, a ceruloplasmin test may uncover copper deficiency. CP is a protein enzyme involved in iron metabolism. Ceruloplasmin is produced as the liver binds copper to a protein. About 95% of the body's copper is bound to ceruloplasmin. In advanced hepatic disease, copper metabolism disorders, nutritional deficiencies, nephrotic syndrome, Wilson's disease, and Menkes kinky hair syndrome, the ceruloplasmin can be low (Bandmann et al. 2015).

Pitfalls of Ceruloplasmin Since CP is an acute—reactant, false normal values can occur in patients with inflammatory conditions and females on the oral contraceptive pill (Bandmann et al. 2015).

8.8.7 Real-Life Example

A 10-year-old female presented with joint pains without swelling of the affected joints. History revealed increasing fatigue over the past 5 months with a history of facial rash on exposure to the sun. Initial testing included a CBC, C-reactive protein (CRP), comprehensive metabolic profile, and an erythrocyte sedimentation rate (sed rate). The results showed mild anemia with a borderline low MCV consistent with microcytic anemia, a sed rate of 55 (normal 5–15), and a mild elevated CRP. Further testing confirmed systemic lupus as the reason for the lab abnormalities. This case illustrates how chronic illness can result in mild microcytosis.

8.9 Normocytosis

The patient with normocytic anemia will have an insufficient number of RBCs of normal size. The underlying reason can be acute or chronic, for example, an acute GI bleed secondary to a congenital problem such as Meckel's diverticulum or chronic anemia due to hemoglobinopathy, RBC membrane or enzyme defect, or monthly menstrual bleeding. A stool guaiac test should be done as part of the workup for normocytic anemia. Gastrointestinal (GI) bleeding, whether from a congenital problem such as Meckel's diverticulum or a polyp of the GI tract, must be considered in the workup of normocytic anemia. The patient may be symptomatic if the underlying process is acute but may be asymptomatic if the anemia occurs over months or if the underlying hematological problem is chronic. Thus, the clinician needs to evaluate the CBC with the previous CBCs in mind.

8.9.1 Hemolysis Overview

When RBC breakdown occurs at an abnormal rate, this is called hemolysis. Three aspects of the immune system contribute to hemolysis—complement, antibodies (usually IgM or IgG), and phagocytic cells (macrophages). The hemolysis of red blood cells can be due to either an acquired or congenital abnormality of the RBC, lack of enzymes critical to forming the RBC membrane, Hb structural problems, or RBC structural problems. Any of the processes above cause a shortened lifespan for the RBC and an increase in erythrocytosis with elevated RC (Hill et al. 2019). The clinical presentation of mild hemolysis is often asymptomatic, while severe hemolysis can cause life-threatening anemia leading to cardiac failure. While congenital anemias generally are picked up in infancy or early childhood, the patient may be diagnosed later with mild hyperbilirubinemia, reticulocytosis, and mild anemia (Haley 2017). In mild levels of hemolysis and normal bone marrow, the patient will compensate with reticulocytosis. During times of stress and infection, the hemolysis can worsen, leading to significant anemia, hyperbilirubinemia, pallor, anemia, reticulocytosis, and occasionally splenomegaly (Haley 2017). These findings during illness or stress alert the clinician to the possibility of hemolytic anemia. Common hemolytic

Table 8.12 Pathophysiology of hemolysis with differential diagnosis

Cellular	Extracellular
Red blood cell membrane disease or membranopathies	Autoimmune disorders
RBC enzyme deficiencies or enzymopathies	Fragmentation due to damage to the RBC
Abnormalities of hemoglobin or hemoglobinopathies	RBC is more susceptible to oxidative damage due to plasma factors. The causes of the plasma factors include liver disease, abetalipoproteinemia, vitamin E deficiency, and Wilson's disease
Direct antibody test will be negative	Direct antibody test will be negative
Extravascular hemolysis	*Intravascular hemolysis*
Due to macrophages in the liver or spleen engulfing the RBC due to abnormalities of the RBC. SCD has both intravascular and extravascular hemolysis Subdued in nature versus intravascular hemolysis Common causes: Warm antibody-type hemolytic anemia, hemolytic disease of the newborn, and non-ABO antibody-mediated allow immune hemolysis as a result of transfusion Hepatosplenomegaly is present	RBC is damaged, releasing hemoglobin. Common causes: Mechanical trauma (i.e., microangiopathy hemolytic anemia or valve disease), complement fixation, or membrane or hemoglobin disorder of the RBC (i.e., SCD, thalassemia) More severe Cold autoimmune hemolytic anemia
The hemoglobin circulates through the liver, and the patient will not have red urine	If the haptoglobin is saturated by hemoglobin, then free unbound hemoglobin is released, causing red or dark urine Hemoglobinuria is more common in cold antibody-type hemolytic anemia; however, it can be present in drug-induced immune hemolytic anemia
Direct antibody test generally is positive	Direct antibody test generally is positive

Adapted from Beris and Picard (2015), Kujovich (2016), Noronha (2016), Siddon, Torney (2019)

disorders include α- and β-thalassemia, glucose-6-phosphate dehydrogenase (G6PD) deficiency, and hereditary spherocytosis (HS) (Kim et al. 2017).

Once hemolysis is established, the next step is to determine the cause of the hemolysis. Hemolysis diagnoses can be divided into non-immune hemolysis and autoimmune hemolysis or cellular or extracellular hemolytic disease (Zhera et al. 2019). Non-immune or hemolysis can be further broken down into hereditary or acquired forms, with each form primarily causing RBC abnormalities. The hereditary forms of non-immune or cellular hemolysis include enzymopathies, membrane disorders, or disorders of Hb structure. Acquired hemolysis can be from a drug (ribavirin or oxidative drugs) or metal intoxication (lead, zinc, copper), intravascular coagulopathy, microangiography, or macro-angiography (associated with mechanical valves).

Another way of looking at hemolysis is from the mechanism of the hemolysis—extravascular or intravascular hemolysis. Extravascular

hemolysis is mediated via the reticuloendothelial system in the spleen and the liver (Noronha 2016). During extravascular hemolysis, the macrophages in the liver or spleen will engulf the RBC due to the RBC's damage. These patients with exclusive extravascular hemolysis will not have red or dark urine since the hemoglobin will circulate into the liver (Khera et al. 2019). The free hemoglobin is bound to plasma haptoglobin and is cleared by the liver. Extravascular hemolysis occurs in SCD, HS, and warm autoimmune hemolytic disease. Heme is released and is converted to biliverdin, ultimately forming bilirubin. Therefore, the patient will present with mild jaundice.

Intravascular hemolysis occurs when the RBC membrane is directly damaged due to toxins, stress, or complement-mediated hemolysis and therefore is found in immune-mediated hemolysis. When the haptoglobin is saturated by hemoglobin, free or unbound hemoglobin will be excreted by the kidney, causing dark urine (Noronha 2016). Table 8.12 helps differentiate the causes of hemolysis based on the pathophysiology.

The differential hemolysis is established using the patient's history and various tests, as listed below.

8.9.2 Tests Used to Establish Hemolysis

8.9.2.1 Reticulocyte Count

Reticulocytosis, as mentioned above, is an important distinguishing feature of hemolysis. Review the section on the RC.

8.9.2.2 Peripheral Smear

In autoimmune hemolytic anemia (AIHA), microspherocytes will occur due to immunoglobulins binding to the RBC (Siddon, Torney 2019). Polychromasia may be seen, and schistocytes or helmet cells may result from toxin or shear stress-mediated hemolysis. Fragmented RBC is consistent with hemolytic anemia. The presence of abnormally shaped RBCs such as spherocytes or elliptocytes, when associated with anemia, puts hereditary spherocytosis/elliptocytosis on the differential (Siddon, Torney 2019). The presence of schistocytes on a smear may indicate thrombotic thrombocytopenic purpura (TTP) or hemolytic uremic syndrome (Kujovich 2016; Siddon, Torney 2019). This test is prone to sampling error, as only 25 to 100 cells are seen. There is considerable overlap between the RBC morphologies leading to alterations of interpretation. Table 8.3 is a complete review of the abnormal RBC that can be present on the peripheral smear and what they may indicate.

8.9.2.3 Haptoglobin

Haptoglobin is a protein that removes free hemoglobin to protect the body from its negative effects. During hemolysis, haptoglobin will bond to the free hemoglobin, and the complex is then removed from the serum by the reticular activating system (Kujovich 2016). Haptoglobin is also an acute-phase reactant, so that it can be falsely elevated during inflammation. A low haptoglobin is sensitive for hemolysis but not specific as other

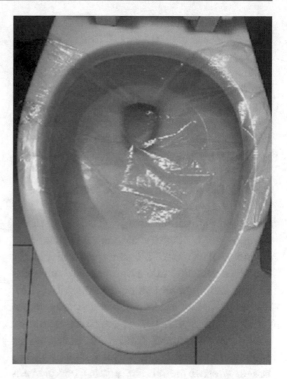

Fig. 8.1 Using plastic wrap to obtain the stool sample

causes of a low haptoglobin include transfusions, regular exercise, and severe liver disease.

A total lack of haptoglobin (anhaptoglobinemia) is found more commonly in countries with a high malaria rate. Haptoglobin is not a useful marker for hemolysis in infants under 2 months (Noronha 2016).

8.9.2.4 Lactate Dehydrogenase (LDH)

LDH, an intracellular enzyme, is plentiful in the RBC. Therefore, it is released during hemolysis, but like haptoglobin, there are other reasons for LDH elevations, including liver disease. The LDH may or may not be a part of a comprehensive metabolic profile. A low haptoglobin with an elevated LDH is 90% sensitive for hemolysis (Kujovich 2016). (The clinician should know whether this test will show up in the comprehensive metabolic profile that they order.)

8.9.2.5 Stool Guaiac

A stool guaiac is an important part of the differential diagnosis of a child with normocytic anemia. As noted, the reticulocyte count may be elevated, and anemia may not be present. The normal bone marrow can compensate for GI losses if the blood loss is mild. The stool can be obtained via rectal exam if the anemia is acute, and it is important to rule out the GI causes of blood loss. If the anemia is mild, the family can easily obtain a stool sample using a plastic wrap draped over the toilet to catch the stool (see Fig. 8.1). The stool can be brought to the lab for testing.

8.9.2.6 Direct Antiglobulin Testing (Direct Coombs)

Direct antiglobulin testing (DAT) or direct Coombs helps identify autoimmune hemolytic anemia (AIHA). DAT is a semiquantitative assay used to detect IgG alloantibodies, IgG autoantibodies, and complement components. The DAT test uses RBCs, unlike IAT, which uses serum (Sidden, Tormey, 2019). The Coombs serum or antihuman globulin is from a rabbit or another animal immunized with purified immunoglobulins to prepare antibodies against complement and IgG. It is used in both the DAT and IAT tests (Sidden, Tormey, 2019). However, for the child with anemia compatible with autoimmune hemolytic disease, the DAT testing is the most important test for determining if the child has an AIHA (Sidden, Tormey, 2019).

It is important to differentiate between immune-mediated (antibody-mediated) and non-immune-mediated hemolysis to properly diagnose the child. A direct antiglobulin test is a method to detect the in vivo coating of a patient's RBC by autoantibodies. When a nonspecific antihuman globulin is added into the patient's RBC, it will bind to the antibodies and cause RBC agglutination. Then, adding antihuman antibodies to the tube can identify the type of immunoglobulin binding to the RBC surface. If there is a binding of the anti-complement antibodies, it points to IgM-bound antibodies or a cold-reactive AIHA. In contrast, if an IgG-binding pattern is seen, this points to a warm autoimmune hemolytic anemia (WAIHA).

DAT-negative AIHA is more likely in cold agglutinin disease (CAD) due to a lack of tight binding to RBCs. The rate of WAIHA with a negative DAT is from 3% to 11% and is likely the result of the DAT's reagent (Segel and Lichtman 2014). More detailed immunological evaluations can be done using a more sensitive Coombs reagent, gel card diagnostic, or flow cytometry outside this text's scope. The possibility of a false-positive reaction is about 1 in 10,000 people and can be the result of antiphospholipid antibodies, spontaneous RBC agglutination, technical issues, cytophilic or nonspecific IgG absorbed from plasma (Segel and Lichtman 2014; Eule et al. 2018), or pharmaceutical processes (antibiotics are the most common) causing RBC agglutination (Sidden, Tormey, 2019). The test tube method is 87% specific for AIHA and only 43% sensitive (Eule et al. 2018). Thus, it is important to order haptoglobins, LDH, RC, urinalysis, and CBC with a smear to increase the likelihood of a correct diagnosis. If a DAT-negative AIHA is suspected, a hematology consult is needed.

In patients with AIHA, false-negative tests may be due to an extremely low antibody coating of the RBC or antibody classes such as IgA, which is not detected by the DAT (Sidden, Tormey, 2019).

In autoimmune hemolysis, the patient's RBCs are destroyed by autoantibodies resulting in weakness, pallor, fatigue, mild jaundice, and mild splenomegaly. The predominant autoimmune hemolysis is divided into (1) cold agglutinin disease (CAD) and (2) warm autoimmune hemolytic anemia (WAIHA), depending on the optimal temperature for reactivity of the autoantibody. WAIHA accounts for 65 to 70% of the cases, and cold antibodies account for 20–25% of the cases (Liebman and Weitz 2017). Warm IgG antibodies will bind to the RBC surface antigens at body temperature, whereas cold IgM agglutinins will find to the RBC and fix complements at temperatures below 37°. The cold IgM can cause cold agglutinin hemolysis (Eule et al. 2018).

The third type of AIHA, known as paroxysmal cold hemoglobinuria (PCH), is much rarer and accounts for 1% to 3% of the cases (Liebman and Weitz 2017). It causes Coombs-negative hemolysis and is associated with thrombosis and pancytopenia (Daughety, De Loughery 2017). PCH is caused by the Donath-Landsteiner (DL) antibody and is complement-mediated. The associated

Table 8.13 Causes of secondary AHIA

Infectious causes	• Epstein-Barr virus • Cytomegalovirus • Parvovirus • Mycoplasma • Pneumococcus
Malignancies	• Hodgkin lymphoma • Allogenic bone marrow transplant
Autoimmune disease and Rheumatological diseases	• Autoimmune lymphoproliferative syndrome (ALPS) • Lupus erythematosus
Drug associated	• Cefotetan • Ceftriaxone • Piperacillin • Fludarabine • Diclofenac
Immune deficiency	• Common variable immunodeficiency
Others	• Solid organ transplant

Adapted from Freedman (2015), Liebman and Weitz (2017), Noronha (2016)

hypercoagulability leads to thrombophilia, causing significant morbidity as well as mortality. Thrombosis of the portal or hepatic vein is associated with PCH, and therefore patients with thrombi in this region should be evaluated for PCH (Daughety, De Loughery 2017). It is seen predominantly in children following an upper respiratory infection. The DL antibody test is not universally available and may even be more problematic in making the diagnosis because the DL antibody test may be negative within a few days (Noronha 2016).

A fourth serologic form of AIHA is the result of warm AIHA-direct antiglobulin in a Coombs negative patient.

In CAD, the autoantibody is usually IgM, whereas in WAIHA, the autoantibody is usually IgG. The IgM antibody is considered complete as it binds to the RBC surface, causing agglutination, whereas the IgG is absorbed to the RBC surface but does not cause complete agglutination (Freedman 2015). Intravascular hemolysis causes an increase in free hemoglobin resulting in red, brown, or tea-colored urine and is more common in CAD. Extravascular destruction of RBC is more common in WAIHA and results in

urine urobilin, causing jaundice with dark yellow urine. Urine and skin color changes are common signs of AIHA. Beyond the neonatal period, AIHA is rare in children.

Autoimmune hemolytic anemias can also be secondary to infections, drugs, malignancy, rheumatological diseases, and common variable immunodeficiency. Table 8.13 outlines the various causes of secondary AHIA.

Key Learning about Hemolysis

- In hemolytic anemia, the LDH, bilirubin, and reticulocyte count will be increased, and the haptoglobin is decreased.
- A reticulocyte count is important in evaluating hemolysis, and the total bilirubin may be slightly to moderately elevated.

8.9.2.7 Antihuman Immunoglobulin Test (Indirect Coombs)

The indirect Coombs test is done at birth to detect infants with hemolytic disease of the newborn due to Rh sensitivity or ABO hemolytic disease of the newborn and transfusion-related alloantibodies. In this test, the patient's serum (not the RBC) is incubated with health donor RBCs. This test's major use is to see if the child has RBC-specific antibodies (Sidden, Tormey, 2019). If agglutination occurs, it indicates RBC autoantibodies pointing to the presence of a circulating antibody. The agglutination is gauged from 0 (no antibodies) to +4 which indicated a strong presence of antibodies (Sidden, Tormey, 2019). If the direct result is negative, but autoimmune hemolytic anemia (AIHA) is suspected, the antihuman immunoglobulin test (indirect Coombs) should be done (Noronha 2016). In hereditary enzymopathies, the peripheral smear may not be helpful, and the patient negative antihuman immunoglobulin test may be negative (Haley 2017).

While this test is highly sensitive, false negatives can occur in severe immunosuppression or antibody-depleting immunotherapies, putting patients at risk for transfusion reactions. False positives will also occur in severe inflammation or if the patient is receiving IVIG (Sidden, Tormey, 2019).

8.9.2.8 Chemistry Panel
An in-depth look at the chemistry panel is presented in the renal and gastrointestinal chapter. However, unconjugated or indirect bilirubin is elevated in the patient with hemolytic anemia.

8.9.2.9 Urinalysis
The urine color may be red, brown, or tea-colored in AIHA due to CAD from the presence of free hemoglobin (intravascular hemolysis). Dark yellow urine and positive urobilinogen are classic of WAIHA due to increased bilirubin in plasma (extravascular destruction of RBC) (Freedman 2015). Additional information about urinalysis is found in Chap. 10.

8.9.2.10 Molecular Technologies for Inherited Hemolytic Anemia (IHA)
Advances in molecular technologies, including next-generation sequencing, may eventually become the first-line approach to identify mutations and to determine the genes responsible for IHA (Kim et al. 2017). Primary providers must

Table 8.14 Types of non-immune congenital hemolytic anemia

Defects in the RBC membrane	• Autosomal dominant forms
	  o Glucose-6-phosphate dehydrogenase deficiency (G6PD)
	  o Pyruvate kinase deficiency
	• Autosomal recessive forms
	  o Rarer forms include phosphoglycerate kinase, glutathione synthetase, glutathione reductase, triosephosphate isomerase, and glucose phosphate isomerase

RBC enzyme defect	• Hereditary spherocytosis • Hereditary elliptocytosis • Southeast Asian ovalocytosis • Rarer forms include dehydrated hereditary stomatocytosis and congenital dyserythropoiesis type II
Hemoglobin defects	• SCD • Thalassemia syndrome • Rarer forms of hemoglobinopathy including CC disease, SD disease, and others

Information derived from Beris and Picard (2015), Noronha (2016)

consider that many insurers will not cover the tests, and the cost of this testing may be prohibitive for first-line use.

8.10 Non-immune Congenital Hemolytic Anemias

Several genetic forms of hemolysis are due to defects in the RBC membrane, RBC enzyme defects, or hemoglobin defects, including thalassemia. Table 8.14 outlines the type of non-immune congenital hemolytic anemia.

8.10.1 Defects in the RBC Membrane-Hereditary Spherocytosis (HS)

HS is a disorder of the RBC membrane that is more common in children with Northern European ancestry (Haley 2017; Wahed et al. 2020). It is transmitted as an autosomal dominant transmission or can be the result of spontaneous mutation. The disease results from the spherocytes' inability to absorb hypoosmotic fluid, causing the RBC to be osmotically fragile and leading to hemolysis in the spleen (Ciepiela 2018). Congenital HS can present in the newborn period with severe anemia or be suspected due to the lower side of normal Hb/Hct with hyperbilirubinemia.

Differential diagnosis of HS includes other RBC membranopathies and enzymopathies and other causes of spherocytosis, including immune hemolytic anemia and Wilson's disease, as seen in Table 8.14.

Several diagnostic tests are used to diagnose HS. The tests are listed below.

8.10.1.1 CBC and Peripheral Smear
HS will present with a normal MCHC in mild cases to an elevated MCHC along with signs of anemia in symptomatic disease (Farias 2017; Haley 2017). Like other congenital hemolytic anemias, increased oxidative stress caused by infections, toxins, or drugs will cause hemolysis to occur, leading to reticulocytosis. Several algorithms can help make the clinician suspect HS,

but they involve measures not typically reported in a CBC (Ciepiela 2018).

8.10.1.2 Direct Antigen Testing (DAT)

DAT is negative in spherocytosis and other congenital hemolytic anemias, including enzymopathies and RBC membrane defects.

8.10.1.3 Flow Cytometry Osmotic Fragility (OF) and Flow Cytometry Eosin-5'-Maleimide Test (EMA Test)

The EMA test is considered the first-line screening test for HS. It causes fluorescent binding to RBC membrane band 3 with reduced intensity seen on flow cytometry in HS, HE, and HP (Farias 2017). While the EMA test is sensitive, it is not specific.

The flow cytometry OF test can achieve up to 85.7% sensitivity and 97.2% specificity. It may be recommended as the test of choice going forward, although present guidelines still recommend the EMA test (Farias 2017). EMA testing has a sensitivity of 92.7–96.6% and a specificity of 99.1%, but labs can have different cut-offs, changing the test's sensitivity and specificity. Hereditary pyropoikilocytosis also causes a decreased fluorescence of EMA-bound RBCs and results in a positive test.

The EMA dye is relatively expensive, and the working solution it uses is unstable. Different labs have different cut-offs, and therefore a positive test may vary from lab to lab (Farias 2017).

8.10.1.4 Incubated Osmotic Fragility (OF) Test

An OF test measures hemolysis in the RBC at different lower sodium chloride concentrations, increasing hemolysis at increasing hypotonic saline solutions. A normal OF test occurs in 10–20% of cases (Farias 2017). Newborns, due to fetal hemoglobin, may have a normal OF test (Farias 2017). A false positive occurs in any severe anemia caused by hemolysis, RBC enzyme deficiencies, recent RBC transfusions, or AIHA (Sidden, Tormey, 2019).

False-negative results occur in obstructive jaundice, in iron deficiency, and in patients with an elevated RC after an aplastic crisis (Farias 2017). There is a false-negative rate of 25% in patients with the disease (Haley 2017). It is also important to remember that secondary reasons for spherocytosis and family history are especially important with both these tests.

8.10.1.5 Confirmatory Tests for HS

Sodium dodecyl sulfate-polyacrylamide gel electrophoresis (SDS-PAGE) and molecular diagnostics are the most sensitive ways to distinguish other hemolytic anemias from HS (Ciepiela 2018). Genetic sequencing evaluates the molecular mutations in genes responsible for encoding one or more plasma membrane proteins—ankyrin, band 3 protein, protein 4.2, and α- or β-spectrin (Ciepiela 2018). Sequencing for red cell skeleton mutations can be done when the results of the above tests are ambiguous.

8.10.2 Hereditary Elliptocytosis (HE) and Hereditary Pyropoikilocytosis (HPP)

The hallmark cell in HE is cigar-shaped elliptical RBC, whereas HPP has severe fragmentation of the RBC frequently seen following thermal burns. Both are rare causes of severe hemolytic anemia, and there is a strong association between HE and HPP. Many HPP patients in childhood evolve into HE patients as adults.

The differential diagnosis includes any primary cause of hemolytic anemia, as seen in Tables 8.12 and 8.13. Typical of the hemolytic anemia discussed, the range of clinical presentation varies from asymptomatic to severe anemia with viral and bacterial infections and malaria inducing marked hemolysis.

The diagnostic tests that are used to diagnose HE and HPP include the same tests used in hemolysis, but the CBC has specific findings as detailed below:

8.10.2.1 CBC and Comprehensive Metabolic Profile

The patient with HPP and HE will have the classic signs of hemolytic anemia—reticulocytosis, elevated LDH, elevated bilirubin, and decreased haptoglobin.

The CBC in HPP should develop extreme hemolytic anemia with marked poikilocytosis and RBC budding, fragmentation, and unusually shaped RBC. The peripheral smear will show microcytosis, poikilocytosis, elliptocytosis, and fragmented RBCs. If the blood is heated from 45 degrees to 46 degrees, HPP RBC fragmentation markedly increases. The workup for diagnosis should be referred to a hematologist.

8.10.3 Real-Life Example

An 11-year-old presented for a well-child visit. The history and exam were unremarkable. The clinician ordered a comprehensive metabolic profile and a CBC as a screen. On reviewing the labs, her abnormal values included a Hct of 34 (normal 35–39%), an MCHC of 38 (normal 33.4–35.5), and an indirect bilirubin of 4.2. An RC, LDH, haptoglobin, and peripheral smear were ordered in the follow-up. The results were consistent with spherocytosis. A family history confirmed early gallbladder disease in the mother, maternal sister, and maternal grandmother. A hematologist confirmed the diagnosis of HS within the family. The affected family members had a positive osmotic fragility test. The family did not know they had HS. A genetic consultation was done in follow-up for further genetic counseling.

8.10.4 RBC Enzyme Deficiencies: Glucose-6-Phosphate Dehydrogenase Deficiency (G6PD)

RBC enzyme deficiencies have a wide clinical presentation ranging from mild or absent anemia to episodic hemolysis to severe anemia. Due to reticulocytosis and relatively mild anemia, the patient may be asymptomatic, but a mildly icteric sclera can be seen. There are two major glucose pathways used by the RBC as a metabolic substrate—the hexose monophosphate (HMP) shunt or protective pathway and the glycolytic pathway

or energy-producing pathway (Grace and Glader 2018). G6PD is the most common HMP shunt, and pyruvate kinase deficiency (PK) is the most common glycolytic pathway. If either enzyme is deficient, hemolysis occurs.

Hemolysis is suspected based on a low HB/Hct, a normal or high MCV, a high RC, a high LDH, and a mildly elevated indirect bilirubin. An enzymopathy should be suspected if the patient has normal hemoglobin electrophoresis, a negative direct Coombs, and no evidence of abnormally shaped cells. A history of prolonged neonatal jaundice and non-immune hemolysis should trigger consideration of a glycolytic enzyme deficiency (Grace and Glader 2018).

G6PD is one of the most common genetic problems since it affects 400 million people globally (World Health Organization [WHO] 2019). Over 300 variations and the clinical manifestations include neonatal jaundice, acute hemolytic anemia triggered by drugs or infection, and a chronic non-spherocytic hemolytic disease (WHO 2019). This enzymopathy is an X-linked recessive disorder that causes hemolytic anemia when the patient has oxidative stress due to fava beans, infection, or certain drugs. Clinicians see patients worldwide and must understand the incidence of G6PD deficiency in the patient's country. In general, patients from a country with a high incidence of malaria have a higher incidence of G6PD deficiency.

It is important to understand the pathophysiology of the enzyme G6PD to understand the tests. RBCs are very vulnerable to oxygen radicals, easily converted to reactive oxygen species like hydrogen peroxide or H_2O_2. These radicals are formed under oxidative stress conditions when the reactive oxygen species overwhelm the antioxidants like glutathione to oppose the radicals. In glutathione assembly, G6PD is an essential enzyme in nicotinamide adenine dinucleotide phosphate (NADPH) production formation, which then forms glutathione. H_2O_2 causes the red cell's hemoglobin to precipitate into Heinz bodies. The spleen pinches off Heinz bodies into bite cells, which can remove the cells. In people without any deficiency of G6PD, glutathione, which is an antioxidant, can prevent the

Table 8.15 Type of G6PD deficiency

Class I	• Severe deficiency with 1% or less • A total absence of G6PD is not compatible with life • Associated with chronic non-spherocytic hemolytic anemia (CNSHA) • Mutation-type G6PD Buenos Aires and G6PD Durham
Class II	• Severe deficiency (less than 10% residual activity, but without CNSHA) • Anemia is induced by certain drugs and ingestion of fava beans • Mutation-type G6PD Mediterranean B form and Santamaria
Class III	• Moderate deficiency (10–60% residual activity) • Can cause an occasional acute hemolytic anemia • Includes the common African G6PD A form and G6PD Canton form
Class IV	• Very mild to moderate deficiency (60% to 90% of residual activity) • Tend to be asymptomatic • G6PD Orissa and G6PD Montalbano
Class V[a]	• Increased activity • Asymptomatic • The mutation is not known

Adapted from Grace and Glader (2018), WHO (2016)

formation of H_2O_2 by giving an electron that oxygen radicals are missing. The extra electrons are made via a metabolic pentose phosphate pathway that G6PD plays an important role. A lack of G6PD limits the rate of formation of the extra electrons since NADPH, which is formed by the mitochondria, cannot be converted into glutathione (Anderle et al. 2018; Ho and John 2015; WHO 2019).

Due to the X-linked pattern of inheritance, males are most affected. In female carriers, random inactivation can occur in the X chromosome in certain cells, creating G6PD-deficient RBCs plus unaffected RBCs. In female carriers, there will be a deficiency of one-half of their RBCs. But in rare cases, including a double X deficiency, the female can be as symptomatic as a male. Table 8.15 shows the different variant types of G6PD based on the amount of residual enzyme activity.

The differential diagnosis for G6PD deficiency includes any of the hereditary hemoglobinopathies, erythrocyte membrane disorders, or other erythrocyte enzyme disorders. Several diagnostic tests are used to diagnose G6PD. The tests are listed below:

8.10.4.1 CBC and Peripheral Smear

During hemolysis, there may be an elevated WBC with hemoglobin that is moderate to severely low. The RDW may be higher due to the presence of an elevated RC. As expected with hemolysis, the haptoglobin is low, and the LDH and indirect bilirubin are elevated.

Heinz bodies or bite cells (poikilocytes) may be reported on the CBC results and should be followed up with pertinent history and physical. Further G6PD-specific testing may be indicated.

8.10.4.2 Qualitative Test for G6PD Activity

Healthy RBCs generate enough G6PD to generate NADPH. Phenotype testing for G6PD is normalized for hemoglobin or the RBC count. Biochemical assays can be either qualitative or quantitative. A qualitative test or a fluorescent spot test looks for NADPH fluorescence after glucose-6-phosphatase and NADPH are combined with RBC hemolysate of RBCs.

Only two states Pennsylvania and the District of Columbia newborn screen for G6PD. The AAP recommends testing the newborn with jaundice to discriminate the infant who is deficient from intermediate and normal persons. A qualitative test, whether a point of care or done in a laboratory, can only differentiate between severe and normal activity levels but does not distinguish among the different intermediate deficiencies. Thus, they can distinguish a G6PD-deficient male and a female with two G6PD-deficient alleles who have G6PD activity that is less than 30% (Anderle et al. 2018). Males with greater than 30% activity are considered normal, but those with less than 30% are considered deficient.

Pitfalls of the qualitative tests include false-negative reactions that occur during hemolysis. Therefore, after a hemolytic episode, the clinician should wait 3 months to repeat the analysis (Grace and Glader 2018). There are problems with sensitivity to this test. For example, in the newborn period, a female with a high RC and low G6PD activity would be considered normal when they risk significant complications from G6PD.

The test will fail to pick up intermediate activity. Females with less than 30% are considered deficient, whereas females with 30–80% activity are considered intermediate. This is problematic as it will miss females with intermediate deficiencies who are at considerable risk for hemolysis if treated with drugs that induce more hemolysis (i. e., the patient treated with primaquine for resistant malaria).

8.10.4.3 Quantitative Tests for G6PD Activity

A quantitative test is done using a quantitative spectrophotometric assay for G6PD activity and reporting the actual degree of deficiency. Newer quantitative point-of-care testing is available and has similar statistics to quantitative laboratory testing for G6PD. For example, in a study by Pal et al., the point-of-care test called the STANDARD test was able to diagnose G6PD less than 30% as compared to a reference assay with a sensitivity of 100% (0.95 confidence interval [CI], 95.7–100) and a specificity of 97% (0.95 CI, 94.5–98.5). It was also able to distinguish females <70% normal G6PD activity with a sensitivity of 95.5% (0.95 CI, 89.7–98.5) and specificity of 97% (0.95 CI, 94.5–98.6) (Pal et al. 2019). Point-of-care testing can be extremely helpful as it is quicker and enables the clinician to develop a plan of care. Point-of-care testing helps the newborn with hyperbilirubinemia to mitigate kernicterus risk (Anderle et al. 2018). In the United States, more than 30% of kernicterus cases are associated with G6PD deficiency (Grace and Glader 2018).

The pitfalls of testing include that qualitative testing may show no G6PD deficiency when an intermediate degree occurs. In the United States, African-American males are at greater risk for this disease, but it is also present in children from Asia, the Mediterranean, Middle East, and India. All screening tests for G6PD must be done when the child does not have active hemolysis.

8.10.4.4 Molecular Analysis for G6PD

Most patients do not need molecular analysis studies if they have episodic hemolysis and normal baseline CBCs. However, if the child has chronic non-spherocytic anemia or a severe deficiency of G6PD, molecular analysis is a complementary test used for confirmation (Grace and Glader 2018). A primary care clinician would refer these children to hematology or genetic clinics for specialty evaluation.

8.10.5 RBC Enzyme Deficiencies: Pyruvate Kinase (PK) Deficiency

PK is an enzyme responsible for the last step of the glycolytic pathway and plays a central role in the cellular energy metabolism producing ATP in the RBC. RBCs lack mitochondria, and without ATP, the RBC would not be viable (Bianchi et al. 2019). PK is transmitted as an autosomal recessive trait and, like G6PD, is protective against malaria. Therefore, the allele is more prevalent in areas of endemic malaria. The degree of anemia, like G6PD, varies from very mild anemia to a fully compensated anemia due to reticulocytosis to life-threatening neonatal anemia. Like G6PD deficiency, neonatal jaundice may be more severe and persistent and require phototherapy and/or exchange transfusions. The anemia improves with age and is better tolerated due to increased red cell 2,3-DPG content increasing oxygen-carrying ability. Splenomegaly is common in 80% of patients, and splenectomy is reserved for transfusion-dependent patients. Gallstones are common, and an aplastic crisis following parvovirus infection can occur along with rarer complications such as kernicterus, leg ulcers, pancreatitis, pulmonary hypertension, and thromboembolic events (Bianchi et al. 2019).

PK is considered a diagnosis after a diagnostic workup for other hemolytic anemias is excluded, including immune-mediated disease, defects in the RBC membrane, and hemoglobin defects. Several diagnostic tests are used to diagnose PK. The tests are listed below:

8.10.5.1 CBC and Peripheral Smears

The peripheral smear in PK deficiency shows signs of hemolysis and accelerated erythropoiesis. The smear will show anisocytosis, poikilocytosis, nucleated RBC, acanthocytes, and echinocytes (Grace and Glader 2018).

8.10.5.2 PK Enzyme Tests

A qualitative enzyme screening can diagnose PK, but it can be problematic due to a high false-negative rate (Grace and Glader 2018). Like G6PD, a direct quantitative assay is available and should be used if the clinician suspects PK deficiency and the qualitative PK screening is negative. The PK enzyme test should also be measured along with another RBC enzyme, such as G6PD or hexokinase. If the PK activity is relatively low compared to other RBC enzymes, a PK deficiency should be suspected. The degree of hemolysis is not related to the measured RBC PK activity measured by direct quantitative testing.

The pitfalls of the spectrophotometric assay of RBC PK activity are related to RBC age, recent transfusion, delay in processing, and specimen contamination. PK activity is influenced by RBC age. If the sample has young RBC and more reticulocytes, it can cause falsely normal levels. Falsely normal levels are also reported in recently transfused patients, the patient whose RBCs express the M2 isozyme, and if the sample contains platelet and leukocyte contamination. Careful RBC purification is needed. False positive occurs if samples are not processed quickly. There are no systematic studies on the sensitivity and specificity of available PK activity assays (Bianchi et al. 2019).

8.10.5.3 Molecular Testing for PK

Molecular testing is useful for prenatal diagnosis and in children with borderline enzyme testing or recently transfused for anemia. Other advantages are less complicated handling, including shipping specimens, which can be done with a smaller amount of blood. DNA analysis is time-consuming and relatively expensive. Not every mutation detected by DNA analysis causes abnormal PK activity (Bianchi et al. 2019). A positive result for a mutation should be considered a variant of uncertain significance (VUS) until it is confirmed by PK enzymatic assay, gene reporter assays, RT-PCR analysis, or Western blot (Bianchi et al. 2019). Mutations can occur in both the PKLR gene and the KLF1 gene. Heterozygous mutations in the PKLR gene can also cause other red cell pathologies, such as HS.

8.10.6 Other Glycolytic and Nucleotide Enzymopathies

Other glycolytic disorders are much rarer than PK deficiency. PK deficiency makes up 80% to 90% of all enzymopathies. Glucose phosphate isomerase makes up 3% to 5% of glycolytic enzymopathies and presents moderate to severe chronic non-spherocytic hemolytic anemia (CNSHA) neurologic defects. Pyrimidine 5'nucleotidase affects nucleotide metabolism and comprises 2–3% of all enzymopathies presenting with CNSHA. Other types of enzymopathies make up less than 1%. A definitive diagnosis in the rarer enzymopathies is obtained by molecular testing.

8.11 Normocytic Hemoglobinopathies

The standard common test to diagnose a hemoglobinopathy is hemoglobin electrophoresis, which involves the separation of hemoglobin based on the size and charge of the different types of hemoglobin. With the decreasing cost of DNA sequencing for the evaluation of hemoglobinopathies, this method can give information about the specific mutation to make an accurate diagnosis.

8.11.1 Sickle Cell Disease (SCD)

SCD affects 1 in 365 African-American births but can be found among people from Southern Europe around the Mediterranean Sea, Hispanic, Middle Eastern, or Asian Indian (National Institute of Health 2020). A patient with SCD has a longer lifespan because of newborn screening leading to earlier identification of patients and early initiation of penicillin, immunizations, and disease-modifying medications such as hydroxyurea. In the United States, 94% of patients survive until adulthood (Azar and Wong 2017). The sickle cell mutation is somewhat protective against malaria (Jayavaradhan and Malik 2018). It is an autosomal recessive condition characterized by abnormally sickle-shaped RBC, which impairs blood flow leading to a vaso-occlusive painful crisis leading to chronic tissue ischemia, splenic autoinfarction, RBC hemolysis causing anemia and hyperbilirubinemia, and organ damage (Meier 2018). The sickled erythrocyte's lifespan is 12 to 16 days, resulting in increased erythropoietin production and placing patients at risk for folate deficiency (Meier 2018). Several diagnostic tests are used to diagnose SCD. The tests are listed below:

8.11.1.1 Newborn Screening
Newborns are screened for a hemoglobinopathy as part of newborn screening. The results of newborn screening for a hemoglobinopathy are followed up by special clinics for sickle cell disease in each state. The primary care clinician should be requesting copies of the newborn screen and ensure the proper follow-up is done. The Agency has recommended three methods for Health Care Policy and Research (AHCPR) hemoglobin electrophoresis, isoelectric focusing, and high-performance liquid chromatography.

8.11.1.2 Hemoglobin Electrophoresis
The test is discussed in the section on thalassemia. The most common hemoglobin variants with clinical significance include hemoglobin S, C, and E. Hemoglobin S gene is found in children with origins from the Caribbean, South and Central Africa, Eastern parts of India, and Arabian countries. Hemoglobin C is found in people living in West Africa. Hemoglobin E is found in East India and Southeast Asia (Wahed et al. 2020).

Isoelectric focusing (IEF) method separates the different hemoglobin types because of their charge on a gel medium. While this method does provide a clearer picture of the different kinds of hemoglobin, it is more expensive and requires laboratory staff that are experienced in this method (Ilyas et al. 2020).

High-performance liquid chromatography (HPLC) is another way to detect hemoglobin disorders, and the preferred way of doing this test is called cation-exchange high-performance liquid chromatography (CE-HPLC). Using CE-HPLC, the hemoglobins are separated by net charges at a particular pH. When HPLC and IEP are both used, the sensitivity and specificity are 99%. This test's pitfalls are difficult to do and expensive (Ilyas et al. 2020).

Hemoglobin electrophoresis's limitations include that the test is expensive, complex, time-consuming, bulky, and difficult to perform due to resource-limited places. The methods require the training of laboratory personnel.

Table 8.16 Diagnostic tests for patients with SCD

Test	When to screen	Reason for screening
CBC with WBC differential, reticulocyte count	3 months– 24 months every 3 months >24 months every 6 months	Establish a baseline and evaluate bone marrow function Important when evaluating the child with SCD who presents with fever or is sick
Percent Hb F	6 months–24 months every 6 months >24 months annually	Hemoglobin F has a stronger affinity for oxygen. If the patient has persistent F hemoglobin, he/she is less likely to have a painful crisis
Renal function (creatinine, BUN, urinalysis)	≥12 months annually	Chronic renal disease needs to be picked up early so treatment with ACE inhibitors can begin and referred for renal transplant (Liem et al. 2019)
Hepatobiliary function evaluation of AST and direct bilirubin	≥12 months annually	Patient's with SCD can develop sickle hepatopathy

Adapted from Liem et al. (2019), Yawn et al. (2014)

8.11.1.3 Point-of-Care (POC) Tests for SCD

These tests are available at a low cost and are helpful in resource-limited countries. There are several kinds of POC under study, which include paper tests, smartphone attachments, lateral flow strips, heme chip, aqueous multiphase system, spatio-temporal dynamics analysis, shear gradient microfluidic adhesion (SIGMA) system, electrical impedance microflow cytometry, and microfluidic paper-based devices (Ilyas et al. 2020).

Screening Tests for the Patient with SCD. The NIH Guidelines for management of SCD (Yawn et al. 2014) recommend the following screening tests as seen in Table 8.16:

CBC with Differential and Reticulocyte Count. Aside from a CBC and RC, an RBC phenotype is recommended by 9 W months in case a phenotypic transfusion is needed. When a child with SCD is ill, the child's normal lab values on the CBC are particularly important. While anemia is common in SCD, a drop of more than 2 g/dL in hemoglobin indicates a hematologic crisis. Patients with SCD normally have leukocytosis, but an elevation of >20,000/mm^3 accompanied by a predominance of neutrophils or a left shift increases the clinician's suspicion for infection. Leukopenia associated with marked anemia and reticulocytopenia is suggestive of parvovirus infection. The child's normal platelet count may be elevated. If the child has a low platelet count, hypersplenism should be on the differential diagnosis.

The child's baseline RC should be available. A normal RC accompanies splenic sequestration, whereas an RC that is less than 0.5 indicates an aplastic crisis. Parvovirus is a likely cause of an aplastic crisis in SCD. This aplasia will last the entire course of the disease rather than in the prodrome when an aplasia occurs. When the reticulocyte count is high, a hyperhemolytic crisis is a probable cause.

When the patient is initially on hydroxyurea, a monthly CBC with differential is done to monitor the ANC and the platelet count. After the therapeutic dosage is reached, drawing a CBC with diff, MCV, ALT, creatinine, and RC is done every 2–3 months is suggested to evaluate for toxicity and compliance (Hoppe and Neumayr 2019). The MCV may be elevated if the child is taking the hydroxyurea, but a recent study reported a sensitivity of 35% and a specificity of 71% for an MCV > 100 in patient's compliance to hydroxyurea using this measure to evaluate compliance (Creary et al. 2020).

Several diagnostic tests are used when following a patient with SCD. The tests are listed below:

Ferritin Level. In patients identified as at high risk for stroke by transcranial Doppler, chronic transfusion therapy can reduce stroke risk. If chronic transfusion therapy is initiated, the serum ferritin is monitored to evaluate for iron overload (Hoppe and Neumayr 2019).

RBC Phenotype. In patients on chronic transfusion therapy, alloimmunization can occur. Therefore, alloantibodies (D, Cc, Ec, Kell, Kidd, and Duffy) are evaluated before any transfusion in children with SCD on chronic transfusion therapy to reduce reaction risk (Hoppe and Neumayr 2019).

Liver Function Tests (LFTs). Chronic hemolysis leads to pigmented gallstones in patients with SCD. Generally, indirect or unconjugated bilirubin will be lower than 4 mg/dl in children with SCD. Gallbladder disease is common, and by age 18, 30% of children with SCD develop cholelithiasis (Yawn et al. 2014).

Iron overload occurs due to chronic transfusion and can cause hepatocyte iron overload. ALT/AST may be elevated in the patient. A hepatic crisis can occur in patients with SCD who presents with abdominal pain (Yawn et al. 2014). Liver function tests are done to evaluate for hepatic disease.

Urinalysis and Microalbuminuria/Creatinine Ratio. Once the child reaches age 10, annual urinalysis and microalbumin/creatinine ratio are needed to evaluate renal function (Hoppe and Neumayr 2019). Isosthenuria, or the ability to concentrate urine, occurs in children with SCD, leading to enuresis. The presence of hematuria means that the child may need a renal ultrasound to look for papillary necrosis (Hoppe and Neumayr 2019). Usually, hematuria is self-limited and can be treated with fluids and pain medication (Hoppe and Neumayr 2019). It is important to look for other causes of proteinuria and hematuria (Hoppe and Neumayr 2019). Regular screening of the urine and creatinine level with the evaluation of glomerular filtration rate helps prevent the renal microvasculature complications by initiating an ACE inhibitor or ARB inhibitor (Azar and Wong 2017).

Blood Cultures. Blood cultures are done in children with SCD and fever. Blood cultures are discussed in the chapter on pediatric infections.

Secretory Phospholipase A2. Secretory phospholipase A2 (sPLA2) is an inflammatory mediator responsible for liberating free fatty acids from triglycerides. The test can identify the patient who is presenting with possible acute chest syndrome in children with SCD. The serum concentration increases before the child develops full-blown acute chest syndrome (ACS) and peaks once the clinical presentation is clear and decreased once the ACS is resolving (Styles et al. 1996).

8.12 Bone Marrow Failure/ Dysfunction and Normocytic Anemia

Bone marrow failure leads to poor production of one or all the lines of cellular components in the blood. A pure red cell aplasia can result from an acquired condition or an inherited bone marrow problem and presents with an elevated MCV and a low RC (Noronha 2016). Poor production across all cell lines will present with an elevated MCV, a marked decrease in the RC with low WBC and platelet count.

8.12.1 Transient Bone Marrow Failure Leading to Normocytic Anemia

Primary red cell aplasia includes TEC (transient erythroblastopenia of childhood) and unknown etiology, whereas secondary red cell aplasia includes infections, paraneoplastic syndromes,

and autoimmune disorders. Parvovirus B19, or fifth disease, is one of the most common reasons for this presentation. Parvovirus has an affinity for the red cell precursors, and therefore aplasia occurs when the child is infected. Patients with hemolysis and HIV are more likely to have more severe anemia as they are dependent on the erythrocyte (Noronha 2016).

There is no clear cause of the transient anemia in TEC, which generally takes between a few weeks to a few months to resolve. Occasionally the WBC, platelet count, and Hb will increase above normal values during recovery from TEC. This disease is most common in infancy.

8.12.2 Normocytic Anemia with Pancytopenia

Aplastic anemia, whether from medications, infections, genetic, paroxysmal nocturnal hemoglobinuria (PNH), or idiopathic, is associated with reduced counts of all blood components. PNH is an acquired hematopoietic stem cell defect that causes hemolysis, anemia, and thrombotic complications. The presentation of PNH tends to occur around the time of an aplastic anemia diagnosis but would respond better to immunosuppressive treatment (Savasan 2018). Acquired aplastic anemia is rare, with an estimated 300 to 600 cases per year (Savasan 2018). Idiopathic is the most common (Ishii and Young 2015). Bone marrow failure is also seen in the disease's genetic forms, such as Fanconi anemia, dyskeratosis congenita, and myelophthisic anemia. Inherited problems of bone marrow function can present at any point during the lifespan with progressive anemia. The inherited disorders of hypoplastic or aplastic anemia may also have associated skeletal abnormalities and short statues. These children are also considered to have cancer predisposition syndromes. For example, Fanconi anemia can present with early-onset head and neck tumors. These patients are referred to hematology for diagnosis and management.

The differential diagnosis of bone marrow failure/dysfunction is listed above as well as leukemias and other oncological problems. It should be remembered that head and neck cancers at an early age may occur before the inherited bone marrow failure occurs (Noronha 2016). In the face of anemia, an RC is critical to the development of appropriate differential diagnoses.

The initial evaluation of a pale, sick child should include a CBC with differential, peripheral smear, and an RC. The RC is a marker of effective erythropoiesis and is important in distinguishing hypoproliferative anemia from other forms of anemia (Ishii and Young 2015). In primary care, children who appear sick should be sent for stat lab work to the hospital-based lab or ED for immediate testing if possible. The importance of history and physical cannot be overstressed to recognize the child who needs urgent care. A bone marrow aspiration must be done to confirm the diagnosis of acute lymphocytic leukemia (ALL) (Kaplan 2019) and other bone marrow failure syndromes.

8.12.3 Real-Life Example

A crying, moderately pale 2-year-old presented with croup to the primary care office. The child had a 2-day history of an upper respiratory infection with croup noted during the office. The child was seen during the fall when it is common to see croup. The mother felt that she was in pain since she was crying more than usual. Due to pallor and concerns of pain, a stat CBC with a peripheral smear with RC was ordered, which showed a WBC of 50,000 and 25% blasts, Hb8, Hct of 24, and a platelet count of 74,500. The RC was 0.01%. The child was referred to the ED after notifying the on-call hematologist. The bone marrow aspirate confirmed acute lymphocytic leukemia, precursor B-cell ALL (Kaplan 2019).

8.13 Macrocytosis

A child with an MCV larger than normal and anemia is considered to have macrocytic anemia. Macrocytic anemia is divided into megaloblastic anemia and nonmegaloblastic anemia (Wang 2016).

8.13.1 Megaloblastic Anemia

In children, megaloblastic anemia is a peripheral blood cytopenia due to ineffective hematopoiesis, usually due to B_{12} or folate deficiency. Other causes include inborn errors of metabolism Lesch-Nyhan disease (Cakmakli et al. 2019), drugs including proton pump inhibitors and metformin, surgical gastrectomy, gastric bypass, ileal resection, chemotherapy, folate antagonist (methotrexate), nitrous oxide exposure, and myelodysplastic syndrome or acute myeloid leukemia (Socha et al. 2020). Copper deficiency should be considered in children without B_{12} or folate deficiency (Green and Dwyre 2015).

B_{12} deficiency occurs due to poor nutrition, malabsorption in the small intestine, pancreatic insufficiency, fish tapeworm infestation, Zollinger-Ellison syndrome (a large amount of hydrochloric acid produced by pancreatic tumor preventing the absorption of $B_{12)}$, blind loop syndrome, or drugs such as hydroxyurea or methotrexate (Green and Mitra 2017). It also causes neuropsychiatric features including paresthesia, decreased vibratory and positional sense, cognitive dysfunction, depression, mania, and hallucination (Socha et al. 2020).

Folate deficiency can result from reduced intake (rare in this country but can be related to poverty), diet-induced (goat milk or synthetic diets), hyperalimentation, and prematurity (Green and Mitra 2017). Folate deficiency can be from decreased absorption due to small bowel inflammation, celiac disease, and tropical sprue. Folate deficiency can be from increased demand, such as puberty, pregnancy, chronic hemolytic anemia, hemodialysis, and eczematous conditions (Socha et al. 2020).

Cobalamin-deficient pernicious anemia or pernicious anemia is rare in children as gastric atrophy occurs after 10–20 episodes of asymptomatic autoimmune gastritis (Toh 2017). It is when there is autoimmune destruction of the parietal cells of the small intestine. Remembering that autoimmune disease travels together, gastric autoimmunity occurs in one-third of patients with thyroid autoimmunity and one-tenth of patients with type 1 diabetes (Toh 2017).

The pathophysiology is the result of the destruction of parietal cells. The screening for this will not be discussed as it is largely an adult disease; however, the pathophysiology is important for the reader to understand.

The parietal cells are responsible for the secretion of an intrinsic factor needed to absorb vitamin B_{12}. Once absorbed, it will bind to transcobalamin II; 50% of the B_{12} is then stored in the liver, and the other 50% goes to other body tissues. As a result of the liver's storage of vitamin B_{12}, it can take at least a year before the manifestation of deficiency is seen.

8.13.2 Nonmegaloblastic Anemia

Macrocytic anemia that is nonmegaloblastic means there is no hypersegmented neutrophils seen on a peripheral smear. The macrocytosis can be due to an elevated reticulocyte count, and the larger size of the reticulocyte causes an elevation of the MCV. On the other hand, the reticulocyte count will be low if the macrocytosis is due to bone marrow disorder, hyperthyroidism, or liver disease (Wang 2016). The causes of macrocytosis can be seen in Table 8.17.

Several diagnostic tests are used to diagnose macrocytic anemia. The tests are listed below.

Table 8.17 Causes of macrocytosis

Type of macrocytosis	Differential diagnosis	CBC findings
Megaloblastic macrocytic anemia (MA)	• Most common • Vitamin B_{12} deficiency • Folate deficiency • Drugs including proton pump inhibitors and metformin, folate antagonists (methotrexate), and nitrous oxide • Surgical procedures involved the stomach and the ilium • Myelodysplastic syndrome or acute myeloid leukemia (Socha et al. 2020) • Rarer causes • Errors of metabolism • Lesch-Nyhan disease (Cakmakli et al. 2019)	• RBC is macrocytic, typical oval in appearance • High MCV that may be >120 fL • Hyperpigmented • Bone marrow shows megaloblastoid erythroid precursors • Hypersegmented polymorphonuclear leukocytes (>6 nuclei) may be seen, but greater than 5% containing five nuclei should also alert the clinician to possible MA (Green and Dwyre 2015)
Normoblastic macrocytic anemia	• Reticulocytosis • Hypothyroidism • Chronic liver disease • Pregnancy • Alcoholism	• RBCs are macrocytic • High MCV that is <120 fL • Bone marrow does *not* show megaloblastoid erythroid precursors

Adapted from Cakmakli et al. (2019), Green and Dwyre (2015), Socha et al. (2020); Wang (2016)

8.13.2.1 Peripheral Smear and RC

A child who presents with an elevated MCV and is suspected of having macrocytic anemia needs a peripheral smear to evaluate for hypersegmented neutrophils. Hypersegmented neutrophils would indicate megaloblastic anemia and call for further evaluation of the child's vitamin B_{12} and folate levels. A reticulocyte count should be done to differentiate between reticulocytosis and other problems for the child without hypersegmented neutrophils.

As stated, a low reticulocyte count plus macrocytic anemia would be suspicious for liver disease, hypothyroidism, pregnancy, or alcoholism (Wang 2016).

8.13.2.2 Vitamin B_{12} Level and Folate Levels

Interpreting vitamin B_{12} (cobalamin) and folate levels can be difficult (Ishii and Young 2015). A fasting serum cobalamin of around 200 is the lower limit of normal. A sensitivity as low as 40% has been reported when a cobalamin of less than 300 is used as the lower limit of normal. Generally, a serum B_{12} level of >400 pg/ML rules out B_{12} deficiency (Green and Dwyre 2015). Also, total serum cobalamin levels may not reflect the activity level of cobalamin. Transcobalamin II-bound cobalamin is the only bioavailable cobalamin, which comprises 20% of the total cobalamin level. The rest of serum cobalamin is metabolic unavailable as it is bound to haptocorrin. Changes in the haptocorrin-binding proteins can change the level of cobalamin. False levels of haptocorrin are seen in multiple myeloma, and falsely high levels are seen in myeloproliferative disease (Green and Dwyre 2015).

Serum folate levels reflect the patient's level for the past few days and do not reflect tissue-level deficiencies. Postprandial increases in folate occur, causing false-negative results. A recent blood transfusion will also cause an increase in folate. It is important to order RBC folate levels since this level reflects the past 3 months' tissue levels. However, this test is also low in B_{12} deficiency, and so this test should be used in conjunction with both folate and plasma B_{12} levels (Green and Dwyre 2015). The disadvantage of this test is a slow turnaround and higher costs.

The pitfalls of B_{12} and folate levels are prone to errors, and therefore methylmalonic acid (MMA) and homocysteine levels (Hcy) are better indicators of these vitamin deficiencies. However, these levels are more expensive, and therefore when the serum cobalamin levels are decreased, this test is cost-effective.

8.13.2.3 Methylmalonic Acid (MMA) and Homocysteine (Hcy) Levels

Methylmalonic acid (MMA) and homocysteine (Hcy) levels are more reliable indicators of vitamin deficiencies. MMA is elevated in cobalamin deficiency and is >90% sensitive for detecting cobalamin deficiency with hematologic manifestations. It is considered the most sensitive test for B_{12} deficiency. HCY is less specific and can be elevated in both folate and cobalamin deficiency, vitamin B_6 deficiency, hypothyroidism, enzyme genetic defects, and methotrexate and phenytoin treatment. Both MMA and Hcy may be elevated in renal insufficiency (Ishii and Young 2015).

8.13.2.4 Circulating Anti-Intrinsic Factor Antibodies (CAFA)

The CAFA looks for the antibodies that cause pernicious anemia. While it is a highly specific test with very few false positives, it is not sensitive as it is positive in only 60% of patients (Green and Dwyre 2015).

> **Key Learning Regarding Macrocytic Anemia**
> - Macrocytic anemia is divided into megaloblastic anemia and nonmegaloblastic anemia.
> - B_{12} and folate levels are prone to errors.
> - Methylmalonic acid (MMA) is the most sensitive test for B_{12} deficiency.

Bleeding Disorders

This section will review platelet disorders and common bleeding disorders. Primary care clinicians may be the first to identify children with bleeding disorders. Advances in X-ray

Table 8.18 Congenital and acquired disorders of platelet size

Congenital disorders associated with small platelets	Congenital disorders associated with large platelets
• Wiskott-Aldrich syndrome—Congenital mutation of WAS, wIPF-1 gene: X-linked mutation associated with eczema, immune deficiency, and thrombocytopenia • X-linked thrombocytopenia similar but milder mutation of the WAS gene • Inherited microthrombocyte	• MYH9 gene mutation-related disease—Autosomal dominant—Variably presents problems including nephritis, growth hormone deficiency, high-frequency hearing loss, glaucoma, cataracts, and familial spastic paraplegia o Epstein syndrome o Fechtner syndrome o Sebastian syndrome o May-Hegglin anomaly • 22q11.2 deletion syndrome o DiGeorge syndrome o Velocardiofacial syndrome (Rosa et al. 2011) – Associated with Bernard-Soulier syndrome due to mutation in GP1b, and if they have this, they will have large platelets • Platelet granule defects o Gray platelet syndrome and Quebec platelet syndrome o Chediak-Higashi syndrome associated with immunodeficiencies and neutropenia

Adapted from Haley (2020), Sharma et al. (2018)

crystallography have deepened our understanding of the interactions between factors, allowing for the development of a host of new anticoagulants. The section has been divided into platelet and bleeding disorders. A review of the function of the platelet is seen at the beginning of the chapter.

Hemostasis involves the formation of a clot at the site of injury. Hemostasis is a collaboration of the endothelial cells of the blood vessels, proteins in the plasma, and blood cells (primarily platelets) (Olson 2015). However, the two major components of clotting are the coagulation components and platelets. These two systems are intimately related (Winter et al. 2020). While the process of coagulation is complex, this review is adequate for this chapter.

Simply put, coagulation and its breakup have three components:

Box 8.1 Key Bleeding History and Physical Exam Points

Key Bleeding History Points

• Is there a family history of bleeding after surgery, childbirth, tooth extraction, and easy bruisability?

• Does the child take any medications, including the use of aspirin or nonsteroidal medications?
• Have you noted any other bleeding, especially when brushing teeth or excessive bruising following falls?
• Is there a history of nose bleeding, including the length of time of bleeding and frequency?
• Has the child had bleeding after dental procedures or pulling out baby teeth?
• In an adolescent female, the use of the pictorial blood loss assessment chart (Fig. 8.2) needs to be done to assess menstrual bleeding. Also, the following questions should help you get a complete picture:
  • How long does your period last from the start of bleeding to the end of bleeding?
    • <7 days
    • ≥7 days
    • Unsure.
  • Do you ever experience "flooding" or "gushing" during your period?
    • Never, rarely, or some periods.
    • Every or most periods.
    • Unsure.

- Do you ever bleed through a tampon or napkin in 2 h or less?
  - Never, rarely, or some periods.
  - Every or most periods.
  - Unsure (adapted from American College of Obstetricians and Gynecologists [ACOG] 2019).
- Do you have liver disease?
- Has anyone in the family been diagnosed with a bone marrow disorder?
- Is there a family or child history of problems with platelets or bleeding?
- Has the child had unexplained anemia?
- Standard bleeding assessment tools can be helpful:
  - International Society on Thrombosis and Hemostasis Bleeding Assessment Tool or ISTH-BAT is a hemostasis bleeding assessment tool found at https://bleedingscore.certe.nl/:
    - This one is shortened and easier to use in a clinical setting.
    - A score greater than 2 is positive in children (Rodeghiero et al. 2019).
  - The Pediatric Bleeding Questionnaire (PBQ) was originally developed for VWD but can assess bleeding in pediatrics. The link is found here: https://www.ahcdc.ca/storage/files/pediatric-bleeding-questionnaire-scoring-key.pdf.
- Does the family have a history of deafness, renal insufficiency, albinism, or immunodeficiency?

Key Physical Examination Pointers
- Assess for hypermobility patients with Ehlers-Danlos (ED) using the Beighton scale (https://ehlers-danlos.com/wp-content/uploads/002513_beighton-score-a-valid-measure-for-generalized-hypermobility-in-children.pdf). Children with ED have easy bruisability (Rodeghiero et al. 2019).
- Assess for hepatomegaly, splenomegaly, and lymphadenopathy.
- Assess for fever.
- Consider child abuse if bruising does not fit the normal pattern or is unusual in appearance:
  - TEN-4:
    - Bruising in a child less than 4 that is on the torso (chest, abdomen, back, genital region, or buttock), ears, or neck.
  - TEN-4 FACESp (more sensitive and specific than TENS-4):
    - Add bruising to the frenulum, the angle of the jaw, the cheek, eyelids, or subconjunctival hemorrhage (Kairys 2020).
- Telangiectasias in nasal mucosa indicate hereditary hemorrhagic telangiectasia.
- Look around pressure areas for petechiae, including bra straps, bookbag straps, and waistband.
- Hematomas around joints are associated with factor deficiencies.

Adapted from Haley 2020; Kairys 2020; Rodeghiero et al. 2019; Sharma et al. 2018

- Primary hemostasis occurs when following injury to the vessel's endothelium, a platelet plug is formed by vasoconstriction, platelet adhesion, and aggregation. Thrombin activates platelets; factors V, VIII, XI, and XII; and von Willebrand factor. These coagulation factors are a series of proteins that control soluble plasma fibrinogen into insoluble fibrin that traps RBC and platelets. Liver hepatocytes primarily produce these coagulation factors except for factor VIII, which is also produced by the lymphatic system (Winter et al. 2020).
- Coagulation occurs (secondary hemostasis).
- Fibrinolysis occurs, breaking up the clot into its degradation products, with plasmin being the central enzyme. Tissue plasminogen activator is plasmin's activator (Van Herrewegen et al. 2012).

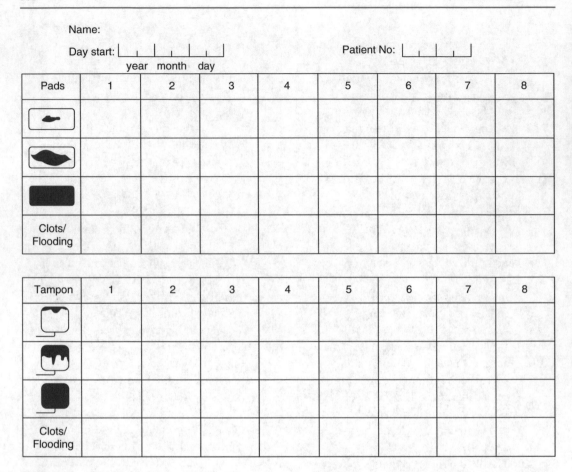

Fig. 8.2 Pictorial blood loss assessment chart for menstruating females

8.14 Disorder of Platelets

Platelet disorders include thrombocytosis, thrombocytopathia (impaired platelet function), and thrombocytopenia. Disorders of platelet frequently present with bleeding of the mucous membranes or under the skin (Sharma et al. 2018). Thus, the presence of petechiae or bleeding when brushing the teeth should alert the clinician to a platelet problem. Congenital problems with platelets present in three ways—congenital thrombocytopenia with small, normal-sized, and large platelets. These will be discussed below and can be seen in Table 8.18.

It is important to take a complete bleeding history as well as do a complete physical exam. A platelet problem can occur as part of a complete cytopenia. Key bleeding history and physical exam points are seen in Box 8.1.

8.14.1 Thrombocytopathia (Impaired Platelet Function)

Impaired functions of platelet can lead to hemorrhage, prolonged bleeding time, and abnormal clot formation. The congenital causes of thrombocytopathia include von Willebrand disease (VWD), Chediak-Higashi syndrome (associated with oculocutaneous albinism (OCA), immune deficiency, neurological dysfunction), Hermansky-Pudlak syndrome (pulmonary fibrosis and OCA), storage pool disorders, secretion defects, and Glanzmann thrombasthenia. The most commonly acquired form of platelet dysfunction is drug-induced thrombocytopathia.

The mean platelet volume (MPV) reflects the size of the platelets. Table 8.18 reviews congenital disorders associated with small or large platelets. Children with normal platelet size, but dysfunctional platelets, may have skeletal abnormalities and have amegakaryocytic thrombocytopenia or thrombocytopenia with absent radii (Sharma et al. 2018). Several other rare congenital genetic disorders present with normal platelet size including autosomal dominant and autosomal recessive (Sharma et al. 2018). Some of the platelet disorders are associated with hematological malignancy. As a result, referral to a hematologist is recommended to diagnose patients with platelet function disorders and decide on follow-up.

8.14.2 Thrombocytopenia

The definition of thrombocytopenia is a platelet count of less than 150,000/L. Pseudothrombocytopenia occurs when platelets clump. Clumping occurs when the patient's blood is mixed with the EDTA found in the CBC tube and can be corrected when the blood is drawn and put in a heparinized or citrated tube. Thrombocytopenia is usually not clinically apparent until the count falls below 50,000, and the risk of clinically important spontaneous bleeding does not occur until this number occurs (Haley 2020). A systematic review points out the most severe bleeding events occurred with a platelet count of less than 30,000 (Neunert et al. 2015).

8.14.2.1 Acquired Thrombocytopenia
Fetal or Neonatal Alloimmune Thrombocytopenia (FNAIT). FNAIT is the most common cause of severe thrombocytopenia in the neonate, with platelet counts less than 50,000. It results from the neonate acquiring paternal antigens that the mother does not have, leading to maternal antibody production. The antibodies then cross the placenta and destroy fetal platelets, which can lead to intracranial bleeding. FNAIT can occur during the first pregnancy, and there is a high rate of recurrence in each subsequent pregnancy (Haley 2020).

Immune-Mediated Thrombocytopenia (ITP). ITP is the autoimmune destruction of platelets that can be primary or secondary to various systemic diseases such as SLE, AIHA, HIV, and CLL (Sharma et al. 2018). It is defined as a platelet count of less than 100,000. It is classified as newly diagnosed when the ITP has lasted between 0 and 3 months and persistent when it lasts from 3 months to 12 months. When the ITP has lasted greater than 12 months, it is considered chronic. Severe disease is characterized by bleeding rather than the actual platelet count (Lo and Deane 2014). It is caused by immune dysregulation, and there is the production of autoantibodies to platelet antigens and megakaryocytes. Typically, the child is well appearing and may have petechiae, bruising, or mucosal bleeding. The child has a normal physical exam, and a bone marrow aspiration is not typically done (Haley 2020). Children tend to have more severe thrombocytopenia, but only 3% will have any clinically significant bleeding, and the risk of intracranial hemorrhage is only 1%. Most children will recover spontaneously and can be managed on an outpatient basis with a CBC done weekly (Lo and Deane 2014).

Drug-Induced Thrombocytopenia. Drug-induced antibodies can induce platelet abnormalities, neutropenia, and autoimmune anemia (Aster and Bougie 2007). In this disease, the thrombocytopenia usually occurs 1 to 2 weeks following a drug's initiation but can occur in the first 2 days or hours (Haley 2020). The medication induces the antibodies, and when the drug is removed, the platelets will return to normal within a week. The most well-known medications to induce thrombocytopenia are nonsteroidal anti-inflammatory drugs (NSAIDs).

Thrombotic Thrombocytopenic Purpura (TTP). TTP is a rare disorder in children characterized by thrombotic microangiopathy and acquired or congenital deficiency in the gene ADAMTS13 (Joly et al. 2018). Lab manifestations of TTP include thrombocytopenia with high reticulocyte count, undetectable levels of haptoglobin, elevated LDH, and schistocytes on the smear (Joly et al. 2018). There are two types of assays available to test for a deficiency in ADAMTS13, functional and immunochemical (Joly et al. 2018). Functional assays using collagen-binding activity are time-consuming and labor-intensive. In contrast, the ELISA-based immunochemical assays are faster but less accurate and cannot be used in an emergency (Joly et al. 2018).

8.14.3 Thrombocytosis

Thrombocytosis or a platelet count over 450,000 per liter can be secondary or primary. The primary disorders are primarily inherited by autosomal dominant fashion. The disorders of primary thrombocytosis are related to alterations of the cells of the bone marrow. They can be essential or reflect a myeloproliferative disorder. The most common secondary thrombocytosis is from an infection, inflammation, iron deficiency, or neoplasms.

Reactive thrombocytosis is the most common type of thrombocytosis. The types and causes include transient elevations due to acute blood loss, infection, inflammation (third phase of Kawasaki disease), and extreme physical exertion or can be more sustained, which is seen in iron deficiency, hemolytic anemia, chronic inflammation, chronic infection, and asplenia or possibly but much rarer drug reaction (Schafer 2015). The underlying causes of thrombocytosis need to be determined.

Clonal thrombocytosis is much rarer, and causes include myeloproliferative neoplasms.

8.14.4 Diagnostic Testing for Platelet Disorders

8.14.4.1 CBC with Peripheral Smear

A CBC with a peripheral smear is important when evaluating the child with petechiae. When the platelet count is elevated, it is important to repeat it the next day (Schafer 2015). A peripheral smear is important to exclude the possibility of a myeloproliferative disorder, aplastic anemia, or malignancy (Sharma et al. 2018).

8.14.4.2 Immature Platelet Fraction (IPF)

Increased turnover of platelets may lead to giant platelet. Increased turnover will be reflected in the immature platelet fraction (IPF). The IPF assesses the bone marrow response to thrombocytopenia. The IPF will increase in peripheral platelet destruction and will be normal or decreased in bone marrow failure (Haley 2020).

8.14.4.3 Standard Platelet Aggregometry

The gold standard of testing platelet function is light transmission aggregometry (LTA). This method is labor-intensive, requires a large amount of blood, and may not be readily available. A platelet function analyzer is more readily available but has definite limitations. The results can show a prolonged platelet time when the patient has anemia, takes NSAIDS, has VWD, or has thrombocytopenia. It excludes the more serious platelet function disorders such as severe von Willebrand disease or Glanzmann thrombasthenia. Still, it fails to rule out less severe VWD and platelet storage pool disorders (Haley 2020).

8.14.4.4 Bleeding Time

Bleeding time has low sensitivity and cannot differentiate between primary hemostatic defects. This test has fallen out of favor.

8.14.4.5 Thromboelastography

This method evaluates clot formation and whole blood strength. It is a point of care in which whole blood is added to an oscillating cup and a transducer detects the clot formation. This test is not used in an outpatient setting and is used primarily in the ED, ICU, or operating room (Haley 2020).

8.14.4.6 Next-Generation Sequencing (NGS)

There are at least 40 identified genes as causes of thrombocytopenia (Nurden and Nurden 2020). However, NGS is more likely to be covered by insurance if ordered from a specialty clinician. There is a separate chapter on the different genetic types of testing.

8.14.4.7 Additional Lab Tests for Autoimmune Platelet Disorders

Renal function, direct antiglobulin testing, prothrombin time, partial thromboplastin time, and immunoglobulins are all tests that should be done to evaluate the child with ITP.

8.14.5 Real-Life Example

A 9-year-old presented for a well-child visit without any complaints. During the physical exam, petechiae were noted at the ankle. The child did not remember any recent injury. A CBC, differential, and peripheral smear were obtained at the lab, which showed normal WBC and RBC indices and a normal peripheral smear. However, the platelet count was 50,000, so immune thrombocytopenia was suspected. The hematologist confirmed the diagnosis. The child's thrombocytopenia resolved with the use of Promacta/romiplostim (TPO-RA).

8.15 Coagulation Disorder: Bleeding

As discussed, coagulation is a cascade that leads to fibrin formation and interactions between protein coagulation factors. Coagulation disorders can be congenital (primary) or acquired (secondary), especially in a sick child. Vitamin K deficiency is common and can result from inadequate intake or malabsorption due to gastrointestinal problems, including cystic fibrosis, biliary atresia, or α-1 antitrypsin deficiency. Vitamin K is important in the production of coagulation factors II, VII, IX, and X.

Bleeding disorders can be due to primary deficiencies of one of the many clotting factors. Children with a bleeding disorder may not present in early childhood. Adolescent girls may not be identified as having a bleeding disorder until the onset of menses. A history of bleeding symptoms or a family history of VWD in a first-degree relative is a red flag, and laboratory assessment for VWD or another bleeding disorder is warranted (Castaman and Linart 2017). A history of menorrhagia in early adolescence in a patient with a bleeding disorder can be associated with acute anemia and hemorrhage (Graham et al. 2018). ACOG (2019) recently recommended that females with menorrhagia be screened for a bleeding disorder.

The differential diagnosis of a child with signs of bleeding in the form of petechiae and purpura on the skin ranges from benign to serious. The child with petechiae above the nipple line is most likely from a benign cause such as severe vomiting or coughing to streptococcal pharyngitis. Petechia or purpura below the nipple line in a sick appearing child is more concerning and can indicate sepsis or Rocky Mountain spotted fever. The child with RMSF usually has a high WBC with bandemia, thrombocytopenia, and/or hyponatremia (Black 2014). The child with hemolytic uremic syndrome will present with renal failure, non-immune Coombs-negative hemolytic anemia, and thrombocytopenia. The child will have an abnormal urinalysis but will also have unexplained petechiae and purpura.

Most epistaxis in children is from the anterior nasal tract. The child who presents with epistaxis most commonly has digital picking of the nasal cavity as the cause. However, other causes include congenital malformation in the nasal cavity such as arteriovenous malformation or hemangioma; infections such as sinusitis or upper respiratory tract infection; neoplasms such as lymphoma or rhabdomyosarcoma; iatrogenic from medications such as NSAIDs; allergic rhinitis; bleeding disorder such as von Willebrand's; or inflammatory effects of systemic lupus or granulomatosis with polyangiitis (Syider et al. 2018).

8.15.1 von Willebrand Disease (VWD)

VWD is the most common inherited bleeding problem, with estimates of incidence ranging from 0.1% to 1% (Castaman and Linart 2017; O'Brien and Saini 2019; Sharma and Flood 2017). It is inherited in an autosomal fashion and is caused by a deficiency or abnormality in the von Willebrand factor (VWF). A gene encodes VWF on the

Table 8.19 Understanding the types of VWD

Type of VWD	Degree and kind of deficiency	Important points
Type 1	• Autosomal dominant • Partial quantitative deficiency of VWF	• Common: 60% to 70% of all cases • Patients with levels of VWF between 30 and 50 IU/dL with bleeding symptoms may fall outside of the strict criteria for type 1 VWD • Mild decrease in VWF/ag and platelet-dependent VWF activity • Normal to mild FVIII
All types of type 2	• Usually autosomal dominant except for 2n, which is autosomal recessive • Qualitative deficiency of VWF	• Qualitative deficiency accounts for 25% to 30% of all cases
Type 2A	• Predominantly autosomal dominant • A decrease in platelet function with defects in dimerization, multimer storage, molecular weight VWF multimer	• Recessive forms are rare • Mild decrease in VWF/ag and a moderate decrease in platelet dependent VWF activity • Normal to mild FVIII
Type 2B	• Autosomal dominant • Increased affinity of VWF for platelet GP1bα with increased clearance of these platelet-VWF aggregates	• Mild thrombocytopenia • Mild decrease in VWF/ag and a moderate decrease in platelet-dependent VWF activity • Normal to mild FVIII
Type 2 M	• Autosomal dominant • Reduced VWF binding to platelet glycoprotein (GP1bα) or collagen	• Mild decrease in VWF/ag and a moderate decrease in platelet dependent VWF activity • Normal to mild FVIII
Type 2 N	• Autosomal recessive • Markedly decreased binding of VWF to factor VIII and decreased half-life of factor VIII • Defective binding of factor VIII to VWF	• This leads to loss of factor VIII abilities to carry VWF • Gets misdiagnosed as mild hemophilia type A due to aPTT prolongation and low factor VIII levels • Mild decrease in VWF/ag and a moderate decrease in platelet-dependent VWF activity • Normal to mild FVIII
Type 3	• Autosomal recessive • Almost complete deficiency of VWF	• Large deletions in VWF • This leads to loss of factor VIII abilities to carry VWF • Severe decrease in VWF/ag and severe decrease in platelet-dependent VWF activity • Mild to moderate FVIII

Adapted from Castaman and Linart (2017), Ng and Di Paola 2018; O'Brien and Saini (2019)

short arm of chromosome 12, leading to a large glycoprotein. VWF is important in primary and secondary hemostasis. The disease presents with easy bruisability, menorrhagia, and mucocutaneous bleeding (Castaman and Linart 2017).

The diagnosis is made by combining the signs and symptoms of bleeding and laboratory evidence of qualitative or quantitative deficiencies (Ng and Di Paola 2018). There is a wide range of bleeding problems depending on the type of von Willebrand. Types 1 and 3 cause a quantitative VWD, where types 2A, 2B, 2 M, and 2 N cause qualitative abnormalities. As the type of VWD increases from 1 to 3, the degree of bleeding is more severe. Several guidelines report that a VWF level of less than 30% is diagnostic for

Table 8.20 Severity of factor VIII and IX deficiencies

Bleeding phenotype	Factor activity
Severe	Factor activity less than 1 IU/dl
Moderate	Factor activity of 1 to <5 IU/dL
Mild	Factor activity 5 to <50 IU/dL

Adapted from Croteau 2018

VWD (Castaman and Linart 2017); however, levels between 30% and 50% are considered low. Table 8.19 outlines the common types of VWD.

8.15.2 Primary Factor Deficiencies

Primary factor deficiencies can range from hemophilia A and B (due to a deficiency of factor

VIII and IX, respectively) to rarer disorders of fibrinogen and factors II, V, VII, X, XI, and XIII or a combination of factors V and VIII (Castaman and Linart 2017). While it is an X-linked disease of males, female carriers can have FVIII or FIX levels around 50 IU/dL, and some have clinically significant bleeding. Females with Turner syndrome, uniparental disomy, skewed lyonization, or variants of compound heterozygous pathogenic variants can have moderate to severe deficiency (Croteau 2018).

The hallmark of FVIII and FIX deficiency is bleeding into the joints or hemarthrosis. The ankles, knees, and elbows are the most commonly affected joints. Excessive bleeding can occur within an organ after minor trauma. While musculoskeletal bleeding is considered characteristic of hemophilia, mucosal bleeding and epistaxis are common. Prolonged bleeding post circumcision, a large cephalohematoma after birth, or intracranial hemorrhage after minimal birth trauma in males with Factor VIII or FIX deficiency can occur (Croteau 2018). If the deficiency is mild, the presentation can occur in school age or adolescence. The severity levels are seen in Table 8.20:

Vitamin K malabsorption or deficiency can lead to bleeding. Newborns are supplemented with 0.5–1 mg of vitamin K at birth to avoid bleeding. Vitamin K is critical for activating coagulation factors II (prothrombin), VII, IX, and X, with normal values not occurring until 6 months of age (Stachowiak and Furman 2020).

Liver disease results in clotting problems by two mechanisms: (1) the decreased bile salt synthesis causes impaired vitamin K absorption and results in deficiency, and (2) clotting factor production occurs in the liver and is impaired in liver disease.

The initial standard screening recommended in the 2019 guidelines by the European Hematology Association (EHA) in a patient who presents with bleeding but a negative screen on the ISTH-BAT with a score less than 2 in children is CBC with differential with a peripheral smear, prothrombin time (PT), activated partial thromboplastin time (aPTT), and fibrinogen. If the ISTH-BAT is >2 or there is unusual bleeding in infancy, the EHA recommends two additional tests—VWF activity and standard platelet aggregometry (Rodeghiero et al. 2019).

Citrated plasma is the most common substrate used for coagulation testing in the lab. Citrate prevents coagulation and allows preservation of the sample. The sample is then centrifuged to

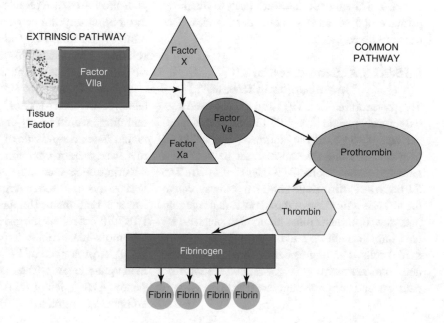

Fig. 8.3 Extrinsic and common pathway of coagulation

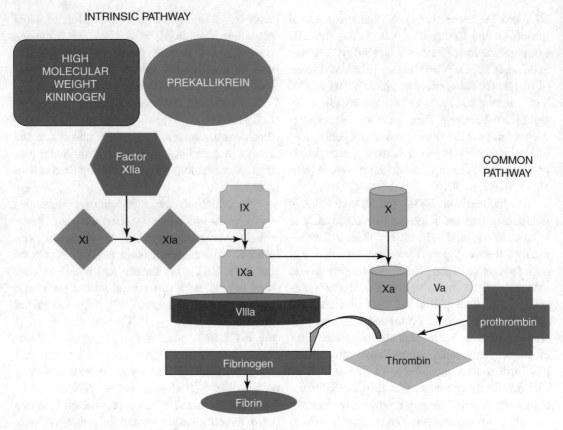

Fig. 8.4 Intrinsic and common pathway of coagulation

generate a platelet-poor plasma before the measurement of the coagulation factors occurs.

Several diagnostic tests are used to diagnose primary and secondary factor deficiencies. The tests are listed below:

8.15.2.1 Activated Partial Thromboplastin Time (aPTT)

The prothrombin time (PT) and the activated partial thromboplastin time (aPTT) measure the functioning of the extrinsic, intrinsic, and common pathway, and their measures must be done in a platelet-free environment (Winter et al. 2020). The PT tests the extrinsic and common pathway, where the aPTT is a function of the intrinsic and common pathway. Both tests must be done in platelet-free environment with no leukocytes, RBCs, or endothelial cells. The figures below show the extrinsic and common pathway (Fig. 8.3) and the intrinsic pathway and common pathway (Fig. 8.4).

An aPTT is done when plasma and negatively charged surfaces such as silica or kaolin with a phospholipid extract free of tissue factor (partial thromboplastin) are activated. This takes several minutes and follows by adding calcium chloride solution to cause a clot formation with the intrinsic pathway (Winter et al. 2020).

An aPTT monitors active concentrations of hemophilia factors (factor VIII and factor IV). It, therefore, would be an important test if the clinician notes deep tissue or joint bleeding. While this was once a common test used to monitor heparin effectiveness, the new chromogenic heparin assays used today target factor Xa, and, to a lesser extent, factor IIa, therefore monitoring the PTT will not reflect the effectiveness of the newer low-molecular-weight heparins (Winter et al. 2020). A prolonged aPTT is usually the result of inadequate levels of factors VIII (antihemophilic factor [AHF]), factor IX (plasma thromboplastin component), or factor XI (plasma thromboplastin antecedent). The plasma levels of factor VIII must be reduced for the aPTT to be prolonged. As shown above, the prekallikrein is a major player in initiating the contact pathway, and when it is absent, the PTT is prolonged. About 75% of prekallikrein is bound to high-molecular-weight kininogen (HMWK) or the "Fitzgerald factor."

The cleavage of HMWK by activated prekallikrein results in the release of bradykinin. Bradykinin increases vascular permeability and vasodilation, leading to angioedema (Winter et al. 2020). While the contact pathway that initiates the intrinsic factor and common pathway that is measured in the APTT is not directly involved in hemostasis, it is important in thrombosis, inflammation, and complement activation.

8.15.2.2 Prothrombin Time (PT)

Tissue factor is a cell surface protein. As shown in Fig. 8.2, the tissue factor is the driver of the extrinsic and common pathway, which forms coagulated plasma within 15 seconds. In determining the PT, an extract rich in tissue factor and phospholipids is added to the patient plasma. By adding the TF and the patient's factor VIIa, there is factor X's activation to factor Xa. This ultimately converts prothrombin to thrombin. Warfarin's effectiveness as a drug is best measured via the PT as this pathway is vitamin K dependent except for factor V and fibrinogen. The PT measures how long it takes for a patient to clot.

The international normalized ratio or INR is standardized for the PT for patients on warfarin using the international sensitivity index (ISI) of the thromboplastin reagent. The ideal reagent has an ISI close to 1.0. If the patient's INR is too low, the patient is at risk for a clot, whereas if the INR is too high, the patient is at risk for bleeding. The INR is directly derived from the patient's PT and is calculated as a ratio of the patient's PT to a control PT standardized for the potency of the thromboplastin reagent developed by the World Health Organization (WHO). The formula is seen below:

$$INR = Patient\,PT \div Control\,PT^{ISI}$$

While a normal INR for a patient on anticoagulants is generally between 2 and 3, this value must be individualized based on the patient's characteristics, prescription and nonprescription medications, comorbid conditions, and diet (Fig. 8.4).

8.15.2.3 Platelet Function Analyzer (PFA)

The PFA has excellent sensitivity for picking up severe VWF deficiency, but it is far less sensitive in the mild type 1 VWD (O'Brien and Saini 2019).

8.15.2.4 von Willebrand Factor Antigen VWF:Ag

VWF:Ag measures the total amount of VWF protein in a sample. It was done by enzyme-linked immunosorbent assay (ELISA) in the past. Today latex immunoassay (LIA) is the usual method used due to its ease of use and speed. Normal levels are between 50 and 200 IU/dL.

8.15.2.5 Functional Assessment of von Willebrand Factor

Ristocetin-based platelet binding testing (VWF:RCo) is used to assess the patient's plasma VWF ability to agglutinate platelets since ristocetin mimics the stress that causes VWF to bind to platelets. This test may be falsely positive in some African Americans. The test is prone to error due to intralaboratory and interlaboratory variability. VWF:PG1bm assays help diagnose type 2 VWD and have greater sensitivity and precision than ristocetin-based tests.

8.15.2.6 von Willebrand Factor Collagen Binding (VWF:CB)

VWF:CB uses ELISA methodology to test VWF binding to collagen, but these assays lack interlaboratory standardization. They are used when the traditional testing falls to identify the patient as having VWD, but the clinical suspicion is strong.

There are several pitfalls for tests involving VWF. Benign variations can occur. VWF is lower in patients with type O blood. Higher VWF/AG levels are higher in people of African-American heritage, but the VWF ristocetin cofactor activity is similar. There is a greater likelihood of a polymorphism in the VWF gene in African Americans that decreases ristocetin-dependent binding of VWF to platelet GP1bα, but this is a laboratory finding rather than a bleeding risk (O'Brien and Saini 2019).

VWF is an acute-phase reactant that may be elevated in patients with an inflammatory condition, exercise, and stress. VWF increases with age, and therefore the levels must be taken into consideration to the patient's clinical presentation (Sharma and Flood 2017).

Early studies reported that VWF might be higher in women taking estrogen, but subsequent studies found it was normal in healthy women who are nonsmokers. If the patient is being evaluated for bleeding due to menorrhagia and is on estrogen therapy, estrogen should not be stopped. However, if the results of the VWF are borderline, then it may be needed (O'Brien and Saini 2019).

Sample collection for all testing involving VWF should be done with a large-bore needle and should be as atraumatic as possible. A struggling or crying child or an anxious older child or adolescent and inflammation or recent exercise can increase VWF and factor VIII. The agitation of the sample by the lab technician or extremes of temperature during transport or storage can lead to false abnormalities (O'Brien and Saini 2019).

8.15.2.7   Other Tests

There are a variety of other tests used by specialists. They include von Willebrand factor propeptide (looking for VWF clearance), stabilizing factor VIII, factor VII-binding capacity, and low-dose ristocetin-induced platelet aggregation.

8.15.2.8   Genetic Analysis

Genetic testing for most patients with type 2 VWD and type 3 is helpful, but in type 1 VWD, the missense mutations are reported within the entire VWF gene. Also, especially with patients with 30% to 50% of the normal levels of VWD, the genetic variant causing the mutation is not clear. The clinician must keep up with changes in the genetic analysis as this field is constantly changing.

8.15.2.9   Mixing Studies

A mixing study evaluates whether 50% of the concerning coagulation factor's activity is present in the patient's serum. If the patient has a clotting factor deficiency, mixing the patient's plasma with 100% of the normal factor will result in at least 50% in the normal. Therefore, the PT or PTT will be normal when run after mixing the patient's serum with the normal plasma indicating a factor deficiency. If there is an inhibitor in the patient's serum, the mixing study will not correct the low factor, and therefore the patient has an inhibitor that is causing the problem. An inhibitor's presence means that the 1:1 mix will yield normal PT and PTT right after the mixing, but if the mixed serum is incubated for 1–2 h, the results will become abnormal. Thus, a mixing study determines the cause of the factor deficiency (Choi et al. 2016).

8.15.2.10   Factor VIII

Factor VIII is one of the essential coagulation proteins. Factors VIII and IX are the two hemophilia factors with deficiencies of either factor, causing deep muscle or joint bleeding. The traditional way of measuring factor VIII activity is a one-stage clot-based assay and is a modified aPTT. Chromogenic or amidolytic two-stage factor VII assay can further clarify limitations in vitro activity measurements (Winter et al. 2020). Chromogenic assays do not use a factor-deficient plasma and do not use an aPTT clot-based reaction. Factor VIII plasma levels can be measured by one- and two-stage chromogenic assays, yet these assays cannot accurately measure factor levels less than 1 IU/L (Peyvandi et al. 2016). In male patients with mild to moderate hemophilia, both assays are recommended to diagnose non-severe hemophilia (Winter et al. 2020).

Decreased or deficient levels of this factor lead to hemophilia A, which can present with mild to severe bleeding. Increased factor VIII levels put patients at higher risk for deep vein thrombosis and pulmonary embolism (Jenkins et al. 2012). Patients with any deficiency in factor VIII should be managed in conjunction with a hematologist.

8.16 Coagulation Disorder: Clotting

A thrombophilia workup may be completed for patients who present with VTE and have a strong family history of VTE or other risk factors (i.e., surgery, oral contraceptives, immobilization for long periods). There are evolving guidelines regarding the initiation of thrombophilia workup (Ashraf et al. 2019), which center around whether the knowledge of an inherited thrombophilia will change the management of the patient. A family history of VTE should be taken before prescribing a drospirenone birth control pill (ACOG 2020). The clinician should refer to US Medical Eligibility Criteria for Contraceptive Use (CDC 2020). A referral to a hematologist should be considered if a thrombophilia workup is needed. College of American Pathologists recommends thrombophilia testing for pediatric patients if they have a personal history of VTE or arterial thrombosis. Both the American College of Medical Genetics and the College of American Pathologists recommend against testing for methyltetrahydrofolate reductase (MTHFR) polymorphism as part of the workup for thrombophilia (Hickey et al. 2013).

8.16.1 COVID-19 and Coagulation

With the recent pandemic caused by COVID-19, coagulopathies have garnered increasing attention due to coagulopathies being reported in even young patients. Several changes in circulating prothrombotic factors, including an increase in factor VIII and fibrinogen, are why there has been an increase in venous thromboembolism (VTE). The hypercoagulable state is called thromboinflammation or COVID-19-associated coagulopathy (Al-Subaie 2021). An elevation of D-dimer is a consistent finding in patients with COVID-19. The inflammation in COVID-19 is likely responsible for activating the coagulation cascade, leading to increased coagulation-related problems in patients with COVID (Al-Subaie 2021). D-Dimer can also be a marker of the severity of the disease in COVID (Lima et al. 2020).

8.16.2 Factor V Leiden

Factor V Leiden (FVL) is a mutation in the FV gene, which leads to a poor response to activated protein C, resulting in increased thrombin generation and placing the patient at increased risk for clotting. FVL is inherited and prevents protein C/protein S complex from inactivating factor V. It is the most common inherited thrombophilia and is the most common genetic risk factor for VTE (Kujovich 2011). This test requires patient or parent consent.

8.16.3 Protein C

Protein C reduces thrombin formation and acts as an anticoagulant. Therefore, decreased plasma levels increase a patient's risk of thromboembolism (Oto et al. 2020). At least 16 different assays are available to test a patient's activated protein C (Oto et al. 2020).

8.16.4 Protein S

Protein S is a vitamin K-dependent plasma glycoprotein found mainly in the liver (ten Kate and van der Meer 2008). It has many functions, including direct inhibition of the tenase and prothrombinase complexes, a cofactor to protein C, and involvement in fibrinolysis (ten Kate and van der Meer 2008). There are two types of protein S assays available: clotting assays that measure activated protein C cofactor activity and immunoassays that measure total and free protein S levels (ten Kate and van der Meer 2008).

8.16.5 Testing for Thrombophilia

The tests below are tests commonly performed as part of a thrombophilia workup and are included in the chapter for the reader's knowledge. They are not recommended to be done in a primary care setting. Testing should only be undertaken in patients at an increased risk and who would benefit from screening for thrombophilia. The tests for thrombophilia screening are not perfect. Therefore, a negative screening should not be interpreted as the patient not having an inherited VTE risk (Ashraf et al. 2019).

8.16.5.1 Prothrombin or Factor II

Prothrombin is a clotting protein important in forming fibrin in the last stage of the clotting cascade when fibrin is formed. Increased production of prothrombin occurs as a result of a single-base pair change. This mutation is present in approximately 2% of the general population, with a slightly higher risk of the mutation in people from Southern Europe.

Antithrombin is an endogenous anticoagulant that is produced in the liver (Corral et al. 2018). Reductions in the levels of antithrombin place patients at increased risk of thrombosis. Lab testing for diagnosis involves either functional or genetic analysis as a majority of the patients with antithrombin deficiency have a defect in SER-PINC1 (Corral et al. 2018).

8.16.5.2 Prothrombin G20210A

Prothrombin G20210A is a mutation in the prothrombin gene that leads to elevated prothrombin activity and prothrombin plasma concentrations (von Ahsen et al. 2000). An abnormal result of this genetic test as either heterozygous or homozygous carrier indicates that a patient is at higher risk for thrombosis. It is the second only to factor V Leiden as the most common cause of inherited thrombosis (Zöller et al. 1999). This test is performed by PCR and requires patient or parental consent.

8.16.5.3 D-Dimer

D-Dimer is a marker of the activation of coagulation and an indirect marker of fibrinolysis. There are at least 30 different assays for D-dimer available, including enzyme-linked immunosorbent assays (ELISA), immunofluorescent assays, and latex agglutination assays (Johnson et al. 2019). Elevated D-dimer levels are found in patients with VTE. Still, they must be assessed in the context of a complete history and physical exam, as D-dimer alone is not diagnostic for

VTE. Elevations do occur during normal pregnancies, reaching two to four times normal by 9 months of gestation. There are variable rises in D-dimers in active malignancy; however, D-dimer's elevation is frequently found in the hospitalized patient, indicating that it can rise in various conditions (Olson 2015). An elevated D-dimer is not specific since moderate elevations can be found in so many conditions. However, levels over 5000 ng/mL can be seen in disseminated intravascular coagulation, ascending aortic dissections, and pulmonary embolism (Olson 2015).

8.16.5.4 Lupus Anticoagulant

Lupus anticoagulant is an antibody that binds to phospholipids and proteins. The term "lupus anticoagulant" is a misnomer. It is often not associated with lupus and is not associated with anticoagulation. This antibody's presence places one at increased risk for coagulation (Teruya et al. 2007). There are at least four different assays commercially available, and none is the gold standard for lupus anticoagulant assays (Teruya et al. 2007). Testing for lupus anticoagulants should not be done if the patient receives rivaroxaban, dabigatran, or enoxaparin (Ashraf et al. 2019).

8.16.5.5 Additional Antiphospholipid Antibodies

Two other antiphospholipid antibodies, anticardiolipin and anti-β2-glycoprotein 1, are commonly tested in a thrombophilia workup. The presence of these antibodies on two or more occasions at least 12 weeks apart is considered a potential laboratory risk factor for thrombosis development. However, this risk is not as high as a positive lupus anticoagulant (Galli et al. 2003). Laboratory testing for these antibodies involves using ELISA, but there is a lack of standardization between laboratories (Zhou et al. 2018). As previously mentioned, the clinician must remember that if the test for any of the antiphospholipid antibodies is positive, it will need to be repeated 12 weeks later since these antibodies may be transient.

8.16.5.6 Fibrinogen

Fibrinogen is synthesized in the liver, and assays measure functional fibrinogen. As shown in Figs. 8.2 and 8.3, fibrinogen, due to thrombin's action, leads to fibrin formation. Thrombin action is inhibited by hirudin without the presence of any cofactors. This binding is irreversible.

8.16.6 Real-Life Example

A 9-month-old presented for a preoperative visit before a VSD repair, including preoperative labs. The child's family history was unremarkable. The child's exam was normal except for a blowing holosystolic, grade 3/6 harsh murmur at the low left sternal border radiating to the back. As the tourniquet was applied, multiple petechiae appeared below the line of the tourniquet. The results of the lab showed elevated PTT and normal PT.

Further testing for VWD was positive. The family was questioned in detail about bleeding following deliveries as they had not had surgery or dental work done involving tooth removal. Both the mother, maternal grandmother, and the 9-month-old sibling were positive for VWD.

Questions

1. Please interpret this CBC.

Test	Result	Normal/high/low
WBC	12.6	Normal
RBC	3.28	Low
Hgb	8.4	Low
Hct	25.2	Low
MCV	60	Low
MCH	20	Low
MCHC	29	Low
RDW	20	High
Platelet	475	High
MPV	7.0	Normal
NRBC	0.0	Normal
% neutrophils	45	Normal
% bands	2	Normal
% lymphocytes	43	Normal
% monocytes	6	Normal
% basophils	1	Normal
% eosinophils	3	Normal

The peripheral smear shows microcytosis, hypochromasia, poikilocytosis, and anisocytosis.

What is the most likely cause of this kind of CBC in a Caucasian toddler?
   (a) Iron deficiency anemia
   (b) Hemolysis
   (c) Thalassemia trait
   (d) Leukemia

2. Using the CBC results above, what is the absolute neutrophil count (ANC) in this patient?
   (a) 5670
   (b) 5922
   (c) 5277
   (d) 4578

3. What is the most common acquired bleeding problem in children?
   (a) Immune thrombocytopenia
   (b) von Willebrand disease
   (c) Hemophilia
   (d) Protein C deficiency

4. What does the term poikilocytosis mean?
   (a) Changes in size
   (b) Changes in shape
   (c) Pale cells
   (d) Small cells

   Review this CBC and answer the question below:

WBC	5.6	5.5–15.0
RBC	5.95	3.7–5.30
Hb	9.0	10.5–13.5
HCT	26.5	33–49
MCV	56	70–86
MCHC	16	23–31
Platelet	450	150–450

5. What is the likely cause of the child's anemia?
   (a) Thalassemia trait
   (b) Iron deficiency
   (c) Hemolysis
   (d) Leukemia

6. What is usually elevated in hemolytic anemia?
   (a) Haptoglobin
   (b) WBC
   (c) Platelet count
   (d) Lactate dehydrogenase (LDH)

7. What is the most likely value of the MCV in macrocytic anemia?
   (a) 85
   (b) 95
   (c) 105
   (d) 145

8. Which of the following children has moderate neutropenia?
   (a) WBC 9.5 with 78 neutrophils, 12 lymphocytes, 2 bands, 3 eosinophils, and 5 monocytes
   (b) WBC 4.5 with 8 neutrophils, 77 lymphocytes, 5 bands, 3 eosinophils, 3 basophils, and 4 monocytes
   (c) WBC 6.7 with 18 neutrophils, 67 lymphocytes, 12 bands, and 1 eosinophil, 1 basophil, and 1 monocyte
   (d) WBC 4.8 with 6 neutrophils, 88 lymphocytes, 2 bands, 1 eosinophil, 1 basophil, and 2 monocytes

9. Which of the following is elevated in iron deficiency anemia?
   (a) Ferritin
   (b) Total iron-binding capacity
   (c) Serum iron
   (d) Transferrin

10. What do you expect to happen 7 to 10 days after iron initiation in a patient with thalassemia trait?
    (a) Reticulocyte count will significantly increase
    (b) Nothing will happen
    (c) The hemoglobin will rise at least 1 gm
    (d) The RDW will increase

11. What does the term anisocytosis mean?
    (a) Different size
    (b) Different shape
    (c) Small cells
    (d) Paleness of the cells

12. A child has microcytic anemia that did not respond to 1 month of iron. What is the next best step?
    (a) Increase the dose of iron to 5 mg/kg/day for 1 month
    (b) Order another reticulocyte count
    (c) Repeat the serum ferritin
    (d) Do a hemoglobin electrophoresis

13. First, calculate Mentzer's index using the following indices:
    RBC is 5.45, Hb is 10.4, and MCV is 56. What is the most likely diagnosis based on the calculated Mentzer's index?
    (a) Iron deficiency
    (b) Normocytic anemia
    (c) Thalassemia trait
    (d) Thalassemia major

14. If the patient is compensating for hemolysis, what will be elevated?
    (a) Reticulocyte count (RC)
    (b) Red cell count
    (c) Creatinine kinase
    (d) White cell count

15. An African-American male newborn has prolonged jaundice. Which of the following is the most likely diagnosis?
    (a) Spherocytosis
    (b) Glucose-6-phosphate dehydrogenase deficiency (G6PD deficiency)
    (c) Elliptocytosis
    (d) Sickle cell disease

16. You note a CBC with normocytic anemia and circulating nucleated red blood cells (nucleated RBCs). Of the following, what is the most likely diagnosis?
    (a) Autoimmune hemolytic anemia
    (b) Moderate iron deficiency
    (c) Thalassemia trait
    (d) Mild lead poisoning

17. Which of the following labs would be consisted of autoimmune hemolytic anemia?
    (a) Decreased haptoglobin, decreased lactate dehydrogenase (LDH)
    (b) Increased haptoglobin, increased LDH
    (c) Decreased haptoglobin, increased LDH
    (d) Increased haptoglobin, decreased LDH

18. A child has normochromic and normocytic anemia with a normal differential. What is the next step in the evaluation of the child?
    (a) Do a uric acid and lactate dehydrogenase (LDH)
    (b) Do a stool guaiac and reticulocyte count
    (c) Repeat the CBC with a differential
    (d) All of the above
    (e) None of the above

19. Why is the 1-month-old neonate with SCD asymptomatic?
    (a) The high levels of fetal hemoglobin
    (b) Maternal transfer of hemoglobin
    (c) The inability of the neonate to mount a response to infection
    (d) The high level of hemoglobin A2
20. You are reviewing the previous day's lab results. One of the CBCs catches your attention as the WBC count is 3.8 with a normal differential. The rest of the CBC is normal. Under what circumstances would this leukopenia be an expected finding?
    (a) A low WBC is never normal
    (b) It may be low in viral illnesses or a small group of African-American males
    (c) It is usually low in a patient with strep pharyngitis
    (d) It is usually low in a patient with sickle cell disease

Rationale

1. Answer: A
   Rationale: The CBC is the classic picture of IDA. The RBC, Hb, Hct, and MCV are low. The RDW is elevated. The level of RDW elevation is usually around 18. If you do Mentzer's index MCV/RBC, the result is 18.29. The approach would be to start the patient on a therapeutic level of iron (3–6 mg/kg) and follow back in 1 week. If you do a reticulocyte count, the result will show reticulocytosis, and the Hb will have already responded by 1 g/dl.
   If the child had thalassemia trait, the RBC would be high, and the RDW would be normal. In hemolysis, the child would have a low Hb and Hct but a normal or slightly elevated MCV. The RDW would either be normal or slightly elevated. The elevation seen in the RDW is the result of reticulocytosis. As you may remember, reticulocytes are much larger in size, and therefore the RDW may be elevated as the cells do not all look like each other.

2. Answer: B
   Rationale: The absolute neutrophil count or ANC is determined by multiplying the

neutrophils and the bands by the WBC. You need to add the bands and the neutrophils together so you would get 47. It would be best if you remembered that 45 neutrophils and 2 bands are a percentage of 100, so you must multiply 0.47. The WBC of 12.6 is actually 12,600. When you carry out the multiplication, the ANC is 5922.

3. Answer: A
   Rationale: This is a memorization question. The most common acquired bleeding problem is immune thrombocytopenia. The rest of the answers are genetic disorders, not acquired.

4. Answer: B
   Rationale: Anisocytosis is a variation in the RBC size, whereas poikilocytosis presents a variation in RBC shape (Cascio and De Loughery 2017). Pale cells are hypochromic, whereas small cells are microcytic.

5. Answer: A
   Rationale: The CBC shows microcytic anemia as the child has a low Hb and Hct with an MCV of 56. Again, Mentzer's index is done by dividing the MCV/RBC. The MCV is 56, and the RBC is 5.95, resulting in a Mentzer's index of 9.41. If Mentzer's index is less than 13, and then thalassemia trait should be considered. The next step in the management is a hemoglobin electrophoresis. Remember that patients born in other countries may not have been screened for a hemoglobinopathy at birth.

6. Answer: D
   Rationale: A low haptoglobin with an elevated LDH is 90% sensitive for hemolysis (Kujovich 2016). Therefore, D is the correct answer. Platelets and WBC are not affected by hemolysis.

7. Answer: C
   Rationale: A macrocytic anemia generally has an MCV greater than 100, but 145 would be out of the range normally seen.

8. Answer: B
   Rationale: To answer question 8, you must remember that an ANC between 1500 and 1000 is mild neutropenia. An ANC of 1000–500 is moderate neutropenia, and an ANC of 500 to 0 is severe neutropenia.

In answer A, the ANC in A is 78 neutrophils +2 bands equal 80% or 0.80. You multiply 0.80 by 9500 to get 7800 as the ANC, well above 1500. In answer B, eight neutrophils and five bands equal 13% or 0.13. You multiply 0.13 by 4500, and this equals an ANC of 585, which is moderate neutropenia. In answer C, 18 neutrophils and 12 bands equal 30% or 0.3. You multiply 0.3 by 6700, and this equals an ANC of 2010, which is normal. In answer D, six neutrophils and two bands equal 0.8% or 0.08. You multiply 0.08 by 4800, and this equals an ANC of 384, which is severe neutropenia. Therefore, B is the correct answer.

9. Answer: B
   Rationale: In IDA, the ferritin is low, and therefore A is not correct. The serum transferrin is also low in IDA. TIBC is an indirect measure of transferrin. It measures the availability of iron-binding sites on the transferrin molecule. The serum iron would also be low in IDA.

10. Answer: B
    Rationale: A patient with the thalassemia trait will not respond to iron therapy. There will be no change in the CBC if the patient has thalassemia trait and not IDA.

11. Answer: A
    Rationale: Anisocytosis is a variation in the RBC size, whereas poikilocytosis presents a variation in RBC shape (Cascio and De Loughery 2017). Pale cells are hypochromic, whereas small cells are microcytic.

12. Answer: D
    Rationale: In this question, the child has not responded to iron therapy, and a hemoglobinopathy should be considered.

13. Answer: C
    Rationale: The first step is to calculate Mentzer's index. The MCV/RBC is 56/5.45, which equals 10.27. This result is significantly less than 13; therefore, hemoglobin electrophoresis would be the next step.

14. Answer: A
    Rationale: When the RBCs break up, causing anemia, the bone marrow will respond by releasing premature RBCs or reticulocytes. These cells can carry oxygen and meet the body's need for oxygen.

15. Answer: B
    Rationale: African-American newborns with prolonged jaundice should be tested for glucose-6-phosphate dehydrogenase deficiency (G6PD deficiency). G6PD deficiency is more common than elliptocytosis or spherocytosis. The high level of hemoglobin F is protective against any symptoms in patients with SCD. The child with SCD will develop mild jaundice as hemoglobin drops, but this usually does not occur until 6 months.

16. Answer: A
    Rationale: In a patient with normocytic anemia with circulating nucleated RBCs (NRBCs), autoimmune hemolytic anemia should be considered. The CBC in moderate iron deficiency and thalassemia trait would show microcytic anemia and no circulating NRBCs. NRBCs are seen when there is a marked increase in erythropoietic activity. In mild lead poisoning, there may not be any CBC changes.

17. Answer: C
    Rationale: See rationale to question 6.

18. Answer: B
    Rationale: The best answer to this question is to do a stool guaiac and RC. It is not routine to repeat a CBC if there is nothing abnormal about the CBC results. Uric acid and an LDH would not be the next step. If the RC were less than 0.5% and indicated hypofunctioning of the bone marrow, then a workup for an oncological problem would be appropriate. A positive stool guaiac may explain the blood loss associated with gastrointestinal bleeding associated with normocytic anemia.

19. Answer: A
    Rationale: The presence of fetal hemoglobin protects the newborn from being symptomatic if they have sickle cell anemia. As the fetal hemoglobin drops, the child becomes symptomatic.

20. Answer: B
    Rationale: The WBC count can be low in a patient with a viral illness or African-American males. It is important to review previous CBCs when evaluating a CBC whenever possible.

References

AlFadhli S, Al-Awadhi A, Alkaldi D. Validity assessment of nine discriminant functions used for the differential between iron deficiency anemia and thalassemia minor. J Tropic Pediatr. 2006;53(2):943–7.

Al-Subaie AM. Coagulopathies in novel coronavirus (SARS-CoV-2) pandemic: Emerging evidence for hematologists. Saudi J Biol Sci. 2021;28(1):956–61.

Amal-Zaghloui A, Al-Bukhari NB, Maged-Shalaby HA, AL-Pakistani SH, Halawani SH, Wassif T, Wassif G. Introduction of new formulas and evaluation of previous red blood cell indices and formulas in the differentiation between beta thalassemia trait and iron deficiency in the Makkah region. Hematology. 2016;6:351–8.

American Academy of Pediatrics [AAP] Recommendations for preventive pediatric health care 2019. Retrieved from: https://downloads.aap.org/AAP/PDF/periodicity_schedule.pdf

American College of Obstetricians and Gynecologists. Screening and management of bleeding disorders in adolescents with heavy menstrual bleeding. ACOG Committee opinion no. 785. Obstet Gynecol. 2019;134:e71–83.

American College of Obstetricians and Gynecologists. Risk of venous thromboembolism among users of drospirenone-containing oral contraceptive pills. Committee Opinion No. 540 reaffirmed 2020. Retrieved December 12, 2020, from https://www.acog.org/clinical/clinical-guidance/committee-opinion/articles/2012/11/risk-of-venous-thromboembolism-among-users-of-drospirenone-containing-oral-contraceptive-pills

Anderle A, Bancone G, Domingo G, Gerth-Guyette E, Pal S, Satyagraha A. Point-of-care testing for G6PD deficiency: opportunities for screening. Int J Neonatal Screen. 2018;4(4):34. https://doi.org/10.3390/ijns4040034.

Ashenden M, Clarke A, Sharpe K, D'Onofrio G, Plowman J, Gore CJ. Stability of athlete passport parameters during extended storage. Int J Lab Hematol. 2013;35:183–92.

Ashraf N, Visweshwar N, Jaglal M, Sokol L, Laber D. Evolving paradigm in thrombophilia screening. Blood Coagul Fibrinolysis. 2019;30(5):249–52.

Aster RH, Bougie DW. Drug-induced immune thrombocytopenia. N Engl J Med. 2007;357(6):580–7.

Azar S, Wong TE. Sickle cell disease: a brief update. Med Clin N Am. 2017;101:375–93.

Bandmann O, Weiss KH, Kaler SG. Wilson's disease and other neurological copper disorders. Lancet Neurol. 2015;14(1):103–13.

Barone, J. Eosinophilia mnemonics. 2020. http://www.baronerocks.com/m/index.php/mnemonics/mnemonics-hematology/471-eosinophilia

Bender M, Yusuf C, Davis T, Dorley MC, del Pilar Aguinaga M, Ingram A, et al. Newborn screening practices and alpha-thalassemia detection—United States, 2016. MMWR Morb Mortal Wkly Rep. 2020;69:1269–72.

Beris P, Picard V. Non-immune hemolysis: diagnostic considerations. Semin Hematol. 2015;52:287–303.

Bianchi P, Fermo E, Glader B, Kanno H, Agarwal A, Barcellini W, et al. Addressing the diagnostic gap in pyruvate kinase deficiency: consensus recommendation of the diagnosis of pyruvate kinase deficiency. Am J Hematol. 2019;94(1):149–61.

Black S. Petechiae and purpura: the ominous and the not-so-obvious? Pediatr Ann. 2014;43(8):297–303.

Boxer L. Neutrophil abnormalities. Pediatr Rev. 2003;24(2):52–63.

Briggs C, Culp A, Davis B, D'Onofrio G, Zini G, Machin SJ. IVSH guidelines for evaluation of blood cell analyzers including those used for differential leucocyte and reticulocyte counting. Int J Lab Hematol. 2014;36:613–27.

Bruno M, DeFalco L, Iolascon A. How I diagnose non-thalassemic microcytic anemias. Semin Hematol. 2015;52(4):270–9.

Buoro S, Mecca T, Seghezzi M, Manenti B, Azzara G, Ottomano C, Lippi G. Validation rules for blood smear revision after automated hematological testing using Mindray CAL-8000. J Clin Lab Anal. 2017;31:322067. https://doi.org/10.1002/jcla.22067.

Cakmakli HF, Torres RJ, Menendez A, Yalcin-Cakmakli G, Porter CC, Puig JG, Jinnah HA. Macrocytic anemia in Lesch-Nyhan disease and its variants. Genet Med. 2019;21(2):353–60.

Cangemi G, Pistorio A, Miano M, Gattorno M, Acquila M, Bichocchi MP, et al. Diagnostic potential of hepcidin testing in pediatrics. Eur J Haematol. 2013;90:323–30.

Cascio MJ, De Loughery TG. Anemia: evaluation and diagnostic tests. Med Clin N Am. 2017;101:263–84.

Castaman G, Linart S. Diagnosis and treatment of von Willebrand disease and rare bleeding disorders. J Clin Med. 2017;6:45–63.

Centers for Disease Control [CDC]. US Medical Eligibility Criteria (US MEC) for Contraceptive Use, 2016. Updated November 2020. Retrieved on December 12, 2020, https://www.cdc.gov/reproductivehealth/contraception/mmwr/mec/summary.html

Chabot-Richards DS, Foucar K. Does morphology matter in 2017? An approach to morphologic clues in non-neoplastic blood and bone marrow disorders. Int J Lab Hematol. 2017;39:23–30.

Choi S, Rambally S, Shen Y. Mixing study for evaluation of abnormal coagulation testing. JAMA. 2016;316(20):2146–7.

Ciepiela O. Old and new insights into the diagnosis of hereditary spherocytosis. Ann Transl Med. 2018;6(17):339–46.

Corral J, de la Morena-Barrio ME, Vicente V. The genetics of antithrombin. Thromb Res. 2018;169:23–9.

Creary S, Chisolm D, Stanek J, Neville K, Garg U, Hankins JS, O'Brien SH. Measuring hydroxyurea adherence by pharmacy and laboratory data compared with video observation in children with sickle cell disease. Pediatr Blood Cancer. 2020;67(8):e28250.

Croteau SE. Evolving complexity in Hemophilia management. Pediatr Clin N Am. 2018;65(3):407–25.

D'Angelo G. Role of hepcidin in the pathophysiology and diagnosis of anemia. Blood Res. 2013;48(1):10–5.

Daugherty MM, De Loughery TG. Unusual anemias. Med Clin N Am. 2017;101:417–29.

De Loughery TG. Iron deficiency anemia. Med Clin N Am. 2017;101:319–32.

Dewaswala N. Eosinophilia mnemonic. 2020. http://immense-immunology-insight.blogspot.com/2013/09/eosinophilia-mnemonic.html

Diez-Silva M, Dao M, Han J, Lim CT, Suresh S. Shape and Biomechanical Characteristics of Human Red Blood Cells in Health and Disease. MRS Bull. 2010;35(5):382–88.

Eule C, Gupta A, Nagalla S. The direct antiglobulin test for evaluating anemia. J Am Med Ass. 2018;320(24):2593–4.

Farias MG. Advances in laboratory diagnosis of hereditary spherocytosis. Clin Chem Lab Med. 2017;55(7):944–8.

Franco RS, Puchulu-Campanella MF, Barber LA, et al. Changes in the properties of normal human red blood cells during in vitro aging. Am J Hematol. 2013;88:44–51.

Freedman J. Autoimmune hemolysis: a journey through time. Transfus Med Hemother. 2015;42:278–85.

Galli M, Luciani D, Bertolini G, Barbui T. Lupus anticoagulants are stronger risk factors for thrombosis than anticardiolipin antibodies in the antiphospholipid syndrome: a systematic review of the literature. Blood. 2003;101(5):1827–32.

Grace RF, Glader B. Red blood cell enzyme disorders. Pediatr Clin N Am. 2018;65:579–95. https://doi.org/10.1016/j.pcl.2018.02.005.

Graham R, Davis J, Corrales-Medina FF. The adolescent with menorrhagia: diagnostic approach to a suspected bleeding disorder. Pediatr Rev. 2018;39(12):588–600.

Green R, Dwyre D. Evaluation of macrocytic anemias. Semin Hematol. 2015;52(4):279–86.

Green R, Mitra AD. Megaloblastic anemia: nutritional and other causes. Med Clin N Am. 2017;101:297–317.

Haley C. Congenital hemolytic anemias. Med Clin N Am. 2017;101:361–74.

Haley KH. Platelet disorders. Pediatr Rev. 2020;41:224–35.

Hermiston ML, Mentzer WC. A practical approach to the anemic child. Pediatr Clin N Am. 2002;49:877–89.

Hickey SE, Curry CJ, Toriello HV. ACMG practice guideline: lack of evidence for MTHFR polymorphism testing. Genet Med. 2013;15(2):153–6.

Higgins J. Red blood cell population dynamics. Clin Lab Med. 2015;35(1):43–57.

Hill BL, Simpson VZ, Higgins JM, Hu Z, Stevens RA, Baseler M. Evaluation of the performance of the Sysex Xt2000i hematology analyzer with whole blood stored at room temperature. Lab Med. 2009;40:709–18.

Hill QA, Hill A, Berentsen S. Defining autoimmune hemolytic anemia: a systematic review of the terminology used for diagnosis and treatment. Blood Adv. 2019;3(12):1897–906.

Ho L, John RM. Understanding and managing Glucose-6-phosphate dehydrogenase deficiency. J NP. 2015;11(4):443–50.

Hoppe C, Neumayr L. Sickle cell disease: monitoring, current treatment, and therapeutics under development. Hematol Oncol Clin N Am. 2019;33:355–71.

Ilkovska B, Kotevska B, Trifunov G, Kanazirev B. Serum hepcidin reference range, gender differences, menopausal dependence and biochemical correlates in healthy subjects. J IMAB. 2016;22(2):1127–31.

Ilyas S, Simonson A, Asghar W. Emerging point-of-care technologies for sickle cell disease diagnostics. Clin Chem Acta. 2020;501:85–91.

Ishii K, Young NS. Anemia of central origin. Semin Hematol. 2015;52(4):321–38.

Jayavaradhan R, Malik P. Genetic therapies for sickle cell disease. Pediatr Clin N Am. 2018;65(3):465–80.

Jenkins PV, Rawley O, Smith OP, O'Donnell JS. Elevated factor VIII levels and risk of venous thrombosis. Br J Haematol. 2012;157(6):653–63.

John R. (2018). Diagnostic laboratory tests. Presentation for students In N 6630 at Columbia University School of Nursing.

Johnson ED, Schell JC, Rodgers GM. The D-dimer assay. Am J Hematol. 2019;94(7):833–9.

Joly BS, Coppo P, Veyradier A. Pediatric thrombotic thrombocytopenic purpura. Eur J Haematol. 2018;101(4):425–34.

Kairys S. Child abuse and neglect: the role of the primary care pediatrician. Pediatr Clin NA. 2020;67(2):325–39.

Kaplan JA. Leukemia in children. Pediatr Rev. 2019;40(7):319–30.

Khera S, Hafeez Z, Padilla A. Case 2: Acute Onset and Worsening of Anemia in a 3-year-old Boy. Pediatr Rev. 2019;40(5):247–50.

Kim Y, Park J, Kim M. Diagnostic approaches for inherited hemolytic anemia in the genetic era. Blood Res. 2017;52(2):84–94.

Kohn J. A cellulose acetate supporting medium for zone electrophoresis. Clin Chim Acta. 1957;2(4):297–303.

Kujovich JL. Factor V Leiden thrombophilia. Genet Med. 2011;13(1):1–16.

Kujovich JL. Evaluation of anemia. Obstet Gynecol Clin N Am. 2016;43:247–64.

Kumar R, Derbigny WA. Cellulose acetate electrophoresis of Hemoglobin. In: Kurien B, Scofield R, editors. Electrophoretic separation of proteins. Methods in molecular biology, 1855. New York, NY: Humana Press; 2019.

Kumar S, Bhatia P, Jain R, Bharti B. Plasma hepcidin levels in healthy children: review of current literature highlights limited studies. J Pediatr Hematol Oncol. 2019;41(3):238–42.

Liebman HA, Weitz IC. Autoimmune hemolytic anemia. Med Clin N Am. 2017;101:351–9.

Liem RI, Lanzkron S, Coates D, DeCastro TL, Desai AA, et al. American Society of Hematology 2019 guidelines for sickle cell disease: cardiopulmonary and kidney disease. Blood Adv. 2019;3(23):3867–97.

Lima WG, Barra A, Brito JC, Nizer W. D-dimer serum levels as a biomarker associated for the lethality of patients with coronavirus disease 2019: a meta-analysis. Blood Coagul Fibrinol. 2020;31(5):1–3.

Lippi G, Simundic AM. Laboratory networking and sample quality: a still relevant issue for patient safety. Clin Chem Lab Med. 2012;50:1703–5.

Litao MK, Kamat D. Red blood cell distribution width: clinical use beyond hematology. Pediatr Rev. 2018;39:204–9.

Lo E, Deane S. Diagnosis and classification of immune-mediated thrombocytopenia. Autoimmun Rev. 2014;13:588–3.

Martin A, Thompson A. Thalassemias. Pediatr Clin N Am. 2013;60:1383–91.

Matos J, Dusse L, Borges K, deCastro R, Coura-Vital W, das Carvalho MG. A new index to discriminate between iron deficiency anemia and thalassemia trait. Rev Bras Hematol Hemoter. 2016;38(3):214–9.

Meier ER. Treatment options for sickle cell disease. Pediatr Clin N Am. 2018;65(3):427–43.

National Institute of Health, Sickle cell disease. U. S. Department of Health and Human Services, National Heart, Lung, and Blood Institute. Retrieved October 11, 2020. From https://www.nhlbi.nih.gov/health-topics/sickle-cell-disease

Neunert G, Noroozi N, Norman G, Buchanan GR, Goy J, Nazi I, et al. Severe bleeding events in adults and children with primary immune thrombocytopenia: a systematic review. J Thromb Haemost. 2015;13(3):457–64.

Ng CJ, Di Paola J. von Willebrand disease: diagnostic strategies and treatment options. Pediatr Clin N Am. 2018;65:527–41.

Noronha S. Acquired and congenital anemia. Pediatr Rev. 2016;37:235–46.

Nurden AT, Nurden P. Inherited thrombocytopenias: history, advances and perspectives. Haematologica. 2020;105(8):2004–19.

O'Brien SH, Saini S. von Willebrand disease in pediatrics: evaluation and management. Hematol Oncol Clin N Am. 2019;33:425–38.

Okan V, Cigiloglu A, Cifci S, Yilmaz M, Pehlivan M. Red cell indices and functions differentiating patients with the beta-thalassemia trait from those with iron deficiency anaemia. J Int Med Res. 2009;37(1):25–30.

Olivares M, Walter T, Osorio M, Chudud P, Schelsinger L. Anemia of a mild viral infection: the measles vaccine as a model. Pediatr. 1989;84(5):851–5.

Olson JD. D-dimer: an overview of hemostasis and fibrinolysis, assays, and clinical applications. Adv Clin Chem. 2015;69:1–46.

Oto J, Fernández-Pardo Á, Miralles M, Plana E, España F, Navarro S, Medina P. Activated protein C assays: a review. Clin Chim Acta. 2020;502:227–32.

Pal S, Bansil P, Bancone G, et al. Evaluation of a novel quantitative test for Glucose-6-phosphate dehydrogenase deficiency: bringing quantitative testing for glucose-6-phosphate dehydrogenase deficiency closer to the patient. Am J Trop Med Hyg. 2019;100(1):213–21.

Peyvandi F, Garagiola I, Young G. The past and future of haemophilia: diagnosis, treatments, and its complications. Lancet. 2016;388(10040):187–97.

Piel FB, Weatherall DJ. The α thalassemias. N Engl J Med. 2014;371(20):1908–15.

Powers JM, Buchanan GR. Disorders of iron metabolism: new diagnostic treatment approaches to iron deficiency. Hematol Oncol Clin. 2019;33(3):393–408.

Priya P, Subhashree AR. Role of absolute reticulocyte count in the evaluation of pancytopenia-a hospital-based study. J Clin Diagn Res. 2014;8(8):FC01–FC3.

Robinson N, Sottas PE, Pottgiesser T, Shumacher YO, Saugy M. Stability and robustness of blood variables in an anti-doping context. Int J Lab Hematol. 2011;33:146–53.

Rodeghiero F, Pabinger I, Ragni M, Abdul-Kadir R, Berntorp E, Blanchette V. Fundamentals for a systematic approach to mild to moderate inherited bleeding disorders: an EHA consensus report. HemaSphere. 2019;3:5–17.

Rosa RF, Rosa RC, Dos Santos PP, Zen PR, Paskulin GA. Hematological abnormalities and 22q11.2 deletion syndrome. Rev Bras Hematol Hemoter. 2011;33(2):151–4. https://doi.org/10.5581/1516-8484.20110037.

Savasan S. Acquired aplastic anemia: what we have learned and what is on the horizon. Pediatr Clin N Am. 2018;65:597–606.

Schafer AI. Thrombocytosis. JAMA. 2015;314(11):1171–2.

Schwartz JT, Fulkerson. An approach to the evaluation of persistent hypereosinophilia in pediatric patients. Front Immunol. 2018;9:1944–50.

Sdogou T, Tsentidis C, Gourgiotis D, Marmarinos A, Gkourogianni A, Papassotiriou I, Anastasiou T, Kossiva L. Immunoassay-based serum hepcidin reference range measurements in healthy children: differences among age groups. J Clin Lab Anal. 2015;29(1):10–4.

Segel GB, Lichtman MA. Direct antiglobulin ("coombs") test-negative autoimmune hemolytic anemia. Blood Cells Mol Dis. 2014;53:152–61.

Sharma R, Flood VH. Advances in the diagnosis and treatment of Von Willebrand disease. Am Soc Hematol. 2017;130:379–84.

Sharma R, Perez Botero J, Jobe SM. Congenital disorders of platelet function and number. Pediatr Clin N Am. 2018;65(3):561–78.

Siddon, AJ, Tormey, CA. Chapter 6. The chemical and laboratory investigation of hemolysis. In: Makowski, GM, Advances in Clinical Chemistry. 1st edition. Academic press; 2019:215–58.

Socha DS, DeSouza SI, Flagg A, Sekeres M, Rogers HJ. Severe megaloblastic anemia: vitamin deficiency and other causes. Cleveland Clin J Med. 2020;87(1):153–64.

Stachowiak A, Furman L. Vitamin K is necessary for newborns. Pediatr Rev. 2020;41(6):305–6.

Styles LA, Schalkwijk CG, Aarsman AJ, Vichinsky EP, Lubin BH, Kuypers FA. Phospholipase A2 levels in acute chest syndrome of sickle cell disease. Blood. 1996;87(6):2573–8.

Syider P, Arianpour K, Mutchick S. Management of epistaxis in children and adolescents: avoiding a chaotic approach. Pediatr Clin N Am. 2018;65:607–21.

ten Kate MK, van der Meer J. Protein S deficiency: a clinical perspective. Haemophilia. 2008;14(6):1222–8.

Teruya J, West AG, Suell MN. Lupus anticoagulant assays: questions answered and to be answered. Arch Pathol Lab Med. 2007;131(6):885–9.

Thom CS, Dickson CF, Gell DA, Weiss MJ. Hemoglobin variants: biochemical properties and clinical correlates. Cold Spring Harb Perspect Med. 2013; 3:a01858.

Toh B. Pathophysiology and laboratory diagnosis of pernicious anemia. Immunol Res. 2017;65:320–30.

Valiya KR, Gidwani RK, Kucha NP, Goswami FJ, Shah MM, Prajapati SA. Applicability of different hematological discrimination indices for differential diagnosis of beta-thalassemia trait and iron deficiency anaemia. Medpulse Int J Pathol. 2019;1293: 145–52.

Van Herrewegen F, Meijer JC, Peters M, van Ommen CH. Clinical practice the bleeding child. Part II: disorders of secondary hemostasis and fibrinolysis. Eur J Pediatr. 2012;171:207–14.

Vehapoglu A, Ozgurhan G, Demir AD, Uzuner S, Nursoy MA, Turkmen S, Kacan A. Hematological indices for differential diagnosis of beta-thalassemia trait and iron deficiency anemia. 2014; https://doi.org/10.1155/2014/576738.

von Ahsen N, Lewczuk P, Schütz E, Oellerich M, Ehrenreich H. Prothrombin activity and concentration in healthy subjects with and without the prothrombin G20210A mutation. Thromb Res. 2000;99(6): 549–56.

Wahed A, Quesada A, Dasgupta A. Hematology and coagulation: a comprehensive review for board preparation, certification and clinical practice. Amsterdam: Elsevier; 2020.

Walters MC, Abelson HT. Interpretation of the complete blood count. Pediatr Clin North Am. 1996;43(3): 599–622.

Wang M. Iron deficiency and other types of anemia in infants and children. Am Fam Physician. 2016;93(4):270–8.

Weiss G. Anemia of chronic disorders: new diagnostic tools and new treatment strategies. Semin Hematol. 2015;52(4):313–20.

WHO. Technical specification series for submission to WHO-diagnostic assessment: in vitro diagnostic medical devices to identify glucose-6-phosphate dehydrogenase (G6PD) activity. Geneva, Switzerland: WHO; 2016.

Willekens FL, Roerdinkholder-Stoewinder B, Groenen-Dropp YA, et al. Hemoglobin loss from erythrocytes in vivo results from spleen-facilitated vesiculation. Blood. 2003;101:747–51.

Winter WE, Greene DN, Beal SG, Isom JA, Manning H, Wilkerson G, Harris N. Clotting factors: clinical biochemistry and their roles as plasma enzymes. Adv Clin Chem. 2020;94:31–84.

Witmer CM. Hematologic manifestations of systemic disease (including iron deficiency, anemia of inflammation and DIC). Pediatr Clin N Am. 2013;60: 1337–48.

World Health Organization [WHO]. Updating the WHO G6PD classification of variants and the International Classification of Disease, 11th revision (ICD-11). 2019. Retrieved from https://www.who.int/malaria/mpac/mpac-october2019-session7-updating-G6PD-classification.pdf?ua=1

Wu DW, Li YM, Wang F. How Long can we Store Blood Samples: A Systematic Review and Meta-Analysis. EBioMedicine. 2017;24:277–85.

Yawn BP, Buchanan GR, Afenyi-Annan AN, Ballas SK, Hassell KL, et al. Management of sickle cell disease: summary of the 2014 evidence-based report by expert panel members. JAMA. 2014;312(10):1033–48.

Yazici KU, Yazici IP, Ustundag B. Increased serum Hepcidin levels in children and adolescents with attention deficit hyperactivity disorder. Clin Psychopharmacol Neurosci. 2019;17(1):105–12.

Yo CH, Hsieh PS, Lee SH, et al. Comparison of the test characteristics of procalcitonin to C-reactive protein and leukocytosis for the detection of serious bacterial infections in children presenting with fever without source: a systematic review and meta-analysis. Ann Emerg Med. 2012;60:591–600.

Zhera S, Hafeez A, Padilla A. Cae 2: acute onset and worsening of anemia in a 3-year-old boy. Pediatr Rev. 2019;40:247–59.

Zhou J, Hou X, Zhang H, Wang T, Cui L. The clinical performance of a new chemiluminescent immunoassay in measuring anti-β2 glycoprotein 1 and anti-Cardiolipin antibodies. Med Sci Monitor: Intern Med J Exp Clin Research. 2018;24:6816–22.

Zöller B, García de Frutos P, Hillarp A, Dahlbäck B. Thrombophilia as a multigenic disease. Haematologica. 1999;84(1):59–70.

Care of the Child with a Gastrointestinal Disorder

9

Anna L. Rundle, Nicole Baron, and Rita Marie John

Learning Objectives

After completing the chapter, the learner should be able to:

1. Interpret common laboratory studies to evaluate the child with diarrhea.
2. Identify and interpret laboratory studies used for evaluation of celiac disease.
3. Develop a plan for a child presenting with possible inflammatory bowel disease.
4. Evaluate a child for possible liver disease.
5. Understand the diagnostic laboratory tests used in patients with liver disease.

Anna L. Rundle: Special Thanks to Dr. Steven Lobritto

A. L. Rundle (✉)
Pediatric Center for Liver Disease and Transplantation, New York-Presbyterian Morgan Stanley Children's Hospital, New York, NY, USA
e-mail: ar2448@cumc.columbia.edu

N. Baron
Pediatric Gastroenterology, Hepatology and Nutrition, Columbia University Medical Center, New York-Presbyterian Morgan Stanley Children's Hospital, New York, NY, USA

R. M. John
School of Nursing, Columbia University, New York, NY, USA

9.1 Introduction

The gastrointestinal system, responsible for digestion and absorption, is essential for lifelong health. It comprises two major parts, the alimentary canal and digestive tract and accessory organs, including the liver, gall bladder, and pancreas. Gastrointestinal symptoms and disorders are common in primary care practice. Pediatric primary care providers play an important role in the initial diagnosis and management of these conditions. However, additional testing is needed when symptoms persist, and referral to a pediatric gastroenterologist or hepatologist may be considered. This chapter will discuss the approach to care for a child with acute diarrhea or a suspected underlying gastrointestinal disorder. Screening and diagnostic testing for celiac disease (CD), liver disease, and inflammatory bowel disease (IBD) are included. Early recognition and diagnosis of underlying conditions are critical to the child's overall growth and development.

9.2 The Child with Diarrhea in Primary Care

Acute infectious diarrhea is common in primary care, and nearly all preschoolers have one episode of diarrhea (Lo Vecchio et al. 2019). Most children and infants do not require any diagnostic testing as these episodes tend to be self-limiting

(Guarino et al. 2014; Thiagarajah et al. 2018). Acute diarrhea typically lasts for less than 2 weeks, and chronic diarrhea lasts for more than 2 weeks (Thiagarajah et al. 2018). Generally, laboratory studies are not done unless the diarrhea is severe, bloody diarrhea with/without mucopus, immunosuppression, severe illness, or a prolonged illness of more than 7 days (Zimmerman et al. 2020).

9.2.1 The Child with Suspected Infectious Diarrhea

An evaluation for an infectious disease should be completed as part of the workup for any patient presenting with acute diarrhea or bloody diarrhea. Many enteropathogens can cause gastrointestinal infections.

9.2.1.1 Macroscopic Evaluation of Stool

The clinician must know the developmental difference in stool characteristics. In infants, it is important to note the developmental changes that occur over time. At birth, once meconium is passed, the newborn's stool will vary depending on whether they are formula or breastfeeding. As the infant is introduced to complementary foods, the stool will become more formed and may have the color of the food that they are fed. Even the school-aged child fed food with artificial ingredients may have a stool that resembles that food's colors.

The stool should be looked at for shape, color, amount, consistency, mucus, and odor. The use of a Bristol stool chart should be used to characterize the shape of the stool. Color is very important as infants with clay or putty-colored stool may have an obstructive biliary disease and need immediate referral to a hepatologist. Green stool may reflect dietary intake of green vegetables. Black color can reflect more than 100 ml of bleeding from the GI tract (Kasırga 2019) but can also reflect iron intake or bismuth intake from Pepto Bismol. While a small amount of mucus is normal, the presence of bloody mucus or copious mucus is abnormal (Kasırga 2019).

9.2.1.2 Microscopic Examination of the Stool

The microscopic examination of the stool will evaluate for protozoa, helminths, and leukocytes. The evaluation for leukocytes in the stools is not a sensitive test for inflammatory diarrhea since the results do vary (Kasırga 2019). Testing the stool for occult blood is usually done by stool guaiac and is discussed in more detail in Sect. 8.9.2.5.

The Sudan III Stain of stool can detect more than 90% of patients with steatorrhea. The Sudan III Staining has a sensitivity and specificity of 77% and 98%, respectively (Simko 1981). This method involves counting fat globules as well as measuring their dimension. When done by an experienced examiner, the results are similar to the 72-hour fecal fat measurement (Kasırga 2019).

9.2.1.3 Stool Culture

The stool culture is the gold standard for identifying stool pathogens (Wyatt and Kellermayer 2018). The main problem with this testing method is labor-intensive and more prone to error, with inconsistent results that take many days (Torres-Miranda et al. 2020; Zimmerman et al. 2020). The use of molecular diagnostic methods such as PCR offers high sensitivity and specificity for the rapid identification of pathogens. The drawback is that it may detect low levels of enteropathogens without a clear clinical significance (Wyatt and Kellermayer 2018).

9.2.1.4 Stool for Ova and Parasites (O&P)

A fresh specimen of stool for microscopic evaluation for ova and parasites (O&P) is part of evaluating children with persistent diarrhea lasting more than 7 days. It should not be done unless there is at least 1 week of diarrhea (Mohapatra et al. 2018). It is commonly done in refugee children, children traveling to underdeveloped countries, and history of ingestion of contaminated food or water (Mohapatra et al. 2018). Parasites like *Giardia* and *Cryptosporidium* are common in the United States. Unfortunately, examination of the stool may not reveal the parasite as the parasite and/or ova tends to shed intermittently; this is why stool for O&P is ordered three times to maximize the test's sensitivity. However, several studies have found that the first specimen may be the only one needed. Therefore, the result of the first study should be obtained before additional samples are submitted to reduce cost (Branda et al. 2006; Morris et al. 1992; Polage et al. 2011).

Clinicians need to be aware that routine O&P stool examinations may not include *Cryptosporidium*, so it is necessary to ask for *Cryptosporidium* specifically. This is especially important in immunocompromised patients who can develop fulminant infection (Mohapatra et al. 2018).

However, multiplex real-time polymerase chain reaction (PCR) can detect the three most common one-cell parasites – *Entamoeba histolytica*, *Giardia lamblia*, and *Cryptosporidium parvum* (Mohapatra et al. 2018).

9.2.1.5 Enzyme Immunoassays for Enteric Pathogens

A review of enzyme immunoassay can be found in Sect. 6.2.1.7. Several EI tests evaluate enteric pathogens such as *Giardia lamblia*, *H. pylori*, adenovirus, norovirus, and rotavirus. The tests enable rapid identification of possible bacterial, viral, or protozoal diseases. As previously stated, they are not as accurate as PCR but are much lower in cost. Enteric adenoviruses (type 40 or 41) can cause prolonged diarrhea, and there is an adenovirus-specific ELISA analysis that is 78% sensitive and 100% specific for adenovirus (Kasırga 2019).

9.2.1.6 Syndromic-Based Molecular Testing for Detection of Gastrointestinal Pathogens

The use of a gastrointestinal pathogen PCR panel allows for simultaneous qualitative detection and identification of nucleic acids from over 20 of the most common pathogens, including bacteria, viruses, and parasites from one stool sample. The use of such testing is rapid and cost-effective (Beal et al. 2018). This rapid turnaround can decide isolation methods and infection control measures (Zimmerman et al. 2020).

There are several drawbacks of this testing. One drawback of PCR molecular methods is

a positive multiplex PCR test in a patient with IBD. The multiplex PCR fecal pathogen testing can return a positive result for a bacterium leading to delayed diagnosis (Wyatt and Kellermayer 2018). Clinicians need to remember that the testing is so sensitive that a small number of bacteria can lead to a positive result. The test is unable to differentiate the carrier state versus an actual infection. Therefore, a PCR test should only be used on symptomatic patients.

Different molecular PCR panels test for different bacteria, so knowing what the test results will include is critical. Multiple studies have shown that PCR panels have an increased sensitivity for the detection of GI pathogens over culture (Beal et al. 2018; Buss et al. 2015; Gingras and Maggiore 2020; Hannet et al. 2019; Sciandra et al. 2020; Stockmann et al. 2017; Torres-Miranda et al. 2020).

The multiplex panels are expensive, and panel compositions vary from company to company. If gastrointestinal pathogen PCR testing is not available, it is important to test for *Clostridium difficile*, *Salmonella*, *Shigella*, *Campylobacter*, and ova and parasites, including *Giardia* and *Cryptosporidium*.

9.2.1.7 Other Diagnostic Laboratory Tests for Parasitic or Helminth Infections

While peripheral eosinophilia is found in some parasitic and helminth infections, this is a nonspecific finding and may be absent in disseminated disease or patients on steroids (Mohapatra et al. 2018). Other available tests can evaluate for a particular parasitic or helminth infection and are seen in Table 9.1.

9.2.2 Evaluation of Fatty Diarrhea

The stool samples of children with prolonged diarrhea that float on the water of a toilet should be seen by the clinician to help them order the right diagnostic testing. Not all diarrhea is related to intestinal parasites or IBD. As noted above, the macroscopic evaluation of stool is important. Pancreatic insufficiency (PEI) causes steatorrhea

Table 9.1 Other diagnostic laboratory tests for parasitic or helminth infections

Name of test and pathogen identified	Sensitivity and specificity	Comments
E. histolytica		
Kits using ELISA, radioimmunoassay, or immunofluorescence methods are used for fecal antigen tests for *E. histolytica*	Superior to stool for O&P but less sensitive and specific than PCR	Distinguishes *E. histolytica* from *E. dispar* and *Entamoeba moshkovskii*
Serological tests for *E. histolytica*		
Giardia lamblia		
Direct smears	Use of light microscopy after iodine staining—52.4 sensitive and 98.27 specific (Alharbi et al. 2020)	It is the most common protozoal intestinal parasite globally and is transmitted via the fecal-oral route by contaminated water and food. Occurs more in summer and early fall (Leung et al. 2019)
Ritchie sedimentation technique	This technique involves emulsifying the stool and staining it—sensitivity is 40.47, and specificity is 100% (Alharbi et al. 2020)	Low sensitivity limits the use of the test
Direct fluorescent antibody tests that detect intact organisms (Leung et al. 2019)	Faster turnaround than microscopy (Leung et al. 2019)	
Antigen detection assays for *Giardia lamblia*, including ImmunoCard STAT! And CerTest	Better than stool for O&P, but PCR methods are superior. The direct immunofluorescence antigen type of test has the highest sensitivity of these tests (Kasırga 2019). The sensitivity is reported at 42.86–59.52, and specificity is reported at 89.65–98.27 (Alharbi et al. 2020) Faster turnaround than microscopy	Serological tests are not appropriate for the evaluation of *G. lamblia* More common among children under 5, hikers, campers, and backpackers who drink undertreated water
Real-time PCR data analysis	Sensitivity is 95.65–98%, and specificity is 74.03–100% (Alharbi et al. 2020; Leung et al. 2019)	Detects levels as low as 10 parasites/100 by detecting specific genes in the parasite within stool (Leung et al. 2019)
Cryptosporidium		
Immunofluorescent assays and enzyme immunoassay assays for *Cryptosporidium*	Are superior to stool evaluation with acid-fast staining under a microscopic	
Enterobius vermicularis (pinworms)		
Scotch tape test or cellulose-tape slide test for *Enterobius vermicularis* (pinworms)	Stool for O&P not recommended	Looks for eggs captured on adhesive cellophane tape placed against the perineum during the night when the worms come out and lay eggs
Strongyloides		
Serological tests for *Strongyloides* include an enzyme-linked immunoassay (EIA)	Sensitivity is greater than 90%	Recommended by the CDC
Schistosoma		
Circulating antibodies in blood or urine tests can identify an infection with *Schistosoma*		Primarily a disease of underdeveloped countries but can be found in travelers returning from those countries or in Latin American immigrants

Adapted from Alharbi et al. (2020), Kasırga (2019), Leung et al. (2019)

and can signify chronic pancreatitis, cystic fibrosis, a problem with the pancreatic duct system, or surgical pancreatic resection. Extra-pancreatic conditions include celiac disease, irritable bowel syndrome, gastric surgery, Zollinger-Ellison syndrome, and HIV infection (Domínguez-Muñoz et al. 2017). PEI is also associated with diabetes.

9.2.2.1 Fecal Elastase (FE-1)
Steatorrhea usually will not occur unless the lipase secretion is decreased by >90%. The pancreatic elastase-1 is very stable in the intestinal tract since proteolytic degradation does not occur (Sziegoleit and Linder 1991). FE-1 assesses the pancreatic output, amylase, lipase, and trypsin (Domínguez-Muñoz et al. 2017). The test for FE-1 can help distinguish between PEI and the infant with a problem of fat absorption. FE-1 is low in PEI. A meta-analysis and systematic review found that the assay for elastase-1 had a pooled sensitivity of 0.77 (95% CI, 0.58–0.89) and specificity of 0.88 (95% CI, 0.78–0.93) (Vanga et al. 2018). The lower the FE-1 levels, the more likely the patient has PEI (Domínguez-Muñoz et al. 2017).

It is prone to false positives in infants with prolonged high-volume diarrhea (Thiagarajah et al. 2018). The level of >200 mcg/g (normal level of FE-1 level) can rule out exocrine pancreatic insufficiency (EPI) in patients who have a low probability of EPI (such as patients who have irritable bowel syndrome and diarrhea) (Vanga et al. 2018).

The FE-1 immunoassay is usually covered by insurance and is relatively inexpensive. It requires <1 gm of stool and is not affected by either diet or fasting status (Domínguez-Muñoz et al. 2017). The stool sample can be used for up to 30 days if refrigerated to 4°, and it should not be diluted (Domínguez-Muñoz et al. 2017). Pancreatic insufficiency can be treated with pancreatic enzymes, and the child will get better once the pancreatic enzymes are replaced. In patients with chronic diarrhea, low FE-1 results point to pancreatic disease and PEI. In patients with pancreatic disease and malnutrition or maldigestion signs such as prolonged diarrhea or weight loss,

a low FE-1 result points to PEI. This test is a screening test, and when positive, a 72-h test for fecal fat remains the gold standard for diagnosing PEI.

9.2.2.2 72-Hour Test for Fecal Fat
The 72-hour test for fecal fact tests for the coefficient of fat absorption (CFA). It requires a strict diet of 100 g fat/day for a minimum of 5 days. All stools must be collected and placed in the refrigerator over 72 hours (Domínguez-Muñoz et al. 2017). Since the test is so time-consuming and unpleasant to do, the test remains difficult for patients. In addition, if the patient is on pancreatic enzyme replacement therapy, they must discontinue it during the testing. More than 6 g/day fat in the stool sample is considered pathological, but in patients with steatorrhea, more than 20 g of fat is usually found (Kasırga 2019). The result does not differentiate the cause of the steatorrhea.

One of the major limitations of the 72-h fecal fat test is that it does not distinguish between hepatobiliary, intestinal, and pancreatic causes of fat malabsorption. If there is less than 60 g of fat consumed daily, the test results are not accurate.

9.2.3 C. difficile

Clostridium difficile infection (CDI) can present without symptoms (asymptomatic colonization) to fulminant colitis and megacolon. It is a gram-positive, anaerobic bacterium that flourishes when the gut flora is altered by antibiotics or chemotherapy (dysbiosis). Carroll and Mizusawa recommend a two-step process for the diagnosis. The first step is a glutamate dehydrogenase (GDH) test followed by a toxin test or a nucleic acid test for confirmation (Carroll, Mizusawa, 2020). Lee, Plechot, Gohil, and Le (2021) recommend either a GDH test or a NAAT test followed by toxin A/B EIA in conjunction with clinical history (diagnostic stewardship). Currently, there is no consensus about the proper testing order.

The overuse of NAAT testing can lead to overdiagnosis as it will identify carriers at a high rate, leading to the overuse of antibiotics. To have a symptomatic CDI, a child must have adequate contact with a toxin-producing strain of *C. difficile* spores, with subsequent colon overgrowth leading to changes in the colon's microbiota (Lee et al. 2021). Antibiotic exposure is a common reason for increased risk of CDI, with clindamycin, cephalosporins, and fluoroquinolones have the highest risk (Brown et al. 2013; Deshpande et al. 2013). The child receiving laxatives or has a known cause of diarrhea should not have routine testing for *C. difficile* (Lee et al. 2021). While the gold standard was toxigenic culture, due to the slow turnaround of up to 7 days (Carroll, Mizusawa, 2020), and a higher incidence of false-positive results due to non-toxigenic results, makes this method is a reference method and not a diagnostic method (Lee et al. 2021). The testing for *C. difficile* and the pitfalls are found below:

9.2.3.1 Glutamate Dehydrogenase (GDH) Screening

GDH EIA, lateral flow membrane, and enzyme-linked fluorescent assay-chemiluminescent immunoassay (ELFA/CLIA) tests detect the metabolic enzyme present in non-toxigenic and toxigenic C. Difficile. The EIA test's sensitivity ranges from 88% to 95%, and the specificity is from 94% to 98% (Carroll, Mizusawa, 2020). Lee et al. (2021) report a lower specificity of 70%. The lateral flow membrane test has a sensitivity reported from 60% to 100% with a 76–100% specificity. The ELFA tests have a sensitivity of 87–99% and a specificity of 91–97% (Lee et al. 2021). However, the tests cannot differentiate between non-toxigenic and toxigenic forms of *C. difficile*. A test is a screening tool, and positive results must be followed up with a toxin A/B EIA or a nucleic acid test. The higher specificity of these tests will help clarify the results of the GDH screen.

9.2.3.2 Toxin A/B EIA

Toxins A and B are the primary virulence factors that cause *C. difficile* infections. EIA detections of toxins A and B were the main ways of *C. difficile* testing for years before nucleic acid testing. The EIA assays are available in various formats, including ELFA, CLIA, microwell, rapid immunoassays using immunocards, lateral flow

membrane, and cassettes. The sensitivity of the tests varies from 41% to 86% for the microwell EIA to a low of 29–79% for the lateral flow membranes (Carroll, Mizusawa, 2020). The specificity is much higher ranging from 89% to 100% for all tests. EIAs are not recommended as a standalone test (Carroll, Mizusawa, 2020; Lee et al. 2021).

9.2.3.3 Nucleic Acid Detection Methods

The first FDA-approved PCR test for *C. difficile* in stool samples was in 2008. There are several FDA-cleared molecular-based platforms to detect toxin A or B in the United States. The tests are more expensive than the assays above. However, when the laboratory changed from EIA toxin verification to NAAT testing, the cost savings of decreasing the number of treated patients resulted in cost savings despite the expense of the test (Bartsch et al. 2015; Xuan et al. 2020). It is important to make sure that the history and physical exam of the patient are appropriate for testing as studies have shown that in adults, up to 50% are inappropriately tested (Dubberke et al. 2011; Buckel et al. 2015).

The laboratory may ask for reasons for the testing and reject specimens where there is no reason for testing. The sensitivity of the tests varies from 62% to 100%, and the specificity varies from 90% to 100% (Carroll, Mizusawa, 2020). As mentioned previously, the test can detect patients with colonization leading to overdiagnosis and treatment (Carroll, Mizausawaka, 2020; Lee et al. 2021).

9.2.4 *Helicobacter pylori*

H. pylori are the most common bacterial infection, and it is estimated to infect around half of the global population (Sabbagh et al. 2019). The gram-negative human pathogen is associated with gastroduodenal diseases such as gastritis, ulcer, and mucosa-associated lymphoid tissue (MALT) (Wang et al. 2015). Fortunately, children and adolescents do not develop these complications often (Jones et al. 2017). As a result, the guidelines for testing for *H. pylori* in children are limited to specific conditions, as seen in

Box 9.1. Since *H. pylori* do not cause symptoms in children unless they have peptic ulcer disease, a noninvasive test to identify and treat *H. pylori* infection is not indicated (Jones et al. 2017). The Joint ESPGHAN/NASPGHAN Guidelines state that the diagnosis of *H. pylori* infection is done based on histopathology in *H. pylori*-positive gastritis plus a minimum of one other positive biopsy-based test or culture that is positive. Thus, even in noninvasive positive diagnostic testing, an endoscopy should be done based on the guidelines. As a result, the noninvasive tests for *H. pylori* include stool antigen test (SAT), serology, ^{13}C or ^{14}C urea breath test, and molecular methods outlined briefly.

Box 9.1 Specific Indications for Endoscopy and/or Noninvasive Evaluation for *H. pylori*
- Children with gastric or duodenal ulcer disease.
- Children with refractory IDA when there are no identified causes and other diagnoses are ruled out.
- Noninvasive diagnostic testing for *H. pylori* infection can be done when exploring the reason for chronic immune thrombocytopenic purpura (ITP).

9.2.4.1 *Helicobacter pylori (H. pylori)* Stool Antigen Test (SAT)

Since *H. pylori* adhere to the gastric epithelial wall, it is excreted in the feces. The stool must be refrigerated after collection to maintain the high sensitivity of the test. If the test is not immediately done, the stool must be frozen.

The two types of SAT are EIA and immunochromatography assay (ICA). The ICA uses either polyclonal antibodies or monoclonal antibodies. If *H. pylori* prevalence is low to moderate, the stool antigen test is cost-effective. The monoclonal immunoassays (EIAs) have a sensitivity of 94% and specificity of 97% (Sabbagh et al. 2019). The pitfalls of the test include that the results are affected by some gastrointestinal problems such as bleeding ulcers and N-acetylcysteine (NAC)

treatments. The test will yield negative results in low bacterial load due to antibiotics, PPIs, and bismuth (Sabbagh et al. 2019).

9.2.4.2 Antibody-Based (IgG, IgA) Tests for *H. pylori*

Antibodies against *H. pylori* can be detected via ELISA, immunoblotting, and EIA. The North American Society for Pediatric Gastroenterology, Hepatology and Nutrition (NASPGHAN) recommends that in children, no antibody-based (IgG, IgA) tests for *H. pylori* in any medium (serum, whole blood, urine, or saliva) should be used (Jones et al. 2017).

9.2.4.3 ^{13}C or ^{14}C Urea Breath Test

The urea breath test (UBT) is regarded as a gold standard noninvasive method for *H. pylori* diagnosis. The sensitivity of UBT is 95.9% and a specificity of 95.7% (Sabbagh et al. 2019).

The patient's condition, the use of proton pump inhibitors, a recent history of bleeding, bacterium, the child's age, and the test itself can cause false-positive and false-negative results. The test is less reliable in young children (Sabbagh et al. 2019). However, it can distinguish between past and current infections. The test is only used in specialty clinics.

9.2.4.4 Molecular Methods

PCR is quick and has high sensitivity and specificity (›95%). Gastric juice, gastric biopsy, saliva, and feces can be used for this method.

9.2.5   Real-Life Examples

A 16-year-old presented with a 1-week history of diarrhea which was described as initially bloody with mucus. The family was traveling during the past week and reported traveling to Spain and Morocco. A careful history revealed that she was the only person that had eaten a special soup in Morocco and had become ill 24 h after ingesting the soup. The rest of the family had no symptoms. A stool for gastrointestinal pathogen PCR panel was sent, and the results were obtained within 36 hours, showing the child had a *Campylobacter* infection. The child was treated appropriately, and all diarrhea was resolved within 5 days. The rapid results enabled the child to receive prompt treatment.

A 3-year-old had recurrent otitis media and a partial antibody deficiency with impaired polysaccharide responsiveness (IPR). His ear infections required several courses of antibiotics. The child presented with 10 days of marked diarrhea. *C. difficile* was suspected. A NAAT test was positive and confirmed by toxin A/B EIA. Due to the severity of diarrhea, the child was treated with fidaxomicin based on the 2018 guidelines with marked improvement (McDonald et al. 2018).

Key Learning about Diarrhea
- The clinician must know the developmental difference in stool characteristics.
- The Sudan III Stain of stool can detect more than 90% of patients with steatorrhea.
- The use of a gastrointestinal pathogen PCR panel allows for simultaneous qualitative detection and identification of nucleic acids from over 20 of the most common pathogens, including bacteria, viruses. and parasites from one stool sample. These tests cost more but are more accurate, and results can be obtained.
- Steatorrhea usually will not occur unless the lipase secretion is decreased by >90%. Fecal elastase can help the pancreatic output, amylase, lipase, and trypsin (Domínguez-Muñoz et al. 2017).
- Antibiotic exposure is a common reason for increased risk of CDI, but two-step testing must be done to avoid identifying normal colonization.
- *H. pylori* testing should be done in specific clinical situations.

9.3 Overview of Celiac Disease

CD is an immune-mediated enteropathy of the small intestine caused by gluten ingestion found in genetically susceptible individuals. The prevalence of CD is 1–3% in North America and Europe and 1% worldwide (Gujral et al. 2012; Guandalini 2017). There is a strong familial recurrence in the range of 10–15%. Among monozygotic twins, the incidence is from 75 to 80% (Caio et al. 2019) and the high concordance of the disease among monozygotic twins (75–80%). A careful family history of autoimmune disease should also raise concern for possible CD (Caio et al. 2019).

Clinical presentation of CD varies considerably. Some individuals may be asymptomatic, while others may experience gastrointestinal and/or non-gastrointestinal manifestations. Symptoms can be vague and nonspecific and vary by age. Younger children often present with diarrhea, anorexia, abdominal distention, abdominal pain, failure to thrive, and irritability. Older children may experience gastrointestinal symptoms depending on the amount of gluten ingested and may include diarrhea, nausea, vomiting, bloating, abdominal pain, weight loss, and constipation. Extraintestinal symptoms in older children and adolescents may include short stature, joint or bone pain, fatigue, rash, headache, or difficulty concentrating, as outlined in Table 9.2 (Madani and Kamat 2006, Moreno 2014).

Table 9.2 Clinical manifestations of CD

Gastrointestinal	Extraintestinal
Diarrhea	Pubertal delay
Abdominal pain	Poor height gain
Constipation	Unexplained weight loss
Abdominal bloating/distention	Body/joint pain
Poor weight gain	Rash of dermatitis herpetiformis
Malodorous fatty stools	Fatigue
Vomiting	Headaches
	Foggy mind

Adapted from Hill et al. (2016)

9.3.1   Pathophysiology of CD

The pathogenesis of CD is a complex interaction between environmental, genetic, and immunologic factors. Gluten-containing proteins in wheat, rye, and barley have many proteolysis-resistant sequences, resulting in the persistence of larger peptides called gliadins in the gut. These peptides are toxic and can trigger an innate immune response, increasing circulating immunoglobulins or activate small intestine mucosal CD4+ T cells in genetically predisposed patients. This immune response results in damage to the small intestine's lining (Abadie et al. 2011; Guandalini 2017).

Malabsorption results from damage of the small intestine mucosa with loss of absorptive surface area and reduced digestive enzymes leading to impaired absorption of micronutrients such as fat-soluble vitamins, iron, vitamin B12, and folic acid. Severe malnutrition and muscle wasting can occur if the diagnosis is delayed (Amerine 2006; Al-Toma et al. 2019).

Primary care providers must understand the clinical indications for CD screening. Results of screening tests will help guide the provider's referral to pediatric gastroenterology. The gold standard in CD diagnosis is endoscopy, with pathology showing small intestinal villous atrophy. Appropriate CD diagnosis in children is critical to ensure physical and cognitive growth (Alrabadi and Porto 2018).

9.3.2   Who Needs Testing for CD?

Screening for CD is recommended for patients with suggestive symptoms. Box 9.2 identifies children in high-risk groups for which clinicians should consider screening regardless of symptoms. If screening is undertaken for asymptomatic individuals in identified high-risk groups, testing should first be performed at 3 years of age or at the time of diagnosis of the associated condition (Hill et al. 2016; Husby et al. 2012). If initial results for asymptomatic individuals are negative, screening tests should be repeated at intervals or when symptoms develop (Hill et al. 2005).

> **Box 9.2 Asymptomatic Individuals and Conditions to Consider CD Screening**
> - First-degree relatives.
> - Trisomy 21.
> - Turner syndrome.
> - William syndrome.
> - IgA deficiency.
> - Type 1 diabetes.
> - Autoimmune thyroid disease.
> - Autoimmune liver disease.
> - Juvenile chronic arthritis.
>
> Adapted from Hill et al. 2016

9.3.3   Celiac Genetics

CD is strongly influenced by genetic factors, with most of the genetic dependence residing in human leukocyte antigen (HLA)-DQ2 and HLA-DQ8 (Lázár-Molnár and Snyder 2018). If a patient with CD ingests gluten, peptides are produced. These peptides have a high attraction for HLA-DQ2 and HLA-DQ8. A complex of HLA-DQ2 and HLA-DQ8/peptide complexes form and are recognized by the T cells with a specific T-cell receptor (TCR). When the complexes attach to the TCR, antibodies are produced by B-cell-derived plasma cells, leading to an inflammatory response in the GI tract. The inflammatory response causes the patient to produce antibodies to autoantigens, including intestinal tissue transglutaminase (TTG) (Lázár-Molnár and Snyder 2018).

Genetic testing for HLA-DQ2 and HLA-DQ8 alone is not diagnostic since there is a higher incidence of alleles among populations than the actual incidence of CD. The absence of HLA-DQ2 and HLA-DQ8 makes the likelihood of the patient having the disease unlikely. The 2020 ESPGHAN guidelines emphasize using these tests in patients with CD symptoms and elevated serological tests for CD.

9.3.3.1 HLA Testing

There have been considerable advances in DNA sequencing that have enabled clinicians to understand the role of HLA in a variety of diseases (Shieh et al. 2018).

Heterodimers DQ2 and DQ8 are necessary for diagnosing CD but not specific to people with the condition. Up to 40% of the general population have HLA-DQ2 and/or HLA-DQ8. There are celiac genetic panels commercially available to evaluate the presence of such genes. If genetic markers are present, the individual is at an increased risk compared to the general population to develop CD. Being homozygous versus heterozygous will increase the risk further, with HLA-DQ2 homozygous individuals at the greatest risk (Rubio-Tapia et al. 2013).

Celiac genetic testing should not be used as an initial diagnostic test (Rubio-Tapia et al. 2013). Testing for HLA-DQ2/HLA-DQ8 is best reserved for patients in whom there is a diagnostic dilemma. For example, if there is a discrepancy between serology and pathology results. Alternatively, genetic testing can be considered if a patient adopted a gluten-free diet weeks before any serologic testing and CD is suspected. If HLA-DQ2 and HLA-DQ8 are not detected, then CD is highly unlikely (Hill et al. 2016).

HLA testing may be used as an initial test for screening asymptomatic patients at increased risk, such as first-degree relatives of patients with medical conditions at higher risk of developing CD (Husby et al. 2012) (see Box 9.2). If the genetic screen is negative, no additional testing is needed (Hill et al. 2016). If celiac genetics are positive, the next step in screening would be serologic testing for antibodies.

The pitfalls of the test are that genetic testing is expensive to perform and DQ2 and DQ8 are not specific to CD.

9.3.4 Diagnostic Laboratory Tests for CD

The gold standard for diagnosing celiac disease has always been doing an endoscopy and obtaining an intestinal biopsy of the duodenum; however, recent ESPGHAN guidelines suggest serological diagnosis using a combination of TTG-IgA and IgA. When the TTG-IgA is greater than or equal to tenfold the upper limit of normal, and the antiendomysial antibodies are positive, then a biopsy is unnecessary. If the TTG-IgA is less than a tenfold increase, then a biopsy should be done. The guidelines do not state that HLA-DQ2/HLA-DQ8 testing is obligatory to diagnose celiac disease (Husby et al. 2020).

The World Gastroenterology Association (WGA) recommends that patients with a high pretest probability of CD should have TTG-IgA testing with endoscopy. In contrast, patients with a low pretest probability of CD should have serological testing done first, and only if the results are positive should endoscopy be done. The WGA advises the use of TTG-IgA as a first-line test (Bai et al. 2016).

Serologic or antibody testing for CD is useful for screening and an important first step in the diagnosis. The accuracy of testing is dependent on the ingestion of gluten, and avoidance of gluten can give false-negative results. To be confident about the interpretation of the TTG test, the clinician should inquire about the child's intake of gluten. For older school-aged children and adolescents, the equivalent of ≥ 10 g of gluten (equivalent to two slices of whole wheat bread) every day for ≥ 8 weeks assures that the TTG antibody test result is accurate (Hill et al. 2016). The initial testing of total IgA and TTG-IgA is the most accurate test combination (Husby et al. 2020).

CD antibodies belong to the immunoglobulin A (IgA) and immunoglobulin G (IgG) classes. IgA antibodies are more sensitive and specific for CD in comparison to IgG antibodies. IgG antibodies can be misleading due to the high percentage of false positives and are usually reserved for IgA deficiency patients (Caio et al. 2019; Villalta et al. 2010).

According to the North American Society for Pediatric Gastroenterology, Hepatology and Nutrition (NASPGHAN), total immunoglobulin A (IgA) and TTG-IgA are the most appropriate tests for CD screening (Hill et al. 2005; Hill et al. 2016).

A celiac panel will likely include the following tests: (1) total IgA, (2) tissue transglutaminase IgA, (3) deamidated gliadin peptide (DGP)

IgA and IgG, and (4) EMA-IgA. A panel may increase the cost of an initial screen without increasing diagnostic yield, thus the recommendations from the NASPGHAN.

9.3.4.1 Total Immunoglobulin A

Immunoglobulin A (IgA) is an antibody that plays a key role in the immune function of mucus membranes and is in high concentrations in the gastrointestinal and respiratory tracts. Total serum IgA concentration measurement is mandatory in CD screening as it allows the provider to screen for selective IgA deficiency (Al-Toma et al. 2019).

One of the pitfalls of CD testing without IgA is that the clinician ignores the fact that approximately 2% of children with CD will have previously unrecognized IgA deficiency. If initial testing suggests IgA deficiency, further screening should be performed with IgG antibodies (Al-Toma et al. 2019; Hill et al. 2016). If testing is performed without total IgA, those with IgA deficiency will not be identified, and they are at risk for false-negative test results. Furthermore, additional screening with IgG antibodies may not be performed.

9.3.4.2 Tissue Transglutaminase IgA

TTG is a ubiquitous enzyme released from intestinal cells during mechanical or cellular stress. In patients with CD, TTG plays at least two critical roles: (1) deamidating enzyme and (2) target autoantigen in the immune response. TTG converts gliadin peptides in the intestinal mucosa to a more toxic peptide leading to an inflammatory cascade as a deamidating enzyme. As an autoantigen, the activity of TTG results in an increased level of circulating IgA antibodies against TTG and endomysium, a connective tissue protein within the gastrointestinal tract (Di Sabatino et al. 2012). It has a sensitivity of 90–100 and a specificity of 95–100% (Hill et al. 2016).

For most patients, the most valuable screening test for CD is TTG-IgA. The test is performed using enzyme-linked immunosorbent assay (ELISA) technology (Husby et al. 2019). It is also automated in the in vitro test system for the quantitative determination of TTG-IgA

in the serum or plasma. TTG-IgA antibody at levels that are ten times the upper limit of normal is considered a reliable and accurate test to diagnose celiac (Husby et al. 2020). Combining the results of a positive TTG with a second blood draw for endomysial antibody-IgA (EMA-IgA) has a positive predictive value of around 100% (Alkalay 2020).

The pitfalls of TTG-IgA are that the presence of a concurrent illness or other chronic conditions such as diabetes, Crohn's disease, and liver disease may result in mild elevations in TTG-IgA (Green and Jones 2016). Such findings may be nonspecific and of no clinical significance (Gidrewicz et al. 2015; De Leo et al. 2015).

Some studies suggest TTG-IgA may not accurately screen the young child (Husby et al. 2012). In this patient population, collection of deamidated gliadin protein, IgA, and IgG may be prudent.

9.3.4.3 Deamidated Gliadin Antibodies: IgA and IgG

As mentioned above, TTG is a deamidating enzyme. Gliadin peptides, rich in the amino acid glutamate, are excellent substrates for TTG, and via a chemical reaction called deamidation, the amino acid glutamine is changed to glutamate. The resulting deamidated gliadin peptides have a greater affinity to specific protein receptors (HLA-DQ2 or HLA-DQ8) found on the surface of antigen-presenting cells. Once the deamidated gliadin peptides are bound to receptors, they activate small intestine mucosal CD4+ T cells resulting in T-cell reactivity, subsequent B-cell stimulation, and antibody production, including deamidated gliadin peptide (DGP) IgA and IgG (Rubio-Tapia et al. 2013).

DGP antibodies have proven to be additional indicators of CD (Prause et al. 2009). Testing for DGP-IgA and DGP-IgG in conjunction with TTG-IgA is recommended in children under 2 years of age. DGP-IgG antibodies combined with TTG-IgG are recommended in patients with IgA deficiency (Hill et al. 2016). The DGP-IgA has a sensitivity of 80–91% and a specificity of 91–95% (Hill et al. 2016). The DGP-IgG has a sensitivity of 88–91% and a specificity of

86–98% (Hill et al. 2016). DGP tests can detect the antibodies against synthetically derived peptides and are more accurate than AGA tests.

DGP-IgA is less sensitive and less specific than TTG-IgA and EMA-IgA. DGP-IgG has comparable specificity but lower sensitivity than the TTG-IgA and EMA-IgA.

9.3.4.4 EMA-IgA

Endomysium is a connective protein found in the smooth muscle of the gastrointestinal tract. EMA-IgA is highly specific in CD and may correlate to the degree of villous atrophy (Green and Jones 2016). Testing for EMA-IgA requires an immunofluorescent technique using monkey esophagus or human umbilical cord as the substrate. It is expensive to perform, and results are read manually by a technician. As results are subject to interobserver variability, they are more prone to error in interpretation (Green and Jones 2016; Hill et al. 2005; Hill et al. 2016). With the identification of TTG as the autoantigen to identify CD, EMA-IgA testing is used as a second-line test to clarify the diagnosis in patients with equivocal results of TTG-IgA (Hill et al. 2016; James and Scott 2000). It has a 93–100% sensitivity and a specificity of 98–100% (Hill et al. 2016). When the test is positive, it is likely the patient with symptoms has the disease. The clinician must be aware that the EMA-IgA test is more specific than the TTG-IgA, but it is less sensitive than the TTG-IgA (Hill et al. 2016).

The major pitfalls of EMA-IgA are that the test is expensive to perform and results are subject to observer error.

9.3.4.5 Antigliadin Antibodies: IgA and IgG

Antigliadin antibodies (ANA) IgA and IgG are no longer used as screening for CD as they are poorly sensitive and specific compared with TTG and EMA antibody testing. Furthermore, testing has been replaced by DGP antibodies that have higher sensitivity and specificity (Alrabadi and Porto 2018; Al-Toma et al. 2019).

The pitfalls of antigliadin IgA and IgG are that the tests are poorly sensitive and specific compared with antibodies to TTG, EMA, and DGP. The antigliadin IgG and IgA tests are known to have too wide variability between laboratories (Hill et al. 2016).

9.3.4.6 Point-of-Care Tests for TTG Antibodies

Point-of-care testing (POCT) for CD is available and used in Europe for over 10 years (Singh et al. 2019). POCTs are easy to perform once the staff has been properly trained and can help diagnose CD. A recent systematic review and meta-analysis by Singh et al. (2019) reported data from six studies. They found that for TTG-IgA-based POCT, the pooled sensitivity was 90.5% (95% CI, 82.3–95.1%) and the pooled specificity was 94.8% (95% CI, 92.5–96.4%). While the specificity of POCT at 94.8% is high, a small bowel biopsy should be used to confirm the diagnosis (Singh et al. 2019). Due to user error in reading faint lines on some of the POCT tests, training is important. The use of these tests in areas where laboratory access is limited may help in the diagnosis. Antigliadin antibody assay POCTs, while available, are not recommended as TTG-IgA antibody testing is the preferred test in children over the age of 2 years (Rubio-Tapia et al. 2013).

9.3.4.7 Celiac-Associated HLA-DQ Alpha 1 DQ and Beta 1 DNA Typing

When a patient has symptoms consistent with CD but has a negative serology for the tests above, celiac-associated human leukocyte antigens (HLA)-DQ alpha 1 DQ and beta 1 DNA should be considered. HLAs are proteins found on the T lymphocyte and other cells. If a patient has the genetic susceptibility to CD, the T lymphocyte may have certain HLA genes in the class II region (DQ alpha 1, DQ beta 1). The HLA-DQ molecule has two chains: DQ alpha and DQ beta. The chains are encoded by the HLA-DQA1 gene and HLA-DQB1 gene, respectively. The testing for HLA-DQ can be done by serology or by molecular methods. The latter is the most common way to do this today as there are different haplotypes of HLA-DQ2 and HLA-DQ8.

Serological Test. Serological tests only test for the DQB1 chain, while the molecular method tests for DQB1 and DQA1 chains.

Polymerase Chain Reaction (PCR). These can be tested with polymerase chain reaction (PCR)/sequence-specific oligonucleotide probe for celiac-associated HLA-DQ alpha 1 DQ and beta 1 DNA typing. Typing these haplotypes is important in celiac disease as they carry different risk associations (Alkalay 2020).

Around 90–95% of patients with CD have one or two copies of the HLA-DQ2 haplotype, while the rest have HLA-DQ8 haplotype. In one study of CD, 0.7% of patients with CD did not have this association. However, around 20% of patients with CD may have these genes and not have CD (Alkalay 2020).

9.3.5 Celiac Screening: Special Considerations

There are certain conditions where screening for CD requires additional testing or requires retesting. Endoscopy may be required to confirm the diagnosis in certain conditions listed below.

9.3.5.1 Screening for Patients with Selective IgA Deficiency

Selective IgA deficiency is more common in individuals with CD than in the general population. In such cases IgG-based TTG, EMA, or DGP is required to screen for CD. A positive IgG-based test for any of these antibodies in an individual with IgA deficiency is an indication for endoscopy with biopsy to confirm or exclude the diagnosis. Furthermore, as IgG tests are less accurate than IgA tests, if there is high clinical suspicion for CD, endoscopy with biopsy should be considered even if the IgG serological testing is negative (Hill et al. 2005).

9.3.5.2 Young Children

Some data suggests that the TTG-IgA and EMA-IgA tests may not be as reliable in children under 2 years of age. Therefore, when testing for CD in a young child, it is suggested that TTG-IgA be collected along with DGP-IgG to improve the accuracy of testing (Husby et al. 2012; Liu et al. 2007).

9.3.5.3 Patients with Autoimmune Conditions

Individuals with other autoimmune conditions associated with CD, such as type 1 diabetes mellitus and autoimmune thyroiditis, can have transient mild elevations in TTG-IgA that are nonspecific and may not be suggestive of CD. It is not known how elevated the TTG-IgA level is in these patient populations before one would consider endoscopy with biopsy. Therefore, obtaining an EMA-IgA can be helpful. If positive, endoscopy with biopsy would be indicated (Gidrewicz et al. 2015).

9.3.5.4 Concurrent Illness

Transient nonspecific elevation of TTG-IgA can be observed during an acute infectious process. Once illness resolves, these levels return to normal. Caution should be taken when interpreting values during a febrile illness (De Leo et al. 2015).

9.3.6 Real-Life Example

A 13-year-old female presents to her pediatrician with a 6-month history of fatigue and shoulder pain. She is an active gymnast who participates in statewide competitions. However, the level of fatigue and shoulder pain had intensified in the past 2 months, such that she opted to sit out this current season. She reports intermittent headaches and abdominal pain, but frequency had not increased with the onset of fatigue and joint pain. Her bowel movement pattern is regular, and she denies weight loss. Family history is positive for an older brother with diabetes type 1 and a mother with CD.

Physical exam revealed an interactive female in no acute distress, afebrile, and stable vital signs. A review of growth charts revealed weight stable at 50th percentile; height chart revealed drop from the 50th percentile to tenth percentile with no growth in the past year. Her exam was positive for a limited range of motion in upper extremities bilaterally and delayed puberty—no breast bud development.

A CBC, comprehensive metabolic panel (CMP), thyroid-stimulating hormone (TSH), hemoglobin A₁C, inflammatory markers (CRP and ESR), iron studies, total IgA, and TTG-IgA were done. Her hemoglobin A₁C, TSH, and CMP were normal. Her hemoglobulin was low at 10.5, her iron level was low at 35 (normal 60 to 170 mcg/dL), and her TTG-IgA was 75 U/mL (normal 1.2–4.0 U/mL). Repeat blood for EMA-IgA was positive. A referral was made to pediatric gastroenterology. She underwent endoscopy with small bowel pathology findings consistent with CD.

Key Learning about CD Diagnostic Testing
- Celiac serology testing needs to be performed on a gluten-containing diet.
- Total IgA must be collected to screen for IgA deficiency.
- For most patients, TTG-IgA is the most valuable screening test for CD.
- HLA-DQ2 and HLA-DQ8 may be good screening tests for asymptomatic high-risk groups.

9.4 Inflammatory Bowel Disease (IBD) Overview

IBD includes both ulcerative colitis (UC) and Crohn's disease and is a chronic immune-mediated condition of the gastrointestinal tract. Ulcerative colitis affects the colon only and is characterized by inflammation of the mucosal layer. Crohn's disease can involve any part of the gastrointestinal tract from the oral cavity to the anus and is characterized by transmural inflammation. IBD is most often diagnosed in adolescents and young adulthood, with a rising incidence in the pediatric population (Benchimol et al. 2017).

The incidence and prevalence of IBD are increasing globally. The peak incidence of IBD occurs in patients between the ages of 15 and 30 years (Johnston and Logan 2008). In Canada and the United States, the incidence of pediatric IBD is approximately 10 per 100,000 children (Loftus Jr. 2016). Although IBD is not common in early childhood, it has been observed as early as infancy (Heyman et al. 2005). Of the estimated 1.6 million Americans with IBD, 25% will have developed their disease before 18 years of age (Griffiths 2004; Benchimol et al. 2011).

Pediatric IBD can present with various symptoms, intestinal and extraintestinal. Table 9.3 reviews the common red flags for a child with suspected IBD. The common symptoms of ulcerative colitis are abdominal pain and bloody diarrhea. Symptoms in Crohn's disease can be more varied and may also include abdominal pain and bloody diarrhea if colitis is present. However, patients can also present with less specific symptoms such as non-bloody diarrhea, poor growth, weight loss, fatigue, malaise, anemia, or fever. The onset of growth failure is usually

Table 9.3 Common red flags in presentation of the child with suspected inflammatory bowel disease

History
Abdominal pain
Increase in stool frequency, diarrhea (present in up to 70–85% of patients) (Dykes and Saeed 2016)
Change in stool consistency
Hematochezia (blood in stool)
Nocturnal awakening to defecate
Urgency to defecate
Tenesmus
Family history: Relatives with IBD, familial growth patterns, or other autoimmune diseases
Growth failure: Weight loss, anorexia, or poor appetite
Psychosocial history, including the impact upon the daily life of patient and parent(s)
Physical examination
Height and weight: Evaluation of trends and growth velocity
HEENT: Oral ulcers, mucosa pallor
Chest: Hemic flow murmur, clubbing
Abdominal examination: Tenderness, mass
Rectal examination: Evaluate for perianal disease, perianal skin tags, and occult blood
Skin: Pallor, rash
Musculoskeletal: Joint swelling, pain on palpation, effusions of the knee
Tanner stage

Adapted from Dykes and Saeed 2016; Shashidhar et al. 2000

Table 9.4 Common extraintestinal manifestations associated with IBD

HEENT	Aphthous ulcers Lesions indicative of vitamin deficiencies
Dermatologic	Erythema nodosum Pyoderma gangrenosum
Musculoskeletal	Growth failure Arthralgias
Rheumatologic	Arthritis Ankylosing spondylitis
Endocrine	Thyroiditis Osteopenia Osteoporosis
Ophthalmologic	Episcleritis Uveitis Iritis
Pulmonary	Fibrosing alveolitis Granulomatous lung disease Bronchitis
Hepatobiliary	Primary sclerosing cholangitis Autoimmune hepatitis Pancreatitis Cholelithiasis
Urologic	Nephrolithiasis Urinary crystal formation
Hematologic	Anemia of chronic inflammation Increased risk for thromboembolic events Venous thrombosis

Adapted from Grossman and Baldassan (2016)

insidious, and any child or adolescent with persistent growth alterations should undergo IBD evaluation. Growth failure can precede intestinal symptoms by years (Liacouras et al. 2008).

Up to 25% of children experience extraintestinal symptoms. Almost every organ system can be affected, but symptoms involving the eyes, skin, liver, and joints are considered primary manifestations (Rosen et al. 2015a; Sairenji et al. 2017). Table 9.4 outlines some common extraintestinal manifestations associated with IBD.

9.4.1   Pathophysiology of IBD

Although the specific cause of IBD is unknown, internal and external environmental factors, genetic predisposition, and an altered immune system play a role in developing the disease. The high incidence of disease among first-degree

relatives of the affected individual supports the concept of genetic predisposition (Conrad and Rosh 2017; Shapiro et al. 2016).

Current theories on the development of IBD involve a cascade of events that leads to the condition. A stimulus that may be microbial, dietary, or environmental prompts the immune system of the intestinal tract. In a non-genetically predisposed individual, the stimulation and subsequent inflammation are self-limited and controlled. However, in a genetically predisposed individual, the inflammation is not self-limited, and inflammatory mediators are continually produced by immune cells leading to tissue injury and fibrosis (Liacouras et al. 2008).

9.4.2   Importance of History and Physical Exam

A thorough social and family history is important in addition to the history of present illness, as approximately 20% of newly diagnosed patients report a first-degree relative with IBD. Additional family history of other autoimmune conditions such as psoriasis or rheumatoid arthritis increases the likelihood of IBD (Shapiro et al. 2016).

Physical examination is critical as findings may further support the suspicion of IBD. A review of growth charts may reveal flattening of weight and height. Abdominal examination may reveal focal tenderness or fullness relating to the distribution of their disease. The perianal region should be examined for tags, fissures, fistulas, or abscesses. If a digital rectal examination is possible, occult blood testing may be performed (Shapiro et al. 2016).

If findings from the history and physical exam are concerning for IBD, further evaluation is warranted. Table 9.5 outlines the common differential diagnosis for IBD.

9.4.3   Noninvasive Testing for IBD

Although there are no pathognomonic laboratory tests for IBD, initial evaluation includes assessing for nonspecific signs of inflammation

Table 9.5 Common differential diagnosis for IBD

Primary presenting symptom	Differential diagnosis considerations
Abdominal pain	Constipation
	Irritable bowel syndrome
	Appendicitis
	Intussusception
	Peptic disease
	Lymphoma
	Mesenteric adenitis
	Ovarian cyst
	Meckel's diverticulum
	Lactose intolerance
Diarrhea	Infection
	C. difficile
	Salmonella
	Shigella
	Campylobacter
	Yersinia
	Cryptosporidium
	Enteroviruses
	Giardiasis
	Other bacterial, viral, or parasitic infections
	Irritable bowel syndrome
	Carbohydrate intolerance
	Laxative abuse
Bloody diarrhea	Infection
	C. difficile
	Salmonella
	Campylobacter
	Yersinia
	Hemolytic uremic syndrome
	Henoch-Schonlein purpura
	Ischemic bowel
Rectal bleeding, no diarrhea	Polyps
	Fissure
	Meckel's diverticulum
	Solitary rectal ulcer
Growth delay	Endocrinopathy
Weight loss	Anorexia nervosa
Arthritis	Juvenile idiopathic arthritis
	Ankylosing spondylitis
	Infection

Adapted from: Grossman and Baldassan (2016); Liacouras et al. (2008)

Table 9.6 Laboratory evaluation for patients with suspected IBD

Blood tests	Possible findings
Complete blood cell count with differential	Leukocytosis, microcytic anemia, thrombocytosis
Hepatic function panel	Hypoalbuminemia elevated AST, ALT
Erythrocyte sedimentation rate	Elevated marker of inflammation
C-reactive protein	Elevated marker of inflammation
Stool tests	
Stool culture	Rule out infectious enteritis causes, including *salmonella*, *Shigella*, *Yersinia*, and *campylobacter*
Ova and parasite	Rule out parasitic infection
C. difficile	Rule out *C. difficile*
Stool calprotectin, lactoferrin	Elevated inflammatory markers

Adapted from Rosen et al. 2015a

laboratory evaluation for the patient with suspected IBD.

Baseline blood tests should include a complete blood cell count (CBC), liver enzymes, albumin, and the inflammatory markers erythrocyte sedimentation rate (ESR) and C-reactive protein.

9.4.3.1 Complete Blood Cell Count

The complete blood cell count may reveal anemia, thrombocytosis, or leukocytosis. Approximately 70% of patients with IBD will be anemic at diagnosis (Aljomah et al. 2018). Serum hemoglobin results should be correlated with certain red blood cell indices such as mean corpuscular volume to assess for chronicity and/or iron deficiency anemia—microcytic anemia. Observed thrombocytosis and leukocytosis are secondary to the inflammatory response (Mack et al. 2007).

The major pitfall of the CBC is that the findings of the complete blood cell count are not specific to IBD. Anemia can be due to other gastrointestinal disorders that may lead to blood loss, such as peptic ulcer disease or non-GI disorders such as an underlying hematologic disorder. Thrombocytosis and leukocytosis can be noted in any inflammatory response.

and chronic disease (Shapiro et al. 2016; Vermeire et al. 2006). Noninvasive tests performed by the primary care provider, including blood or fecal markers, can assist in ruling out IBD along with identifying patients that would benefit from further workup or referral to a pediatric gastroenterologist. Table 9.6 reviews the

9.4.3.2 Liver Enzymes: Alanine Transaminase and Aspartate Transaminase

The hepatobiliary disease is one of the most common extraintestinal manifestations seen in IBD and may precede the onset of IBD or accompany the active disease. Children may present with liver disease before any clinical signs of IBD. Alanine transaminase (ALT) and aspartate transaminase (AST) are enzymes found in the liver that assist in the metabolism of amino acids. ALT is more specific to the liver, while AST can be found in other organs such as the muscle. An increase in either AST or ALT may be suggestive of liver damage. Abnormal elevations in ALT and/or AST are common during the disease and may be observed in a child suspected to have IBD. However, such enzyme elevations are transient and related to disease activity (Liacouras et al. 2008).

Liver enzyme elevation is not specific to IBD and may suggest underlying hepatic pathology not related to IBD. Other etiologies of liver enzyme elevation can include an acute infection or an adverse event of medication.

9.4.3.3 Albumin

Albumin is another objective marker of chronic intestinal inflammation. Serum albumin can be low in children with more aggressive or extensive disease. Albumin is a negative acute-phase reactant, and hypoalbuminemia may be due to chronic intestinal inflammation resulting in malabsorption and fecal losses combined with poor oral intake. Approximately 40% of patients with IBD have depressed albumin levels at diagnosis (Mack et al. 2007; Vermeire et al. 2006).

Hypoalbuminemia is not a specific finding in IBD and can be found in other conditions such as malnutrition, liver disease, kidney disease, and heart disease.

9.4.3.4 Erythrocyte Sedimentation Rate

Erythrocyte sedimentation rate (ESR) is an acute-phase reactant. Section 6.3.1 of Chap. 6 reviews ESR. During an inflammatory reaction, higher concentrations of fibrinogen cause the erythrocytes to aggregate, resulting in a faster than normal rate for them to settle through plasma. An elevation in ESR may be noted in patients with IBD. However, ESR can be affected by many factors such as albumin levels, characteristics of erythrocytes, and immunoglobulins. Approximately 65 to 75% of patients have an elevated ESR at the time of IBD diagnosis (Mack et al. 2007).

The nonspecificity of ESR may result in false positives in an inflammatory response. Conversely, ESR can be slow in the acute-phase reaction and may result in false-negative results early in an inflammatory process.

9.4.3.5 C-Reactive Protein

C-reactive protein (CRP) is a protein that is made by the liver. Like ESR, CRP is also an acute-phase reactant and rises in response to inflammation throughout the body. Under normal circumstances, CRP is produced in low quantities. However, following an acute-phase stimulant such as inflammation, the production of CRP is rapidly increased in response to the release of cytokines, including interleukin-6, tumor necrosis factor-alpha, and IL-1 beta. CRP has a short half-life compared to other acute-phase reactants and therefore rises early after the onset of inflammation and rapidly decreases after the resolution of inflammation (Tsampalieros et al. 2011). Approximately 85% have elevated CRP at the time of IBD diagnosis (Beattie et al. 1995).

CRP elevation is not specific to IBD. Acute infection results in very high CRP levels that decrease with the treatment of the infection. Furthermore, CRP levels are elevated in many autoimmune conditions, including lupus, rheumatoid arthritis, cancer, and obesity.

Of note, ESR and CRP are more sensitive in detecting Crohn's disease than ulcerative colitis, with CRP found to be more sensitive than ESR (Vermeire et al. 2006).

9.4.3.6 IBD Serologies

Chronic inflammation in the intestinal tract with IBD may change immune response toward microbial flora. Antibodies against such microorganisms or against self-antigens have been detected in IBD populations. They are used as biomarkers in predicting disease course, complications, and response to treatment (i.e., medications or surgery). Furthermore, the presence of specific antibodies demonstrated to be useful in distinguishing patients with Crohn's disease from those with ulcerative colitis. Markers include immunoglobulin A (IgA) and immunoglobulin G (IgG) antibodies against the yeast *Saccharomyces cerevisiae* ([ASCA] IgA and IgG), perinuclear anti-neutrophil cytoplasmic antibody (p-ANCA), anti-chitobioside carbohydrate antibody IgG(ACCA), anti-laminaribioside carbohydrate antibody IgG (ALCA), anti-mannobioside carbohydrate IgG antibody (AMCA), and antibodies to the outer membrane protein of *Escherichia coli* (anti-OmpC) (Malickova et al. 2010; Mitsuyama et al. 2016; Sabery and Bass 2007).

The diagnostic role of serology is considerably less sensitive than C-reactive protein and ESR for the presence of IBD (Benor et al. 2010; Khan et al. 2002). A proportion of children with IBD will have negative tests; the sensitivity of such testing ranges from 65% to 75% (Zholudev et al. 2004). Furthermore, IBD serology testing or IBD panels are expensive to perform and not cost-effective in the diagnosis (Sabery and Bass 2007). Currently, the utility of serologic biomarkers is to assess risks associated with disease phenotype, predict prognosis, and distinguish Crohn's disease from UC. There is a limited value in the initial diagnosis of IBD (Malickova et al. 2010).

9.4.4 Stool Testing

Infectious diarrhea and testing for this are discussed in detail in Sect. 9.2. It is important to remember that the identification of an infectious pathogen does not exclude an IBD diagnosis. If symptoms persist or worsen despite treatment, further evaluation is needed.

9.4.4.1 Fecal Occult Blood

There are two ways to test for fecal occult blood: (1) guaiac fecal occult blood test (gFOBT) and the immunochemical FOBT. The gFOBT uses guaiac, which is produced from the resin of the guaiacum tree. The gFOBT detects heme or the iron component of hemoglobin that might be present in the stool. When the stool containing blood is mixed with a reagent of hydrogen peroxide, which is on guaiac paper, the paper

turns blue when the test is positive. gFOBT is a common way to test stool for blood in primary care as it is a POCT approved for office use. It can detect both upper and lower gastrointestinal bleeding (Bechtold et al. 2016). It is cheaper than immunochemical FOBT but is affected by dietary intake.

The immunochemical FOBT uses antibodies that detect human globin (Bechtold et al. 2016). This kind of test is used primarily in adults to detect colon cancer. It is not affected by dietary intake.

Rectal bleeding presents at least 80% of patients with UC and 40% of those with CD (Kugathasan et al. 2003). If clinical suspicion for IBD is high, but there is no history of rectal bleeding, a stool guaiac test may be useful. Crohn's disease should be strongly considered in a child with weight loss, anemia, and hematochezia as this combination of symptoms has a cumulative sensitivity of 94% for Crohn's disease (El-Chammas et al. 2013).

The results of a stool guaiac or fecal occult blood must be interpreted with caution as dietary intake of certain medications and food can lead to a positive stool test for blood. Table 9.7 reviews

Table 9.7 Causes of false-positive and false-negative results for testing fecal occult blood

Type of error	Reasons
False-negative results	• Both methods ○ Intermittent bleeding that is not present at the time of testing • Immunochemical FOBT ○ upper GI bleeding since globin will be digested by pancreatic enzymes • Guaiac FOBT ○ Ascorbic acid can block an oxidative guaiac reaction since it is a strong reducing agent (Sawhney et al. 2010)
False-positive results	• Extraintestinal blood such as epistaxis • Red meat • Fruit that contains peroxidase such as horseradish (Bangaru and Agrawal 2019) • medications ○ antiplatelet agents (e.g., low-dose aspirin) ○ nonsteroidal anti-inflammatory drugs ○ Oral anticoagulants (Wu 2019)

Adapted from Bangaru and Agrawal (2019); Sawhney et al. 2010; Wu (2019)

the list of medications and food that can cause a false-positive result.

Blood in stool is not diagnostic for IBD, although it may support suspicion or guide the next steps in evaluation. If able, an inspection of the perianal region at the time of testing is important as anal fissures can cause false-positive results.

9.4.4.2 Fecal Calprotectin (FCal)

Calprotectin is a calcium and zinc-binding neutrophilic cytosolic protein that can be detected in stool as an indicator of intestinal inflammation. Fecal calprotectin (FCal) closely correlates with the endoscopic activity of IBD and, as such, is a useful screening tool. FCal is highly sensitive but not specific to IBD (Conrad and Rosh 2017). In a population of children referred to primary care centers, fecal calprotectin had a pooled sensitivity of 92% (95% CI, 84%–96%) and a pooled specificity of 76% (95% CI, 62%–86%) for IBD (Van Rheenen et al. 2010). The negative likelihood ratio = 0.01 (95% CI, 0.00–0.13), so if the test is negative, it is unlikely that the child has IBD (Holtman et al. 2016). Another meta-analysis of ten studies showed that FCal had a pooled sensitivity of 0.99 with a range of 0.92–1.00 and a specificity of 0.65 with a range of 0.54–0.74 (Holtman et al. 2016).

The test for fecal calprotectin must be interpreted with caution as elevated levels of fecal calprotectin can be observed in other causes of intestinal inflammation, including bacterial and viral enteritis, intestinal lymphoma, CD, food allergy, and immunodeficiency. Other conditions such as juvenile polyps, oncologic processes, and NSAID use can result in elevated fecal calprotectin (Conrad and Rosh 2017).

9.4.5 Real-Life Example

A 10-year female was seen with a sore throat and abdominal pain in the spring. The child was brought to the office by her father, who reported a sore throat for 2 days accompanied by fever, abdominal pain, and without any signs of a cold. The child had an RST done by the nursing assistant as per protocol due to a lack of URI symptoms. The clinician was informed of the positive test on entering into the room. A HEENT exam showed pharyngeal erythema with +3 erythematous tonsils with a small number of petechiae. Palatal petechiae were observed. There were 1 cm nodes along the anterior cervical chain, and the tonsillar nodes were 1.5 cm. A prescription for Amoxil was written, and standard teaching was done. As per the clinician's practice, the father was asked if he had any other concerns. The father then reported that the abdominal pain was on and off for 2 months and that he thought she had lost weight.

Further examination revealed perianal tags. Initial diagnostic laboratory tests included a CBC with differential, a sedimentation rate, and a C-reactive protein. The CBC showed mild normocytic anemia, a sedimentation rate of 100 (normal 5–15), and a CRP of 10.5. The child was referred to a pediatric gastroenterologist for possible IBD workup and a colonoscopy with biopsy-confirmed Crohn's disease.

Key Learning for IBD
- Negative findings in blood or stool testing do not rule out IBD.
- Laboratory tests can help guide further evaluation; however, 20% of children with IBD can present normal laboratory values.
- ESR and CRP are not specific to IBD.
- IBD panels are not more effective in diagnosis.
- Endoscopy colonoscopy is the gold standard for diagnosis.

9.5 Evaluation of Liver Disease

Liver chemistries can be abnormal for reasons ranging from self-limiting viral illnesses to structural abnormalities, metabolic disorders, autoimmune diseases, congenital conditions, and oncologic processes. The hepatic function panel is composed of markers of liver injury [aspartate transaminase (AST), alanine transaminase (ALT), alkaline phosphatase (ALP)], markers of liver metabolism (bilirubin), and markers of liver synthetic function (albumin). Additionally, prothrombin time (PT)/international normalized ratio (INR) is a marker of liver function that is not included in the hepatic function panel. To understand what abnormal values in the hepatic function panel indicate, each test will be discussed separately. Then they will be grouped to aid in understanding the possible differential diagnoses.

9.5.1 Markers of Liver Injury

Transaminases are enzymes that are present within cells that catalyze the transfer of an amino group from an amino acid to a keto acid (transamination). In hepatocyte injury and rupture, these transaminases are released into the serum leading to elevations in proportion to liver damage. Suppose this process has either been acutely severe (massive necrosis) or chronic. In that case, the degree of transaminase "leak" may reduce due to a reduction in hepatocyte mass (stromal collapse or replacement by fibrosis). Therefore, a patient with a significant liver injury can present with minimally elevated or even normal enzymes.

9.5.1.1 Aspartate Transaminase (AST)

Aspartate transaminase is a predominately intracellular enzyme involved in amino acid metabolism (to produce oxaloacetic acid). It is present in hepatocytes, muscle cells, kidneys, brain, and red blood cells. Because AST is present in cells when there is damage to these cells, it is released, and the serum levels of this enzyme become elevated. The half-life of AST is 17 ± 5 h (Woreta and Alqahtani 2014). In many injuries to the liver, an elevated AST may be one of the earliest changes noted.

Since AST is not specific to the liver, AST serum elevations can be caused by liver injury, muscle damage (injury or myopathies), kidney disease, or hemolysis. In small children, phlebotomy can be difficult, and serum AST elevation can be caused by hemolysis during the blood draw itself. One clue to this is an elevated serum

potassium from the same sample with a notation from the lab that the sample is hemolyzed, as potassium is also released from cells in the setting of injury. When there is AST elevation without ALT elevation, an extrahepatic cause for AST elevation should be considered.

9.5.1.2 Alanine Transaminase (ALT)

ALT is an enzyme found mostly in liver cells involved in amino acid metabolism (producing pyruvic acid). It is also present in smaller amounts in other tissues, including the kidney, muscle, and heart. Therefore, ALT is more specific to the liver than AST. When hepatocytes are injured, ALT is released and becomes elevated in the serum. The half-life of ALT is 47 ± 10 h (Woreta and Alqahtani 2014). In general, AST elevations tend to peak earlier and are higher than ALT in the setting of acute liver injury.

While an elevated ALT is more specific for liver disease, it is also present in muscle cells. It can be elevated in patients with muscular dystrophy (Veropalumbo et al. 2012) and myositis. ALT baseline values are also be affected by age, BMI, sex, and puberty (Bussler et al. 2018), with different normal ranges established for these groups.

9.5.1.3 Alkaline Phosphatase (ALP)

ALP is an enzyme found primarily in the bone and liver and in lesser amounts in kidneys and intestines. ALP can be fractionated into isoenzymes (liver fraction, bone fraction, and intestinal fraction). It has a half-life of 7 days (Lowe et al. 2021). To determine if the source is the liver, generally, you correlate other lab values (e.g., gamma-glutamyl transferase). The ALP can also be fractionated, and an elevated bone ALP can indicate growth (in children) or bone disease (healing fractures, bone metastasis, hyperparathyroidism, hyperthyroidism) (Lowe et al. 2021). ALP can be low in Wilson's disease, particularly when it presents as fulminant with hemolysis (Lowe et al. 2021). ALP can also be low with hypothyroidism, pernicious anemia, zinc deficiency, and congenital hypophosphatasia (Lowe et al. 2021).

Baseline ALP is elevated in children secondary to bone growth and must be interpreted using established normal ranges in the pediatric population. In addition, a benign entity is known as transient hyperphosphatasemia (TH) that can cause significantly elevated ALP in the setting of an otherwise normal hepatic function panel in children typically 5 years or younger with normalization within 4 months (Otero et al. 2011). TH is a diagnosis of exclusion. Hepatobiliary, renal disease, and bone disease must be ruled out before making this diagnosis (Otero et al. 2011). Workup would include a detailed history, physical, and diagnostic laboratory tests such as GGT, calcium, phosphorus, parathyroid hormone, vitamin D level, blood urea nitrogen (BUN), and creatinine (Otero et al. 2011). People with blood types O and B can have increased ALP for up to 12 hours after a fatty meal (Lowe et al. 2021).

9.5.1.4 Gamma-Glutamyl Transferase (GGT)

GGT is an additional test used to evaluate the hepatobiliary tree for injury. It is not typically included in a hepatic function panel. GGT is an enzyme present predominately in the hepatobiliary system but is also present in the heart, pancreas, lungs, and seminal vesicles. GGT is involved in leukotriene and glutathione metabolism. Because ALP can vary greatly in childhood due to its presence in bone, GGT is more specific to and sensitive for obstructive jaundice, cholecystitis, and cholangitis in children than ALP (Cabrera-Abreu and Green 2002).

It is important to note that newborns normally have serum GGT that is five to seven times higher than the upper limit of normal for adults in the early months of life. After 4 months of age, serum GGT values start to decline, reaching normal adult levels by 5–7 months of age (Cabrera-Abreu and Green 2002). Some liver diseases present with a normal GGT despite profound cholestasis, such as progressive familial intrahepatic cholestasis types 1 and 2 and bile acid synthesis disorders. Table 9.8 reviews normal liver enzymes and their interpretation.

9.5.2 Evaluation of an Abnormal Hepatic Function Panel

Generally, when evaluating liver disease, it is helpful to look for patterns of injury. The patterns of injury include predominately hepatocellular in nature (AST/ALT is disproportionately higher than ALP/GGT), predominately cholestatic in nature (GGT/ALP is disproportionately higher than AST/ALT), and mixed picture (Kwo et al. 2017). One example of a mixed pattern of injury is a primary cholestatic disease associated with elevated AST/ALT secondary to the detergent effect of poor bile flow leading to damage to the liver cells (chemical hepatitis). Because of confounding variables, a workup for abnormal liver tests should begin broadly with an age-appropriate screen and focus as more information is available.

Table 9.8 Liver enzymes (11 months to 16.0 years)

Test	Median (girls)	97th percentile (girls)	Median (boys)	97th percentile (boys)	Interpretation
ALT	14.0 and 20.3 U/L	24.2–31.7 U/L	17.1 and 21.1 U/L	29.9–38.0 U/L	Elevated with hepatocyte injury, sometimes with myopathies
AST	23.1–46.1 U/L	35.2–62.9 U/L	25.7–47.6 U/L	41.5–68.7 U/L	Elevated with hepatocyte injury, heart or muscle injury, or hemolyzed specimen
ALP					Elevated in cholestatic liver disease, bile duct obstruction, bone disease, renal disease, or TH
GGT	9.5–12.0 U/L	14.5–18.1 U/L	9.4–14.8 U/L	14.1–27.4 U/L	Elevated in cholestatic liver disease or bile duct obstruction

Adapted from Bussler et al. (2018)

Note: ALP varies so much by age it does not fit into ranges in these categories

The next important consideration is the extent of liver injury. Elevations in AST/ALT can be defined as borderline, mild, moderate, severe, or massive. Borderline elevation of transaminases is defined as <2x the upper limit of normal (ULN) for age and gender (Kwo et al. 2017). This should prompt a history and physical to uncover any potential toxins, medications/supplements/alcohol use, infection risks, inborn errors of metabolism, autoimmunity, risk factors for fatty liver, or other multisystemic disorders. The physical exam should focus on stigmata of chronic liver disease (palmar erythema, spider telangiectasias, gynecomastia) and portal hypertension (hepatomegaly, splenomegaly, ascites, caput medusa) to establish acuity and chronicity. If the patient has signs of chronic liver disease, the workup should not be delayed regardless of the degree of serum values for liver enzymes. This is important because patients with chronic hepatitis and cirrhosis can present with normal to mildly elevated liver enzymes (Johnston 1999). Additional laboratories to consider include a complete blood count (CBC) with platelet count, AST/ALT, ALP, total bilirubin, albumin, PT/INR, HBsAg, HBcAb, HBsAb, and HCV total Ab with PCR confirmation if positive and abdominal ultrasound with Doppler (Kwo et al. 2017). If labs and the exam are negative and AST/ALT is stable, one can consider observation with repeat laboratories in 3–6 months. If liver test anomalies are persistent, then the workup can be broadened to include ANA, ASMA, anti-LKM, IgG, ceruloplasmin, alpha-1 antitrypsin phenotype, and additional tests based on patient history and physical exam findings [TSH, celiac panel (see section on CD), tick-borne disease, creatine kinase, and aldolase] (Kwo et al. 2017). If liver enzymes remain elevated, consider referral to a specialist for further workup/biopsy (Kwo et al. 2017).

For patients with mild elevation of AST/ALT (defined as 2–5x ULN), the workup is the same except for initiating further workup after confirmed abnormal AST/ALT or after sustained abnormalities on repeat labs 3 months later (Kwo et al. 2017).

Patients with moderate (5–15 × ULN), severe (>15× ULN), or massive (ALT > 10,000) elevation of AST/ALT require an immediate workup for liver disease and need to be evaluated for signs of acute liver failure (Kwo et al. 2017). Immediate transfer to a hospital that offers pediatric liver transplant should also be considered. In addition to the previously mentioned workup, one would check HAV IgM, HAV IgG, HBcAB IgM, HBcAB IgG, EBV/CMV serologies, serum drug panel, urine toxicology, and acetaminophen level (Kwo et al. 2017). If the patient has signs of acute liver failure, they need an immediate liver consult with consideration of transfer to a facility that offers pediatric liver transplant (Kwo et al. 2017). AST has a shorter half-life than ALT; therefore, the ALT may remain elevated longer than AST during recovery (Woreta and Alqahtani 2014).

The differential diagnosis of patients with elevations of liver enzymes has several possible diagnoses. Table 9.9 reviews the possible variations of elevations along with possible diagnoses.

If a patient has significant elevations of LFT beyond the third standard deviation, the following is a list of possible tests to consider. Box 9.3 reviews the evaluation of a child with abnormal LFTs.

Table 9.9 Lab patterns in abnormal liver tests

Developing cirrhosis	– AST/ALT ratio increases and becomes >1 – Platelets <150 (in the absence of an underlying hematologic disorder)
– Acute ischemic injury – Toxic/drug-induced hepatitis – Acute viral hepatitis – Autoimmune hepatitis – Acute liver failure due to Wilson's disease	AST/ALT > 1000
– Extrahepatic source (i.e., rhabdomyolysis, strenuous exercise)	AST/ALT ratio > 5
– NAFLD	Often < 300 IU/L ALT > AST

Adapted from Woreta and Alqahtani (2014)

Box 9.3 Workup for Abnormal LFTs
Abdominal ultrasound with Doppler
  Adjunct testing in patients with elevated
liver enzymes

1. PT/INR (to assess liver function and or vitamin K deficiency)
2. GGT
3. Bilirubin (fractionated to include direct bilirubin)
4. Albumin

  Hepatitis workup

- Hepatitis A total and IgM (if not immune revaccinate)
- Hepatitis B cAb
- Hepatitis B sAg
- Hepatitis B sAb (if not immune revaccinate)
- HCV Ab
- EBV/CMV IgG/IgM

  Autoimmune liver disease workup

- ANA (anti-nuclear Ab)
- ASMA (anti-smooth muscle Ab)
- LKM (liver kidney microsomal)
- SLA (soluble liver antigen)

  Aldolase (to look for muscle source of elevated transaminases)
  Creatine kinase (to look for muscle source of elevated transaminases)
  Wilson's disease

- Ceruloplasmin (if low, obtain a 24-hour urine copper and slit-light exam for Keyser-Fleischer rings to look for evidence of Wilson's disease) can be elevated in acute hepatitis and may need to be repeated, can test for genetics, and obtain 24-hour urine if there is a question.

  TSH, free T4.
  CD

- EMA Ab IgA, tissue transglutaminase (TTG) IgA, total IgA.

  Alpha-1 antitrypsin deficiency

- Alpha-1 antitrypsin phenotype.

  Alagille syndrome

- If Alagille syndrome is suspected (high GGT/bilirubin/triangular facies), obtain an x-ray of the spine to rule out butterfly vertebrae, as well as an ophthalmology appt to look for posterior embryo toxin and cardiology to rule out associated congenital heart disease.

  Metabolic diseases

- Plasma amino acids, urine organic acids (inborn error of metabolism), lysosomal acid lipase.

  If the patient has not had a newborn screen, consider a sweat test if the clinical picture warrants it.

9.5.3   Other Markers of Liver Metabolism

Markers of liver metabolism can be elevated both in cholestatic diseases and in hepatocellular dysfunction. Conjugated bilirubin is excreted into the intestine via the bile, where it is then either excreted in feces, urine, or reabsorbed via enterohepatic circulation. In cholestatic diseases, the drainage of bile is impaired or blocked, which leads to a decrease in the excretion of bilirubin. This decreased excretion of bilirubin leads to elevated serum bilirubin. However, the lack of jaundice does not exclude cholestatic liver disease; patients can also have compromised bile drainage, pruritus, and elevated bile salts without elevated bilirubin.

9.5.3.1 Bilirubin

Bilirubin is a product of heme metabolism from the breakdown of hemoglobin (approximately 80–85%) and in lesser amounts from myoglobin, other hemoproteins and free heme (Yazigi and Balistreri 1995). It is present in the blood either as bound (direct) or unbound (indirect) to various sugar moieties as a function of glycosylation in hepatocytes. When interpreting laboratories, often just the total bilirubin is provided. Whenever the total bilirubin is abnormal, it must be fractionated into direct and indirect bilirubin to clarify the source of dysfunction. Table 9.10 reviews common causes of indirect hyperbilirubinemia, and Table 9.11 gives the formulas for bilirubin calculations.

9.5.3.2 Indirect (Unconjugated) Bilirubin

Unconjugated bilirubin is toxic to cells and circulates in blood predominantly bound to albumin. This form of bilirubin is not water-soluble and can distribute into fatty tissues such as the brain leading to direct toxicity (kernicterus).

When the albumin-indirect bilirubin complex is transported to the liver, unconjugated bilirubin dissociates from albumin and enters the hepatocyte for conjugation. Indirect bilirubin can accumulate in the setting of disorders of hepatic conjugation, increased heme breakdown (hemolysis leading to increased bilirubin production),

or impaired hepatic bilirubin uptake. When albumin becomes saturated, there is unbound bilirubin available to cross the blood-brain barrier leading to brain toxicity (Brierley and Burchell 1993). The maximum binding capacity of albumin is approximately 20 µmol bilirubin/g albumin (Carragher 2014).

9.5.3.3 Direct Bilirubin

In the liver, indirect (unconjugated) bilirubin is covalently bonded to glucuronic acid by glucuronyl transferase through a process known as conjugation leading to a water-soluble form of bilirubin (direct bilirubin). Although direct bilirubin is often used interchangeably with conjugated bilirubin, direct bilirubin is not entirely correct, as direct bilirubin is conjugated bilirubin + delta (δ) bilirubin. Delta bilirubin is generally not measured, and direct bilirubin is thought of as a general measurement of conjugated bilirubin. Delta bilirubin is albumin-bound and increases with chronic bilirubin elevations.

Table 9.11 Bilirubin lab value calculations

Total bilirubin = unconjugated (indirect) bilirubin + (δ bilirubin + conjugated bilirubin) Direct bilirubin = conjugated bilirubin + δ bilirubin Indirect (unconjugated) bilirubin = total bilirubin – Direct bilirubin
δ bilirubin = delta bilirubin

Table 9.10 Common causes of indirect hyperbilirubinemia

	Findings	Diagnosis
Impaired conjugation		
Crigler-Najjar syndrome	Type 1: Severe indirect hyperbilirubinemia can quickly lead to kernicterus Type 2: Can be asymptomatic and can become more severe during times of illness, fasting, or stress Hyperthyroid Physiologic neonatal jaundice	Genetic testing for known mutations (exons 2 to 5 in UGT1A1) Type 2 bilirubin is usually <15 mg/dL, and there is >30% decrease in serum bilirubin after administration of phenobarbital
Reduced hepatic uptake		
Gilbert's syndrome	Mild, intermittent elevated indirect bilirubin, normal LDH, and haptoglobin	Diagnosis of exclusion (liver disease and hemolysis) Genetic testing can confirm
Excess production of bilirubin		
Hemolytic anemias (thalassemia, sickle cell disease, G6PD deficiency, pyruvate kinase deficiency)	Increased LDH and reticulocyte count, low haptoglobin (see "Hematology" chapter for detailed workup)	Newborn screen, hemoglobin electrophoresis (see "Hematology" chapter for detailed workup)

Adapted from Ramakrishnan et al. (2020)

Conjugated bilirubin is actively transported into canicular bile for excretion in stool. When the amount of conjugated bilirubin exceeds the hepatic excretory capacity, some conjugated bilirubin may accumulate in the serum, covalently bound to albumin (delta bilirubin). The capacity to secrete conjugated bilirubin is exceeded in cases of prolonged biliary obstruction or intrahepatic cholestasis (Kalakonda et al. 2020). Albumin has a half-life of 2–3 weeks (Giannini et al. 2005). Therefore, instead of the usual half-life of bilirubin (2–4 h), δ bilirubin can persist for up to several weeks after a biliary obstruction is resolved (Kalakonda et al. 2020).

Both bilirubin and conjugated bilirubin are water-soluble and non-toxic, and therefore neither can significantly bind to tissues or cause damage (e.g., the brain). In this water-soluble state, conjugated bilirubin can be excreted in the bile and to some degree in urine. Conjugated bilirubin is excreted via the biliary system into the intestine, where it is broken down into urobilinogen. It is either reabsorbed via enterohepatic circulation, excreted in the stool (giving feces a brown pigment), or reabsorbed and excreted by the kidneys in urine (McDaniel 2019).

Serum bilirubin elevations can also occur in patients without liver disease. When faced with elevated indirect bilirubin alone, hemolysis should be considered (see "Hematology" chapter).

Elevated δ total bilirubin must always be fractionated to differentiate between hepatobiliary disease and extrahepatic causes of jaundice. However, patients with chronic hemolysis, such as sickle cell disease (SCD), can develop liver disease for a variety of reasons, including sinusoidal obstruction (sickled red blood cells) and iron overload (from repeated red blood cell transfusions) (Banerjee et al. 2001). Therefore, it should not be assumed that jaundice in patients with SCD is from hemolysis alone.

9.5.4 Other Markers of Liver Function

Patients with liver disease can have profoundly abnormal labs, but they are not in liver failure without abnormal markers of liver function. Any patient with evidence of liver failure (low albumin, elevated INR > 2.0, hypoglycemia, signs of encephalopathy) requires immediate transfer to a center that does liver transplantation in the case that it is needed. A patient with acute liver failure can deteriorate quite rapidly.

9.5.4.1 Albumin

Albumin is the predominant circulating protein in the serum manufactured by hepatocytes. It serves many functions, including a molecular transporter (for bilirubin as described above, copper, zinc, thyroxine, cholesterol, and some medications). It is responsible for about 75% of plasma oncotic pressure (Walayat et al. 2017). A low albumin level is correlated with an almost certain development of ascites in cirrhotic patients (<3 g/dL), while those with albumin >4 g/dL do not develop ascites (Wood et al. 1987). The half-life of albumin is 14–18 days (Walayat et al. 2017).

While low albumin can be a marker of impaired liver function, it can also be a sign of poor nutrition, a protein-losing enteropathy, or kidney disease. The half-life of albumin can also be affected by catabolic states (sepsis, end-stage liver disease, and states of inflammation). The liver can increase its production of albumin tenfold when under extreme stress (Walayat et al. 2017). These factors make serum albumin a poor marker of acute liver injury.

9.5.4.2 International Normalized Ratio (INR)

One of the many functions of the liver is to produce clotting factors. Unlike the other laboratory tests discussed, the INR is not a direct measurement of a protein or enzyme. Rather, it is a calculation derived from calculated prothrombin time (PT) and reported as a ratio to normal coagulation controls. It is a measure of liver function because the liver produces most clotting factors (all except factor XIII produced by endothelial cells) that affect this value. When the liver function is compromised (generally when concentrations of clotting factors fall below 10% of normal), INR becomes elevated (Kwo et al. 2017). The short half-life of some of these factors makes the INR a good marker of liver synthetic function (acute and chronic). By consensus definition, patients with acute liver failure have an INR > 1.5 with encephalopathy or INR > 2.0 without encephalopathy (Bhatt and Rao 2018).

The INR reflects coagulation down the intrinsic pathway. Factors II, VII, IX, and X are within this pathway and require vitamin K as a cofactor (Kwo et al. 2017). Therefore, INR becomes elevated with significant liver dysfunction, with vitamin K deficiency, and in the setting of the administration of certain medications (coumadin, vitamin K analog). Vitamin K is a fat-soluble vitamin. Deficiency can occur with poor dietary intake or vitamin K malabsorption secondary to cholestasis and steatorrhea (Kwo et al. 2017). Vitamin K given orally, subcutaneously, or intravenously will correct an elevated INR due to vitamin K deficiency or coumadin but not secondary to significant liver dysfunction. With ongoing cholestasis, vitamin K supplementation will need to continue.

9.5.5 Other Tests Affected by Liver Disease

The tests below are not a direct function of liver metabolism but can be abnormal in liver disease. Abnormal results of these tests may enable the clinician to consider liver disease in a pediatric patient who may have vague complaints or may have these tests done for other reasons.

9.5.5.1 Platelets

Cirrhosis can result in a low platelet count due to decreased thrombopoietin synthesis by the liver and splenic sequestration of platelets due to portal hypertension. A platelet count of <150 is highly suggestive of cirrhosis in the absence of a primary hematologic disorder (Woreta and Alqahtani 2014). Platelets are instrumental in primary hemostasis. They react to tissue factors released at a site of vascular injury to form a plug and expose activated clotting factors to help stimulate additional aspects of clotting (Northup and Caldwell 2013). Studies have shown that the minimum number of platelets needed to initiate

this thrombin burst and produce adequate end products for coagulation in cirrhotic patients is 50–60 × 109/L (Northup and Caldwell 2013).

Patients can occasionally have a normal platelet count in the setting of cirrhosis, such as in the case of patients with polysplenia, asplenia, or a myeloproliferative disorder. There are also numerous alternative etiologies for thrombocytopenia other than cirrhosis (see chapter on hematology). Dysfibrinogenemia and peripheral increase platelet consumption (infection, bleeding), leading to low platelets related to primary liver disease. One important note is that platelet count reflects the number of platelets present but does not reflect platelet function (Northup and Caldwell 2013) and risk of bleeding.

9.5.5.2 Alpha-Fetoprotein (AFP)

Alpha-fetoprotein is a protein that is produced in the liver of the developing fetus. Therefore, it is elevated at birth and generally is <8 ng/mL when a child is 2 years old (Blohm et al. 1998). Since AFP is produced by immature tumor cells, it is useful as a tumor marker for germ cell tumors, hepatoblastoma, hepatocellular carcinomas (HCC), and certain bowel malignancies (Blohm et al. 1998). The most common liver malignancy in children is hepatoblastoma, which is usually diagnosed before the age of 3 years (Hiyama 2014). In patients with hepatoblastoma, AFP is one of the most important clinical markers for clinical change, response to treatment, and relapse (Hiyama 2014). The second most common pediatric liver malignancy is HCC, which can be seen in patients with preexisting liver disease. Liver diseases leading to cirrhosis such as biliary atresia, type I glycogen storage disease, chronic viral hepatitis, and type 2 progressive familial intrahepatic cholestasis (Walther and Tiao 2013) as well as Fanconi's syndrome (Marrero et al. 2018) are examples of conditions that put patients at increased risk of HCC. Hepatitis B virus (HBV) predisposes to HCC, with or without cirrhosis (Tajiri et al. 2016). Viral hepatitis is discussed in more detail in the infectious disease chapter.

AFP is not a perfect test for pediatric liver tumors, and sensitivity varies based on the associated disease and disease state. It is important to note that many of these liver diseases warrant AFP monitoring every 6–12 months in combination with regular abdominal ultrasound for HCC screening, as guided by a pediatric hepatologist or gastroenterologist.

9.5.6 Real-Life Example

A 16-year-old female was seen on the third day of illness with a sore throat and fever. Cervical adenopathy to 2 cm was noted, but the child's strep testing was negative. The mother was told to return if the child did not get better. On day 10 of illness, she returned with a chief complaint of "yellow skin for the last 2 days." The mother also noted dark yellow urine and right upper quadrant abdominal pain. The child was noted to have a 4-cm spleen and a liver edge that was 8 cm below the right costal margin on the exam. The child was sent to the lab for stat lab work. The CBC was remarkable for 15 atypical lymphocytes. Her monospot was positive. The EBV IgM AB to VCA > 0.91 (normal, <0.91), a slightly positive IgG AB to VCA >1.10 (normal, <0.91), and a negative antibody to nuclear Ag. The AST was 700 U/L (normal, 13–26 U/L), and the ALT was 650 U/L (normal, 8–22 U/L). A diagnosis of EBV hepatitis was made, and the child recovered after 3 weeks.

Key Learning about Liver Disease Diagnostic Laboratory Tests
- Markers of hepatocyte injury include the AST, ALT, PT, albumin, and glucose. The glucose will fall when there is severe hepatocyte injury.
- Markers of cholestasis include ALP, GTT, bilirubin, and urobilinogen (urine).
- The prothrombin time (PT) and the international normalized ratio (INR) are markers of liver function not included in the hepatic function panel.
- Besides liver damage, other possible causes for elevated ALT include rhabdo-

myolysis, hemolysis, muscular dystrophy, and liver cancer.
- An elevated AST can be caused by heart and skeletal muscle damage.
- Hemochromatosis can cause significant liver damage, but usually, this is delayed until adulthood. It should be considered in older adolescents, and iron studies will show markedly elevated serum ferritin.

9.6   Hepatitis

Hepatitis is inflammation of the hepatocytes or injury to the liver parenchyma. This is reflected in bloodwork by an elevated AST/ALT, which is released from hepatocytes with inflammation. If this process has either been severe (massive necrosis) or long-term enough, the liver cells can burn out, and there could be too few hepatocytes left to release these enzymes as healthy tissue has been replaced by fibrosis. Therefore, it is possible for a patient whose liver disease is primarily hepatitis to present with minimally elevated or even normal enzymes. Additionally, if the damage is severe enough, it can lead to cholestasis. Hepatitis can be acute, chronic, or acute on chronic (when there is chronic inflammation with an acute flare). The cause of hepatitis can vary greatly from toxic to viral, autoimmune in nature, to a mixed cholestatic picture, and to poor perfusion and metabolic diseases. Hepatitis A through D and their associated labs are discussed in the infectious disease chapter, Section 6.3.6. Box 9.4 reviews the common causes of hepatitis.

Box 9.4 Common Causes of Hepatitis
- Autoimmune hepatitis.
- Extrahepatic autoimmune disease [lupus, CD, juvenile rheumatoid arthritis (JRA), hypothyroidism, others].

- Viral infection [HAV, HBV, HCV, HEV, HDV, EBV, CMV, adenovirus, HSV, SARS CoV2 (Saeed et al. 2020), varicella, enterovirus, others]. See infectious disease chapter for a review of viral hepatitis.
- Other infections (Fitz-Hugh-Curtis syndrome, abscess, amebiasis, others).
- Drug-induced liver injury (DILI).
- Biliary atresia.
- Metabolic [alpha-1 antitrypsin deficiency, Wilson's disease, glycogen storage disease, tyrosinemia, lysosomal acid lipase deficiency (Wolman's syndrome), others].
- Hemodynamic (shock, congestive heart failure, Budd-Chiari syndrome, others).
- NAFLD (nonalcoholic fatty liver disease) (see Chap. 4 for further workup).
- Toxins (acetaminophen, alcohol, iron overdose, anabolic steroids, others).

Adapted from Fawaz and Jonas 2021

9.7 Autoimmune Liver Diseases

Autoimmune liver diseases in childhood can be challenging to diagnose and treat. Autoimmune hepatitis (AIH) is the most common cause of liver disease in the pediatric population (Sheiko et al. 2017), accounting for 12% of referrals to pediatric liver specialists. AIH is thought to occur from a genetic predisposition that is secondarily triggered by an environmental factor (Sokollik et al. 2018). AIH has a female predominance of 75%, with 40% of patients positive for a family history of other autoimmune disorders (Mieli-Vergani and Vergani 2009). The presentation of AIH is extremely variable and can range from mild transaminase elevations to acute liver failure or acute hepatitis with a similar presentation to acute viral hepatitis. Laboratory results can wax and wane without intervention, and symptoms may include jaundice, fatigue, anorexia, or weight loss. Less commonly, about 10% of patients can present with advanced liver disease

and complications of portal hypertension (splenomegaly, variceal bleeding, ascites, malnutrition, diarrhea) (Mieli-Vergani and Vergani 2009). AIH can be supported by nonspecific serum antibodies (seropositive AIH), or serum markers may be absent (seronegative AIH).

Type 1 AIH (AIH-1) is characterized by positive anti-nuclear antibody (ANA) and/or positive smooth muscle antibody (SMA). Type 1 is more common and usually presents around puberty. Patients with a positive SMA are more likely to relapse after withdrawal for AIH and are more likely to require a liver transplant than patients without positive SMA (Himoto and Nishioka 2013).

Type 2 AIH (AIH-2) can present as early as infancy and is associated with a positive liver-kidney microsomal Ab type 1 (anti-LKM-1) and/or anti-liver cytosol Ab type 1 (anti-LC1) and can be associated with IgA deficiency (Mieli-Vergani and Vergani 2009). Type 2 AIH accounts for about one-third of juvenile AIH and generally presents more acutely (Sokollik et al. 2018). Both AIH-1 and AIH-2 often have elevated immunoglobulin G (IgG) (Mieli-Vergani and Vergani 2009). One of the difficulties in diagnosing AIH is the fluctuating course of the disease, with liver enzymes rising and falling over time. If left untreated, AIH will lead to cirrhosis and liver failure. Some patients are more difficult to treat and will progress to cirrhosis despite recognition and treatment. Because autoimmune hepatitis can be treated with immunosuppression, the prognosis for AIH is better than for patients with PSC. However, patients with AIH/PSC overlap have a better prognosis than patients with PSC alone (Nayagam et al. 2019).

9.7.1 Testing for Autoimmune Liver Disease

In general, patients with one autoimmune disease are more likely to develop other autoimmune diseases. Approximately 20% of patients with autoimmune hepatitis have other autoimmune disorders (e.g., thyroiditis, vitiligo, type 1, diabetes, IBD, CD) (Mieli-Vergani and Vergani 2009). Patients with autoimmune hepatitis should also be screened for primary sclerosing cholangitis (PSC), as about 12.5% of patients with AIH and PSC have AIH/PSC overlap syndrome (Laborda et al. 2019).

The following are tests done when the clinician is faced with a patient with unknown jaundice or elevation of liver enzymes without an explanation. These should be seriously considered when there is a family or patient history of autoimmunity.

9.7.1.1 Anti-Nuclear Antibody (ANA)

Anti-nuclear antibodies (ANA) include antibodies that attach to the nucleus of a cell. Antibodies usually attach to foreign antigens, but ANA attaches itself to autoantigens (self-antigens). There are subcategories of ANA, but they are not routinely tested for liver disease (see chapter on "Rheumatology"). ANA is nonspecific and can be seen in healthy adults and children and associated with many other diseases, particularly other autoimmune disorders.

9.7.1.2 Anti-Smooth Muscle Antibody (SMA)

Anti-smooth muscle antibodies are antibodies that are formed against smooth muscle proteins (actin, myosin, vimentin, desmin, and tubulin). In AIH-1, they attach to filamentous actin (F-actin) (Himoto and Nishioka 2013).

9.7.1.3 Immunoglobulins (IgG)

Immunoglobulins (IgG) are the antibody fraction of serum proteins, and patients with autoimmune hepatitis tend to have nonspecific elevations in total IgG. Immunoglobulins can be measured directly or estimated within standard hepatic function panels reflected as the value obtained by subtracting the serum albumin from the total serum protein, the globulin fraction. When the globulin fraction is elevated in autoimmune hepatitis, it reflects an elevated gamma globulin pool (immunoglobulin).

9.7.1.4 Anti-Liver-Kidney Microsomal Type-1 (Anti-LKM-1)

Anti-liver-kidney microsomal type-1 (anti-LKM-1) is associated with AIH-2. There are other LKM antibodies (types 2 and 3) associated

with other diseases, so type 1 has been differentiated (Bogdanos et al. 2009).

9.7.1.5 Anti-Liver Cytosol Type-1 (Anti-LC1)

Anti-liver cytosol type-1 (anti-LC1) is an antibody that frequently appears with anti-LKM-1 in patients with AIH-2 and is less commonly tested (Mieli-Vergani and Vergani 2009).

9.7.1.6 Anti-Soluble Liver Antigen (Anti-SLA)

Anti-soluble liver antigen (anti-SLA) has been found in patients with AIH-1, AIH-2, and AIH/PSC overlap syndrome. It is correlated with a more severe disease course (Sokollik et al. 2018). Anti-SLA is very specific for autoimmune liver diseases (Bogdanos et al. 2009).

9.7.1.7 Anti-Mitochondrial Antibody (AMA)

Anti-mitochondrial antibody (AMA) is found in 90–95% of patients with PBC, but titers are not correlated with disease severity (Himoto and Nishioka 2013). It is not frequently tested in pediatrics and can be seen in AIH as well.

9.7.1.8 Immunoglobulin 4 (IgG4)

Immunoglobulin 4 is a subset of immunoglobulins (can be checked by ordering IgG subclasses 1–4) that have been associated with autoimmune diseases of the pancreas, biliary tract, lymph nodes, kidney, and lungs, to name a few (Dorn et al. 2012). Gastrointestinal diseases involving elevated IgG4 are primarily autoimmune pancreatitis (AIP) and IgG4-related sclerosing cholangitis (Dorn et al. 2012).

Most autoimmune markers for autoimmune liver disease are relatively nonspecific. Additionally, autoimmune antibodies may be absent despite biopsy and treatment proved AIH (seronegative AIH). Treatment tends to involve prolonged immunosuppressive regimens and chronic monitoring for progressive disease and disease complications. For these reasons, an experienced specialist needs to be involved in diagnosis, which involves a combination of liver enzymes, autoimmune markers, liver biopsy results (histology), and response to treatment.

In healthy pediatric patients, autoantibodies are rare (Mieli-Vergani and Vergani 2009). Therefore, antibody levels 1: 10 (anti-LKM) and 1:20 (ANA and SMA) should be considered positive in children, while in adults, it is generally 1:40 (Mieli-Vergani and Vergani 2009). In some labs, the cutoff value for positivity is higher than the cutoff for significance in pediatrics (Sokollik et al. 2018). Seronegative patients may become seropositive later in their disease course (Manns et al. 2010). The autoantibodies most used in pediatrics are ANA, anti-LKM-1, and anti-SMA.

9.8   Primary Sclerosing Cholangitis

Primary sclerosing cholangitis is a chronic liver disease that causes stricturing and sclerosing of the biliary tree. Although it is rare in the general population, it occurs in at least 10% of children who have ulcerative colitis (Laborda et al. 2019). PSC can lead to significant liver damage, with 50% of patients developing complications within 10 years of diagnosis and 30% requiring liver transplantation (Laborda et al. 2019). Stricturing and scarring in the bile ducts can lead to cholestasis, poor nutrient absorption, pruritus, hepatobiliary fibrosis, cirrhosis, end-stage liver disease (ESLD), and carries an elevated risk of cholangiocarcinoma (CCA). There is currently no pharmacological treatment to delay the progression of PSC. Patients are treated with supportive care (ursodiol to potentially improve bile flow, anti-pruritic medication, fat-soluble vitamin supplementation, antibiotics, and nutritional supplementation) and screening for complications. Portal hypertension screening includes serial physical exams (spleen size, stigmata of chronic liver disease), imaging, serum platelet values, elastography, and endoscopy to screen for esophageal varices. Given diminished bile flow, affected patients are predisposed to cholangitis with low thresholds for antibiotic treatment and interventional approaches to augment bile drainage. If PSC is suspected, the diagnosis is made by magnetic resonance cholangiopancreatography (MRCP), endoscopic retrograde cholangiopancreatography (ERCP), or liver biopsy. If patients progress to ESLD, the only treatment is a liver transplant. Unfortunately, there is a risk of recurrent PSC after liver transplantation, which has been found to occur in up to 26% of children (Martinez et al. 2019). Additionally, about one-quarter of patients who do not have known IBD before transplantation will develop IBD post-transplant, making screening for IBD an important part of post-transplant care (Laborda et al. 2019).

9.8.1   Diagnostic Laboratory Screening in Primary Sclerosing Cholangitis

CCA is rare in childhood. Tumor screening includes serial tumor markers (CA19–9), serial imaging (sonogram, CT, MR), as well as ERCP to brush bile duct strictures to screen for CCA. Patients with PSC who have developed cirrhosis should get HCC surveillance (see Sect. 9.5.5.2) (Bowlus et al. 2022). In addition, screening for IBD is important and is found in Sect. 9.4.3.

9.8.1.1 Carbohydrate antigen 19-9 (CA19–9)

CA19-9 (carbohydrate antigen 19-9) is a protein found to be a biomarker for CCA in patients with PSC. There are pitfalls to using CA19-9 in screening for CCA: about 7% of the population has undetectable CA19-9 levels due to being Lewis antigen negative; it is also associated with pancreatic, colorectal, gastric or gynecologic cancers (Liang et al. 2015); the sensitivity and specificity is highly variable related to different cut-off values (Bowlus et al. 2022). CA19-9 can also be elevated in patients with bacterial cholangitis (Chapman et al. 2010). The AASLD practice guidelines do not recommend routine surveillance in patients under the age of 18 years (Bowlus et al. 2022), though CA-19-9 and cross-sectional imaging might be useful in patients who have stricturing disease (Chapman et al. 2010).

9.9   Other Autoimmune Liver Diseases

Primary biliary cirrhosis (PBC) is another autoimmune cholestatic liver disease with elevated liver tests and pruritus. This condition is exceedingly

Table 9.12 Autoimmune markers in liver disease

Lab	Associated autoimmune liver disease	Notes
Anti-nuclear antibody (ANA)	AIH-1, primary sclerosing cholangitis (PSC), PBC	It can also present in other non-autoimmune liver diseases (HCV, NAFLD, viral hepatitis, HCC) (Himoto and Nishioka 2013)
Anti-smooth muscle antibody (anti-SMA)	AIH-1	Unfavorable prognosis for AIH-1 (Sokollik et al. 2018) It can be used to monitor disease activity in patients with AIH-1 (Sokollik et al. 2018)
Anti-liver-kidney microsomal type-1 (anti-LKM-1)	AIH-2	It can be used to monitor disease activity in patients with AIH-2 (Sokollik et al. 2018)
Anti-liver cytosol type-1 (anti-LC1)	AIH-2	It can be used to monitor disease activity in patients with AIH-2 (Sokollik et al. 2018)
Anti-soluble liver antigen (anti-SLA)	AIH-1 and AIH-2, PSC/AIH overlap syndrome	Defines a more severe course (Sokollik et al. 2018)
Atypical perinuclear anti-neutrophil antibody (p-ANCA)	AIH-1, PSC/AIH overlap syndrome	Virtually absent in AIH-2 (Sokollik et al. 2018)
Anti-mitochondrial antibody (AMA)	PBC, AIH-1	PBC is very rare in children and is not routinely screened

Adapted from Sokollik et al. (2018); Himoto and Nishioka (2013)

rare to present in childhood, but there have been isolated case reports (Dahlan et al. 2003). PBC is associated with a positive anti-mitochondrial antibody (AMA), but this is rarely screened because it is rare in the pediatric population. Table 9.12 reviews the autoimmune markers along with the associated autoimmune liver disease.

9.10   IgG4-Related Sclerosing Cholangitis

IgG4-related sclerosing cholangitis is most common in men over the age of 60. However, a handful of pediatric patients have fit this diagnosis (Hsu et al. 2019). The picture can be similar to PSC because it is an autoimmune disease that affects the bile ducts. However, it is important to distinguish it from PSC because IgG4-related sclerosing cholangitis is responsive to immunosuppressive therapy and treatment can lead to remission (Rosen et al. 2015b).

9.10.1   Real-Life Example

A 5-year-old African-American male with no significant past medical history presents to the office with his father. His father reports the patient's school notified him that the patient had yellow eyes. The patient's father reports the patient

had two to four episodes of non-bloody, yellow vomiting for the past 3–4 days. The patient had one to two episodes of vomiting today. No diarrhea. The patient's father reports that his urine is being more yellow than usual. There is no history of fever. He is complaining of mild right-sided abdominal pain but is unable to describe or rate it further.

The patient reports travel to Ghana July–August last summer. The patient's father reports that the patient received malaria prophylaxis before, during, and after the trip. No visitors from Africa since his trip. No other complaints, no known sick contacts, and no treatment before ED presentation. No known allergies. The direct bilirubin is 7.5 (normal, <0.3 mg/dL), and the total bilirubin was 11.3 (normal, 0.1–1.2 mg/dL). The ALT was 2610 (normal, 4–36 IU/L), the AST was 3167 (normal, 8–33 IU/L), and the alkaline phosphatase was 449 (normal, 38–126 IU/L). The GGT was 79 (normal, 7–50 IU/L). The hepatitis panel for A, B, and C was unremarkable. The lipase and amylase were within normal limits. The PT was 20.8 (normal, 9.6–11.6 s), the INR was 2.0 (normal, 0.9–1.1 ratio), and the PTT was 27.5 (normal, 21.0 to 30.0). The thick and thin smear for malaria was negative. The ceruloplasmin was 36 (normal, 29–56 mg/dL). EBV titers did not show an acute infection. All markers for autoimmune hepatitis were negative, but a liver biopsy confirmed seronegative autoimmune hepatitis.

Key Learning about Autoimmune Liver Disease

- Autoimmune hepatitis (AIH) is the most common cause of liver disease in the pediatric population.
- A family history of autoimmunity may be elicited. Remember, a child with one autoimmune disease is predisposed to other autoimmune diseases.
- Primary sclerosing cholangitis (PSC) is a chronic liver disease that causes stricturing and sclerosing of the biliary tree. PSC can progress to end-stage liver disease.
- Most autoimmune markers for autoimmune liver disease are relatively nonspecific.
- Autoimmune antibodies may be absent despite biopsy, and this type of autoimmune hepatitis is called seronegative AIH.
- A complete workup should be done if a child or neonate presents with jaundice and/or elevated transaminases.

9.11 Wilson's Disease

Wilson's disease (WD) is an autosomal recessive disorder of copper excretion with a prevalence of approximately 1:30,000 (Socha et al. 2018). The ATP7B gene encodes an enzyme used in hepatocytes to transport copper. In Wilson's disease, this protein is missing or diminished, leading to decreased excretion of copper into the bile by hepatocytes and failure to incorporate copper into ceruloplasmin (Roberts and Schilsky 2008). Once copper-containing solid foods are introduced in infancy, progressive copper accumulation begins (Socha et al. 2018). Over time, copper accumulates and deposits in organs such as the brain, cornea, liver, and kidneys. WD can present at any age. Given that the damage from WD occurs over time from the accumulation of copper, it is rare that it presents before the age of 5 years; however, symptomatic WD has been diagnosed in children under 5 years (Roberts and Schilsky 2008).

WD can present as liver disease, hemolysis, neurological disease, eye disease, or psychiatric disease (Roberts and Schilsky 2008). Neurologic symptoms in childhood include changes in behavior, a decline in school performance, or difficulty with tasks requiring hand-eye coordination, deterioration in handwriting with micrographia, tremor, drooling dysarthria, dystonia, spasticity, and dysphagia (Roberts and Schilsky 2008). Psychiatric conditions seen in WD include depression, anxiety, and psychosis (Roberts and Schilsky 2008). Other extrahepatic manifestations of WD can include renal disease (aminoaciduria, nephrolithiasis), premature osteoporosis and arthritis, cardiomyopathy, pancreatitis, and hypoparathyroidism (Roberts and Schilsky 2008).

In childhood, 30% of patients with WD present with chronic liver failure, 25% present with acute hepatitis, and 12% present with fulminant liver failure (Warner and Kelly 2021). Treatment consists of zinc supplementation to prevent copper accumulation, with or without chelation to chelate excess copper that has already accumulated. Care must be taken with close monitoring to prevent over chelation. In patients who have progressed to liver failure, the only treatment is a liver transplant.

9.11.1 Diagnostic Laboratory Workup for WD

The patient with WD needs a careful diagnostic laboratory evaluation. The patient with classic Kayser-Fleischer rings confirmed by an ophthalmologist should receive an immediate referral to a liver specialist. As mentioned above, there are subtle symptoms and signs in which WD should be considered, and the diagnostic workup started.

9.11.1.1 Ceruloplasmin

Ceruloplasmin is a copper-carrying protein that is secreted by hepatocytes; it accounts for 90% of circulating copper in normal patients (Roberts and Schilsky 2008). The majority of reports show that 90–100% of patients with WD have low ceruloplasmin (Roberts and Schilsky 2008). Ceruloplasmin is very low in early infancy, peaks in early childhood, and then settles to the adult range (Roberts and Schilsky 2008). Serum ceruloplasmin of <20 mg/dL is consistent with WD; it is diagnostic if the patient also has Kayser-Fleischer rings.

It is important to note that ceruloplasmin is an acute-phase reactant. Therefore, during states of acute inflammation, it can be normal or high (Roberts and Schilsky 2008). This is particularly important to consider in the patient with acute liver failure, as normal ceruloplasmin can be falsely reassuring. Additionally, patients with hyperestrogenemia (e.g., pregnancy or birth control) can elevate ceruloplasmin (Roberts and Schilsky 2008). Low ceruloplasmin can also be caused by copper deficiency and in patients with Menkes disease (Roberts and Schilsky 2008).

9.11.1.2   Serum Copper

The total serum copper is a combination of non-ceruloplasmin-bound ("free") copper and copper bound to ceruloplasmin. The copper level is usually low in WD but can be markedly elevated in acute liver failure (Roberts and Schilsky 2008). The non-ceruloplasmin copper may be more useful in the diagnosis and is usually >25 µg/dL in most untreated patients with WD. The non-ceruloplasmin copper is a calculation made using the serum copper level and ceruloplasmin.

Pitfalls of Serum Copper. The non-ceruloplasmin copper can become elevated in acute liver failure in general, as well as in cholestasis (Roberts and Schilsky 2008). Additionally, because it is a calculation, it is dependent on the accuracy of the copper and ceruloplasmin. The copper level is more useful in guiding treatment (with zinc and or chelators) in patients with known WD than in diagnosis (Roberts and Schilsky 2008).

9.11.1.3   24-Hour Urine Copper

The 24-hour urinary excretion of copper reflects the amount of non-ceruloplasmin-bound copper in circulation (Roberts and Schilsky 2008). The diagnostic level for WD has been >100 µg/day; however, 16%–23% of patients diagnosed with

WD have a 24-hour urine copper level < 100 µg/day, and > 40 µg/day could be considered a better threshold (Roberts and Schilsky 2008).

It is important to note the volume of the 24-h urine because if the sample is not truly a 24-h sample, it will not be accurate. Additionally, patients who are heterozygous for WD may have intermediate levels, and patients with another liver disease (including autoimmune hepatitis) may have 24-h urine copper levels of 100–200 µg/day (Roberts and Schilsky 2008). In pediatric patients, measuring urinary copper excretion in the setting of D-penicillamine (a copper chelator) administration may be helpful to distinguish other liver diseases from WD (Roberts and Schilsky 2008). This was only found to be helpful in patients with active hepatitis (92% sensitivity) but not in screening asymptomatic siblings (46% sensitivity) (Roberts and Schilsky 2008). Box 9.5 summarizes the recommendations to diagnose WD.

Box 9.5 Wilson's Disease Diagnosis Recommendations
1. Consider WD in any child >1 year of age with signs of liver disease (asymptomatic elevated liver enzymes, cirrhosis, or acute liver failure) (Socha et al. 2018).
2. WD must be excluded in any teenager with unexplained cognitive, psychiatric, or movement disorder (Socha et al. 2018).
3. When WD is suspected, refer to a skilled examiner for a slit-light exam to rule out Kayser-Fleischer rings. However, the absence of Kayser-Fleischer (KF) rings does not rule out Wilson's disease (KF rings are usually absent in patients presenting with liver disease, present in 44–62% of patients with mainly hepatic disease at the time of treatment, and may be absent in 5% of patients with neurologic presentation) (Roberts and Schilsky 2008).
4. A very low ceruloplasmin (<5 mg/dL) is a very strong evidence for

WD. Modestly subnormal levels warrant further investigation. A normal ceruloplasmin does not exclude the diagnosis of WD (Roberts and Schilsky 2008).

5. A 24-h urine copper should be obtained in all patients considered for WD. A 24-h urine copper in symptomatic patients with WD is typically >100 μg/day, but findings of >40 μg require further investigation (Roberts and Schilsky 2008).

6. Genetic testing (whole genome sequencing) should be considered in patients for whom it is difficult to establish a diagnosis. It can be done on first-degree relatives of patients with WD, and a clinical geneticist should be consulted to interpret results (Roberts and Schilsky 2008).

7. All first-degree relatives of patients with newly diagnosed WD must be screened for WD (Socha et al. 2018).

Adapted from Socha et al. 2018; Roberts and Schilsky 2008

9.12 Alpha-1 Antitrypsin Deficiency (A1ATD)

Alpha-1 antitrypsin deficiency (A1ATD) is the most common genetic cause of pediatric liver disease (Mitchell and Khan 2017). In infancy, A1ATD can present as neonatal hepatitis (with jaundice, failure to thrive, pruritus, hepatosplenomegaly) and can look like other common causes of neonatal cholestasis. A patient can present later in childhood with previously unrecognized liver disease manifesting in decompensated liver disease (gastrointestinal bleeding, ascites, liver failure) (Patel and Teckman 2018). The AAT mutant Z protein accumulates and causes damage to the liver; however, given the vast variety of liver disease presentations in these patients, there are likely environmental and genetic disease

modifiers that determine the severity of liver disease (Patel and Teckman 2018). A1ATD is also associated with chronic obstructive pulmonary disease that presents later in life, and therefore parents should be screened for A1ATD.

9.12.1 Diagnostic Laboratory Evaluation

The clinical picture of liver disease in pediatric patients with A1AT deficiency ranges from asymptomatic to developing the life-threatening liver disease (3–5%) (Patel and Teckman 2018). The diagnostic laboratory evaluation must be done quickly in the patient with decompensated liver disease.

9.12.1.1 Alpha-1 Antitrypsin Levels

This test should not be the first-line test in a patient with suspected A1ATD. The AAT level is not considered a gold standard for diagnosis because it is an acute-phase reactant and can be falsely elevated during systemic inflammation. Therefore, the phenotype should be ordered (Patel and Teckman 2018).

9.12.1.2 Alpha-1 Antitrypsin (AAT) Phenotype

The gold standard of diagnosis is testing for AAT phenotype. Patients are diagnosed with A1ATD when their phenotype is ZZ or compound heterozygotes (SZ) (Patel and Teckman 2018).

9.13 Cholestatic Diseases

The liver performs many vital body functions, including lipid and fat-soluble vitamin digestion and absorption, cholesterol metabolism, blood sugar regulation, excretion of toxins, maintenance of oncotic pressure, and production of clotting factors and infection prevention/protection. The liver must excrete bile, which is composed of bile acids, phospholipids, cholesterol, water, bilirubin, electrolytes, metabolized drugs, and xenobiotics (Harb and Thomas 2007). Not only are products of liver metabolism excreted through the bile, but with insufficient bile flow (cholestasis), the bile backs up into the liver and causes damage to the liver itself. If the damage is significant enough, it can lead to scar tissue and potentially liver failure. Cholestasis can be present with or without jaundice. Jaundice becomes visible once total bilirubin reaches 2.5–3.0 mg/dL (Fawaz et al. 2017).

The bile allows for the breakdown and absorption of dietary fat and absorption of fat-soluble vitamins; therefore, nutrition assessment is particularly important in patients with cholestasis, with particular attention paid to fat-soluble vitamin levels (A, D, E, and K – INR, which may reflect low vitamin K levels if elevated and correctable with vitamin K administration).

Cholesterol levels may be significantly elevated in patients with cholestatic disease due to the excess of bile salts, which are the building blocks of cholesterol. On a lipid panel, the LDL can be markedly elevated. Still, the elevation is often caused by lipoprotein X (Lp-X), which is not associated with accelerated atherosclerosis (Nemes et al. 2016). Cholestasis can also lead to profound pruritus that can affect the quality of life significantly. Bile salts can be measured on lab draws to determine if itching in a cholestatic patient is due to cholestasis. Box 9.6 reviews the common differential diagnoses for cholestasis in children, and Box 9.7 reviews the common differential diagnosis for neonatal cholestasis.

- Viral infection (herpes viruses; parvovirus; hepatitis A, B, and C; enteroviruses; adenovirus; HIV).
- Other infections (sepsis, UTI, listeria, tuberculosis).
- Autoimmune [gestational alloimmune liver disease, primary sclerosing cholangitis (PSC), primary biliary cholangitis (PBC), autoimmune cholangiopathy].
- Bile duct obstruction (choledocholithiasis, choledochal cyst, tumor).
- Mitochondrial disease.
- Endocrine (hypothyroidism, panhypopituitarism, others).
- Infiltrative disorders [Langerhans cell histiocytosis (LCH)].
- Progressive familial intrahepatic cholestasis (PFIC) types 1–6.
- Sickle cell anemia.
- Toxic (parenteral nutrition, fetal alcohol syndrome, others).

Adapted from Loomes and Emerick 2021

9.13.1 Neonatal Cholestasis

Physiologic neonatal jaundice is characterized by an elevation in the total bilirubin with a normal direct bilirubin; it is discussed in detail in the newborn section. In contrast, neonatal cholestasis is jaundice caused by elevated conjugated bilirubin and is pathologic. While neonatal jaundice is relatively common, neonatal cholestasis only occurs in 1 in every 2500 infants (Fawaz et al. 2017). Any infant that is not well-appearing or has concerning findings (lethargy, poor tone, failure to thrive, fever, hepatosplenomegaly, ascites, acholic stools, dark urine) should be evaluated expeditiously. Biliary atresia (BA) is the most commonly known cause of neonatal cholestasis, followed by genetic disorders and neonatal cholestasis of unknown etiology (Fawaz et al. 2017). The number of idiopathic neonatal hepatitis cases has decreased as diagnostic and genetic testing improves (Fawaz et al. 2017).

Box 9.6 Common Differential Diagnoses for Cholestasis

- Biliary atresia.
- Neonatal giant cell hepatitis.
- Cystic fibrosis.
- Alagille syndrome.
- Metabolic disorders (alpha-1 antitrypsin deficiency, glycogen storage disease type IV, urea cycle defects, galactosemia, tyrosinemia type I, citrin deficiency, others).
- Bile acid synthesis defects.

According to the North American Society for Pediatric Gastroenterology, Hepatology and Nutrition (NASPGHAN) guidelines, infants who are still jaundice by 2 weeks of age should have a fractionated bilirubin to assess for direct hyperbilirubinemia. Any infant with a direct bilirubin >1.0 mg/dL should be considered pathologic (Fawaz et al. 2017), necessitating additional assessment. It is important to assess urine and stool color during the visit, and any infant with dark urine and acholic stool warrants a prompt evaluation.

Biliary atresia is a rare congenital liver disease (~1:10,000 live births) of unknown etiology that leads to progressive sclerosing/destruction of the extrahepatic bile ducts, progressive liver fibrosis, progressive liver failure, and death without intervention. Biliary atresia is treated with a surgical procedure called the Kasai portoenterostomy, a surgery that attaches the jejunum directly to the liver edge after removal of the affected extrahepatic biliary tree and may reestablish bile flow. Without a functioning Kasai or a liver transplant, BA is fatal by 1–2 years of age. Since the Kasai procedure's timing has implications for outcomes (better below 45 days of age—70% of patients will establish bile flow), there is a time pressure to ensure early diagnosis. After 90 days of life, outcomes yield less than 25% reestablished bile flow (Fawaz et al. 2017), leaving liver transplant as the only option for cure.

When an infant is jaundiced at 14 days, they require a full family history, gestational history, physical examination (including stool sample for color), and a fractionated bilirubin to determine if this is direct hyperbilirubinemia (Fawaz et al. 2017). The initial workup for neonatal cholestasis can be started in primary care. This workup aims to narrow the differential diagnoses and to establish the extent of the liver involvement. The work up should start with a CBC with differential, INR, transaminases, alkaline phosphatase, direct bilirubin, glucose, albumin and -1 antitrypsin phenotype should be done. A TSH and T4 should be done if the newborn screen is not available (Fawaz et al. 2017) or the clinician feels they want to recheck the result. Urine evaluation should include a urinalysis, urine culture, and reducing substances to check for galactosemia. If the infant has a fever or looks sick, bacterial cultures of blood, urine, and spinal fluid should be considered. As stated in other chapters, the newborn screen should also be checked, and the results put into the chart. Some states require two newborn screens, and that should be initiated if not previously done. A fasting ultrasound is also part of the initial workup (Fawaz et al. 2017). The child should be referred to a liver specialist with the results of the initial workup. Other specialists involved in the care of these patients include ophthalmology, pediatric surgery, metabolic geneticist, nutritionist, and cardiology (Fawaz et al. 2017).

> **Box 9.7 Common Differential Diagnoses for Neonatal Cholestasis**
> - Biliary atresia.
> - Neonatal hepatitis.
> - Neonatal sclerosing cholangitis.
> - Alagille syndrome.
> - Alpha-1 antitrypsin deficiency.
> - Caroli's disease.
> - Viral infection (CMV, HIV).
> - Bacterial infection (urinary tract infections, sepsis, syphilis).
> - Parenteral nutrition-associated cholestasis.
> - Genetic/metabolic disorders [citrin deficiency, alpha-1 antitrypsin deficiency, tyrosinemia, galactosemia, hypothyroidism, PFIC (types 1, 2, or 3), cystic fibrosis, panhypopituitarism].
> - Lipid metabolism (Niemann-Pick type C, lysosomal acid lipase deficiency).
>
> Adapted from Fawaz et al. 2017

9.13.2 Real-Life Example

A firstborn 3-week-old full-term neonate was seen for the first time in the office with a chief complaint of continued jaundice. The child was delivered via NSVD, weighing 8 pounds and 3 ounces after an uneventful 40-week pregnancy.

The mother noted jaundice on the first day of life. The mother reported that the last provider told her that her neonate's jaundice was due to breast-feeding. A careful history revealed a history of jaundice down to the lower abdomen since birth and clay-colored stools four times a day. The exam was remarkable for jaundice to the lower abdomen with a firm liver edge at 3 cm below the right costal margin. The rest of the exam was unremarkable. A stat total and direct bilirubin were 11.4 mg/dl (normal, 0.05–0.68) and 4.3 (normal, 0.05–0.30), respectively. A TSH and T4 were normal from the newborn screen. The AST was 236 (normal, 20–67 U/L), and the ALT was 289 (normal, 5–33 U/L). The GGT was 507 (normal for age, 0–130 U/L), and ALP was 732 (normal for age, 150–420 U/L). The glucose was 79, and albumin was normal. An α-1 antitrypsin phenotype was planned if the ultrasound was negative; however, the ultrasound showed a choledochal cyst. The child was referred to pediatric surgery the same day.

Key Learning about Neonatal Cholestasis

- Physiologic neonatal jaundice is characterized by an elevation in the total bilirubin with a normal direct bilirubin.
- A direct bilirubin should be repeated if there is concern about continuing jaundice.
- An infant who is jaundiced at 14 days should have a complete history, physical exam, an evaluation of stool for color, and a fractionated bilirubin to determine if this is direct hyperbilirubinemia.
- It should never be assumed that a breastfeeding infant with jaundice who is breastfed has breastfeeding jaundice.

Questions

1. In hepatocellular liver disease, which of the following is the most likely to be elevated?
   (a) Alanine transaminase (ALT).
   (b) Gamma-glutamyl transferase (GTT).
   (c) Direct bilirubin.
   (d) Iron.

2. A 30-month-old child presents with a 2-week history of diarrhea. The mother reports that the stools are yellow, floating on the toilet bowel, and occur four to five times a day. The child was recently traveling in the national park. The mother reports that they were hiking when they ran out of water. She gave the child a few sips of water from a stream. The child has lost 1 pound but otherwise has a normal physical exam. What is the best initial diagnostic laboratory test to order?
   (a) CBC with differential and comprehensive metabolic profile.
   (b) Stool for ova and parasites.
   (c) Multiplex PCR stool that includes testing for giardiasis.
   (d) Stool culture.

3. Out of the following tests, which of the following is the most specific for autoimmune hepatitis?
   (a) Anti-nuclear antibody (ANA).
   (b) Anti-mitochondrial antibody (AMA).
   (c) Immunoglobulin 4 (IgG4).
   (d) Anti-smooth muscle antibody (SMA).

4. Which of the following lab results is most indicative of chronic liver disease?
   (a) Direct bilirubin of 14 mg/dL.
   (b) INR of 2.0.
   (c) Platelet count of 45.
   (d) ALT of 5000.

5. Which of the following diagnoses is most consistent with a total bilirubin of 14 mg/dL and direct bilirubin of 0.8 mg/dL?
   (a) Biliary atresia.
   (b) Crigler-Najjar type 2.
   (c) Primary sclerosing cholangitis (PSC).
   (d) Autoimmune hepatitis (AIH).

6. What is the single most important risk factor for celiac disease (CD)?
   (a) Age.
   (b) Race.
   (c) Gender.
   (d) Family history of a first-degree relative with CD.

7. Which of the following is *not* an antibody blood test used to screen for celiac disease?
   (a) Anti-nuclear Antibody (ANA).
   (b) Tissue transglutaminase antibody IgA.

(c) Endomysial antibody IgA.

(d) Total serum IgA.

8. For most patients, what is the most valuable screening test for patients with celiac disease?

(a) Deamidated gliadin peptide IgG.

(b) Deamidated gliadin peptide IgA.

(c) Tissue transglutaminase IgA.

(d) Antigliadin IgA.

9. If a patient is found to have selective IgA deficiency, which of the following would you screen for next?

(a) Deamidated gliadin peptide IgA and IgG.

(b) Endomysial antibody IgA and tissue transglutaminase IgG.

(c) Deamidated gliadin peptide IgG and antigliadin IgG.

(d) Tissue transglutaminase IgG and deamidated gliadin peptide IgG.

10. Which of the following patients need a screen for celiac disease?

(a) A 2-year-old female with congenital heart decease.

(b) A 4-year-old male with trisomy 21.

(c) A 10-year-old male with precocious puberty.

(d) A 5-year-old female with a seizure disorder.

11. Which of the following tests would be the best choice when you are screening a patient for IBD?

(a) CBC, hepatic function panel, hemoglobin A1C, ANA.

(b) CBC, basic metabolic panel, total IgA, TTG-IgA.

(c) CBC, hepatic function panel, ESR, CRP.

(d) CBC, basic metabolic panel, ESR, ANA.

12. A patient reports 4 weeks of bloody diarrhea and weight loss. Which of the following stool test results are most suggestive of IBD?

(a) *C. difficile* negative, GID PCR negative, fecal occult blood negative.

(b) *C. difficile* positive, fecal occult blood positive, fecal calprotectin <16 – within normal range.

(c) *C. difficile* negative, GID PCR positive for norovirus, fecal occult blood negative.

(d) *C. difficile* negative, GID PCR negative, fecal calprotectin 432 (<16 is within normal range).

13. Which of the following is not an extraintestinal manifestation associated with IBD?

(a) Precocious puberty.

(b) Growth failure.

(c) Aphthous ulcers.

(d) Primary sclerosing cholangitis.

14. Which of the following group of results are most suggestive of IBD?

(a) ESR normal, CRP elevated CBC with thrombocytosis and microcytic anemia and low albumin.

(b) ESR normal, CRP normal, CBC with thrombocytosis, elevated albumin.

(c) ESR normal, CPR normal, CBC with macrocytic anemia and thrombocytopenia.

(d) ESR normal CRP normal, CBC within normal range, elevated albumin.

Rationale

1. Answer: A

In hepatocellular disease, the ALT and AST are elevated. The ALP, GTT, bilirubin, and urobilinogen are more likely to be elevated in cholestatic liver disease. Iron is not an indicator of hepatocellular disease.

2. Answer: C

The history of traveling in the national park and drinking from a stream points to the need to rule out an enteric pathogen. Giardiasis can give malabsorption-type stools and is a likely culprit, but there are other one-cell pathogens and bacteria to consider. Traditional microscopy for stool parasites has a lower sensitivity and specificity than newer PCR molecular methods. The latter may provide a more accurate diagnosis (Mero et al. 2017). Therefore, in this case, C would likely give the clinician the quickest and most efficient option.

3. Answer: D

SMA is more specific for AIH than the other tests. ANA is a nonspecific marker for autoimmune hepatitis and can be found in healthy patients and patients with other auto-immune diseases. AMA is rarely checked in pediatrics; it is mostly associated with PBC, primarily an adult disease. IgG4 elevation is associated with IgG4-related sclerosing cholangitis (or autoimmune pancreatitis).

4. Answer: C

A patient with liver disease with a low platelet count may have a low platelet count due to portal hypertension, a manifestation of chronic liver disease. An elevated direct bilirubin can be seen with either acute or chronic liver disease. INR can be elevated due to either medication, liver failure (acute or chronic), or vitamin K deficiency, but it does not necessarily reflect chronicity. A markedly elevated ALT is seen more commonly with acute hepatitis than in chronic liver disease.

5. Answer: B

Biliary atresia presents with elevated direct bilirubin. Crigler-Najjar type 2 is the milder form of the disease; can be asymptomatic but becomes symptomatic during times of stress, illness, or fasting, usually with total bilirubin <15 mg/dL; and therefore fits this picture. PSC is a cholestatic disease that may or may not lead to jaundice, in which case it would primarily be direct hyperbilirubinemia. Autoimmune hepatitis is primarily a hepatocellular disease, but it would be primarily direct hyperbilirubinemia if it were advanced enough to lead to jaundice.

6. Answer: D

Celiac disease is a genetic component, and it is recommended that siblings of celiac patients above the age of 3 should be screened even if asymptomatic.

7. Answer: A

ANA is not part of the screening for celiac disease, while all of the other antibodies listed may be on the screening panel for celiac disease

8. Answer: C

For most patients, the TTG-IgA is the most valuable screening test. In patients with CD, TTG plays at least two critical roles: (1) deamidating enzyme and (2) target autoantigen in the immune response.

9. Answer: D

If a patient is IgA deficient, you will screen for IgG-specific antibodies to tissue transglutaminase and deamidated gliadin peptide.

10. Answer: B

Patients with trisomy 21 are included in the high-risk group and as such, even if asymptomatic, should be screened once they are 3 years of age or older.

11. Answer: C

CBC may have thrombocytosis and/or anemia findings. The hepatic function panel may reveal an elevation in liver enzymes or hypoalbuminemia, and inflammatory markers such as ESR and CRP may be elevated.

12. Answer: D

Chronic bloody diarrhea with weight loss with negative infectious stool studies but with elevation in fecal calprotectin is concerning for an inflammatory process in the GI tract.

13. Answer: A

Growth failure, aphthous ulcers, and primary sclerosing cholangitis are extraintestinal manifestations that can be seen in IBD, and delay in puberty can be seen in IBD patients as well versus precocious puberty.

14. Answer: A

Although patients with IBD can have normal blood results, findings of an elevation of an inflammatory marker (CRP) coupled with anemia, thrombocytosis, and hypoalbuminemia suggest IBD.

References

Abadie V, Sollid LM, Barreiro LB, Jabri B. Integration of genetic and immunological insights into a model of CD pathogenesis. Annu Rev Immunol. 2011;29: 493–525.

Alharbi A, Toulah FH, Wakid MH, Azhar E, Farraj S, Mirza AA. Detection of Giardia lamblia by microscopic examination, rapid chromatographic immunoassay test, and molecular technique. Cureus. 2020;12(9):e10287.

Aljomah G, Baker SS, Schmidt K, Alkhouri R, Kozielski R, Zhu L, Baker RD. Anemia in pediatric inflammatory bowel disease. J Pediatr Gastroenterol Nutr. 2018;67(3):351–5.

Alkalay MJ. Update on celiac disease. Curr Opin Pediatr. 2020;32(5):654–60.

Alrabadi LS, Porto AF. Assessment of community pediatric providers' approach to a child with celiac disease and available serological testing associated with a large tertiary care center. Clin Pediatr (Phila). 2018;57(10):1199–203.

Al-Toma A, Volta U, Auricchio R, Castillejo G, Sanders DS, Cellier C, et al. European Society for the study of Coeliac Disease (ESsCD) guideline for coeliac disease and other gluten-related disorders. United European Gastroenterol J. 2019;7(5):583–613.

Amerine E. Celiac disease goes against the grain. Nursing. 2006;36(2):46–8.

Bai JC, Fried M, Corazza GR, Schuppan D, Farthing M, Catassi C, et al.; World Gastroenterology Organization. World Gastroenterology Organisation global guidelines on celiac disease. 2016 Retrieved on June 10, 2021, https://www.worldgastroenterology.org/UserFiles/file/guidelines/celiac-disease-english-2016.pdf

Banerjee S, Owen C, Chopra S. Sickle cell hepatopathy. Hepatology. 2001;33(5):1021–8.

Bangaru S, Agrawal D. Medication effects on fecal occult blood testing-reply. JAMA Intern Med. 2019;179(4):591–2.

Bartsch SM, Umscheid CA, Nachamkin I, Hamilton K, Lee BY. Comparing the economic and health benefits of different approaches to diagnosing Clostridium difficile infection. Clin Microbiol Infect. 2015;21(1):77. e1–9.

Beal SG, Tremblay EE, Toffel S, Velez L, Rand KH. A gastrointestinal PCR panel improves clinical management and lowers health care costs. J Clin Microbiol. 2018;56(1):e01457-17.

Beattie RM, Walker-Smith JA, Murch SH. Indications for investigation of chronic gastrointestinal symptoms. Arch Dis Child. 1995;73(4):354–5.

Bechtold ML, Ashraf I, Nguyen DL. A clinician's guide to fecal occult blood testing for colorectal cancer. South Med J. 2016;109(4):248–55.

Benchimol EI, Bernstein CN, Bitton A, Carroll MW, Singh H, Otley AR, et al. Trends in epidemiology of pediatric inflammatory bowel disease in Canada: distributed network analysis of multiple population-based provincial health administrative databases. Am J Gastroenterol. 2017;112(7):1120–34.

Benchimol EI, Fortinsky KJ, Gozdyra P, Van den Heuvel M, Van Limbergen J, Griffiths AM. Epidemiology of pediatric inflammatory bowel disease: a systematic review of international trends. Inflamm Bowel Dis. 2011;17(1):423–39.

Benor S, Russell GH, Silver M, Israel EJ, Yuan Q, Winter HS. Shortcomings of the inflammatory bowel disease serology 7 panel. Pediatrics. 2010;125(6):1230–6.

Bhatt H, Rao GS. Management of acute liver failure: a pediatric perspective. Curr Pediatr Rep. 2018;6(3):246–57.

Blohm ME, Vesterling-Hörner D, Calaminus G, Göbel U. Alpha 1-fetoprotein (AFP) reference values in infants up to 2 years of age. Pediatr Hematol Oncol. 1998;15(2):135–42.

Bogdanos DP, Mieli-Vergani G, Vergani D. Autoantibodies and their antigens in autoimmune hepatitis. Semin Liver Dis. 2009;29(3):241–53.

Bowlus CL, Arrivé L, Bergquist A, Deneau M, Forman L, Ilyas SI, et al. AASLD primary sclerosing cholangitis and cholangiocarcinoma guidance. hepatology. 2022. Pending publication.

Branda JA, Lin TY, Rosenberg ES, Halpern EF, Ferraro MJ. A rational approach to the stool ova and parasite examination. Clin Infect Dis. 2006;42(7):972–8.

Brierley CH, Burchell B. Human UDP-glucuronosyl transferases: chemical defense, jaundice and gene therapy. BioEssays. 1993;15(11):749–54.

Brown KA, Khanafer N, Daneman N, Fisman DN. Meta-analysis of antibiotics and the risk of community-associated Clostridium difficile infection. Antimicrob Agents Chemother. 2013;57(5):2326–32.

Buckel WR, Avdic E, Carroll KC, Gunaseelan V, Hadhazy E, Cosgrove SE. Gut check: clostridium difficile testing and treatment in the molecular testing era. Infect Control Hosp Epidemiol. 2015;36(2):217–21.

Buss S, Leber A, Chapin K, Fey PD, Bankowski MJ, Jones MK, et al. Multicenter evaluation of the BioFire FilmArray gastrointestinal panel for etiologic diagnosis of infectious gastroenteritis. J Clin Microbiol. 2015;11(3):915–25.

Bussler S, Vogel M, Pietzner D, Harms K, Buzek T, Penke M, Händel N, Körner A, Baumann U, Kiess W, Flemming G. New pediatric percentiles of liver enzyme serum levels (alanine aminotransferase, aspartate aminotransferase, γ-glutamyltransferase): effects of age, sex, body mass index, and pubertal stage. Hepatology. 2018;68(4):1319–30.

Cabrera-Abreu J, Green A. (Gamma)-glutamyltransferase: value of its measurement in paediatrics. Ann Clin Biochem. 2002;39:22–5. Retrieved from http://ezproxy.cul.columbia.edu/login?url=https://www.proquest.com/docview/201681943?accountid=10226

Caio G, Volta U, Sapone A, Leffler DA, De Giorgio R, Catassi C, Fasano A. Celiac disease: a comprehensive current review. BMC Med. 2019;17(1):142.

Carragher F. Chapter 25—paediatric clinical biochemistry. In: Marshall W, Lapsley M, Day A, Ayling R, editors. Clinical biochemistry: metabolic and clinical aspects. 3rd ed. Illinois: Churchill Livingstone; 2014. p. 484–96.

Carroll KC, Mizusawa M. Laboratory tests for the diagnosis of clostridium difficile. Clin Colon Rectal Surg. 2020;33(2):73–81.

Chapman R, Fevery J, Kalloo A, Nagorney DM, Boberg KM, Shneider B, et al. American Association for the Study of Liver Diseases. Diagnosis and management of primary sclerosing cholangitis. Hepatology. 2010;51(2):660–78. https://doi.org/10.1002/hep.23294. PMID: 20101749

Conrad MA, Rosh JR. Pediatric inflammatory bowel disease. Pediatr Clin N Am. 2017;64(3):577–91.

Dahlan Y, Smith L, Simmonds D, Jewell LD, Wanless I, Heathcote EJ, Bain VG. Pediatric-onset primary biliary cirrhosis. Gastroenterol. 2003;125(5):1476–9.

De Leo L, Quaglia S, Ziberna F, Vatta S, Martelossi S, Maschio M, Not T. Serum anti-tissue transglutaminase antibodies detected during febrile illness may not be produced by the intestinal mucosa. J Pediatr. 2015;166(3):761–3.

Deshpande A, Pasupuleti V, Thota P, Pant C, Rolston DD, Sferra TJ, Hernandez AV, Donskey CJ. Community-associated Clostridium difficile infection and antibiotics: a meta-analysis. J Antimicrob Chemother. 2013;68(9):1951–61.

Di Sabatino A, Vanoli A, Giuffrida P, Luinetti O, Solcia E, Corazza GR. The function of tissue transglutaminase in celiac disease. Autoimmun Rev. 2012;11(10):746–53.

Domínguez-Muñoz JE, Hardt D, Lerch PMM, Löhr MJ. Potential for screening for pancreatic exocrine insufficiency using the fecal Elastase-1 test. Dig Dis Sci. 2017;62(5):1119–30.

Dorn L, Finkenstedt A, Schranz M, Prokop W, Griesmacher A, Vogel W, Zoller H. Immunoglobulin subclass 4 for the diagnosis of immunoglobulin subclass 4-associated diseases in an unselected liver and pancreas clinic population. HPB (Oxford). 2012;14(2):122–5.

Dubberke ER, Han Z, Bobo L, Hink T, Lawrence B, Copper S, Hoppe-Bauer J, Burnham CA, Dunne WM Jr. Impact of clinical symptoms on interpretation of diagnostic assays for Clostridium difficile infections. J Clin Microbiol. 2011;49(8):2887–93.

Dykes SM, Saeed S. Inflammatory bowel disease. In: McInerny T, editor. AAP textbook of pediatric care. Elk Grove Village, IL: AAP Press; 2016. p. 2199–203.

El-Chammas K, Majeskie A, Simpson P, Sood M, Miranda A. Red flags in children with chronic abdominal pain and Crohn's disease—a single center experience. J Pediatr. 2013;162(4):783–7.

Fawaz R, Baumann U, Ekong U, Fischler B, Hadzic N, Mack CL, et al. Guideline for the evaluation of cholestatic jaundice in infants: joint recommendations of the North American Society for Pediatric Gastroenterology, Hepatology, and Nutrition and the European Society for Pediatric Gastroenterology, hepatology, and nutrition. J Pediatr Gastroenterol Nutr. 2017;64(1):154–68.

Fawaz R, Jonas MM. Acute and chronic hepatitis. In: Wyllie R, Haymes JS, Kay M, editors. Pediatric gastrointestinal and liver disease. 6th ed. Philadelphia, PA: Elsevier; 2021. p. 819–37.

Giannini EG, Testa R, Savarino V. Liver enzyme alteration: a guide for clinicians. CMAJ. 2005;172(3):367–79.

Gidrewicz D, Potter K, Trevenen CL, Lyon M, Butzner JD. Evaluation of the ESPGHAN celiac guidelines in a North American pediatric population. Am J Gastroenterol. 2015;110(5):760–7.

Gingras BA, Maggiore JA. Performance of a new molecular assay for the detection of gastrointestinal pathogens. Access Microbiol. 2020;2 https://doi.org/10.1099/acm:0.000160.

Green PR, Jones R. Chapter: how do I know if I have it? The diagnosis of celiac disease. In: Celiac disease: a hidden epidemic. New York: William Morrow, an imprint of HarperCollins Publishers; 2016. p. 40–63.

Griffiths AM. Specificities of inflammatory bowel disease in childhood. Best Pract Res Clin Gastroenterol. 2004;18(3):509–23.

Grossman AB, Baldassan RN. Inflammatory bowel disease. In: Kliegman R, Stanton B, St. Geme JW, Schor NF, Behrman RE, editors. Nelson textbook of pediatrics. 20th ed. Philadelphia, PA: Elsevier; 2016. p. 1819–31.

Guandalini S. The approach to celiac disease in children. Int J Pediatr Adolesc Med. 2017;4(3):124–7.

Guarino A, Ashkenazi S, Gendrel D, Lo Vecchio A, Shamir R, Szajewska H, et al. European Society for Pediatric Gastroenterology, Hepatology, and Nutrition/European Society for Pediatric Infectious Diseases evidence-based guidelines for the management of acute gastroenteritis in children in Europe: update 2014. J Pediatr Gastroenterol Nutr. 2014;59(1):132–52.

Gujral N, Freeman HJ, Thomson AB. Celiac disease: prevalence, diagnosis, pathogenesis and treatment. World J Gastroenterol. 2012;18(42):6036–59.

Hannet I, Engsbro AL, Pareja J, Schneider UV, Lisby JG, Pružinec-Popović B, Hoerauf A, Parčina M. Multicenter evaluation of the new QIAstat gastrointestinal panel for the rapid syndromic testing of acute gastroenteritis. Eur J Clin Microbiol Infect Dis. 2019;38(11):2103–12.

Harb R, Thomas DW. Conjugated hyperbilirubinemia: screening and treatment in older infants and children. Pediatr Rev. 2007;28(3):83–91.

Heyman MB, Kirschner BS, Gold BD, Ferry G, Baldassano R, Cohen SA, et al. Children with early-onset inflammatory bowel disease (IBD): analysis of a pediatric IBD consortium registry. J Pediatr. 2005;146(1):35–40.

Hill ID, Dirks MH, Liptak GS, Colletti RB, Fasano A, Guandalini S, et al. Guideline for the diagnosis and treatment of celiac disease in children: recommendations of the North American Society for Pediatric Gastroenterology, Hepatology and Nutrition. J Pediatr Gastroenterol Nutr. 2005;40(1):1–19.

Hill ID, Fasano A, Guandalini S, Hoffenberg E, Levy J, Reilly N, Verma R. NASPGHAN clinical report on the diagnosis and treatment of gluten-related disorders. J Pediatr Gastroenterol Nutr. 2016;63(1):156–65.

Himoto T, Nishioka M. Autoantibodies in liver disease: important clues for the diagnosis, disease activity and prognosis. Auto Immun Highlights. 2013;4(2):39–53.

Hiyama E. Pediatric hepatoblastoma: diagnosis and treatment. Transl Pediatr. 2014;3(4):293–9.

Holtman GA, Lisman-van Leeuwen Y, Reitsma JB, Berger MY. Noninvasive tests for inflammatory bowel disease: a meta-analysis. Pediatrics. 2016;137(1):e20152126.

Hsu D, Leyva-Vega M, D'Mello S, Josyabhatla R, Liebling M, Shtilbans T. Autoimmune pancreatitis and IgG4-associated cholangitis in a toddler. Pediatrics. 2019;144(2):2. Meeting Abstract 826

Husby S, Koletzko S, Korponay-Szabó I, Kurppa K, Mearin ML, Ribes-Koninckx C, et al. Hepatology and nutrition guidelines for diagnosing coeliac disease 2020. J Pediatr Gastroenterol Nutr. 2020;70(1):141–56.

Husby S, Koletzko S, Korponay-Szabó IR, Mearin ML, Phillips A, et al. ESPGHAN Working Group on Coeliac Disease Diagnosis; ESPGHAN Gastroenterology Committee; European Society for Pediatric Gastroenterology, Hepatology, Nutrition. European Society for Pediatric Gastroenterology, Hepatology, and Nutrition guidelines for the diagnosis of coeliac disease. J Pediatr Gastroenterol Nutr. 2012;54(1):136–60.

Husby S, Murray JA, Katzka DA. AGA clinical practice update on diagnosis and monitoring of celiac disease-changing utility of serology and histologic measures. Expert Rev Gastroenterol. 2019;156(4):885–9.

James MW, Scott BB. EMA antibody in the diagnosis and management of coeliac disease. Postgrad Med J. 2000;76(898):466–8.

Johnston DE. Special considerations in interpreting liver function tests. Am Fam Physician. 1999;59(8):2223–30. PMID: 10221307

Johnston RD, Logan RF. What is the peak age for onset of IBD? Inflamm Bowel Dis. 2008;14(Suppl 2):S4–5.

Jones NL, Koletzko S, Goodman K, Bontems P, Cadranel S, Casswall T, et al. ESPGHAN, NASPGHAN. Joint ESPGHAN/NASPGHAN guidelines for the management of Helicobacter pylori in children and adolescents (update 2016). J Pediatr Gastroenterol Nutr. 2017;64(6):991–1003.

Kalakonda A, Jenkins BA, John S. Physiology, bilirubin. [updated 2020 Mar 29]. In: Stat pearls [internet]. Treasure Island (FL): Stat Pearls Publishing; 2020. Available from: https://www.ncbi.nlm.nih.gov/books/NBK470290/.

Kasırga E. The importance of stool tests in diagnosis and follow-up of gastrointestinal disorders in children. Turk Pediatri Ars. 2019;54(3):141–8.

Khan K, Schwarzenberg SJ, Sharp H, Greenwood D, Weisdorf-Schindele S. Role of serology and routine laboratory tests in childhood inflammatory bowel disease. Inflamm Bowel Dis. 2002;8(5):325–9.

Kugathasan S, Judd RH, Hoffmann RG, Heikenen J, Telega G, Khan F, et al. Epidemiologic and clinical characteristics of children with newly diagnosed inflammatory bowel disease in Wisconsin: a statewide population-based study. J Pediatr. 2003;143(4):525–31.

Kwo PY, Cohen SM, Lim JK. ACG Clinical Guideline: evaluation of abnormal liver chemistries. Am J Gastroenterol. 2017;112(1):18–35.

Laborda TJ, Jensen MK, Kavan M, Deneau M. Treatment of primary sclerosing cholangitis in children. World J Hepatol. 2019;11(1):19–36.

Lázár-Molnár E, Snyder M. The role of human leukocyte antigen in celiac disease diagnostics. Clin Lab Med. 2018;38(4):655–68.

Lee HS, Plechot K, Gohil S, Le J. Clostridium difficile: Diagnosis and the consequence of over diagnosis. Infect Dis Ther. 2021;10(2):687–97.

Leung AKC, Leung AAM, Wong AHC, Sergi CM, Kam JKM. Giardiasis: an overview. Recent Patents Inflamm Allergy Drug Discov. 2019;13(2):134–43.

Liacouras CA, Piccoli DA, Jacobstein D, Baldassano R. Inflammatory bowel disease. In: Bell LM, editor. Pediatric gastroenterology: the requisites in pediatrics. Philadelphia, PA: Mosby. Elsevier Health Sciences; 2008. p. 131–41.

Liu E, Li M, Emery L, Taki I, Barriga K, Tiberti C, et al. Natural history of antibodies to deamidated gliadin peptides and transglutaminase in early childhood celiac disease. J Pediatr Gastroenterol Nutr. 2007;45(3):293–300.

Lo Vecchio A, Buccigrossi V, Fedele MC, Guarino A. Acute infectious diarrhea. Adv Exp Med Biol. 2019;1125:109–20.

Loftus EV Jr. Update on the incidence and prevalence of inflammatory bowel disease in the United States. Gastroenterol Hepatol (N Y). 2016;12(11):704–7.

Loomes KM, Emerick KM. Pediatric cholestatic liver disease. In: Wyllie R, Haymes JS, Kay M, editors. Pediatric gastrointestinal and liver disease. 6th ed. Philadelphia, PA: Elsevier; 2021. p. 769–85.

Lowe D, Sanvictores T, John S. Alkaline phosphatase. [updated 2021 Aug 11]. In: Stat pearls [internet]. Treasure Island (FL): Stat Pearls Publishing; 2021. Available from: https://www.ncbi.nlm.nih.gov/books/NBK459201/.

Mack DR, Langton C, Markowitz J, LeLeiko N, Griffiths A, Bousvaros A, et al. Laboratory values for children with newly diagnosed inflammatory bowel disease. Pediatrics. 2007;119(6):1113–9.

Madani S, Kamat D. Clinical guidelines for celiac disease in children: what does it mean to the pediatrician/family practitioner? Clin Pediatr (Phila). 2006;45(3):213–9.

Malickova K, Lakatos PL, Bortlik M, Komarek V, Janatkova I, Lukas M. Anticarbohydrate antibodies as markers of inflammatory bowel disease in a central European cohort. Eur J Gastroenterol Hepatol. 2010;22(2):144–50.

Manns MP, Czaja AJ, Gorham JD, Krawitt EL, Mieli-Vergani G, et al. Diagnosis and management of autoimmune hepatitis. Hepatology. 2010;51(6):2193–213.

Martinez, et al. Primary sclerosing cholangitis immune reactivity pre-transplant is a predictor of recurrent disease after liver transplantation. Oral abstracts (abstracts 1–288). Hepatology. 2019;70:1–187. https://doi.org/10.1002/hep.30940.

Marrero JA, Kulik LM, Sirlin CB, Zhu AX, Finn RS, Abecassis MM, et al. Diagnosis, Staging, and Management of Hepatocellular Carcinoma: 2018 Practice Guidance by the American Association for the Study of Liver Diseases. Hepatology. 2018;68(2):723–50. https://doi.org/10.1002/hep.29913. PMID: 29624699.

McDaniel M. Hepatic function testing: the ABCs of the liver function tests. Physician Assistant Clin. 2019;24:541–50.

McDonald LC, Gerding DN, Johnson S, Bakken JS, Carroll KC, Coffin SE, et al. Clinical Practice Guidelines for Clostridium difficile infection in adults and children: 2017 update by the Infectious Diseases Society of America (IDSA) and Society for Healthcare Epidemiology of America (SHEA). Clin Infect Dis. 2018;66(7):e1–e48.

Mero S, Kirveskari J, Antikainen J, Ursing J, Rombo L, Kofoed PE, Kantele A. Multiplex PCR detection of Cryptosporidium sp, *Giardia lamblia* and *Entamoeba histolytica* directly from dried stool samples from Guinea-Bissauan children with diarrhoea. Infect Dis (Lond). 2017;49(9):655–63.

Mieli-Vergani G, Vergani D. Autoimmune hepatitis in children: what is different from adult AIH? Semin Liver Dis. 2009;29(3):297–306.

Mitchell EL, Khan Z. Liver disease in Alpha-1 antitrypsin deficiency: current approaches and future directions. Curr Pathobiol Rep. 2017;5(3):243–52.

Mitsuyama K, Niwa M, Takedatsu H, Yamasaki H, Kuwaki K, Yoshioka S, Yamauchi R, Fukunaga S, Torimura T. Antibody markers in the diagnosis of inflammatory bowel disease. World J Gastroenterol. 2016;22(3):1304–10.

Mohapatra S, Singh DP, Alcid D, Pitchumoni CS. Beyond O&P times three. Am J Gastroenterol. 2018;113(6):805–18.

Moreno M. Celiac disease in children and adolescents. JAMA Pediatr. 2014;168(3):300.

Morris AJ, Wilson ML, Reller LB. Application of rejection criteria for stool ovum and parasite examinations. J Clin Microbiol. 1992;30:3213–6.

Nayagam J, Miquel R, Joshi D. Overlap syndrome with autoimmune hepatitis and primary sclerosing cholangitis. Euro Med J Hepatol. 2019;7(1):95–104.

Nehls O, Gregor M, Klump B. Serum and bile markers for cholangiocarcinoma. Semin Liver Dis. 2004;24(2):139–54. https://doi.org/10.1055/s-2004-828891. PMID: 15192787

Nemes K, Åberg F, Gylling H, Isoniemi H. Cholesterol metabolism in cholestatic liver disease and liver transplantation: from molecular mechanisms to clinical implications. World J Hepatol. 2016;8(22):924–32.

Northup PG, Caldwell SH. Coagulation in liver disease: a guide for the clinician. Clin Gastroenterol Hepatol. 2013;11(9):1064–74.

Otero JL, González-Peralta RP, Andres JM, Jolley CD, Novak DA, Haafiz A. Elevated alkaline phosphatase in children: an algorithm to determine when a "wait and see" approach is optimal. Clin Med Insights Pediatr. 2011;22(5):15–8.

Patel D, Teckman JH. Alpha-1-antitrypsin deficiency liver disease. Clin Liver Dis. 2018;22(4):643–55.

Polage CR, Stoddard GJ, Rolfs RT, et al. Physician use of parasite tests in the United States from 1997 to 2006 and in a Utah cryptosporidium outbreak in 2007. J Clin Microbiol. 2011;49:591–6.

Prause C, Ritter M, Probst C, Daehnrich C, Schlumberger W, Komorowski L, et al. Antibodies against deamidated gliadin as new and accurate biomarkers of childhood coeliac disease. J Pediatr Gastroenterol Nutr. 2009;49(1):52–8.

Ramakrishnan N, Bittar K, Jialal I. Impaired bilirubin conjugation. [updated 2020 Jul 27]. In: StatPearls [internet]. Treasure Island (FL): StatPearls Publishing; 2020. https://www.ncbi.nlm.nih.gov/books/NBK482483/.

Roberts EA, Schilsky ML. American Association for Study of Liver Diseases (AASLD). Diagnosis and treatment of Wilson disease: an update. Hepatology. 2008;47(6):2089–111.

Rosen D, Thung S, Sheflin-Findling S, Lai J, Rosen A, Arnon R, Chu J. IgG4-sclerosing cholangitis in a pediatric patient. Semin Liver Dis. 2015b;35(1):89–94.

Rosen MJ, Dhawan A, Saeed SA. Inflammatory bowel disease in children and adolescents. JAMA Pediatr. 2015a;169(11):1053–60.

Rubio-Tapia A, Hill ID, Kelly CP, Calderwood AH, Murray JA. American College of Gastroenterology. ACG clinical guidelines: diagnosis and management of celiac disease. Am J Gastroenterol. 2013;108(5):656–76.

Sabbagh P, Mohammadnia-Afrouzi M, Javanian M, Babazadeh A, Koppolu V, Vasigala VR, Nouri HR, Ebrahimpour S. Diagnostic methods for Helicobacter pylori infection: ideals, options, and limitations. Eur J Clin Microbiol Infect Dis. 2019;38(1):55–66.

Sabery N, Bass D. Use of serologic markers as a screening tool in inflammatory bowel disease compared with elevated erythrocyte sedimentation rate and anemia. Pediatrics. 2007;119(1):e193–9.

Saeed A, Shorafa E, Shahramian I, Afshari M, Salahifard M, et al. An 11-year-old boy infected with COVID-19 with presentation of acute liver failure. Hepat Mon. Online ahead of Print. 2020;20(6):e104415.

Sairenji T, Collins KL, Evans DV. An update on inflammatory bowel disease. Prim Care. 2017;44(4):673–92.

Sawhney MS, McDougall H, Nelson DB, Bond JH. Fecal occult blood test in patients on low-dose aspirin, warfarin, clopidogrel, or non-steroidal anti-inflammatory drugs. Dig Dis Sci. 2010;55(6):1637–42.

Sciandra I, Piccioni L, Coltella L, Ranno S, Giannelli G, Falasca F, Antonelli G, Concato C, Turriziani O. Comparative analysis of 2 commercial molecular tests for the detection of gastroenteric viruses on stool samples. Diagn Microbiol Infect Dis. 2020;96(1):114893.

Shapiro JM, Subedi S, LeLeiko NS. Inflammatory bowel disease. Pediatr Rev. 2016;37(8):337–47.

Shashidhar H, Integlia MJ, Grand RJ. Clinical manifestations of pediatric inflammatory bowel disease. In: Kirsner JB, editor. Inflammatory bowel disease. Philadelphia: WB Saunders; 2000.

Sheiko MA, Sundaram SS, Capocelli KE, Pan Z, McCoy AM, Mack CL. Outcomes in pediatric autoimmune hepatitis and significance of azathioprine metabolites. J Pediatr Gastroenterol Nutr. 2017;65(1):80–5.

Shieh M, Chitnis N, Monos D. Human leukocyte antigen and disease associations: a broader perspective. Clin Lab Med. 2018;38(4):679–93.

Simko V. Fecal fat microscopy. Acceptable predictive value in screening for steatorrhea. Am J Gastroenterol. 1981;75:204–8.

Singh P, Arora A, Strand TA, Leffler DA, Mäki M, Kelly CP, Ahuja V, Makharia GK. Diagnostic accuracy of point of care tests for diagnosing celiac disease: a systematic review and meta-analysis. J Clin Gastroenterol. 2019;53(7):535–42.

Socha P, Janczyk W, Dhawan A, Baumann U, D'Antiga L, Tanner S, et al. Wilson's disease in children: a position paper by the hepatology Committee of the European Society for Paediatric Gastroenterology, Hepatology and Nutrition. J Pediatr Gastroenterol Nutr. 2018;66(2):334–44.

Sokollik C, McLin VA, Vergani D, Terziroli Beretta-Piccoli B, Mieli-Vergani G. Juvenile autoimmune hepatitis: a comprehensive review. J Autoimmun. 2018;95:69–76.

Stockmann C, Pavia AT, Graham B, Vaughn M, Crisp R, Poritz MA, Thatcher S, Korgenski EK, Barney T, Daly J, Rogatcheva M. Detection of 23 gastrointestinal pathogens among children who present with diarrhea. J Pediatr Infect Dis Soc. 2017;6(3):231–8.

Sziegoleit A, Linder D. Studies on the sterol-binding capacity of human pancreatic elastase 1. Gastroenterol. 1991;100(3):768–74.

Tajiri H, Takano T, Tanaka H, Ushijima K, Inui A, Miyoshi Y, et al. Hepatocellular carcinoma in children and young patients with chronic HBV infection and the usefulness of alpha-fetoprotein assessment. Cancer Med. 2016;5(11):3102–10.

Thiagarajah JR, Kamin DS, Acra S, Goldsmith JD, Roland JT. Lencer WI,…PediCODE Consortium. Advances in evaluation of chronic diarrhea in infants. Gastroenterology. 2018;154(8):2045–2059.e6.

Torres-Miranda D, Akselrod H, Karsner R, Secco A, Silva-Cantillo D, Siegel MO, et al. Use of BioFire FilmArray gastrointestinal PCR panel associated with reductions in antibiotic use, time to optimal antibiotics, and length of stay. BMC Gastroenterol. 2020;20(1):246.

Tsampalieros A, Griffiths AM, Barrowman N, Mack DR. Use of C-reactive protein in children with newly diagnosed inflammatory bowel disease. J Pediatr. 2011;159(2):340–2.

Van Rheenen PF, Van de Vijver E, Fidler V. Faecal calprotectin for screening of patients with suspected inflammatory bowel disease: diagnostic meta-analysis. BMJ. 2010;341:c3369.

Vanga RR, Tansel A, Sidiq S, El-Serag HB, Othman MO. Diagnostic performance of measurement of Fecal Elastase-1 in detection of exocrine pancreatic insufficiency: systematic review and meta-analysis. Clin Gastroenterol Hepatol. 2018;16(8):1220–1228.e4.

Vermeire S, Van Assche G, Rutgeerts P. Laboratory markers in IBD: useful, magic, or unnecessary toys? Gut. 2006;55(3):426–31.

Veropalumbo C, Del Giudice E, Esposito G, Maddaluno S, Ruggiero L, Vajro P. Aminotransferases and muscular diseases: a disregarded lesson. Case reports and review of the literature. J Paediatr Child Health. 2012;48(10):886–90.

Villalta D, Tonutti E, Prause C, Koletzko S, Uhlig HH, Vermeersch P, et al. IgG antibodies against deamidated gliadin peptides for diagnosis of celiac disease in patients with IgA deficiency. Clin Chem. 2010;56(3):464–8.

Walayat S, Martin D, Patel J, Ahmed U, Asghar MN, Pai AU, Dhillon S. Role of albumin in cirrhosis: from a hospitalist's perspective. J Commun Hosp Intern Med Perspect. 2017;7(1):8–14.

Walther A, Tiao G. Approach to pediatric hepatocellular carcinoma. Clin Liver Dis. 2013;2(5):219–22.

Wang YK, Kuo FC, Liu CJ, Wu MC, Shih HY, Wang SS, et al. Diagnosis of helicobacter pylori infection: current options and developments. World J Gastroenterol. 2015;21(40):11221–35.

Warner S, Kelly DA. Liver failure. In: Wyllie R, Haymes JS, Kay M, editors. Pediatric gastrointestinal and liver disease. 6th ed. Philadelphia, PA: Elsevier; 2021. p. 852–71.

Wood L, Colman J, Dudley F. The relationship between portal pressure and plasma albumin in the development of cirrhotic ascites. J Gastroenterol Hepatol. 1987;2(6):525–31.

Woreta TA, Alqahtani SA. Evaluation of abnormal liver tests. Med Clin North Am. 2014;98(1):1–16.

Wu PE. Medication effects on fecal occult blood testing. JAMA Intern Med. 2019;179(4):591.

Wyatt A, Kellermayer R. PCR-based fecal pathogen panel testing should be interpreted with caution at diagnosis of pediatric inflammatory bowel diseases. Ann Clin Lab Sci. 2018;48(5):674–6.

Xuan S, Zangwill KM, Ni W, Ma J, Hay JW. Cost-effectiveness analysis of four common diagnostic methods for Clostridioides difficile infection. J Gen Intern Med. 2020;35(4):1102–10.

Yazigi N, Balistreri WF. Bilirubin. In: Fernandes J, Saudubray JM, Van den Berghe G, Tada K, Buist

NRM, editors. Inborn metabolic diseases. Berlin, Heidelberg: Springer; 1995.

Zholudev A, Zurakowski D, Young W, Leichtner A, Bousvaros A. Serologic testing with ANCA, ASCA, and anti-OmpC in children and young adults with Crohn's disease and ulcerative colitis: diagnostic value and correlation with disease phenotype. Am J Gastroenterol. 2004;99(11):2235–41.

Zimmerman S, Horner S, Altwegg M, Dalpke A. Workflow optimization for syndromic diarrhea diagnosis using the molecular Seegene Allplex GI-bacteria assay. Eur J Clin Microbiol Inf Dis. 2020;39:1235–50.

Care of the Child with a Renal Problem

Deanna Schneider and Clare Cardo McKegney

10

Learning Objectives

After completing the chapter, the learner should be able to:

1. Interpret common laboratory studies to evaluate the child with a urinary complaint, including point-of-care dipstick, urinalysis, urine culture, and serum metabolic profile.
2. Outline the diagnostic laboratory approach to the child with proteinuria, hematuria, or both proteinuria and hematuria.
3. Understand the significance of abnormalities of calcium, phosphorus, and vitamin D.
4. Interpret lipid levels and abnormalities of renal function.
5. Identify and interpret laboratory studies used for the evaluation of renal tubular acidosis.
6. Identify and interpret laboratory studies used for the evaluation of the nephrotic syndrome.

10.1 Introduction

The child with a kidney and urinary tract problem or both needs careful evaluation and follow-up in the primary care office. During a routine prenatal scan, the neonate may have been identified as

D. Schneider (✉) · C. C. McKegney
Columbia University School of Nursing,
New York, NY, USA
e-mail: ds2453@cumc.columbia.edu

having vesicoureteral reflux (VUR) and may require follow-up. It is now felt that lower-grade reflux is a normal physiological state that tends to resolve spontaneously (Kaufman et al. 2019). A urinalysis and urine culture are important in evaluating a urinary complaint, and a complete or comprehensive metabolic profile may be done when there is concern about renal disease. The clinician needs to be aware of the reasons for false-negative and false-positive results. Understanding the presentation of rheumatological diseases with kidney involvement and disorders of the kidneys is important for the clinician as they see patients with fatigue, pallor, joint pain, bone pain, or nonspecific complaints.

10.2 The Child with a Urinary Complaint

There are many indications for urinalysis with a urine dipstick in the pediatric primary care office. Interpretation of the urine dipstick will guide the practitioner to a diagnosis. Situations that warrant the use of a spot dipstick urinalysis include suprapubic pain, gross hematuria, periorbital or peripheral edema, urinary frequency, dysuria, nocturnal enuresis, polydipsia, polyuria, and suspected renal disease. A thorough history and physical exam is required for timely and correct diagnosis in addition to the laboratory findings.

10.2.1 Recommendations for Urinalysis

At one time, the American Academy of Pediatrics (AAP) recommended the urinalysis at specific health supervision intervals as documented as standards of practice (Primack 2010). Following recommendations from the AAP Committee on Nephrology in 2007, urinalysis, including the dipstick, was removed from routine health supervision visits in pediatrics due to a high false-positive rate, leading to increased costs, family anxiety, and excessive testing. The AAP reserves the urinalysis only when indicated by health and family history or in a symptomatic patient (Filice et al. 2014). However, many pediatric practices still do office dipsticks for well-child visits (Viteri and Reid-Adam 2018) despite the guidelines.

The AAP recommends yearly urinalysis in children who were born <32 weeks, have a very low birth weight or umbilical artery lines, congenital heart diseases whether repaired or unrepaired, transplant of solid organ or bone marrow, malignancy, prolonged use of nephrotoxic drugs, recurrent episodes of acute kidney injury, family history of renal disease, or a known history of renal disease (Viteri and Reid-Adam 2018). Flynn et al. (2018) suggests that children with a body mass index (BMI) of greater than 95% should have a urinalysis as part of their well-child evaluation.

10.2.1.1 Urinalysis

Urinary frequency, dysuria, urinary accidents in a toilet-trained child, and fever are all patient complaints that warrant further investigation for a urinary tract infection (UTI), which will be discussed further in the chapter. A urine dipstick plus a microscopic is considered a urinalysis.

The dipstick. The urine dipstick is an extremely sensitive test, and therefore the results need to be correlated with the historical and physical findings of the patient (Cyriac et al. 2017). It is a quick and inexpensive test that can be done in the office. When the dipstick results indicate further evaluation, the urine sample is sent to the lab for microscopy. While the dipstick can be done quickly, evidence suggests the rate of

false-positive results in unwarranted laboratory evaluation reduces cost-effectiveness (Mambatta et al. 2015). Therefore, in-depth history and physical exam need to be performed when assessing children during routine and interval visits to determine when appropriate to use the dipstick urinalysis as a screening tool.

The urine dipstick evaluates multiple components and breakdown products found in urine. Urine can be obtained in many ways: midstream, nonsterile voided, voided clean catch, or sterile specimen collection. The results of a dipstick evaluate the appearance, pH, odor, and presence of protein, glucose, ketones, blood, and leukocyte esterase. Urine volume is not measured in a dipstick or spot urinalysis. The dipstick reactant pads give clinicians a wealth of information (Cyriac et al. 2017). While a dipstick urinalysis is the most affordable, accessible, and widely used form of urinary evaluation in primary care, the finding on a dipstick cannot diagnose a UTI (Schmidt and Copp 2015). Table 10.1 reviews the components of the laboratory urinalysis and dipstick.

Microscopic analysis of urine. A microscopic exam studies red blood cells (RBCs), white blood cells (WBCs), casts, crystals, and bacteria. Microscopic analysis of urine done in laboratories is done by automated systems. There are two different kinds of systems used today, digital imaging and flow cytometry. As a result, the thresholds for significant pyuria are different. Urinary casts are made up of cells, fat bodies, or microorganisms with a Tamm-Horsfall protein matrix. Table 10.2 reviews the microscopy results and the clinical significance.

A gram stain can be done to determine whether gram-negative or gram-positive bacteria are present, Gram-negative rods, streptococci, and staphylococci have a characteristic appearance (Simerville et al. 2005).

10.2.2 Urinary Tract Infection (UTI)

UTI is a common occurrence in the pediatric population. The accuracy of diagnosis is crucial for proper management and prevention of long-

Table 10.1   Interpretation of the components of the dipstick

Test pad chemistry components	Normal values	What does the information yield?
Color	Clear, yellow	• Changes in the color of the urine can be related to infection, foods, medications, metabolic products • Cloudy urine can be caused by pyuria, but, in alkaline urine, precipitated phosphate crystals is a more common reason (Simerville et al. 2005) • Endogenous causes of dark urine include amorphous urates (brick-dust sediment), erythrocytes, myoglobin, hemoglobin, metabolic products, homogentisic acid (alkaptonuria), and porphyrins (Utsch and Klaus 2014) • Exogenous causes of dark urine include food products such as red beets, rhubarb blackberries, and food dyes; *Serratia marcescens*; and medications (nitrofurantoin, rifampicin, phenolphthalein, chloroquine, deferoxamine, ibuprofen, metronidazole, phenothiazines, phenytoin, and imipenem/cilastatin (Utsch and Klaus 2014)
Specific gravity (SG)	1.003–1.030	• Dilute urine (SG <1.010) can give both false-positive and false-negative (Mazaheri and Assadi 2019) • SG identifies the patient's hydration status. ○ Low SG – The patient is well hydrated (<1.010) ○ High SG – The patient may be dehydrated (>1.020) ○ Note: When the SG is equal to the plasma osmolarity, this indicates disease affecting the ability to concentrate urine • SG will be high with: ○ Significant proteinuria ○ Glucosuria ○ Inappropriate antidiuretic hormone secretion • SG will be low with: ○ Diuretic use ○ Diabetes insipidus ○ Adrenal insufficiency ○ Aldosteronism ○ Impaired renal tubular function (Cyriac et al. 2017)
pH	4.5–8	• Acidic urine indicates dehydration and uric stones • pH >5.5 in the face of acidosis indicates renal tubular acidosis, type 1 (Hechanova 2020) • Alkaline urine is found in ○ Urinary tract infections are secondary to urea-splitting bacteria/organisms ○ Presence of calcium phosphate stones
Leukocytes	Negative	• This test detects the presence of WBC, which can indicate urinary tract infection (pyuria) or vaginitis/urethritis • False-positive results will occur in the presence of contamination in the vaginal or penile area without proper hygiene • Sensitive (67%–84%) but less specific (64%–92%) for UTI (Utsch and Klaus 2014)
Blood	Negative	• A positive test for blood detects the presence of hemoglobin or RBC ○ Test pad highlights uniformly are consistent with hemoglobin ○ Test pads that have a spotted appearance suggest RBC are present • Extremely sensitive test: Negative means no presence of blood • RBC morphology is not detected in the dipstick; therefore, urine will need microscopy for cell configuration • False-positive tests occur when ○ Ascorbic acid is present in the urine ○ There is an elevated SG, pH >5, and proteinuria ○ If the patient is taking captopril (Cyriac et al. 2017)

(continued)

Table 10.1 (continued)

Test pad chemistry components	Normal values	What does the information yield?
Nitrites	Negative	• Detected secondary to the presence of bacteria with nitrate reductase enzyme reduces normal nitrates to nitrites (Cyriac et al. 2017) • A positive test only means there are bacteria in the urine (Cyriac et al. 2017) • Specific 98% (90–100%) but not sensitive 53% (15%–82%) for UTI (Utsch and Klaus 2014) • Vaginal secretions and contamination may yield a false positive • False negatives result from • Less than 4 hours in the bladder as this is the time needed for the conversion of nitrate to nitrite • Inadequate dietary nitrate • Infection caused by non-nitrate-reducing bacteria such as *enterococcus* or *pseudomonas* spp. or *staphylococcus saprophyticus* • If that patient is on antimicrobials that inhibit bacterial metabolism • A large volume of dilute urine • Ascorbic acid in the urine (Leung et al. 2019)
Ketones	Negative	• Ketones are a result of fat metabolism and are not normally present in the urine • Ketones can be positive in diabetes, pregnancy, and a ketogenic diet and ketotic hypoglycemia • Ketonuria indicates starvation, cold exposure, or extended periods of rigorous exercise (Cyriac et al. 2017)
Bilirubin	Negative	• Trace amounts need investigation • The most likely cause is hepatocellular disease such as hepatitis • The prehepatic cause is related to hemolysis
Urobilinogen	Trace	• Urobilinogen is a product of bacterial action of direct bilirubin in the intestines

Protein	Negative	• Test pads are most sensitive for albumin with specificity and sensitivity of more than 99%, but it is not sensitive for other proteins (Leung and Wong 2010)
		• The dipstick pad gives a semiquantitative result (refer to the section in this chapter discussing the investigation of proteinuria)
		• False positives if the
		  ○ Urine is alkaline
		  ○ SG results greater than 1.030
		  ○ pH above 8.0
		  ○ Gross hematuria, pyuria, or bacteremia
		  ○ The patient is on penicillin or sulfonamides
		  ○ Within 3 days of receiving IV radioactive dyes
		• False negative if the
		  ○ Urine is acidic
		  ○ The protein is not albumin
		• Proteinuria results
		  ○ 1+ = 30 mg of protein per dL
		  ○ 2+ corresponds to 100 mg per dL
		  ○ 3+ to 300 mg per dL
		  ○ 4+ to 1000 mg per dL

Glucose	Negative	• Glycosuria is most commonly present in diabetes mellitus and Cushing's syndrome • Fanconi's syndrome, cystinosis, and Wilson's disease can also cause glycosuria due to tubular dysfunction and altered threshold for reabsorption of glucose in the kidney (Cyriac et al. 2017)

Adapted from Cyriac et al. (2017), Hechanova (2020), Leung et al. (2019), Mazaheri and Assadi (2019), Simerville et al. (2005), Leung and Wong (2010)

Table 10.2 Microscopy results and clinical significance

Finding	Clinical significance
Bacteria	• Sensitivity of 81% with a range of 16–99 and specificity of 83% with a range of 11–100% (Utsch and Klaus 2014)
RBCs	• Dysmorphic RBCs, suggesting glomerulonephritis (Brown and Reidy 2019)
WBCs	• For digital imaging, 2 WBC/HPF is significant, and for flow cytometry, 25 to 50 WBC per microliter is significant (Chaudhari et al. 2016) • When the WBC count is done by hemocytometer, the gold standard for pyuria is ≥5 WBCs per HPF in centrifuged urine or ≥ 10 WBC in uncentrifuged urine (Leung et al. 2019) • Using an automated system with uncentrifuged urine, 3 WBC/HPF in urine with a SG <1.015 suggests pyuria. In urine with an SG of ≥1.015, 6 WBC/HPF suggests pyuria and a presumptive UTI In children less than 2 years (Chaudhari et al. 2016) • Presence of pyelonephritis, glomerulonephritis, interstitial nephritis, and renal inflammatory processes
Types of epithelial cells	• Present in the urinary sediment • Squamous epithelial cells: Large, irregularly shaped, small nucleus, fine granular cytoplasm o Suggests contamination • Transitional epithelial cells—Presence is normal
Cellular casts	
WBC casts	• WBC cases indicate tubular disease, which is found in acute pyelonephritis and interstitial nephritis
RBC casts	• RBC cast cells can be present with an upper limit threshold of no more than 0–5 per low-power field (LPF) • RBC cast cells are noted after strenuous exercise in a healthy patient • When more than five casts are present in LPF, one must consider pathology (Brown and Reidy 2019) • RBC casts suggest glomerulonephritis (Brown and Reidy 2019)
Renal tubular epithelial casts	• Epithelial cell casts are the result of damage and death of the tubule cells. It is an indication of tubular necrosis, nephritis syndrome; interstitial nephritis; eclampsia, in transplant patients, kidney rejection; and possible heavy metal ingestion including lead poisoning
Noncellular casts	
Hyaline casts	• Nonspecific finding • The most common type of urinary cast • Clear tiny tubular particles that are easily missed on urine microscopy unless a stain is used • A hyaline cast are usually not indicative of renal disease • Hyaline casts may be due to strenuous exercise, diuretic medications, severe vomiting, or fever which causes sluggish urine flow
Fatty casts	• It can be found in renal disease, nephrotic syndrome, and hypothyroidism
Granular or waxy casts	• Suggests advanced renal disease (Simerville et al. 2005)
Broad casts	• Found in advanced renal disease (Simerville et al. 2005)
Crystals	
Crystals	• Found in the urinary sediment of healthy children • Cystine crystals – Colorless, hexagonal shape. Found in acidic urine – Diagnostic of cystinuria • Uric acid crystals – Yellow to orange-brown and diamond- or barrel-shaped • Triple phosphate crystals may be normal but can be associated with alkaline urine and UTI (commonly associated with *Proteus* sp. (Simerville et al. 2005)

Adapted from Brown and Reidy (2019), Chaudhari et al. (2016), Leung et al. (2019), Simerville et al. (2005)

term sequelae. UTI is defined as the presence of abnormal urinalysis that suggests infection (pyuria and bacteremia) and a positive culture of at least 50,000 colony forming units (CFU) per mL of a pathogen from a specimen obtained by catheterization and/or suprapubic aspirate (Taib and Jamal 2015). The estimated incidence is 7–8% of girls, and 2% of boys will have a UTI. UTI can be of the upper tract or pyelonephritis (PN) or limited to the lower tract or cystitis. It is difficult to distinguish between the location in young children. Sixty percent of febrile UTIs in the first year of life are PN; a scar at the site of the infection is present around 30–40% of the time (Montini et al. 2011). The incidence of PN in the first 6 months of life is 12-fold higher in uncircumcised boys; however, from 6 to 12 months, the incidence is higher in girls from 6 months to 12 months (Leung et al. 2019).

A clinician's level of suspicion regarding the diagnosis of a UTI should be high in children under the age of 2 with fever and no other source of infection. This specific group of children, because they are nonverbal, often have indistinct complaints. Therefore, poor feeding, lethargy, prolonged jaundice, vomiting, fever, and malodorous urine are all symptoms that require careful consideration for UTI. Preschoolers and older children can verbalize symptoms localized to the urinary tract and express the classic historic findings of dysuria, frequency, and incontinence in toilet-trained children. The severity and occurrence of a pediatric UTI are dependent on innate host immunity and bacterial virulence factors (Simões E Silva et al. 2020).

10.2.2.1 Urine Culture

When evaluating a patient for presumed infection, a culture should be obtained. Urine specimen collection in the pediatric population is divided into two categories: nontoilet-trained and toilet-trained children. The practitioner must obtain the sample in the child who cannot collect a urine sample with a sterile or "clean catch" approach. Although the most invasive form of urine collection is the suprapubic aspirate (SPA), it remains the most accurate. SPA is contraindicated in children with an abdominal wall defect or coagulopathy (Leung et al. 2019). In a nontoilet-trained child with high suspicion of UTI, catheterization is commonly used for accurate urine collection. Urine obtained by the bagged specimen is susceptible to contamination with periurethral flora in both girls and uncircumcised boys (Leung et al. 2019). The false-positive rate from bagged urine is 30–75%, leading to the need for another specimen done by clean catch, catheterization, or suprapubic aspiration (Doern and Richardson 2016; Desai et al.

2016; Verliat-Guinaud et al. 2015). As a result, this form of urine collection has lower diagnostic utility (Schmidt and Copp 2015). The AAP recommends that the urine specimen for culture in children between 2 months and 24 months be obtained through suprapubic aspiration or catheterization only (Subcommittee On Urinary Tract Infection 2016).

The diagnostic evaluation is not complete until the sample undergoes urinalysis and urine culture. The most clinically significant findings for the presumed diagnosis of UTI are the presence of leukocyte esterase and nitrates. RBCs may be seen, and symptoms may worsen if the SG is high (Utsch and Klaus 2014). Table 10.3 reviews diagnostic laboratory tests in UTI.

Once the urine is obtained, it is plated in blood agar, and bacterial growth is generally available within 24 h with sensitivities in 48 h. If the routine culture is negative, but the child is still symptomatic and the gram stain shows bacteria, an anaerobic culture should be considered (Leung et al. 2019). If there are unusual bacteria or multiple bacteria in the same specimen, malformation in the kidney and urinary tract or immunodeficiency should be ruled out. Table 10.4 reviews the possible results of urine culture and the clinical significance.

UTI occurs via the blood in newborns, but the ascendant route is responsible for UTIs after the neonatal period (Simões E Silva et al. 2020). Pyelonephritis or a preexisting congenital renal anomaly predisposes a child to URI and can result in renal insufficiency. Renal insufficiency can lead to electrolyte and acid-base disturbances. One study of 80 children reported that 75% of them had electrolyte or acid-base derangement. Hewitt and Montini (2021) reported that antenatal ultrasound shows two kinds of kidney damage when there is VUR: (1) congenital maldevelopment of the hypoplastic or dysplastic kidney associated with a high-grade IV–V VUR and (2) scarring of the kidney secondary to VUR. The former is most likely to be a male and has a greater risk of renal dysfunction, and the latter is more common in females, and renal insufficiency is less likely to occur. Renal scarring can occur in up to 5% of girls and 13%

Table 10.3 Urinary tract infection and diagnostic labs

Dipstick urinalysis	Microscopic analysis	Urine culture
• Leucocyte esterase is noted in the presence of inflammation and white blood cells and is 78% specific for UTI diagnosis (Schmidt and Copp 2015)* • The presence of nitrates is consistent with gram-negative bacteria** • Leukocyte plus nitrites are 80–90% sensitive for a UTI (Schmidt and Copp 2015)	• Requires more skill to perform and is more expensive • WBCs, RBCs, and bacteria are 66% sensitive and 99% specific for UTI in centrifuged samples (Schmidt and Copp 2015) • Microscopic samples with pyuria and leucocyte esterase consistent with UTI have a noted decreased SG. Therefore, urine concentration needs to be evaluated in UTI diagnosis (Chaudhari et al. 2016)	• Recognized as the gold standard for the diagnosis • 50,000 CFU noted in a sterile sample (catheterization or aspirate) is indicative of UTI • 100,000 CFU noted in a "clean catch" sample is indicative of UTI (Schmidt and Copp 2015)

*Leukocyte esterase is commonly seen in inflammatory conditions. False-negative leukocyte esterase may indicate the urine is collected too early in the course of the disease
**False-negative nitrates are clinically significant when the urine has been in the bladder for less than 4 h
Adapted from Chaudhari et al. 2016; Schmidt and Copp 2015

Table 10.4 Urine culture and clinical significance of finding

Results	Clinical significance
More than two organisms	• The specimen should be recollected as this likely represents contamination unless it is collected by SPA
Escherichia coli (*E. coli*)	• The most common uropathogen • *E. coli* causes approximately 80% of UTIs in children • Fimbriae attach to uroepithelial walls, which help overcome normal host defenses (Kaufman et al. 2019) • *E. coli* is dominant in the first 6 months in healthy girls • *Proteus mirabilis* is the dominant bacteria in boys after 6 months
Streptococcus agalactiae	• More common in the neonate (Leung et al. 2019)
Klebsiella, Proteus, Enterobacter, and *Enterococcus* species (Kaufman et al. 2019)	• Common pathogens • Colonization with gram-negative bacteria is common before the development of a UTI (Simões E Silva et al. 2020)
Streptococcus pneumoniae, streptococcus viridians, Staphylococcus aureus, Staphylococcus epidermidis, haemophilus influenzae, Streptococcus agalactiae	• These species are more common if the child has an anomaly of the urinary tract (neurologic, anatomical, or functional) or a compromised immune system (Leung et al. 2019)
Staphylococcus saprophyticus	• Is responsible for ≥15% of UTI in sexually active female adolescents (Schlager 2016)
Staphylococcus aureus, streptococcus Agalactiae, Proteus mirabilis, Pseudomonas aeruginosa, Nontyphoidal salmonella	• It can be caused by hematogenous spread, and hematogenous spread is uncommon after the neonatal period (Leung et al. 2019)
Viruses such as adenoviruses, enteroviruses, echoviruses, and coxsackieviruses usually cause lower urinary tract infections	• Usually, cause a lower tract infection • Adenovirus most commonly causes a hemorrhagic cystitis
Polyomaviruses such as BK virus	• In immunocompromised children can cause hemorrhagic cystitis

Adapted from Kaufman et al. (2019), Leung et al. (2019), Schlager (2016), Simões E Silva et al. (2020)

of boys after the first UTI (Larcombe 2015). Predisposing factors for scarring include high-grade VUR, urinary obstruction, pyelonephritis in infancy, bacterial virulence, individual host factors, delay of treatment, and increased number of upper urinary tract infections or pyelonephritis (Karavanaki et al. 2017). The risk is higher in the first 2 years of life, and by 8, the risk is markedly reduced.

New tests to improve the sensitivity and specificity of UTI evaluation are under development (Davenport et al. 2017). Urinary biomarker platforms (interleukin 6 and neutrophil gelatinase-associated lipocalin) and droplet microfluidic platforms have been proposed to expedite the correct diagnosis and help differentiate actual infections from asymptomatic bacteriuria. The use of PCR fluorescence in situ hybridization and mass spectrometry can expedite a timely diagnosis of common uropathogens such as *E. coli* (Fritzenwanker et al. 2016); however, PCR has drawbacks. It can identify common uropathogens, but it may miss uncommon species since it looks for specific targets. It also cannot differentiate between asymptomatic bacteriuria and contamination (Kaufman et al. 2019).

10.2.3 Real-Life Example

A 7-year-old female presents to the office with complaints of pain when urinating. Upon further evaluation, the clinician elicits that the girl has been complaining of pain for 3 days. The patient reports that she has also had two episodes of incontinence. The patient presents to the office today with complaints of abdominal pain, nausea, and a fever of 102.3°F. The child's past medical history is unremarkable. She reports that she held her urine 5 days ago for 3 h while in a line at an amusement park. The physical exam is normal except for a mild amount of tenderness in the suprapubic region. She is well-appearing and, on the exam, has no costal vertebral angle tenderness. The result of a point-of-service midstream clean catch urine dipstick reveals a SG 1.030, pH 7, leukocytes 125, blood trace, nitrates ++, ketones negative, bilirubin negative, protein neg-

ative, and glucose negative. In addition to the history and physical exam, the patient's urine sample suggests an acute UTI. A urine sample for microscopy showed WBCs >25 HPF, RBCs 5–10, and multiple bacteria, but no red cell casts. The culture was positive for *E. coli* which was sensitive to amoxicillin.

Key Learning about Urine Evaluation
- The AAP reserves the urinalysis only when indicated by health and family history or in a symptomatic patient (Filice et al. 2014).
- The AAP recommends that urine specimen for culture in children between 2 months and 24 months should be obtained through suprapubic aspiration or catheterization only.
- A positive urine culture indicative of a UTI occurs when there are 50,000 CFU noted in a sterile sample (catheterization or aspirate), or 100,000 CFU noted in a "clean catch" sample (Schmidt and Copp 2015).
- *E. coli* is the most common pathogen found in a positive culture.
- The presence of two or more bacteria most often indicates contamination.

10.3 The Child with Proteinuria

The presence of protein in a routine urine sample is noted in approximately 10% of children, decreasing to 0.1% when repeated (Leung and Wong 2010). When proteinuria is benign, the cause is often orthostatic proteinuria or transient proteinuria (Ranch 2020). When considering the amount of protein noted on the spot urine, the clinician also needs to evaluate the entire sample. The SG, presence of blood, nitrates, etc. can alter the decision-making process. The differential diagnoses associated with proteinuria are varied. Clinical features of renal disease include hypertension, edema, and growth failure (Leung and Wong 2010). Proteinuria is a critical finding associated with renal disease and/or damage.

Table 10.1 reviews the components of the urinalysis, including protein.

Small amounts of protein in the urine are considered acceptable but vary by age. In neonates and infants, clinically significant proteinuria is greater than 100 mg/m^2 per day or more than 0.2 mg protein/mg on a spot urine collection. In older children, up to 300 mg/m^2 is considered significant (Viteri and Reid-Adam 2018). Although commonly found in insignificant amounts on random urine samples, protein in the urine can be associated with chronic renal disease. The clinician should perform a thorough history with a complete physical exam to determine the laboratory studies needed to evaluate proteinuria.

10.3.1 Pathophysiology and Proteinuria

Understanding the physiology of the kidney clarifies proteinuria. Little plasma protein crosses the glomerular capillary membranes in a healthy kidney. The glomerular barrier is composed of the fenestrated endothelium, basement barrier, and podocytes. When insulted by injury, infection, and/or inflammation, the barrier can weaken and disrupt the electrostatic filter. Proteinuria can be a result of glomerular damage (Viteri and Reid-Adam 2018). Glomerular damage can further result in dysfunction of the nephron and tubular malfunction. This malfunction can lead to the reabsorption of protein in the proximal tubules causing an oversecretion of certain protein and overflow of proteinuria.

When protein is found in the urine, it can be due to a mixture of plasma proteins and renal tubular proteins. Lower urinary tract infections can also cause proteinuria. As previously noted, <100 mg/m$_2$/day is the normal threshold for the presence of protein noted in the urine. Tamm-Horsfall protein accounts for approximately 50% of the protein molecules found in benign proteinuria; albumin accounts for approximately 30%. The remainder is made of immunoglobulins, tubular proteins, and other low-molecular weight (LMW) proteins. The type of protein excreted correlates with the type of kidney disease. The primary care clinician needs to understand that albuminuria is strongly associated with chronic kidney disease (CKD) as a marker for glomerular disease and is a long-term complication of hypertension and diabetes. Urinary loss of LWM protein is more suggestive of tubulointerstitial disease (Viteri and Reid-Adam 2018).

When protein concentrations of LMW proteins exceed the capacity threshold of the tubule, proteinuria is the manifestation. When this damage occurs, both large and small protein particles can permeate the barrier and seep into the urine. If this occurs at high rates, hypoalbuminemia can occur. This will cause a disturbance in the capillary osmotic pressure, which is responsible for fluid stabilization in the vasculature. The ultimate finding of hypoalbuminemia is edema. Proteinuria and edema are the cardinal signs of nephrotic syndrome, discussed further in this chapter. Children often present with periorbital edema that can be mistaken for allergies; however, the clinician should consider evaluation with a urinalysis. Often, with time, more severe edema ensues in the case of nephrotic syndrome, and the diagnosis is more obvious (Baum 2008).

10.3.2 Orthostatic Proteinuria

Before discontinuing the routine UA in pediatric health maintenance, transient and orthostatic proteinuria accounted for most cases of proteinuria in the pediatric population. Both are diagnoses of exclusion and, therefore, a thorough evaluation needs to occur when protein presents in any urine sample. Transient proteinuria is noted in fever, strenuous exercise, extreme exposures to cold, dehydration, heart failure, and seizure. Once proteinuria is considered clinically isolated proteinuria, a clinician can be assured it is not associated with adverse clinical outcomes, and further evaluation is unnecessary (Ranch 2020).

In the face of persistent proteinuria, a patient needs further evaluation. Initial evaluation of persistent proteinuria includes a thorough history, physical exam, and laboratory assessment. Clinical manifestations of renal disease can vary.

Providers must inquire about family history of renal disease, hematuria, deafness, vision impairment, and hypertension. The clinician should also elicit from the patient a recent history of vigorous exercise, tea-colored urine, respiratory illness, febrile illness, rash, arthralgia, or swelling (Pomeranz et al. 2016c). The physical exam is a crucial part of the assessment. The provider should assess for signs of renal disease. The presence of edema, malar or pruritic rash, growth failure, and hypertension all warrant a more detailed laboratory investigation in the presence of spot urine consistent with 1+ protein. A protein greater than 2.0 or persistent proteinuria less than 3.0 on any urine sample should be considered clinically significant and evaluated with further testing (Viteri and Reid-Adam 2018).

In adolescents, orthostatic proteinuria is a benign reason for proteinuria and occurs when the patient is upright. Upon a spot test dipstick, the protein level is generally less than 1+. Orthostatic proteinuria accounts for 60% of all cases of proteinuria in primary care, resulting in a benign clinical course (Pomeranz et al. 2016b). A repeat first-morning spot urine should be obtained if protein is picked up on a routine dipstick or an incidental finding. A urine sample after being in a recumbent position with no evidence of protein can resolve the issue. The patient can then be noted as having orthostatic proteinuria. It is best practice to repeat a urine sample in the orthostatic patient within 6 months to a year. This step-wise approach and investigation reduce harmful or invasive tests and unnecessary costs to the patient (Leung and Wong 2010). Significant proteinuria is a well-known hallmark of glomerulopathy (McIntyre and Taal 2008).

10.3.2.1   Dipstick Proteinuria

The urine dipstick is the test most frequently used for screening a patient for proteinuria in primary care. Table 10.1 reviews the reading of a dipstick. The literature has noted that high SG or very alkaline urine can interfere with the dipstick reactant and cause a false-positive result (Viteri

and Reid-Adam 2018). However, newer research suggests that high alkalinity and SG do not play a role in false-positive results of proteinuria (Robinson et al. 2019). Therefore, it is important to recognize that the SG and pH of the urine may alter the protein dipstick results; however, these traditional beliefs are being challenged (Ranch 2020). The dipstick test primarily detects albumin and generally does not identify LMW protein.

If the protein is trace, the urine needs a repeat test using the first-morning sample. If that result is either negative or trace, a repeat should be done 1 year later to check for proteinuria. However, if the protein is ≥1+, the dipstick and P/C ratio should be repeated using the first-morning sample (Leung et al. 2017). A dipstick read greater than 1+ (30 mg/dL) is considered an abnormal result. In children <2 years, if the spot urine P/C ratio is ≤20 mg/mmol (0.2 mg/mg) or ≤ 50 mg/mmol (0.5 mg/mg) and everything else on the dipstick is negative, then orthostatic or functional proteinuria is the most likely diagnosis. Urine testing can be repeated in 1 year (Leung et al. 2017).

A false-positive proteinuria can occur if SG results are greater than 1.030, the pH is above 8.0, or with gross hematuria, pyuria, or bacteriuria. A false positive can occur if the urine sits on the dipstick for a long time or if the patient is taking penicillin or sulfonamides. A false positive can also occur within 3 days after administering radiographic dyes (Leung and Wong 2010). This data calls for the spot urine to be sent for albumin/creatinine ratio (ACR) as the alternative for accurate diagnosis and quantification of proteinuria (Parker et al. 2020).

10.3.2.2   Spot Urine Protein/ Creatinine Ratio

When protein is discovered as an incidental finding, a first-morning void for spot urine protein/creatinine (P/C) ratio and urinalysis is indicated. The P/C ratio is calculated by dividing the protein concentration by the creatinine concentration. The enzymatic assays have a better specificity, sensitivity, and precision compared to the Jaffe assays (Cobbaert et al. 2009; Panteghini and IFCC Scientific Division 2008). The enzymatic assay is preferred in pediatric patients and patients with hyperfiltration or jaundice or keto-acidosis where the Jaffe method results would be affected (Delanaye et al. 2017). Due to different methods used by different labs, the spot P/C ratio should be done in the same laboratory.

The spot urine P/C ratio is reported in different units such as mg/mg, mg/g, mmol, or a numerical value without any units (more commonly done when the value is mg/mg) (Leung and Wong 2010). Results from the spot urine P/C ratio are interpreted differently by different authors. Generally, a spot urine P/C ratio of <0.2 mg/mg is considered normal in children over 2 years (Ranch 2020; Kamińska et al. 2020). Guidelines from the International Society of Nephrology's Kidney Disease Improving Global Outcomes (KDIGO) (2013) Work Group defines proteinuria in children under 2 as normal/minimal when the P/C ratio is <50 mg/mmol (0.5 mg/mg), increased when it is 50–200 mg/mmol (0.5–2.0 mg/mg), and nephrotic when it is >200 mg/mmol (2.0 mg/mg). An abnormal spot urine P/C ratio in a child under 2 years but over 6 months is >50 mg/mmol or > 500 mg/g or > 0.5 mg/mg. In a child over the age of 2 years, an abnormal spot urine P/C ratio is >20 mg/mmol or >200 mg/g or >0.2 mg/mg (Kamińska et al. 2020). Nephrotic syndrome ranges are >220 mg/mmol or >2200 mg/g or >2.2 mg/mg (Kamińska et al. 2020).

A main limitation of the spot P/C ratio is that the variability of urinary protein excretion during the day and from day to day is not accounted for with spot urine. African-Americans have lower values because they secrete more creatinine to urine than Caucasians of similar weight and height. If the urine creatinine levels are very low (≤3.45 mmol/L (39 mg/dL) or high (≤3.45 mmol/L (39 mg/dL) or ≥ 5.48 mmol/L (62 mg/dL), the protein concentration may be over or underestimated. If the glomerular filtration rate (GFR) levels are ≤10 mL/1.73m², the spot urine P/C is overestimated. There is also a poor correlation between the spot urine P/C ratio and 24-hour urine collection in patients

with nephrotic syndrome. The spot P/C ratio is inaccurate when the patient is malnourished or protein-deprived because the test depends on muscle mass (Kamińska et al. 2020).

10.3.2.3   12–24-Hour Urine for Quantitative Testing of Protein and Creatinine

The "gold standard" of proteinuria is obtaining a total protein/albumin excretion in a 24-hour urine collection (Leung and Wong 2010). Further investigation for proteinuria includes quantitative testing for creatinine clearance. While this can be done via a timed 12–24-hour urine collection, this may be a difficult task for the pediatric patient and their family; therefore, the spot first-morning void for the albumin/creatinine ratio (ACR) or protein/creatinine ratio (PCR) is an adequate alternative. One advantage of measuring the untimed urine PCR over a 24-hour urine protein measurement is that the urinary concentration of dilution does not affect its values because it compares the urinary protein concentration with urinary creatinine concentration (Mazaheri and Assadi 2019). The 24-hour urine can also consider the various activities and vital sign fluctuation during 24 hours (Leung and Wong 2010). There are several reasons why the 24-hour urine collection is problematic, as seen in Box 10.1.

Box 10.1 Causes of Diagnostic Inaccuracy of a 24-Hour Urine Collection
- Collection timing is inaccurate
- Patient missing a sample collection
- Poor storage causing alkaline bacteria to grow, leading to inaccurate protein results
- Incomplete bladder emptying
- Collecting two first-morning urines, instead of throwing out the first day's morning urine
- Not returning the sample in a timely fashion
- Difficult to do in children

Adapted from Kamińska et al. 2020

10.3.2.4 Spot Urine for Urine Albumin/Creatinine (a/C) Ratio

Urine albumin measurements are required to detect microalbuminuria. Patients with diabetes who are at risk for diabetic nephropathy should have a urine A/C ratio measurement on early-morning specimens. This test has largely replaced timed urine collection. A/C ratios are not routinely used to evaluate proteinuria in well children (McIntyre and Taal 2008). Albuminuria can be classified as microalbuminuria when the A/C ratio is 30–300 mg/g creatinine or as macroalbuminuria when the A/C ratio is >300 mg/g creatinine (Guh 2010).

10.3.3 Persistent/Abnormal Proteinuria

Further evaluation is always warranted when persistent proteinuria is present or the patient presents with clinical symptoms. Proteinuria is considered persistent when found on two or more first-morning urine samples (Ranch 2020). Several diagnostic tests are used to aid the clinician caring for the patient with an abnormal protein/creatinine ratio. The tests include the complete metabolic profile for serum electrolytes, blood urea nitrogen (BUN), and creatinine, albumin, complement levels of C3 and C4, anti-streptolysin antibodies, antinuclear antibody (ANA), double-stranded DNA (dsDNA), anti-neutrophil cytoplasmic antibodies (ANCA), and all hepatitis antibodies and antigens. Utilizing such laboratory studies helps a practitioner focus their evaluation. Some tests are reviewed here, and the remainder are discussed in Sect. 10.5.3.

10.3.3.1 Complete Metabolic Profile

Serum electrolytes, blood urea nitrogen (BUN), and creatinine levels give the practitioner a window into the functioning of the kidney. The kidneys play an integral role in maintaining electrolyte homeostasis in the body, particularly sodium, potassium, chloride, calcium, and phosphorous. They are also active in maintaining the acid-base balance of the body, particularly through the regulation of bicarbonate. Interpretation of bicarbonate regarding acid-base balance is discussed in Sect. 10.6.1.1, as is the calculation of renal function in Sect. 10.7.1.2. Sodium, potassium, chloride, calcium, phosphorous, BUN, and creatinine will be discussed here.

Sodium. Sodium is an abundant and important electrolyte for carrying out basic metabolic functions, and any deviations from normal should be evaluated closely. Sodium, the major cation in extracellular fluid, is tightly linked to fluid balance. Because the total body water varies by age, normal ranges for sodium vary by age and are shown in Table 10.5. The body's ability to maintain a sodium-water balance relies on the complex interplay of the adrenal glands, kidneys, and pituitary gland via the renin-angiotensin-aldosterone system (Bianchetti et al. 2017).

When faced with abnormal sodium levels, the clinician must evaluate the patient's sodium value and overall fluid status. Abnormal sodium levels are typically classified by variation from normal, hyponatremia or hypernatremia, and overall volume status, hypovolemia, normovolemia, or hypervolemia. The causes of abnormal sodium levels in children are broad and involve the renal and neurologic, cardiovascular, and gastrointestinal systems. In particular, children with renal disorders can present with both elevated or decreased sodium levels, depending upon the underlying disease and the pathology within the kidney (Bianchetti et al. 2017). Common causes of abnormal sodium levels in children of renal and other etiologies can be seen by classification in Table 10.6. It should be noted that sodium values may also be spurious and should be carefully evaluated if there is hyperlipidemia, which can cause a false decrease and severe hyperprotein-

Table 10.5 Normal serum sodium values by age

Age	Value (mmoL/L)
Birth to <7 days	132–147
≥7 days to <2 years	133–145
≥2 years to <12 years	134–145
≥12 years to adult	135–145

Adapted with permission from Oxford Press from Colantonio et al. (2012)

Table 10.6 Common causes of abnormal sodium levels in children

Hyponatremia	Hypernatremia
Extracellular hypovolemic "depletional"	Hypovolemic
• Intestinal salt wasting from vomiting, diarrhea, or suction of gastric contents • Salt loss through the skin from cystic fibrosis or sustained vigorous exercise • Renal sodium loss from mineralocorticoid deficiency/resistance, diuretic use, salt-wasting renal failure, salt-wasting tubulopathies, and cerebral salt wasting (Bianchetti et al. 2017)	• Inadequate intake • Diarrhea resulting in the intestinal salt loss • Renal water and salt wasting: Post-obstructive polyuria, diuretic use, diabetes insipidus, and damage to the renal medulla
Extracellular normo-hypervolemic "dilutional"	Normovolemic
• Increased body water: Increased intake • Abnormal antidiuretic hormone release: cardiac failure, liver disease, nephrotic syndrome, glucocorticoid deficiency, and medications cause renal water retention (Bianchetti et al. 2017) • Syndrome of inappropriate antidiuretic hormone • Chronic renal failure and oliguric renal failure	• Essential hypernatremia • Hyperventilation • Fever
	Hypervolemic
	• Inappropriate intravenous fluid administration • Salt poisoning • Primary aldosteronism and conditions that cause low-renin hypertension

Adapted from Bianchetti et al. (2017)

emia, which can cause a false elevation (Liamis et al. 2013).

Potassium. Potassium is distributed throughout the body, with approximately 98% being intracellular, particularly in the skeletal muscle. Intracellular potassium levels range from 140 to 150 millimole per liter (mmol/L). The sodium-potassium-adenosine triphosphate (ATP) pump is responsible for moving potassium into the cell in exchange for sodium. Through this mechanism, extracellular potassium levels are typically kept between 3.5 and 5 mmol/L, but normal values can range from 3.2 to 6.2 mmol/L depending on age (Noone and Langlois 2017). Neonates have potassium levels on the higher end because fetal concentration is typically 5 mmol/L or greater and they tend to retain more potassium (Bianchetti et al. 2017). After the initial postnatal period, infants and children up to 5 years of age have slightly higher potassium concentrations to facilitate growth and, by 5 years old, have adult values (Loh and Metz 2015).

The intracellular-to-extracellular potassium gradient is essential to the proper functioning of many physiologic and metabolic processes in the body, including regulating the osmotic balance between cellular and interstitial fluid, skeletal and cardiac muscle contraction, and carbohydrate metabolism (Daly and Farrington 2013). Under normal physiologic conditions, approximately 80–90% of daily potassium intake is excreted in the urine, with the remainder lost in sweat and feces. The kidneys play an integral role in maintaining potassium balance. A large proportion of potassium is filtered from the blood via the glomerulus and then reabsorbed in the proximal tubule and loop of Henle. Serum concentration is further adjusted via potassium secretion in the distal tubule and finally reabsorption in the collecting tubule. Altogether, this process is primarily regulated by aldosterone, and any abnormalities in the structural components or functional regulation can alter potassium levels (Oh and Briefel 2017).

Causes of altered potassium levels in children are vast. Potassium abnormalities can result from alterations in intake, excretion, and a wide variety of conditions that change the extracellular-to-intracellular potassium gradient. Table 10.7 lists the common causes of both elevated and decreased potassium levels in children. Hyperkalemia is defined as a serum concentration of greater than 5.5 milliequivalents per liter (mEq/L), with moderate elevation being 6–7 mEq/L and severe being greater than 7 mEq/L. Hyperkalemia is generally considered

Table 10.7 Common causes of abnormal potassium levels in children

Hypokalemia	Hyperkalemia
Intracellular shifts of potassium	Extracellular shifts of potassium
• Metabolic alkalosis • β-adrenergic agonists: Albuterol, insulin, theophylline, caffeine, and epinephrine • Hyperthyroidism • Barium poisoning	• Acidosis, especially inorganic • Hyperkalemic familiar periodic paralysis • Hyperglycemia
Increased losses of potassium	Increased endogenous potassium load
• Medications: Sodium polystyrene sulfonate, and corticosteroids • Therapy for renal failure: Hemodialysis and renal replacement therapy	• Extensive tissue injury, burns, heatstroke, and trauma • Hemolysis • Rhabdomyolysis • Tumor lysis syndrome • Tissue necrosis • Hemolytic uremic syndrome
Gastrointestinal losses	Increased exogenous potassium load
• Diarrhea • Vomiting • Increased ostomy output • Nasogastric drainage	• Diet, salt substitutes • Banked blood transfusions • Gastrointestinal hemorrhage • Poisoning • Medications: Potassium-sparing diuretics, cyclosporine, NSAIDs, heparin, tacrolimus, pentamidine, trimethoprim, ACE inhibitors, and potassium-containing medications such as supplements and potassium penicillin
Urinary losses	Decreased excretion +/− increased intake
• Diuretics: Loop, thiazide, and osmotic such as mannitol • Antibiotics: Amphotericin B, cisplatin, and aminoglycosides such as piperacillin and ticarcillin • Diabetic ketoacidosis • Hypomagnesemia • Cushing syndrome • Primary mineralocorticoid excess • Hyperaldosteronism • Renal tubular disorders: Fanconi's, Bartter's, and Gitelman's syndrome	• Acute renal failure and severe chronic renal failure • Mineralocorticoid deficiency (Addison's disease, selective aldosterone deficiency, congenital adrenal hyperplasia) • Hyporeninemic hypoaldosteronism • Hereditary enzyme deficiencies • Tubulointerstitial disease • Type IV renal tubular acidosis • Obstruction • Sickle cell disease • Systemic lupus erythematosus
Inadequate intake	Pseudohyperkalemia
• Poor diet • Eating disorders	• Use of tourniquet when drawing blood • Hemolysis of drawn blood • Leukocytosis (WBC count >50 K) or thrombocytosis (platelet count >1,000,000) • Pneumatic tube transport of a highly leukocytic or thrombotic specimen

Adapted from Daly and Farrington (2013); Noone and Langlois (2017), Lehnhardt and Kemper (2011), Liamis et al. (2013)

more clinically significant than hypokalemia owing to the increased risk for abnormal cardiac conduction, which is most often seen in the setting of severely elevated levels. Still, any abnor-mal value requires careful consideration by the clinician.

The most common cause of hyperkalemia in infants and children is "pseudohyperkalemia," which results from hemolysis that occurs when a blood sample is obtained via a heel stick, a small intravenous line, or otherwise inadequate venipuncture (Daly and Farrington 2013). Pseudohyperkalemia can also be seen if the sample is processed greater than 1 hour after venipuncture, which can deplete the glucose in the sample and therefore slow the function of the sodium-potassium-ATP pump, or is stored at lower than room temperature because the lower temperature inhibits the pump and potassium and then leaks out of the cells (Noone and Langlois 2017).

Children with impaired renal function, acute or chronic, can also present with hyperkalemia in the setting of reduced glomerular filtration rate with low urine flow, which causes decreased renal excretion of potassium (Lehnhardt and Kemper 2011). Hypokalemia is defined as a serum concentration less than 3.5 mEq/L and that can become life-threatening when less than 2.5 mEq/L. Because serum levels do not reflect intracellular potassium, they are also not reflective of total potassium stores. True hypokalemia is relatively rare in healthy persons and is primarily seen in pediatric patients due to excessive gastrointestinal losses due to vomiting or diarrhea (Daly and Farrington 2013).

Chloride: Chloride is found throughout the body, particularly in gastric secretions, sweat, urine, lymph, connective tissue, bone, and cartilage. As the primary extracellular cation, it is the chief counter ion for sodium. As a result, chloride concentrations change in proportion to sodium concentrations and play an important role in regulating the body's volume status, osmolality, and acid-base balance (Greenbaum 2020). Chloride is a key component in evaluating acid-base disorders, especially when calculating the serum anion gap, as discussed in Sect. 10.6.1.2. Elevated levels are associated with acidosis, while decreased levels are associated with alkalosis. The kidney is primarily responsible for regulating chloride homeostasis, where it is freely filtered and reabsorbed in parallel with sodium. Serum chloride concentrations are typically maintained between 97 and 110 mmoL/L in newborns and 98 and 106 mmol/L thereafter (Lo 2020). Altered chloride levels can result from abnormalities in renal function and other extrarenal causes. They typically occur in the setting of altered sodium concentrations and acid-base disorders, although they can occur in isolation in rare circumstances (Greenbaum 2020).

Hypochloremia is, in general, encountered infrequently. When present, it is most often associated with loss of chloride-rich gastric secretions either through vomiting or diarrhea. Hypochloremia is classically associated with both cystic fibrosis and hypertrophic pyloric stenosis. Due to changes in diagnostic processes, hypochloremia associated with hypertrophic pyloric stenosis does not always bear out clinically (Glatstein et al. 2011; Tutay et al. 2013). Hypochloremia can also be seen with decreased chloride intake. A relatively rare entity, as sodium chloride is abundant in most diets, infants who are fed unconventional formulas with inadequate chloride can develop hypochloremic metabolic alkalosis (Signorelli et al. 2020). A good nutrition history is critical in these patients, who present with failure to thrive, constipation, food refusal, muscle weakness, and delayed development.

Hyperchloremia can be encountered for a wide variety of clinical reasons, including excessive administration, a net loss of water as in diabetes insipidus, excessive loss of electrolytes as seen in diarrhea and osmotic diuresis, and conditions that cause metabolic acidosis such as certain forms of diarrhea, renal tubular acidosis, and some types of chronic kidney disease (Nagami 2016). Elevated chloride levels and a resultant metabolic acidosis are often encountered in the setting of aggressive intervenous hydration, particularly when normal saline is administered for fluid resuscitation in the setting of septic shock. This is associated with acute kidney injury and poorer outcomes in critically ill children (Stenson et al. 2018). Clinicians caring for patients in this context must choose appropriate fluids for resuscitation and monitor for electrolyte imbalances carefully.

Carbon dioxide. Carbon dioxide will be discussed in Sect. 10.6.1.1.

Blood urea nitrogen (BUN) and creatinine. Renal function is expressed in the serum electrolyte panel as BUN and creatinine. An elevation in either of these numbers suggests impaired renal function. Urea is the main waste product from the breakdown of protein compounds in the body. It is functionally measured and expressed in relation to its nitrogen content, thus the BUN value. Urea is produced at a variable rate; it increases with high dietary protein intake, tissue breakdown, hemorrhage, or trauma and decreases in a low-protein diet or liver disease. Urea is freely filtered by the glomerulus and reabsorbed in the proximal tubule and inner medullary collecting duct of the kidney. The amount of urea reabsorbed in the proximal tubule depends on vascular volume; reabsorption is especially increased in depletion states. Urea reabsorption also increases in the inner medullary collecting duct when urine osmolality is high due to a high urea concentration. Because of the variable rate of production and reabsorption in the kidney, BUN is not considered a good laboratory reflection of the GFR in the healthy kidney. Of note, in advanced renal failure, BUN is more closely reflective of GFR and is, therefore, a more reliable marker (Oh and Briefel 2017).

BUN is generally increased in conditions with decreased renal clearance but can also be increased in upper gastrointestinal bleeding and high-protein diets. While it is not a good reflection of glomerular filtration on its own, BUN's physiologic properties with respect to vascular volume give BUN some clinical utility in evaluating dehydration, where it is elevated (Hoxha et al. 2014; Shaoul et al. 2004). More recently, BUN elevation in children has also been shown to be a reliable marker for severe acute pancreatitis (Vitale et al. 2019). Decreased BUN is seen infrequently but may be seen in low-protein diets, starvation, and liver disease. Reference values for serum urea levels, by age and sex, can be seen in Table 10.8.

Creatinine is an endogenous substance derived from muscle cells (Noone and Langlois 2017). It is generated at a relatively constant rate and, in the setting of normal renal function, creatinine excretion is almost equal to its production. It is not bound to plasma proteins, is freely filtered by the glomerulus, and is only reabsorbed in the renal tubules in a small amount. For these reasons, it is the most widely used laboratory marker of GFR and is also employed to calculate renal function, as discussed in Sect. 10.7.1.2. Creatinine is measured in the laboratory typically via one of two methods: enzymatic reactions with amidohydrolase or creatine iminohydrolase or the Jaffe reaction, which uses trinitrophenol (also known as picric acid or picrate) (Oh and Briefel 2017). Normal serum creatinine levels for children by age and sex, using both methods, can be seen in Tables 10.9 and 10.10.

Like BUN, serum creatinine is increased in the setting of impaired renal clearance. Any abnormalities in creatinine values should be evaluated closely and prompt the primary care clinician to consider a consultation with a pediatric nephrologist. Creatinine levels can be falsely increased when there is significantly elevated glucose, particularly when the value is obtained using the Jaffe method. Picrate can also react with glucose, fructose, protein, urea, and ascorbic acid. A falsely elevated creatinine is most pronounced in diabetic ketoacidosis (Oh and Briefel 2017).

Table 10.8 Normal serum urea values by age and sex

Age	Urea (mg/dL)	
	Females	Males
0 to <14 days	2.5–24.9	2.5–24.9
15 days to <1 year	3.1–17.6	3.1–17.6
1 to <10 years	8.7–23.2	8.7–23.2
10 to <19 years	6.4–19.6	6.4–21.8

Adapted with permission from Oxford Press from Colantonio et al. (2012)

Table 10.9 Normal serum creatinine values for children by age and sex[a]

Age	Creatinine (mg/dL)	
	Females	Males
0 to 14 days	0.27–0.98	0.27–0.98
15 days to <2 years	0.1–0.38	0.1–0.38
2 to <5 years	0.18–0.45	0.18–0.45
5 to <12 years	0.29–0.62	0.29–0.62
12 to <15 years	0.38–0.85	0.38–0.85
15 to <19 years	0.47–0.88	0.53–1.11

Adapted with permission from Oxford Press from Colantonio et al. (2012)
[a] Using the enzymatic method

Table 10.10 Normal serum creatinine values by age and sex[a]

Age	Creatinine (mg/dL)	
	Females	Males
0 to 14 days	0.32–1.06	0.32–1.06
15 days to <1 year	0.31–0.55	0.31–0.55
1 to <4 years	0.38–0.55	0.38–0.55
4 to <7 years	0.43–0.67	0.43–0.67
7 to <12 years	0.52–0.71	0.52–0.71
12 to <15 years	0.56–0.86	0.56–0.86
15 to <17 years	0.58–0.87	0.63–1.08
17 to <19 years	0.59–0.9	0.66–1.13

Adapted with permission from Oxford Press from Colantonio et al. (2012)
[a] Using the Jaffe method

Table 10.12 Normal serum calcium levels by age

Age	Serum total calcium		Ionized calcium	
	mg/dL	mmol/L	mg/dL[a]	mmol/L
0–3 months	8.8–11.3	2.2–2.83	4.88–5.6	1.22–1.4
1–5 years	9.4–10.8	2.35–2.7	4.88–5.28	1.22–1.32
6–12 years	9.4–10.3	2.35–2.57	4.6–5.28	1.15–1.32
13–20 years	8.8–10.2	2.2–2.55	4.48–5.2	1.12–1.3

Adapted from Noone and Langlois (2017), KDIGO (2009); KDIGO (2017)
[a] Calculated using a conversion factor of 0.25 as recommended by KDIGO (2017)

Table 10.11 Forms of calcium in the body and their function

Calcium form	Function
Free or ionized portion	• Biologically active form • Approximately 50% of total serum calcium
Complex calcium	• Bound closely to anions such as bicarbonate and citrate • Approximately 10% of total serum calcium
Plasma-bound calcium	• Primarily found bound to albumin • Must recalculate calcium in patients with low albumin • Accounts for the remaining 40%

Adapted from Klemm and Klein (2017)

10.3.3.2 Calcium

In conjunction with the intestines, bones, and parathyroid, the kidneys play a vital role in the body's metabolism and regulation of calcium levels. Calcium levels are sensed in the parathyroid gland, kidney, and bones. Hypocalcemia prompts the release of parathyroid hormone, which stimulates calcium release from bones and increases intestinal calcium absorption (Bianchetti et al. 2017). Through vitamin D metabolism, the parathyroid hormone also stimulates increased calcium reabsorption in the kidneys (Lietman et al. 2010). Abnormalities at any step in this process can result in altered calcium homeostasis.

Calcium, the most prevalent cation in the body, is primarily stored in the skeleton. Total calcium measurement includes both ionized calcium and protein-bound calcium. Table 10.11 reviews the forms of calcium in the body and their function.

The plasma-bound calcium must be corrected for low albumin. Alternatively, ionized calcium levels can be measured (Klemm and Klein 2017), although this is not routinely done.

Normal serum calcium concentrations are greater in children than adults. Normal levels by age are presented in Table 10.12 and are derived from clinical guidelines developed by the KDIGO Work Group in 2009 and updated in 2017. Owing to the role nutritional intake plays in calcium levels, any patient with abnormal calcium levels should prompt the clinician to obtain a thorough dietary history. Hypercalcemia is less common in children than adults, but when it is present, it is clinically significant. Hypercalcemia may be discovered in infants and neonates when a routine chemistry panel is ordered to evaluate failure-to-thrive. In small infants, the use of enriched formulas that provide excess calcium can quickly result in hypercalcemia. Neonates and infants can also present with hypercalcemia due to hyperparathyroidism, phosphate depletion, inborn errors of metabolism, and genetic conditions such as familial hypocalciuric hypercalcemia and Williams syndrome. Older children develop hypercalcemia for various reasons, the most common being hyperparathyroidism, immobilization, and malignancy (Lietman et al. 2010). Hypocalcemia is also commonly encountered in the pediatric population. It is frequently seen in acute critical illness, including acute and chronic renal failure but may also be associated with deficiencies in both calcium and vitamin D intake and hypoparathyroidism (Nadar and Shaw 2020).

It should also be noted that calcium levels are intricately connected with vitamin D levels. Not only do vitamin D metabolites regulate calcium reabsorption in the kidney but also in the intestines. Altered vitamin D levels can greatly affect calcium levels and should be evaluated in the setting of both hypo- and hypercalcemia. The measurement of vitamin D levels is discussed in Sect. 10.7.1.3.

10.3.3.3 Phosphorous

The vast majority of phosphorous, 80–85%, is stored in the skeleton as inorganic phosphate. The remaining 15–20% is present intracellularly as organic phosphate is an essential component of nucleic acids, phospholipids, and ATP. Only inorganic phosphate is routinely measured clinically. Inorganic phosphate levels are highest during the neonatal period and early childhood and then decline because children readily retain phosphate (Bianchetti et al. 2017). Table 10.13 denotes normal inorganic phosphate levels by age.

Phosphorous is abundant in food, and most of the phosphate is derived from dietary intake. The kidney plays the primary role in regulating phosphate levels and generally ensures that output is equivalent to the net intake by the intestines

(Bianchetti et al. 2017). The glomerulus freely filters it; more than 80% is reabsorbed in the proximal tubule and a small amount in the distal tubule. Phosphorous levels are influenced by parathyroid hormone, which, when released, decreases phosphorous reabsorption in the proximal tubule, thus lowering serum concentrations (Klemm and Klein 2017). It is this mechanism that causes an increase in calcium reabsorption and results in a decrease in phosphorous.

Children can develop alterations in inorganic phosphate levels in various conditions listed in Table 10.14. In the setting of acute or chronic impaired renal function, children often present with hyperphosphatemia due to decreased glomerular filtration rate. Children who ingest large amounts of phosphate-containing laxatives may also develop mild renal insufficiency due to volume contraction in the setting of diarrhea, which can further exacerbate the problem (Bianchetti et al. 2017). It should also be noted that hyperphosphatemia secondary to the use of phosphate enemas has been described in children (Ladenhauf et al. 2012), with the risk increased in children under 2 years of age (Bianchetti et al. 2017). Spurious elevated levels of phosphate can be seen in hyperbilirubinemia and hyperlipidemia, and sample contamination with heparin or recombinant tissue plasminogen activator pseudohypophosphatemia is associated with mannitol administration (Liamis et al. 2013).

Calcium and phosphorous levels, particularly in the patient with altered renal function, should be evaluated closely. As previously noted, calcium and phosphorous typically have an inverse relationship; however, this is not always seen in children with impaired renal function. Children with kidney disease typically develop hyperphosphatemia as their renal function decreases and impair excretion. Hyperphosphatemia results in an increased release of parathyroid hormone and subsequent increased calcium release from the bones and absorption from the intestines. This is evident in labs as hypercalcemia and hyperphosphatemia, which become especially problematic if the concentrations are high enough to cause precipitation of the two in the blood and subsequent injury to vessels and organs. In children,

Table 10.13 Normal inorganic phosphate levels by age

Age	Level	
	mg/dL[a]	mmol/L
0–3 months	5–7.44	1.62–2.4
4–6 months	5.5–6.85	1.78–2.21
6–12 months	4.28–6.66	1.38–2.15
1–2 years	4.1–5.98	1.32–1.93
3–4 years	3.16–5.95	1.02–1.92
5–6 years	4.5–5.36	1.13–1.73
7–8 years	3.28–5.58	1.06–1.8
9–10 years	3.5–5.27	1.13–1.7
11–12 years	3.22–5.55	1.04–1.79
13–15 years	3–5.58	0.97–1.8

Adapted from Bianchetti et al. 2017
[a]Calculated using a conversion factor of 3.1 as recommended by Bianchetti et al. (2017)

Table 10.14 Causes of abnormal inorganic phosphate levels in children

Hypophosphatemia	Hyperphosphatemia
Low dietary intake or poor intestinal absorption	*Increased phosphate load*
• Severe cases of malnutrition	• High dietary intake or increased intestinal absorption
• Very-low-birth weight infants during rapid postnatal growth	• Newborns fed with cow's milk
• Chronic use of phosphate binders	• Total parenteral nutrition
Internal redistribution	• Phosphate-containing laxative use
• Refeeding syndrome	• Vitamin D intoxication
• Respiratory alkalosis	• Tumor lysis, rhabdomyolysis, lactic, and ketoacidosis
• Severe diabetic ketoacidosis after insulin therapy	*Decreased renal phosphate excretion*
Urinary loss	• Reduced renal function
• Hyperparathyroidism	• Increased renal tubular reabsorption
• Rickets	• Hypoparathyroidism
• Tumor-induced osteomalacia	• Idiopathic childhood nephrotic syndrome
• Gitelman's and Bartter's syndromes	• Medications: Growth hormone, bisphosphonates, dipyridamole
	• Familiar hyperphosphatemic tumoral calcinosis

Adapted from Bianchetti et al. (2017)

this can also result in fractures, skeletal deformities, and poor growth (Hanudel and Salusky 2017). The Kidney Disease Outcomes Quality Initiative (K/DOQI) of the National Kidney Foundation, in their Clinical Practice Guidelines for Bone Metabolism and Disease in Chronic Kidney Disease, recommended the calcium-phosphate product be calculated and kept below 55 mg²/dL² in patients with chronic renal failure to prevent these complications (K/DOQI 2003). Calcium-phosphorous product is commonly used in clinical practice; however, in their updated clinical practice guidelines endorsed by the National Kidney Foundation, the KDIGO Work Group noted that this calculation is not necessarily clinically relevant in the setting of progressing renal failure. They recommend evaluating the values together, but not necessarily as a calculated product (KDIGO 2009, KDIGO 2017).

10.3.3.4 Serum Albumin
Albumin in abnormal levels can indicate glomerular filtration problems with the kidney and therefore is a more specific test when faced with proteinuria. Albumin is especially useful in the evaluation of nephrotic syndrome, which is discussed in Sect. 10.7.1.

10.3.3.5 Complement Levels
A complement system is a complex group of plasma proteins that play an essential role in the immune system. They act as enzymes that facilitate immunologic and inflammatory activation in the body. The protein components of the complement system are primarily synthesized in the liver. Once activated, the proteins are distributed throughout the body. Most of the complement system is categorized into major components of C1 to C9, with subcategories identified on a deeper cellular level. The most common complement test evaluated by nephrologists is the C3 and C4 protein levels, immunostaining of biopsy specimens for complement proteins, and hemolytic potential in the patient's serum (CH50 and AH50) (Thurman 2015).

The complement system can be activated by antibody-antigen, bacterial endotoxin, or lectin pathways. The system aids in removing damaged cells and acts as an important line of defense against fungi, bacteria, and viruses (Thurman 2015). Although it has defensive properties, the complement system also causes kidney injury in various diseases; therefore, a clinical evaluation of the complement system is an important part of the diagnostic evaluation in patients with glomerulonephritis (Thurman 2015). When the complement system is overly activated, the serum levels fall since the component has been used up. In renal disease associated with an increase of antibody-antigen activation, the complement serum levels will be low. Low complement is also seen within the bacterial-endotoxin pathway when the system is activated in an immune response. Serum measurement of C3 and C4 can narrow a diagnosis in patients with nephrotic syndrome. Low serum complement levels are seen in systemic renal diseases such as SLE, "shunt nephritis," atypical hemolytic uremic syndrome (aHUS), and post glomerulonephritis. Normal complement levels are seen in IgA nephropathy, basement membrane disease, and renal-limited antineutrophil cytoplasmic antibody vasculitis. For the clinician, assessing the complement system in the acute phase of a renal inflammation or immunologic-related illness will guide the clinician's differential and management (Thurman 2015).

10.3.3.6 Antistreptolysin Antibodies

Elevated antistreptolysin in the bloodstream indicates a recent streptococcal infection and can help with the epidemiology of glomerulonephritis. Serological testing is discussed in further detail in Sect. 6.6.4.4.

10.3.3.7 Screening for Hepatitis

Hepatitis screening is done on patients with proteinuria as it is a common finding when the virus caused glomerular inflammation and/or damage. Membranoproliferative glomerulonephritis is often associated with hepatitis B and C (Leung and Wong 2010). Therefore, in the presence of persistent proteinuria, the patient should be screened for hepatitis. Hepatitis screening is discussed in further detail in Sect. 6.3.6 and the liver section in Chap. 9.

10.3.3.8 Rheumatologic Tests

If the ANA, dsDNA, and ANCA are abnormal, a rheumatologic indication for proteinuria should be considered. Diagnostic testing for rheumatological diseases is discussed in further detail in Chap. 12.

10.3.4 Real-Life Example

A 14-year-old male presents to the office for a well-child physical exam and a sports clearance physical. He will compete for his high school cross-country team later in the coming months. Upon initial triage in the office, the nurse makes the clinician aware that the routine screen of his urine on dipstick has 1+ protein and an SG of 10.30. The urine is also noted to be dark in color. The patient's family history is benign, with no renal or kidney disease noted. His physical exam is unremarkable. When discussing the patient's exercise regimen, he reports to the clinician he runs 5–10 miles a day to prepare for his upcoming cross-country season. Before his visit, he ran a 6-mile run. The clinician orders first-morning spot urine. The specimen is received, and it is negative for protein, has an SG of 10.10, and is noted to be clear yellow. The clinician can safely discuss the findings of protein in the prior sample as secondary to orthostatic proteinuria.

10.4 Evaluation of the Child with Isolated Hematuria

Unlike proteinuria, the presence of blood in the urine can be a chief complaint of a patient seeking medical attention. Hematuria can also be an incidental occurrence on routine urinalysis. For the diagnosis of hematuria to be made, red blood cells (RBCs) on dipstick or urinalysis must be present. Microscopic hematuria is often defined as the presence of 5 or more RBCs per high-powered field in the sediment of freshly voided urine (Pomeranz et al. 2016c). On the contrary, macroscopic hematuria is the presence of gross blood in the urine; however, it must be noted that discolored or red-tinged urine is not synonymous with gross hematuria. Discolored urine must have the presence of RBCs for it to be clinically significant for macroscopic or gross hematuria. Many conditions can cause red or brown urine; therefore, the presence of RBCs must be confirmed in discolored urine (see Table 10.15 for the causes of discolored urine). The evaluation of hematuria can be split into two different categories: microscopic and macroscopic.

Table 10.15 Common causes for discolored urine with a negative dipstick for hematuria

Ingestion of foods	• Food coloring (analine)
	• Beets
	• Blackberries, rhubarb, paprika
Ingestions of toxins	• Lead (benzene) and metabolites
	• Homogentisic acid, tyrosinosis, urates
Ingestions of drugs	• Sulfonamides
	• Nitrofurantoin
	• Salicylates, ibuprofen,
	• Pyridium, phenytoin, rifampin, chloroquine
	• Deferoxamine
	• Iron
	• Sorbitol
Common endogenous causes of dark urine	• Erythrocytes
	• Hemoglobin
	• Myoglobin
	• Metabolites
	• Amorphous urates

Adapted from Pomeranz et al. (2016c), Utsch and Klaus (2014); Viteri and Reid-Adam (2018)

10.4.1 Microscopic Hematuria

Microscopic hematuria is often found on routine screening. Most children with isolated microhematuria do not have a treatable or serious cause (Kaplan and Pradhan 2013). Within the literature, isolated microhematuria is noted in 1–2% of children between the ages of 6 and 15 years. It is often spontaneous and resolves without consequence (Brown and Reidy 2019). When evaluating a patient with microscopic hematuria, the clinician must obtain a detailed history and physical exam. The history should evaluate for the presence of key elements to suggest etiology. Urinary symptoms such as dysuria, frequency, urgency, and flank pain and a recent history of vigorous exercise and trauma (including foreign body, catheterization, and sexual/physical abuse) may indicate the need for further workup (Pomeranz et al. 2016c). Medication history and in-depth family history, including renal disease, must also be obtained. If the child is asymptomatic and the history reveals no known etiology, the patient can repeat the urine two to three times over a 2–3-month period. If subsequent urinaly-ses are negative for the presence of RBCs, microscopic hematuria can be considered idiopathic and transient (Pomeranz et al. 2016c).

Most children present with asymptomatic microscopic hematuria. A history of group A streptococcal skin infection 2–6 weeks earlier or throat infection 1–2 weeks earlier should prompt the clinician to include post-strep glomerulonephritis (GN) in their differential (Baum 2008). Post-strep GN has a wide range of presentations, from asymptomatic, microscopic hematuria to the acute nephritic syndrome. The acute nephritic syndrome presents with red-brown urine, proteinuria, edema, hypertension, and acute kidney injury. Although it often subsides on its own, if the diagnosis is delayed or the disease is more severe, the child may have more significant findings on the exam, such as hypertension, peripheral edema, or pulmonary edema. Laboratory investigation may reveal low complement protein C3 but normal C4 levels. Low C3 levels that persist beyond 3–4 weeks after the infection may warrant a renal biopsy, especially if there is continued hematuria and/or proteinuria (Baum 2008; Primack 2010; Viteri and Reid-Adam 2018).

A positive dipstick can also indicate hemoglobin and/or myoglobin; therefore, microscopic urinalysis is essential in determining the presence of RBC and/or hemoglobin in these patients. When distinguishing between hemoglobin and myoglobin, often these substrates need to be measured in the urine. Hemoglobinuria is the result of hemolysis. Myoglobinuria occurs in rhabdomyolysis after viral myositis in healthy children. It can also be noted in children with inborn errors of metabolism often occurring after exercise (Pomeranz et al. 2016c).

If there is a familial history of microscopic hematuria, evaluation by a genetic counselor should be considered because microscopic hematuria is a soft finding in familial chronic kidney disease. The patient with persistent asymptomatic hematuria should be evaluated further.

Continued evidence of microscopic hematuria and/or microscopic hematuria in the presence of proteinuria requires further laboratory evaluation and referral to nephrology.

10.4.2 Macroscopic/Gross Hematuria

Gross hematuria can originate from both the upper and lower urinary tract. The most common causes of gross hematuria in children include UTI, trauma, and perianal irritation (Brown and Reidy 2019). UTIs are often associated with hematuria; therefore, renal disease can be excluded in the presence of a positive bacterial component on urine culture. The occurrence of gross hematuria in children in the United States is estimated to be 1.3 of 1000 outpatient visits (Brown and Reidy 2019). It is the clinician's responsibility to determine the source of the hematuria. Again, this begins with a thorough history and physical exam.

When evaluating a patient who presents with dark-colored or blood-tinged urine, the presence of RBCs must be noted on microscopy assessment of spun sediment. This laboratory evaluation will exclude other material that may be the root cause of dark-colored or blood-tinged urine (see Table 10.15 for common sources that can discolor urine). Urine microscopy should be done, and the results are outlined in Table 10.2.

Once a clinician has determined the presence of RBCs in the urine through dipstick, further microscopy can aid in differentiating between upper and lower tract root causes. The history and physical exam should direct all laboratory assessments. Red urine, clots, dysuria, frequency, urgency, flank, abdominal pain, and costovertebral angle tenderness (Brown and Reidy 2019) show blood is more than likely coming from the lower tract. Upper urinary tract causes for gross hematuria associated are with red, brown, cola−/ tea-colored urine, painless, hypertension, proteinuria, impaired renal function, dysmorphic RBCs cast cells, and systemic symptoms such as fever, malaise, arthralgia, and rash (Brown and Reidy 2019). Added diagnostics are needed and should include urinalysis, urine culture, urine calcium creatinine, and 24-hour urine for the presence of stone formation. In the setting of stone formation, calcium, phosphate, uric acid, oxalate, and cysteine could be present in the 24-hour sample. A basic metabolic panel, complete blood count, and coagulation studies should be done when a coagulopathy or kidney malfunction is suspected. Consultation with nephrology and urology must be made to consider imaging such as renal bladder ultrasound with Doppler, computed tomography scan, magnetic resonance imaging, and/or cystoscopy.

10.4.3 Common Causes for Hematuria in the Pediatric Patient

The causes of hematuria found on dipstick can range from benign to significant renal disease. The pediatric clinician must understand the common causes of hematuria and how hematuria presents in primary care. When a child presents with hematuria, the clinician should consider fever, excessive exercise, UTI, and trauma as a cause for the finding. In the presence of persistent hematuria (greater than 6 months), the clinician must evaluate further. The history and physical findings aid in the diagnosis in deciding pathology.

Hypercalciuria is often associated with persistent asymptomatic hematuria. Patients 2 years and above with a urine calcium/creatinine ratio of >2.0 have levels consistent with hypercalciuria. This finding is often benign however can lead to stone formation. Nephrolithiasis may be associated with micro- or macrohematuria. In some patients, the stone formation is found as an incidental finding, while in other patients, the child presents with abdominal and/or flank pain (Viteri and Reid-Adam 2018). Table 10.16 outlines the upper and lower tract causes for hematuria.

Lee et al. (2006) found that 461 children with abnormal urinalysis underwent renal biopsy, half demonstrated normal findings. Among the abnormal results, the most common pathologies were thin basement membrane neprhopathy (TBMN), followed by IgA nephropathy. IgA nephropathy presents with microscopic hematuria with non-nephritic proteinuria. It also can present with gross hematuria (Brown and Reidy 2019). This disease, also known as Berger's disease, is triggered by an upper respiratory or gastrointestinal disease. It becomes clear within days of the infec-

Table 10.16 Upper and lower tract causes for hematuria

Lower tract causes for hematuria	Non-glomerular causes for upper tract hematuria	Glomerular causes for upper tract hematuria
• Exercise (micro)[a] • Fever (micro)[a] • UTI (micro/macro)[a] • Trauma (macro) • Urethritis (micro) • Bladder calculus/mass (macro) • Schistosomiasis (macro) • Adenovirus hemorrhagic cystitis (macro)	• Nephrolithiasis (micro/macro)[a] • Hypercalciuria (micro) • Nutcracker syndrome (micro/macro)[a] • Sickle cell trait (micro) • Coagulation disorders (micro/macro) • Polycystic kidney disease (micro/macro)[a] • Wilms tumor (micro/macro)[a] • Structural abnormalities (micro)	• IgA nephropathy (micro/macro)[a] • Henoch-Schönlein purpura (micro/macro)[a] • Alport syndrome (micro/macro)[a] • Thin basement membrane disease (micro/macro) • Postinfectious glomerulonephritis (micro/macro)[a] • Hemolytic uremic syndrome (micro)[a]

Adapted from Viteri and Reid-Adam (2018)
[a] Protein may be present

tion. The diagnosis is made by renal biopsy. The prognosis of patients with IgA nephropathy varies, with 40% of patients progressing to end-stage renal disease (Brown and Reidy 2019).

Another disease process in the pediatric population is IgA vasculitis. Although rare, with an incidence of 23 per 100,000 children under 17 years (Brown and Reidy 2019), pediatric providers must consider these diseases when faced with hematuria and proteinuria. The most common IgA vasculitis known as Henoch-Schönlein purpura (HSP) has a definitive rash (palpable purpuric lesions without thrombocytopenia), arthritis (oligoarticular, transient, and nondeforming), abdominal pain, and renal disease. In addition to the physical findings, laboratory urinalysis will demonstrate hematuria with or without RBC casts and no or mild proteinuria (Viteri and Reid-Adam 2018).

The diagnosis of postinfectious glomerulonephritis (GN) can often be associated with microscopic hematuria. Therefore, it is important to investigate the possibility of its presence in a child with microscopic hematuria on a routine dipstick. The historical findings associated with asymptomatic microscopic hematuria related to GN typically reveal either a skin infection (2–6 weeks prior) or a throat infection (1–2 weeks prior). However, if a diagnosis is delayed, patients may present with significant findings of brown cola-colored urine, hypertension, proteinuria, edema, and in severe cases, fluid overload (hypertension, edema, pulmonary edema) (Viteri and

Reid-Adam 2018). In addition to hematuria on urine microscopy, complement levels C3 and C4 may be low. It is important to note that children may continue to have microscopic hematuria for up to 6 months secondary to inflammation once recovered.

10.4.4 Real-Life Example

A 13-year-old well female presents to the office with a rash. The rash began on her bilateral ankles and spread to her calves. She recently started playing field hockey and first thought of the rash from being hit with a hockey stick. She seeks medical attention because the rash has spread to her thigh and buttocks, and she reports generalized abdominal pain. Upon examination, the patient has palpable purpura diffusely noted to the buttocks, hips, upper thighs, and lower legs. She denies any other symptoms. She denies medications and allergies. Her initial laboratory reveals a CBC within normal limits and no thrombocytopenia present. A dipstick in the office is dark yellow, clear, SG 10.40, and greater than 10 RBC. While there is no definitive test to aid in the diagnosis of HSP, the following labs should be ordered: CBC (hemoglobin, RBC, and platelets should be normal), ESR (should be normal or slightly elevated), PT/PTT (should be normal), IgA (often elevated in the acute phase), C3 (normal or low), ANA (negative), throat swab (to consider post-strep complication), BUN/

creatinine (in advanced renal disease will be elevated), urinalysis (microscopic hematuria or macroscopic hematuria in nephritis), and stool guaiac (positive if gastrointestinal involvement has occurred).

Key Learning about Isolated Proteinuria or Isolated Hematuria
- Causes for both isolated proteinuria and hematuria can be benign or can be a result of renal disease.
- Proteinuria needs to be evaluated with a first-morning void.
- Isolated hematuria also needs microscopic evaluation.

10.5 Proteinuria and Hematuria

In rare instances, children will present with proteinuria and hematuria. When combined, the risk for potential renal disease is higher. Patients who present with combined hematuria and proteinuria have a significant risk for IgA nephropathy and other renal diseases (Quigley 2008).

When hematuria and proteinuria occur together without symptoms, a repeat urinalysis with urine protein/creatinine (P/C) ratio should be sent for laboratory evaluation. If the urine is not normalized, the threshold for repeat testing lies within the protein/creatinine ratio where 0.2 mg/mg indicates referral to nephrology. If a child has a urine P/C ratio value of >350 mg/mmol (3.5 mg/mg), the result is consistent with nephrotic proteinuria.

Children with microscopic hematuria and proteinuria also require a thorough history and physical exam. Findings suggestive of renal disease include edema, hypertension, decreased urinary output, rash, arthralgias, loss of appetite, and weight loss (Viteri and Reid-Adam 2018). Referral to pediatric nephrology is typically required, and renal biopsy should be considered (Plumb et al. 2018). Table 10.17 indicates the most common diagnoses clinicians should consider when a patient presents with hematuria and proteinuria combined.

10.5.1 Genetic Diseases Presenting with Hematuria and Proteinuria

In patients presenting with hematuria and proteinuria, one must consider a family or hereditary history of persistent hematuria and associated symptoms. Family members with dialysis or chronic renal disease must be highlighted as a risk factor when assessing a patient with hematuria. Thin basement membrane nephropathy (TBMN) is a result of genetic alterations in type IV collagen chains. TBMN is often noted in patients with asymptomatic-persistent microscopic hematuria. Family history will reveal a history of microscopic hematuria. Although this is often a benign disease, subsets of patients with TBMN have progressed to chronic kidney disease (CKD). Mutations in the genetic alterations of type IV collagen have led researchers to link a spectrum of nephropathies (Brown and Reidy 2019), with the most severe being Alport syndrome (AS). Specific attention with a patient history of deafness and renal disease should alert the clinician to the possibility of Alport syndrome. AS is a hereditary disease that is associated with both microscopic and macroscopic hematuria. This syndrome can progress to end-stage renal disease. AS is often associated with high-frequency sensorineural hearing loss and ocular abnormalities (Viteri and Reid-Adam 2018). Long-term prognosis of Alport syndrome is poor (Brown and Reidy 2019). To further evaluate a child with TBMN and progressive renal disease, a renal biopsy is needed.

10.5.2 Diagnostic Laboratory Tests

Several diagnostic tests aid the clinician with both proteinuria and hematuria, as these findings require a diagnostic evaluation. The tests are listed below:

Table 10.17 Common causes of hematuria with proteinuria by system/drugs

System	Possible causes of hematuria with proteinuria
Renal	• Nephritis • Diffuse proliferative nephrotic syndrome • Acute post-streptococcal glomerulonephritis • Interstitial glomerulonephritis • Membranoproliferative glomerulonephritis • IgA nephropathy
Gastrointestinal	• Inflammatory bowel disease
Rheumatological	• Nephritis of systemic lupus erythematous • Thrombotic microangiopathy • Cryoglobulinemia • IgA vasculitis (Henoch-Schönlein purpura) • Antineutrophil cytoplasmic antibody (ANCA)-associated vasculitis • Granulomatosis with polyangiitis (GPA; formerly known as Wegener's granulomatosis) • Eosinophilic granulomatosis with polyangiitis (EGPA; previously known as Churg-Strauss syndrome) • Microscopic polyangiitis (MPA) (Yates and Watts 2017)
Genetic causes	• Alport syndrome or hereditary nephritis • Thin basement membrane nephropathy with alteration in type IV collagen chains (subtype of hereditary-persistent hematuria)
Infectious causes	• Virus • HIV • Hepatitis B and C • Epstein-Barr infections • Adenovirus • Hantavirus • Polyomavirus • Bacteria • *Mycoplasma pneumoniae* • *Salmonella, streptococcus, Yersinia* • *Yersinia pseudotuberculosis* • *Leptospira shermani* (Joyce et al. 2017)
Drugs	Tubulointerstitial nephritis can be caused by antimicrobials, NSAIDS, neuropsychiatric drugs, diuretics (Joyce et al. 2017)

Adapted from Brown and Reidy (2019), Joyce et al. (2017), Quigley (2008), Yates and Watts (2017), Viteri and Reid-Adam (2018)

10.5.2.1   24-Hour Urine for Protein and Creatinine

The 24-h urine for protein and creatinine is discussed in Sect. 10.3.2.3.

10.5.2.2   Complete Metabolic Profile

The information about the comprehensive metabolic profile can be found in Sect. 10.3.3.1.

10.5.2.3   Assessments of Inflammatory Markers

The common inflammatory markers include ESR, CRP, amyloid A, ferritin, and procalcitonin. The information regarding this is found in Sect. 6.3.

10.5.2.4   Urinalysis with Microscopy

Urinalysis with microscopy is reviewed in Sect. 10.2.1.1.

10.5.3 Serological Testing

When the clinician suspects that hematuria and/or proteinuria may be related to a rheumatologic or immunologic process, serological testing can be helpful. In particular, diagnosis of antineutrophic cytoplasmic antibody (ANCA)-associated vasculitis such as granulomatosis with polyangiitis (GPA), eosinophilic granulomatosis with polyangiitis (EGPA), and granulomatosis with polyangiitis (MPA) can be aided by serological diagnostics. These relatively rare autoimmune conditions are characterized by the infiltration of inflammatory cells into the blood vessels causing necrosis and, when affecting the renal system, the subsequent clinical presentation of hematuria, proteinuria, and renal dysfunction. Although they are multisystem diseases, renal involvement contributes significantly to their morbidity (Plumb et al. 2018), and clinicians must consider them in their evaluation. Diagnosis of these conditions can be challenging, and they are often mistaken for other conditions, including IgA vasculitis (also known as Henoch-Schönlein purpura) (Plumb et al. 2018), nephrotic involvement in systemic lupus erythematosus, and Goodpasture's syndrome (Yates and Watts 2017). A thorough serologic evaluation of hematuria and proteinuria includes studies to rule in ANCA-associated vasculitis and exclude other conditions.

Enzyme-linked immunosorbent assay and indirect immunofluorescence testing for ANCA are both sensitive and specific diagnostics for GPA and MPA, specifically cytoplasmic (cANCA) staining for GPA and perinuclear (pANCA) staining for MPA (Plumb et al. 2018). If positive, these would rule in ANCA-associated vasculitis. Plumb et al. (2018) also suggest additional serologic tests to exclude more common causes of hematuria and proteinuria, including antinuclear antibodies, anti-extractable nuclear antibodies, and anti-double-stranded DNA antibodies, which, if present, would suggest an etiology related to systemic lupus erythematous. Further discussion of these studies can be found in section ****. Complement function (C3, C4, and CH 50) should also be assessed and, if abnormal, would lead the clinician to consider a variety of other conditions, including postinfectious glomerulonephritis. Interpretation of complement levels is discussed in detail in Sect. 10.3.3.5. The presence of anti-glomerular basement membrane antibodies would suggest Goodpasture's syndrome (Gulati and McAddo 2018). A celiac screen should also be considered as celiac disease is associated with autoimmune inflammatory disorders, specifically IgA nephropathy, and

may present with hematuria and proteinuria (Costa et al. 2018).

10.5.4 Infectious Disease Testing

Depending on the clinical presentation, patients with suspected ANCA-associated vasculitis should have blood cultures, urine microscopy and cultures, mycoplasma serology, antistreptolysin serology, and anti-DNase B titers drawn (Plumb et al. 2018). These are discussed in Sects. 6.6.1 and 6.6.4.4.

10.6 Evaluation of the Child with Mild Acidosis in the Primary Care Setting

Maintaining the body's acid-base balance is a complex process that requires the cooperative interaction of the respiratory, gastrointestinal, and renal systems. While the respiratory system controls acid-base balance by regulating carbon dioxide (CO_2^+) levels, the kidneys regulate long-term acid-base homeostasis by managing the reabsorption of bicarbonate (HCO_3^-) and secretion of hydrogen (H^+). Disturbances in the acid-base equilibrium are often discovered in the primary care setting through routine evaluation of CO_2^+ in the blood and urine pH. Although mild acidosis is most frequently encountered in the child with transient gastrointestinal conditions such as vomiting and diarrhea, persistent acidosis without a gastrointestinal component should alert the clinician to consider a renal etiology such as renal tubular acidosis (RTA).

10.6.1 Renal Tubular Acidosis (RTA)

RTA is a group of disorders characterized by defective renal acid-base regulation. In RTA, the kidney cannot acidify urine, resulting in acid retention and a normal anion gap metabolic acidosis (Yaxley and Pirrone 2016). This imbalance is evident in both blood and urine studies. The resulting persistent acidic state manifests clinically in the child as poor oral intake, vomiting, diarrhea, dehydration, polyuria, and failure to thrive. Prompt identification and adequate treatment of the acidosis via supplementation can prevent poor growth and even allow catch-up growth in some children (Lopez-Garcia et al. 2019).

RTA can occur as both a primary and acquired condition, but most cases of children with RTA result from a genetic defect (Santos et al. 2017; Santos et al. 2015). RTA is classified into four major types: distal (type 1), proximal (type 2), mixed (type 3), and hyperkalemia (type 4). Each subtype is defined by specific pathophysiologic, genetic, molecular, and clinical features. Proximal (type 1) RTA is the most common subtype in Western countries. Owing to the genetic etiology, many children present with RTA within the first weeks or months of life (Santos et al. 2017; Santos et al. 2015). Although the specific genetic and molecular features are beyond the scope of this chapter, they are well described in the literature (Alexander and Bitzan 2019; Santos et al. 2017; Santos et al. 2015). The specific underlying pathophysiology, defining laboratory studies, and notable etiologies and clinical features associated with each main subtype can be seen in Table 10.18.

RTA is a relatively heterogeneous condition, and multiple subtypes exist. Partial distal (type 1) RTA is a condition where, under normal physiologic circumstances, the individual can maintain their acid-base balance; however, they cannot acidify their urine when presented with an acid load. Children with distal RTA can present with hypercalciuria and nephrolithiasis (Alexander and Bitzan 2019). These conditions are rare in children, and RTA should be considered as an etiology when children have hypercalciuria and nephrolithiasis (Marra et al. 2019). Fanconi's syndrome, a global disorder of the proximal tubule that prevents the reabsorption of electrolytes and other substances, is associated with proximal (type 2) RTA. In addition to the standard features of proximal (type 2) RTA, children with this condition present with hypophosphatemia, glucosuria, low-molecular-weight proteinuria, and aminoaciduria (Foreman 2019).

All subtypes of RTA result in net acidification of the blood and alkalinization of the urine. This pathophysiology is most frequently reflected in laboratory values in the blood as decreased serum total CO_2^+ (TCO_2) with a normal anion gap and in the urine as decreased pH.

Table 10.18 reviews the types of RTA along with their key clinical features and diagnostic laboratory values.

Several diagnostic tests are used to aid the clinician in evaluating the patient with acidosis. The tests are listed below:

10.6.1.1 Total CO_2

Serum electrolytes, some of the most frequently obtained diagnostic studies, play an important role in maintaining acid-base homeostasis in the body. Clinicians recognize many acid-base disorders by evaluating TCO_2 on routine electrolyte panels (Kraut and Madias 2018). RTA, in particular, is often identified incidentally in this manner when TCO_2 returns are reduced during investigations for other purposes (Yaxley and Pirrone 2016). It should be noted that children may also present with mildly reduced TCO_2 in the setting of prolonged crying, a common occurrence surrounding venipuncture in children. The clinician needs to exclude this cause of decreased TOC_2 when considering potential diagnoses. In the setting of type 1 RTA, TCO_2 is typically less than 17.5 mEq/L (Chan et al. 2001).

Measurement of TCO_2 in serum includes both ionized and nonionized fractions. Ionized fractions include bicarbonate (HCO_3^-), carbonate (CO_3^{2-}), and carbamino compounds. The nonionized fraction includes carbonic acid (H_2CO_3) and physically dissolved carbon dioxide ($PaCO_2$) (Noone and Langlois 2017). Approximately 95% of TCO_2 is bicarbonate; therefore, TCO_2 is frequently thought of as a "surrogate" for HCO_3^- in venous blood (Kraut and Madias 2018; Noone and Langlois 2017). Of note, both dissolved carbon dioxide ($PaCO_2$) and bicarbonate (HCO_3^-) can be obtained individually by obtaining an arterial blood gas, with HCO_3^- being a calculated value. Both are important values when evaluating the role of the respiratory system in acid-base homeostasis. Because of the invasive nature of

Table 10.18 Types of RTA with their clinical features and diagnostic laboratory findings

Type	Pathophysiology	Defining laboratory findings	Notable etiologies and clinical features
Distal (type 1)	The inability of the distal convoluted tubule and collecting tubule to secrete H^+ in the urine	*Serum:* Hypokalemia *Urine:* Hypercalciuria	• Nephrocalcinosis and nephrolithiasis from hypercalciuria • Some genetic mutations also have sensorineural hearing loss or hemolytic anemia • Associated with autoimmune disorders, nephrotoxic medications, renal tubule interstitial disorders, and other systemic disorders (Alexander and Bitzan 2019).
Proximal (type 2)	Impaired HCO_3^- reabsorption in the proximal tubule resulting in HCO_3^- loss in the urine	*Serum:* Hypokalemia *Urine:* Can have pH <5.5 if plasma HCO_3^- is below urinary excretion threshold	• Rare in isolation • Component of Fanconi's syndrome, Lowe syndrome, and Wilson's disease • Associated with autoimmune disorders, exposure to nephrotoxic medications, and disorders of the tubular interstitium.
Mixed (type 3)	Combined features of distal (type 1) and proximal (type 2)	*Serum:* Hypokalemia *Urine:* Hypercalciuria	• A rare, primarily autosomal recessive inherited condition • Clinical presents with osteopetrosis, cerebral calcifications, nephrocalcinosis and nephrolithiasis, facial dysmorphisms, conductive hearing loss, and cognitive impairment.
Hyperkalemic (type 4)	Aldosterone deficiency or resistance results in defective production of ammonium (NH_4^+) and failure of H^+ reabsorption	*Serum:* Hyperkalemia, hypoaldosteronism *Urine:* Hyperammonemia	• Wide variety of etiologies • Associated with adrenal insufficiency, autoimmune conditions, medications, and intrinsic renal disease (Alexander and Bitzan 2019).

Adapted from Alexander and Bitzan (2019), Santos et al. (2015), Yaxley and Pirrone (2016)

Table 10.19 Normal serum TCO_2 values for pediatric patients by age and sex

Age	Normal serum TCO_2 value (mmoL/L)	
	Females	Males
0 to 14 days	5–25	5–25
15 days to <1 year	9–25	9–25
1 to <5 years	13–25	13–25
5 to <15 years	17–27	17–27
15 to <19 years	16–27	17–29

Adapted with permission from Oxford Press from Colantonio et al. (2012)

the test, they are rarely obtained in the primary care setting and are therefore beyond the scope of this chapter.

Reference ranges for normal TCO_2 levels, as shown in Table 10.19, vary depending on age (Loh and Metz 2015; Noone and Langlois 2017). Normal TCO_2 in infants is lower than in adults, averaging 22 mEq/L, due to the decreased ability

of the neonatal proximal tubule to reabsorb HCO_3 (Baum and Quigley 1995; Quigley 2012).

Serum TCO_2, which roughly represents the body's metabolic acid-base balance, is reduced in the presence of acidosis and elevated in alkalosis. When acidosis is discovered, the next step for the clinician is to determine the serum anion gap. The differentials for metabolic acidosis in pediatric patients are broad and are frequently characterized by their anion gap. Calculating a serum anion gap assists the clinician in developing an appropriate differential diagnosis list to guide diagnosis and management further.

Key Learning About Total CO_2

- Total CO_2 levels a few points below normal may result from prolonged crying in the pediatric patient.
- RTA should be considered in a patient with persistent low TCO_2.

10.6.1.2 Serum Anion Gap

The body maintains its neutral pH status by carefully balancing the concentrations of positively charged cations and negatively charged anions. It would be impractical to measure all the various anions and cations in the body to evaluate for causes of acid-base disturbances. Fortunately, in acidosis, the serum anion gap is a simple value available to aid clinicians in diagnosis. Four of the most abundant freely circulating electrolytes in the body include the cations sodium (Na^+) and potassium (K^+) and the anions chloride (Cl^-) and bicarbonate ($HCO3^-$). The serum anion gap measures the difference between these key cations and anions to estimate the unmeasured anions contributing to the acidosis.

Serum anion gap can be calculated as follows: $(Na^+ + K^+) - (Cl^- + HCO_3^-)$. As previously noted, in the absence of arterial blood gas, TCO_2 acts as a surrogate for HCO_3. Potassium (K^+) is frequently omitted because it is a quantitatively minor component of serum electrolytes, and fluctuations in its concentration have little effect on the overall calculation (Oh and Briefel 2017). Therefore, the serum anion gap in venous blood is most frequently calculated as follows: $Na^+ - (Cl^- + TCO_2^-)$.

A normal serum anion gap is 8–16, with a mean of 12 ± 2 (Oh and Briefel 2017; Sharma et al. 2015). Reference ranges vary based on the instrument used to measure the various components; therefore, it is important to know the reference range of the analyzer when possible (Berend 2017). The nomenclature used to discuss and interpret anion gap can be confusing for expert clinicians and novice students alike. The terms "normal anion gap," "non-gap," and "hyperchloremic" have all been used to describe the same disorder of hyperchloremia and acidosis with an anion gap within normal limits. The preferred terminology, which best reflects the underlying physiology, is normal anion gap metabolic acidosis (Berend 2017). Several online anion gap calculators are available for the busy clinician to quickly calculate the anion gap while also avoiding math mistakes. MDCalc, Medscape, Omni calculator, and others are easy-to-use resources.

Because there is such a wide range of normal values, interpretation of the anion gap should include comparing the patient's baseline when possible (Ayala-Lopez and Harb 2020; Berend 2017; Kraut and Nagami 2013). Albumin and phosphate are the major unmeasured ions contributing to the anion gap (Sharma et al. 2015). While phosphate concentration has a small impact on the anion gap, hypoalbuminemia can skew results (Noone and Langlois 2017). Correction for hypoalbuminemia improves the sensitivity of the serum anion gap value, particularly in the presence of a high anion gap (Kraut and Nagami 2013). Noone and Langlois (2017) recommend correcting for hypoalbuminemia to prevent missing diagnoses by using the Figge equation, where SAG indicates serum anion gap:

$$SAG + \mathbf{0.25} \times (\text{normal albumin} - \text{measured albumin}\left(g/\mathbf{L}\right)$$

OR

$$SAG + \mathbf{2.5} \times (\text{normal albumin} - \text{measured albumin}\left(g/\mathbf{dL}\right)$$

The above-noted online anion gap calculators are readily available, easy to use, and correct for abnormal albumin levels. In the setting of pathology, it is more common to see an increased anion gap versus a decreased gap because organic and inorganic anions typically accumulate in the blood in pathologic states. Table 10.20 lists the common causes of acidosis with both a normal anion gap and an elevated anion gap encountered in pediatric primary care.

Table 10.20 Common causes of metabolic acidosis encountered in pediatric primary care

Acidosis with normal anion gap	Acidosis with increased anion gap
Gastrointestinal loss of bicarbonate	Lactic acidosis
• Diarrhea	• Tissue hypoxia
• Loss of gastric secretions	• Excessive
Medications	muscular activity
• Acidifying agents: Sodium chloride, potassium chloride, enteral supplements	• Inborn errors of metabolism
• Magnesium chloride	Ketoacidosis
• Cholestyramine	• Fasting or
• Spironolactone	starving state
Renal retention of hydrogen	• Diabetic
• Distal (type 1) RTA	ketoacidosis
Renal loss of bicarbonate	Toxic ingestions
• Proximal (type 2) RTA	• Methanol
• Hyperparathyroidism Hypoaldosteronisms	• Ethanol, ethylene glycol
• Hyperkalemic (type 4) RTA iatrogenic saline infusion	• Salicylates
	• Iron, isoniazid
	Renal failure
	• Uremia

Adapted from Berend (2017), Nitu et al. (2011)

The child with RTA presents with a normal anion gap metabolic acidosis. From a pathophysiologic perspective, the patient with RTA cannot acidify their urine, resulting in a decreased serum TCO2. The body compensates by increasing serum chloride to maintain a normal pH. RTA is reflected in the diagnostic laboratory studies as hyperchloremia, decreased TCO_2, and a normal anion gap.

Diarrhea is the most common cause of normal anion gap metabolic acidosis among children, and the clinician must take care to exclude this differential when considering RTA. RTA should also be considered in children who present with persistent acidosis and poor growth. Renal performance in isolated RTA is otherwise unaffected, and glomerular filtration rate is typically within normal limits (Santos et al. 2017; Santos et al. 2015; Yaxley and Pirrone 2016); however, RTA may be accompanied by other renal pathology (Yaxley and Pirrone 2016).

Key Learning about Mild Acidosis
- Anion gap should be calculated in the presence of acidosis to narrow differentials and further guide diagnosis and management.
- The anion gap is calculated as $Na - (Cl + TCO_2)$.
- Diarrhea is the most common cause of normal anion gap metabolic acidosis in children.
- The child with RTA presents with a normal anion gap metabolic acidosis.

10.6.1.3　Urine pH

Urine pH reflects the concentration of hydrogen ions in the urine and measures the urinary acidification mechanism in the distal tubule (Sharma et al. 2015). The test is frequently obtained via routine urinalysis, the mechanics of which are discussed in Sect. 10.2.1.1. While the gold standard for assessment of pH is measurement via pH electrodes, dipsticks are frequently used because they are convenient, easy to use, and cost-effective (Berend 2017).

Urinary pH varies greatly depending on the body's acid-base balance and usually ranges from 5.0 to 8.0. In the metabolically acidotic state, patients with normal renal function and intact urinary acidification systems will excrete hydrogen into their urine and generate a urinary pH <5.3 to restore a neutral plasma pH. Those with RTA, in the setting of metabolic acidosis, will be unable to acidify their urine and instead produce abnormally alkaline urine suggested by a urine pH >5.3 (Sharma et al. 2015; Yaxley and Pirrone 2016).

Although dipsticks are readily available in the primary care setting, their limitations in evaluating pH should be noted. The pH values of standard dipsticks range from 5.0 to 8.5 or 9.0, but significant deviations from the true pH have been observed for values below 5.5 and above 7.6 (Delanghe and Speeckaert 2016). It is essential to keep this in mind when evaluating urine pH in the setting of RTA. Analysis with a pH meter in certain circumstances may be warranted (Berend 2017).

Urine pH as a diagnostic value is relatively limited as it is affected by many factors, including time of day, prandial state, medications, various illness states, and diet, among others. Indeed, urine pH is a poor diagnostic tool in diagnosing RTA when used alone (Yaxley and Pirrone 2016). Recent research, however, suggests an association between urine pH and common pathogens in children with urinary tract infections (Lai et al. 2019). In particular, infection by urea-splitting organisms is notable because these can elevate urine pH and cause a normal anion gap metabolic acidosis mimicking RTA and is further exacerbated when combined with intravascular depletion (Finer and Landau 2018; Sharma et al. 2015; Yaxley and Pirrone 2016). Obtaining a fresh, midstream, clean catch sample when possible can decrease the ability of urea-splitting microorganisms to further contaminate a standing sample as the organisms alkalinize the urine and skew results (Berend 2017). High protein diets, which acidify urine, and vegetarian diets, which produce more alkaline urine, can also alter results (Berend 2017). A fresh morning urine sample should be obtained when possible to avoid alterations in serum bicarbonate levels related to food intake (Finer and Landau 2018; Sharma et al. 2015).

Urine pH can also be greatly affected by other illness states, especially diarrhea with chronic metabolic acidosis. Diarrhea, particularly if it is chronic, can result in hypokalemia and chronic metabolic acidosis. In this state, the body shifts potassium out of cells and moves hydrogen and sodium inside. In response to this, the kidneys secrete hydrogen and increase the secretion of ammonia into the urine. The ammonia binds with the regularly secreted hydrogen-producing urine with a pH >5.5 despite the proper function of the urinary acidification system. The findings of metabolic acidosis, alkaline urine, and hypokalemia

suggest distal (type 1) RTA. Administration of potassium arrests this process, and the urine then becomes appropriately acidic, excluding RTA (Yaxley and Pirrone 2016).

Regarding RTA, it is also important to note that urine pH is of limited utility in children with proximal (type 2) RTA, particularly when TCO_2 rises above 17 mEq/L (Finer and Landau 2018).

Key Learning about Urine pH
- A fresh, midstream, clean catch sample should be obtained in the morning for the most accurate results.
- Dipsticks are limited in evaluating pH, particularly if below 5.5 and above 7.6. Measurement via pH electrode versus dipstick may be warranted for the most accurate results.

10.6.2 Real-Life Example

A 23-month-old was seen for a well visit for the first time after 1 year. The family reported that they were concerned about her weight as she had only gained 2 pounds over the past year. They reported a picky appetite, but she had good days when the mother said, "She ate more than she usually did." The rest of her history was unremarkable, and her development was normal. She was bilingual but spoke in sentences in both languages. The child's physical exam was unremarkable except for a height, weight, and weight-for-height less than the fifth percentile. A CBC and metabolic profile were ordered. Her CBC showed a very mild iron deficiency, and the metabolic profile was remarkable for a CO_2 of 13 with a normal anion gap. The mother denied prolonged crying during the venipuncture. A repeat metabolic profile was done, along with a urinalysis. The CO_2 was again 13 with a normal anion gap, and her urine pH was 8. A referral to nephrology was made, and the diagnosis of RTA, type 1, was confirmed. The child was placed on Bicitra with marked improvement in her failure to thrive.

10.7 Evaluation of the Child with Edema

Edema, the excess accumulation of interstitial fluid in the body, is associated with a wide variety of pathologic states. It can present as a localized fluid collection or a generalized accumulation, typically referred to as anasarca. Differential diagnoses for edema, a selection of which can be seen listed in Table 10.21, are extensive and represent various organ systems and degrees of illness severity. Edema can develop due to increased hydrostatic capillary pressure, as seen in congestive heart failure, or decreased plasma protein concentration, as seen in nephrotic syndrome.

Initial evaluation of the child who presents with edema requires a focused but thorough evaluation. First, acute life-threatening conditions such as anaphylaxis and angioedema threatening airway patency must be excluded. Once excluded, the clinician should complete a history and physical examination to determine the character of the edema, associated symptoms and physical exam findings, and notable historical findings. The patient who presents with edema and findings concerning hypertension should prompt the clinician to evaluate the urine for proteinuria and consider nephrotic syndrome (NS) as a differential diagnosis.

10.7.1 Nephrotic Syndrome

The classic presentation of NS is a child aged 3–9 years with a chief complaint of sudden-onset gravity-dependent edema; however, children can present at any age (Andolino and Reid-Adam 2015). Periorbital edema, a classic finding that typically presents as worse in the morning and improves throughout the day, might be mistaken for seasonal allergies (Andolino and Reid-Adam 2015; Wang and Greenbaum 2019). After ambulation, edema becomes more prominent in the lower extremities and may also be notable in the penis and scrotum of males or the labia of females. Although edema is thought of as a classic presenting symptom, some patients may only present with significant proteinuria (Andolino and Reid-Adam 2015). History might reveal a recent illness, such as an upper respiratory tract infection (Andolino and Reid-Adam 2015). Hypertension might also be present (Wang and Greenbaum 2019).

NS can be classified as a clinical entity in several different ways: age of presentation, genetic versus acquired, primary versus secondary, histologic findings on biopsy, and response to steroid therapy. The age at which the child presents dictates the likely cause. NS that develops in the first year of life is likely genetic, while in older children, NS is likely acquired (Wang and Greenbaum 2019). Primary NS exists in the absence of systemic disease, while secondary NS is associated with a systemic disease. Histologic classifications include minimal change disease (MCD), focal segmental glomerulosclerosis (FSGS), membranoproliferative glomerulonephritis (MPGN), and membranous nephropathy (MN) (Wang and Greenbaum 2019). The primary pathophysiologic mechanism is an injury to the

Table 10.21 Common causes of edema in children

Localized	Generalized
Angioedema	*Sepsis*
Lymphedema	*Cardiovascular*
Venous thrombosis/ obstruction	• Congestive heart failure
	• Congenital heart disease
Pleural effusions	• Acquired heart disease
Ascites	(cardiomyopathy, myocarditis,
Response to tissue injury	etc.)
	• Arteriovenous malformations
	Hematologic
	• Severe anemia
	• Kasabach-Merritt syndrome
	Endocrine
	• Hypothyroidism
	• Severe thyrotoxicosis
	Renal
	• Nephrotic syndrome
	• Tubulointerstitial disease
	• Glomerulonephritis
	• Renal failure
	Hepatic
	• Liver failure
	• Metabolic disease
	Gastrointestinal
	• Kwashiorkor malnutrition
	• Protein-losing enteropathy
	Dermatologic
	• Severe burns

Adapted from Pomeranz et al. (2016a)

podocyte and glomeruli (Ding and Saleem 2012; Greenbaum et al. 2012).

Most children with NS between 2 and 7 years of age have a primary idiopathic disease. In these children, biopsy most commonly reveals MCD, and they go on to be responsive to steroid treatment. Frequently, MCD is presumed, and treatment with steroids proceeds without biopsy. The patient is monitored for proteinuria, and MCD is confirmed if a response is seen to steroids. Older children and adolescents are more likely to have primary FSGS, MN, and MPGN. NS is also more likely to develop in older children secondarily in the setting of systemic diseases such as sickle cell disease and systemic lupus erythematosus, infections such as hepatitis B and C, exposure to medications such as nonsteroidal anti-inflammatories, and malignancies (Andolino and Reid-Adam 2015).

Regardless of the specific etiology or histopathologic findings, all forms of NS involve an increased glomerular permeability to proteins resulting in the classic constellation of laboratory findings: proteinuria, hypoalbuminemia, and hyperlipidemia. Additional laboratory findings associated with NS of note to the clinician include renal function assessment via glomerular filtration rate (GFR), vitamin D studies, and evidence of anemia and thrombocytosis on the complete blood count (CBC).

Several diagnostic tests aid the clinician in caring for the patient with possible nephrotic syndrome. The tests are used to evaluate the patient with possible nephrotic syndrome are outlined below:

10.7.1.1   Serum Albumin

Albumin, the most abundant protein in normal plasma, usually constitutes approximately two-thirds of total plasma protein (McPherson 2017). It is responsible for storing amino acids for incorporation into other proteins and acts as a general transport or carrier protein throughout the body. As one of the largest molecules in plasma, it is the main determinant of colloid oncotic pressure. Low albumin levels in the vasculature trigger fluid accumulation in the inter-

stitial space and the clinical manifestation of edema (McPherson 2017).

Measurement of albumin, often paired with total protein measurement, is frequently conducted as part of a routine serum chemistry profile. Clinicians also commonly obtain albumin as a component of a test panel, such as a comprehensive metabolic or hepatic panel, where it is paired with total protein or a renal function panel. Serum albumin levels are used to evaluate and monitor renal and hepatic disease, assess nutritional status, and monitor some electrolytes and medications. The patient who presents to pediatric primary care with edema, particularly if it is periorbital and/or dependent in nature, should prompt the clinician to obtain an albumin level to evaluate NS.

Albumin is measured in the serum via electrophoresis, where it binds with high affinity to cationic dyes, frequently bromocresol green and bromocresol purple (Pincus et al. 2017). Normal albumin levels by age and sex can be seen using both dyes in Tables 10.22 and 10.23. Interpretation of albumin levels is rather straightforward and based on reference values. Hypoalbuminemia is a

Table 10.22 Serum albumin reference values by age and sex using bromocresol green

Age	Serum albumin value (g/dL)	
	Females	Males
0 to 14 days	3.2–4.6	3.2–4.6
15 days to <1 year	2.6–5.3	2.6–5.3
1 to <8 years	3.8–4.7	3.8–4.7
8 to <15 years	4.1–4.9	4.1–4.9
15 to <19 years	3.9–4.9	4.1–5.2

Adapted with permission from Oxford Press from Colantonio et al. (2012)

Table 10.23 Serum albumin reference values by age and sex using bromocresol purple

Age	Serum albumin value (g/dL)	
	Females	Males
0 to 14 days	2.6–4.2	2.6–4.2
15 days to <1 year	2.1–4.7	2.1–4.7
1 to <8 years	3.5–4.6	3.5–4.6
8 to <15 years	3.7–4.7	3.7–4.7
15 to <19 years	3.5–4.9	3.7–5

Adapted with permission from Oxford Press from Colantonio et al. (2012)

key diagnostic criterion for NS, and guidelines from the KDIGO Work Group define albumin levels in NS as <2.5 mg/L (Gipson et al. 2009; Lombel et al. 2013).

Although elevated serum albumin levels are infrequently encountered, they can be seen in conditions with decreased plasma water, such as dehydration or the setting of a high-protein diet (Mutlu et al. 2006). Decreased albumin levels are much more common and clinically relevant. Conditions classically associated with hypoalbuminemia include NS and protein-losing enteropathy (Al Balushi and Mackie 2019). Hypoalbuminemia has also long been associated with poor nutrition in children. Clinicians have been using decreased albumin levels as markers for malnutrition for some time, but this practice is not recommended. Albumin falls in critical and chronic illness settings due to inflammation (Gabay and Kushner 1999), not necessarily because of malnutrition. In a 2020 White Paper, the American Society of Parental and Enteral Nutrition states that "serum albumin and prealbumin…should not be used as nutrition markers" (Evans et al. 2020). While no longer clinically relevant in terms of malnutrition assessment, decreased levels of albumin have been shown to have predictive value in outcomes for critically ill children (Leite et al. 2016) and adults (Touma and Bisharat 2019), likely in part due to albumin's relationship with inflammation.

> **Key Learning about Albumin**
> - Hypoalbuminemia is a poor marker for nutritional status.
> - Albumin level < 2.5 mg/L is consistent with NS when paired with hyperlipidemia and proteinuria.

10.7.1.2 Renal Function

Accurate, precise, and efficient assessment of renal function in children is essential to identify early acute kidney injury (AKI), monitor nephrotoxic medications, ensure safe administration of contrast-enhanced imaging, and stage and monitor chronic kidney disease (CKD). The pediatric clinician is most likely to encounter these measurements in managing children with chronic renal conditions.

Glomerular filtration rate (GFR), generally considered the best indicator of renal function, is commonly used in children (Levey 2015; Mian and Schwartz 2017; Noone and Langlois 2017). "Conceptually, it represents the volume of plasma that can be completely cleared of a substance per unit of time" (Mian and Schwartz 2017). Measurement of GFR requires introducing a substance, either endogenous or exogenous, which then undergoes renal filtration. While the "gold standard" substance of GFR measurement is the exogenous starch inulin, the measurement process with this substance requires a continuous infusion of the agent with frequent blood draws and urinary catheter placement for evaluation. The test is cumbersome, particularly in pediatric patients, making it of little use in the inpatient setting, let alone primary care. Instead, GFR is typically estimated using predictive formulas and endogenous markers that are primarily cleared by the kidneys, typically urea, creatinine, and cystatin C (Levey 2015).

As previously stated, creatinine is generated at a relatively constant rate via muscle metabolism, and, in the setting of normal renal function, its excretion is almost equal to its production. The Schwartz formula uses this relationship between muscle mass, reflected by body length, and the relatively stable rate of metabolism and production of creatinine to estimate GFR (eGFR) (Noone and Langlois 2017). The Schwartz formula was initially developed in the 1970s by Schwartz, Haycock, Edelmann, Spitzer (Schwartz et al. 1976), and Counahan (Counahan et al. 1976). The formula was updated in 2009 to reflect advancements in the laboratory measurement of serum creatinine (Schwartz et al. 2009). To date, it is the most widely used method of assessing kidney function in children (Mian and Schwartz 2017). Box 10.2 shows the revised or "bedside" Schwartz formula to calculate eGFR which is as follows, where Scr indicates serum creatinine level:

> **Box 10.2 Schwartz Formula**
> eGFR (ml/min/1.73 m²) = **36.2** × [(height (cm)/Scr (**mmol/L**)].
>   OR
> eGFR (ml/min/1.73 m2) = **0.413** × [(height (cm)/Scr (**mg/dL**)].

It is important to note that GFR is a "dynamic variable" that can vary significantly based upon age, gender, body size, hydration status, protein consumption, and activity levels (Mian and Schwartz 2017). The revised Schwartz formula accounts for body size, but values should be interpreted through the lens of these other variables, especially age. GFR at birth is particularly low, ~20 mL/min/1.73 m², and increases until reaching adult levels of ~120 mL/min/1.73 m² by 2 years of age (Heilbron et al. 1991). GFR is also typically higher in males than females (Pasala and Carmody 2017). Normal GFR values for age can be seen in Table 10.24.

Assessment of GFR has several important clinical applications, particularly for the evaluation of renal disease. GFR that falls outside the normal range expected for age and/or gender should prompt the primary care clinician to refer to nephrology for further guidance. Most renal pathologies that the primary care clinician will encounter, such as NS and RTA, generally have a

renal function within normal limits. Children with primary idiopathic NS do not typically experience renal dysfunction. A minority of children with MCD histology may experience moderately impaired renal function, but this is typically evidenced by elevation of serum creatinine thought to be related to intravascular volume depletion versus true glomerular damage (Meyrier and Niaudet 2018). The clinician caring for children with CKD should know that GFR is a key component in evaluating and staging CKD. The KDIGO, in their Clinical Practice Guideline for the Evaluation and Management of Chronic Kidney Disease, defines chronic kidney disease as a GFR <60 ml/min/1.73 m² (KDIGO 2013). Also of note, the Schwartz formula is most accurate in children with CKD, but it has been validated in a non-CKD population (Staples et al. 2010).

> **Key Learning about Glomerular Filtration Rate**
> • GFR is typically within normal limits in NS but should be evaluated in children with CKD.
> • GFR in children should be calculated using the revised Schwartz formula.
> • Proper GFR interpretation requires evaluating obtained values against age and/or gender norms.

10.7.1.3 Vitamin D

Vitamin D, an essential building block for bone growth, is of particular interest to the pediatric provider. Persistent, severe deficiency results in a failure of bone mineralization and presents clinically as rickets. A significant problem until the beginning of the twentieth century is that an understanding of the condition resulted in nutritional supplementation and the near disappearance of the condition. Recent studies, however, indicate that deficiency has both increased in occurrence (Misra et al. 2008) and has been associated with a wide variety of disease states, including infections (Facchini et al. 2015;

Table 10.24 Normal GFR values in children by age

Age (and sex delineation as appropriate)	Average GFR	Range
2–8 days[a]	30	17–60
4–28 days	47	26–68
37–95 days	58	30–86
1–6 months	77	39–114
6–12 months	103	49–157
12–19 months	127	62–191
2–12 years	127	89–165

With permission from Springer Nature from Heilbron et al. (1991)
[a] Term infant

Poowuttikul et al. 2013), autoimmune conditions (Alharbi 2015; Dong et al. 2013), cardiovascular diseases (de la Guía-Galipienso et al. 2020), and cancer (Heath et al. 2019). Children with NS have been found to have decreased vitamin D levels (Weng et al. 2005) and are also at further at risk for developing osteoporosis and difficulties with bone mineralization due to the frequent therapeutic use of corticosteroids (Lombel et al. 2013).

The primary circulating form of vitamin D is 25-hydroxy vitamin D (25(OH)D), which is most commonly obtained as a serum value (Banerjee et al. 2020; Herrmann et al. 2017). Vitamin D has several metabolites with biological activity, 25-hydroxy D_3 (cholecalciferol) and 25-hydroxy D_2 (ergocalciferol) being the two of the major ones. Typically, serum 25(OH)D includes measurement of a total 25(OH)D and both metabolites (Banerjee et al. 2020).

The majority of vitamin D is stored in the body bound to protein: 85–90% tightly bound to vitamin D-binding protein (VDBP), 10–15% more loosely bound to albumin, and 0.03–0.04% in its free state (Bikle et al. 2017; Herrmann et al. 2017; Schwartz et al. 2018). The vitamin D bound to VDBP is thought to be biologically inactive, and the bioavailability of the albumin-bound portion is unclear. Still, the free portion is thought to be the biologically active component (Bikle et al. 2017). Vitamin D deficiency, observed via a total 25(OH)D measurements (Nielsen et al. 2015; Weng et al. 2005), is commonly seen in children with NS. The majority of serum 25(OH)D is bound to either a vitamin D-binding protein or albumin, both of which are lost in the urine of patients with NS, and total 25(OH)D levels are low in NS relative to the degree of proteinuria (Banerjee et al. 2020), contributing to poor bone health in children with NS (Banerjee et al. 2013; Biyikli et al. 2004; Freundlich et al. 1986; Huang et al. 1992; Weng et al. 2005), and it has been suggested that supplementation with 25(OH)D can protect against the development of osteoporosis among these patients (Bak et al. 2006; Chen et al. 2015; Gulati et al. 2005).

While it is not recommended to routinely screen well children for adequate vitamin D lev-

els, the Drug and Therapeutics Committee of the Lawson Wilkins Pediatric Endocrine Society recommends screening children at risk for deficiency (Misra et al. 2008). However, determining true vitamin D deficiency can be challenging because of a lack of consensus regarding what constitutes an abnormal level. Table 10.25 describes the recommended classification of vitamin D status based on a total 25(OH)D levels from two prominent organizations: the Lawson Wilkins Pediatric Endocrine Society's 2008 recommendations on Vitamin D Deficiency in Children and Its Management (Misra et al. 2008) and the Endocrine Society's 2016 Global Consensus Recommendations for the Prevention and Management of Nutritional Rickets (Munns et al. 2016).

Clinicians should consider these results when evaluating vitamin D status in children and recommending supplementation; however, it should be noted that the interpretation of vitamin D levels in children with NS is a changing landscape. In their study evaluating the effects of vitamin D and calcium supplementation in children with steroid-sensitive NS, Banerjee et al. (2017) noted an improvement in total 25(OH)D levels but no effect on bone mineralization. Recent studies by Banerjee et al. (Banerjee et al. 2020) suggest an emerging utility for evaluating free 25(OH)D levels, as opposed to a total 25(OH)D levels, to assess for vitamin D deficiency and guide therapy in children with NS and other proteinuric diseases.

Table 10.25 Vitamin D classification in relation to 25(OH)D Levels

Classification	Lawson Wilkins Pediatric Endocrine Society (nmol/L)	Endocrine Society on the Prevention and Management of Nutritional Rickets (nmol/L)
Severe deficiency	<12.5	
Deficiency	<37.5	<30
Insufficiency	37.5–50	30–50
Sufficient	50–250	>50
Excess	>250	
Intoxication	>375	

Adapted from Misra et al. (2008), Munns et al. (2016)

The authors suggest that cutoff levels for free 25(OH)D levels be between 3.75 and 3.9 pg/mL for sufficiency and 2.85 pg/mL for deficiency (Banerjee et al. 2020). Further research in this area is required to both confirm these values and determine appropriate vitamin D supplementation dosage and regimens for children with NS.

The AAP advises against the universal screening of well children or screening of obese or dark-skinned individuals. The AAP recommends increasing the dietary intake of vitamin D with vitamin D supplements if the RDA cannot be met. If an adolescent has a chronic medical illness associated with increased fracture risk, serum 25(OH)D levels should be done (Golden and Carey 2016). There has been an increase in the identification of vitamin D deficiency.

> **Key Learning about Vitamin D**
> - Vitamin D deficiency is commonly encountered in the NS patient.
> - Consider obtaining free 25(OH)D levels to evaluate for true deficiency in the NS patient, if available.
> - Routine vitamin D levels in well children or children with obesity should not be done (Golden and Carey 2016).

10.7.1.4 Lipids

Hyperlipidemia is a characteristic finding of NS (Agrawal et al. 2018). Due to urinary loss of serum proteins such as albumin and immunoglobulins, decreased oncotic pressure causes the liver to compensate by increasing protein production and decreasing catabolism. There is also impaired clearance of lipids and lipoproteins, the latter of which are proteins that both combine with and transport fats and lipids throughout the body (Agrawal et al. 2018). Together, this increases the number of circulating lipids. An increase in the quantity of lipid, combined with further alterations in the lipid metabolic pathway (Andolino and Reid-Adam 2015), results in the characteristic hyperlipidemia associated with NS.

Table 10.26 Interpretation of lipid studies in the patient with NS

Laboratory value	Result
Total cholesterol	Elevated
HDL	Normal to reduced
LDL	Elevated
Triglycerides	Elevated
VLDL	Elevated
IDL	Elevated
Lipoprotein (a)	Elevated
Total cholesterol: HDL	Elevated

Adapted from Agrawal et al. (2018), Vaziri (2016)

Routine screening of healthy children for lipid abnormalities is not recommended (Lozano et al. 2016); however, abnormal lipid metabolism is a common finding in children with renal disease and should be assessed. Routine lipid panels typically measure total cholesterol, high-density lipoprotein (HDL), low-density lipoprotein (LDL), and triglycerides. Some laboratories may also measure very-low-density lipoprotein (VLDL), lipoprotein (a), intermediate-density lipoprotein (IDL), and the ratio of total cholesterol to HDL. Table 10.26 describes the interpretation of lipid studies in the patient with NS.

Lipid metabolism, particularly in the NS patient, is a complex process. Although beyond the scope of this chapter, it is well described in the literature (Agrawal et al. 2018; Hari et al. 2020; Vaziri 2016). Alterations involve the metabolic pathway affecting both lipids and lipoproteins. In NS, the changes in the composition of lipoproteins further mediate changes in key proteins involved in the "biosynthesis, transport, remodeling, and catabolism of lipids and lipoproteins" (Vaziri 2016). Notable alterations include the following: The coenzyme responsible for cholesterol synthesis increases while the enzyme responsible for cholesterol catabolism decreases. Laboratory studies will show elevated total cholesterol and low-density lipoprotein (LDL). In response to nephrotic range proteinuria, various tissues secrete angiopoietin-like-4, a glycoprotein that decreases the conversion of triglycerides to free fatty acids, resulting in hypertriglyceridemia (Andolino and Reid-Adam 2015). Additional alterations include the elevation of apolipoprotein B-containing lipoproteins, specifically

VLDL, IDL, and lipoprotein(a). High-density lipoprotein (HDL) levels are typically normal (Agrawal et al. 2018).

Clinically it is of note that, in NS, the degree of altered lipid metabolism parallels with the degree of proteinuria (Agrawal et al. 2018; Vaziri 2016). Also, due to hyperlipidemia, NS patients are at an increased risk for atherosclerosis, thromboembolism, and cardiovascular and renal dysfunction (Agrawal et al. 2018; Vaziri 2016), particularly those with steroid-resistant NS (Hari et al. 2020). Data describing the treatment of dyslipidemia in children with NS is limited. Lipid-lowering agents are less frequently used in the pediatric NS population than adults, owing to the lack of long-term medication safety data (Agrawal et al. 2018).

Key Learning about Lipid Profile and NS
- Hyperlipidemia is a characteristic finding in NS.
- Most components of the lipid profile are elevated, but HDL may remain normal to reduced.

10.7.1.5 CBC Changes: Anemia

Although elevated hemoglobin can be seen in patients with NS, particularly in the presence of significant edema resulting in intravascular volume depletion (41), anemia is occasionally encountered (Park and Shin 2011). While albumin is the primary protein lost in the urine, NS can lose proteins of various molecular weights, including coagulation factors, immunoglobulins, hormone-binding proteins, minerals, and macronutrients. Significant loss of any of the necessary substrate building blocks for red blood cell formation can manifest on the CBC as anemia in the patient with NS. The etiologies of the anemia in NS are varied. Those of note include deficiencies in iron, erythropoietin, copper, and vitamin B12 (cobalamin). Although prevalence data is currently lacking, anemia has been seen in children with NS, particularly those with persistent disease. The complete pathophysiologic mechanisms of anemia in the setting of normal renal

function, as is the case with most subtypes of NS, are poorly understood at present. It is suspected that many factors contribute to anemia in NS (Iorember and Aviles 2017).

Iron deficiency anemia is the most common form of anemia seen in both children and adults with NS and presents, as expected, as microcytic and hypochromic. The anemia results from urinary loss of both iron and transferrin, although significant transferrin loss alone may be sufficient to develop anemia. Studies have shown that urinary transferrin loss correlates with total urinary protein loss in both adults and children. Anemia can also develop from a clinically significant loss of erythropoietin in the urine. Children who lose erythropoietin in urine are typically responsive to supplementation with erythropoietin and iron, but they may experience a blunted response to therapy if they continue with significant proteinuria (Iorember and Aviles 2017).

Copper, which plays an essential role in erythropoiesis, is transported throughout the body via the protein ceruloplasmin. Loss of ceruloplasmin in the urine can result in anemia in the NS patient. Although not thought to be a common cause of anemia in NS patients, it should be considered if patients are refractory to anemia treatment. If suspected, serum copper levels should be obtained. Cobalamin's essential role in erythropoiesis is also well established. Both cobalamin and transcobalamin, the vitamin's transporter protein, can be lost in the urine. Cobalamin deficiency can manifest on the CBC as macrocytic anemia. Serum cobalamin levels should be obtained if this is suspected (Iorember and Aviles 2017).

Suggested diagnostic studies to evaluate for anemia in the setting of NS include a CBC, reticulocyte count, serum iron level, total iron-binding capacity, transferrin saturation, and transferrin and ferritin levels. The reticulocyte count remains a good indicator of marrow response to anemia and will be low if the anemia is due to erythropoietin, B12, folate, or copper deficiency. Children with iron deficiency anemia will also have a decreased mean corpuscular volume in addition to decreased serum iron, ferritin, and transferrin saturation. If the NS patient with iron deficiency anemia fails to respond appropriately to iron supplementation, the clinician should consider obtaining urine and serum erythropoietin levels to evaluate deficiencies further. An elevation in the mean corpuscular volume indicates macrocytic anemia and suggests a cobalamin or folate deficiency. Treatment for anemia in NS depends upon the cause; supplementation with the deficient component is usually successful (Iorember and Aviles 2017).

10.7.1.6 CBC Changes: Platelets

NS is a known risk factor for both arterial and venous thrombotic events (Eneman et al. 2016; Park and Shin 2011). Although data is limited, it is estimated that 1–27% of children with NS will experience a thrombotic event, most commonly venous in nature. The risk of developing thromboembolism increases severe proteinuria and steroid-resistant NS (Park and Shin 2011). The precise pathophysiologic mechanisms of thrombocytosis and increased thrombotic risk for patients with NS are not well understood but are thought to be multifactorial in nature. An increase in platelet count and activity, specifically aggregability and adhesiveness, is presumed to play a role (Eneman et al. 2016).

Although more variable in adults, platelet counts in children with NS are typically greater than the normal range of 150–450 10^9/L (Eneman et al. 2016). Thrombocytosis is more likely to be present early in therapy, and platelet counts return to normal when long-term remission is reached. The quantity of platelets increases as albumin decreases (Eneman et al. 2016). There is no consensus on the utility of testing platelets for specific abnormalities in the setting of NS. If done before initiation of therapy, results may show an elevated mean platelet volume and decreased platelet distribution width. Platelet activity also increases. Hepatic hyperfunction, in response to hypoalbuminemia, increases platelet-activating substances and thus platelet activity. Hypercholesteremia is also thought to play a role in increasing platelet activity (Eneman et al. 2016).

Platelet function is also affected in NS. Proteins responsible for platelet inhibition are lost in the urine. The degree of proteinuria correlates with platelet hyperaggregability and adhesiveness. Although the underlying rationale for some of these changes is understood and described in the literature, these changes are not easily demonstrated on laboratory studies. The prognostic value of platelet count for determining prognosis in NS is being explored, but further studies need to be conducted to understand better their relationship to risk factors for thrombosis in NS (Eneman et al. 2016).

10.7.2 Real-Life Example

A 2-year-old female was seen in the office with a chief complaint of "being swollen." The 19-year-old mother reported a 2-week history of fatigue, taking long naps, and a poor appetite. She thought she had a viral infection. She brought her to the office when she noticed that her fingerprint could be seen when she pressed on her ankles. She also wondered if she had been voiding less than usual. The mother reported that she had been treated for strep throat 2 weeks ago. The urinalysis showed 4+ protein in the urine. Nephrotic syndrome was considered, and the child was sent to the ED for stat laboratory diagnostic testing. The urine protein/creatinine ratio was found to be high at 7.6 (normal <0.2). The child's serum albumin was low at 2.0 g/dL, and her sodium level was also low at 130 (normal 136–145) with chloride of 96 (normal 98–107). Her total cholesterol was 334, with an LDL of 199, and her triglycerides were 331. A diagnosis of nephrotic syndrome was confirmed. The child responded to treatment.

Key Learning about NS
- Platelets are increased in NS, and anemia is a common finding.
- Hyperlipidemia is an associated finding with NS.
- Children with NS are at increased risk for thrombotic events.
- Serologic testing for infections should be considered as children with NS are susceptible to infections.

Questions

1. A 12-year-old patient is seen for a well check and a negative history except for questionable urinary frequency. Her physical exam is normal. Her urine dipstick has 1+ protein and a specific gravity of 1.020. What is the next best step for her management?
   - (a) Send urine for spot protein/creatinine ratio.
   - (b) Obtain the first-morning void and repeat the dipstick.
   - (c) Send that sample to the lab for urinalysis with microscopic analysis.
   - (d) This is a normal finding.

2. What change indicates remission in a patient with nephrotic syndrome?
   - (a) The disappearance of protein from the urine.
   - (b) Decrease in serum albumin.
   - (c) Increase in serum lipid levels.
   - (d) The disappearance of blood from the urine.

3. Which of the following is the most appropriate test to use to evaluate for persistent proteinuria in a 2-year-old patient?
   - (a) Urine dipstick.
   - (b) 24-hour urine for protein and creatinine
   - (c) Spot first-morning void for urine protein/creatinine ratio.
   - (d) Urinalysis.

4. Which of the following is a laboratory finding consistent with common idiopathic nephrotic syndrome?
   - (a) Polycythemia.
   - (b) Increased 25(OH)D levels.
   - (c) Thrombocytosis.
   - (d) A decreased glomerular filtration rate.

5. A healthy 11-year-old male presents to the office for a routine well-child visit. His medical history is significant for prematurity of 31 weeks with umbilical catheter placement. A routine annual urinalysis is completed for this patient. Which of the following results indicate that no further testing is required?

   - (a) Specific gravity of 1.010, pH 5, and 1+ protein.
   - (b) Specific gravity of 1.005, pH of 9, and 3+ protein.
   - (c) Specific gravity of 1.010, pH of 6, and no protein.
   - (d) WBC > 10,000, pH of 6, and + nitrates.

6. Which of the following would you expect to find in a patient with post-streptococcus glomerulonephritis?
   - (a) Significantly high C3 levels with improvement in 6–8 weeks.
   - (b) Transient hypercalciuria and hematuria improving in 3–6 months.
   - (c) Hematuria in the setting of normal complement levels.
   - (d) Significantly low C3 levels with improvement in 6–8 weeks.

7. In a patient with renal tubular acidosis (RTA), you would expect to see which of the following diagnostic study results?
   - (a) Increased urine pH, decreased serum bicarbonate.
   - (b) Decreased urine pH, decreased serum bicarbonate.
   - (c) Increased urine pH, increased serum bicarbonate.
   - (d) Decreased urine pH, increased serum bicarbonate.

8. An 8-year-old boy with a history of prematurity has a first-morning urinalysis yield +2 proteinuria. You obtained the first-morning urine for spot protein/creatinine ratio which results as 0.18 mg/mg protein/creatinine ratio. What do you tell his caregiver about the results?
   - (a) These results are mildly elevated. We should obtain a renal ultrasound.
   - (b) This result is within the normal range for the child's age.
   - (c) These results are low. "I'm concerned the sample may have been too diluted."
   - (d) This result is approaching the nephrotic range. "I am concerned he may have nephrotic syndrome".

9. When assessing discolored urine for blood, what is the "gold standard" to detect actual hematuria?
   (a) Microscopic examination of spun urine sediment.
   (b) Urine dipstick.
   (c) Urine culture.
   (d) Urine for reducing substances.

10. A child presents to a rural health clinic with periorbital edema and lethargy. He has no past medical history and is otherwise acting normally. Upon examination, you appreciate periorbital edema and lower extremity swelling. Which of the following laboratory results would prompt immediate nephrology referral?
    (a) Low serum albumin.
    (b) Low serum cholesterol.
    (c) High complement 4 level.
    (d) Urine protein/creatinine ratio of 0.19.

11. A 9-year-old female presents to the office with microscopic hematuria and proteinuria. Before the visit, another practitioner assumed the protein noted in the urine was from the RBC in the urine. Today a spot urine protein/creatinine ratio (U p/c) is reviewed for the patient. Which findings would be suggestive of renal disease and require a prompt referral to nephrology?
    (a) U p/c of 0.01.
    (b) U p/c of 0.3.
    (c) U p/c of 0.18.
    (d) U p/c of 0.16.

12. A 17-year-old male presents to the office with a history of alcohol and drug abuse in the past. Today he reports feeling slightly fatigued, with periorbital edema and discolored urine. He reports having had a mild "cold and cough" last week that resolved on its own. Over the past 2 days, he has been involved in a "tough runner" marathon event. He has no fever. Which of the following should the practitioner include in the laboratory evaluation?
    (a) White blood count.
    (b) Serum IgA.
    (c) Urinalysis for nitrates.
    (d) Liver function test.

Questions 13 and 14 are based on the following scenario:

A 3-year-old female presents for evaluation with a 2-day history of vomiting and diarrhea. She has otherwise been growing and developing normally. You obtain a set of serum electrolytes, with results as follows:

Laboratory value	Result
Sodium (mmoL/L)	134
Potassium (mmoL/L)	5.1
Chloride (mmoL/L)	109
TCO$_2$ (mmoL/L)	12

Use the reference values and information provided in the chapter to answer the following questions.

13. What is her serum anion gap?
    (a) 10
    (b) 12
    (c) 13
    (d) 15

14. What is your interpretation of these laboratory results?
    (a) She has pseudohyperkalemia and an increased anion gap. This is likely related to tourniquet placement and/or inadequate venipuncture.
    (b) She has increased TCO$_2$ and a normal anion gap metabolic alkalosis. This is most likely due to prolonged crying during venipuncture.
    (c) She has decreased TCO$_2$ and an increased anion gap metabolic acidosis, most likely due to renal tubular acidosis.
    (d) She has decreased TCO$_2$ and a normal gap metabolic acidosis, which is consistent with her history of vomiting and diarrhea.

Rationale

1. Answer: b
   It is important to evaluate for orthostatic proteinuria in this patient. The next best step for this patient is to obtain a dipstick after being in a recumbent position, which would be best done after sleeping. If proteinuria were present on the first-morning void, the

urine protein/creatinine ratio would be the next best step. Urinalysis with microscopic analysis would be more appropriate for evaluating red blood cells, white blood cells, casts, crystals, and bacteria. If the specific gravity is >1.030, trace or + 1 of protein is likely a false positive.

2. Answer: a

Nephrotic syndrome is characterized by proteinuria, hypoalbuminemia, and hyperlipidemia; therefore, the disappearance of proteinuria indicates disease remission. A decrease in serum albumin would suggest the continued presence of disease. Serum lipid levels increase in nephrotic syndrome; therefore, an increase in serum lipid levels would not indicate remission. Blood is typically not present in the urine in nephrotic syndrome.

3. Answer: c

Although the "gold standard test" for evaluating for proteinuria is a 24-hour collection and evaluation (Kamińska et al. 2020), this is difficult to do in many pediatric patients. A spot first-morning void for urine protein/creatinine ratio is the most appropriate test. A spot first-morning void for albumin/creatinine ratio would also be appropriate. Urine dipstick and laboratory urinalysis can tell the presence of protein in the urine but do not measure creatinine are unable to do the necessary quantitative analysis of protein and creatinine.

4. Answer: c

In addition to the classic laboratory manifestations of nephrotic syndrome, children can also experience anemia (Park and Shin 2011) and decreased vitamin D levels (Weng et al. 2005). Children with nephrotic syndrome, specifically the most common primary idiopathic form, typically do not experience renal dysfunction (Meyrier and Niaudet 2018). Children with nephrotic syndrome are at increased risk for clotting due to thrombocytosis, especially early in therapy, and return to normal once remission is reached (Eneman et al. 2016). Thrombocytosis is, therefore, consistent with nephrotic syndrome.

5. Answer: c

Recall, routine urinalysis in the pediatric well-child visit is recommended only for specific patients. This patient will have annual urinalysis secondary to his prematurity and umbilical lines. Urinalysis results that show any amount of protein, as in choices A and B, should be evaluated with a first-morning void for the protein/creatinine ratio. The urinalysis that reveals signs of infection such as elevated WBCs and nitrates, as in choice D, needs to be sent for microscopy and culture.

6. Answer: d

In patients with confirmed post-streptococcal glomerulonephritis, serum complement 3 is usually reduced. It often takes 6–8 weeks for the C3 level to normalize.

7. Answer: a

Regardless of the subtype, all forms of RTA result in net acidification of the blood and alkalinization of the urine. This is evident in diagnostic studies as increased urine pH and decreased serum bicarbonate.

8. Answer: b

The normal range for spot protein/creatinine ratio in children greater than 2 years of age is less than 0.2 mg/mg protein/creatinine (Ranch 2020; Kamińska et al. 2020).

9. Answer: a

The urinalysis via dipstick is a practical and cost-effective test in primary care offices; however, it cannot be replaced with microscopic analysis. Dipstick results cannot differentiate between the number of RBCs when a dipstick reveals 0–3+ blood (Viteri and Reid-Adam 2018).

10. Answer: a

Children with nephrotic syndrome often present to the office with facial swelling, which is mistaken for allergies, and this patient also has lower extremity swelling. The laboratory finding most suggestive of advanced kidney involvement is the low serum albumin. This patient needs a prompt referral for the management of the presumed nephrotic syndrome. In nephrotic syndrome, serum cholesterol would be elevated. Low serum cholesterol suggests another etiology for his symptoms.

11. Answer: b

When hematuria and/or proteinuria is noted in an isolated event, the findings are not as concerning as when hematuria and proteinuria are combined. The spot U p/c is the most frequent and reliable test when assessing a pediatric patient. A level greater than 0.2 is suggestive of renal disease.

12. Answer: b

IgA nephropathy is noted in children older than 10 years of age. It is often accompanied by micro−/macroscopic hematuria post an infectious process. Elevated serum IgA will assist in the proper management of this patient. The history of extreme exercise might lead a practitioner to believe the protein and/or blood is from rhabdomyolysis; however, with the physical findings suggestive of nephrotic syndrome, one must consider IgA nephropathy as well.

13. Answer: b

The serum anion gap is calculated as follows: sodium − (chloride + TCO$_2$). For this patient, that would be 134 − (109 + 12), which comes to 12.

14. Answer: d

This patient has sodium, potassium, and chloride levels within normal limits for her age. Her TOC$_2$ is decreased, consistent with metabolic acidosis, and should prompt the clinician to calculate a serum anion gap. Her serum anion gap, as previously calculated, is 12. This is normal. Vomiting and diarrhea are the most common cause of normal anion gap acidosis in the pediatric patient, which is consistent with this patient's history. If she had prolonged crying during venipuncture, the clinician would expect her TCO$_2$ to be slightly decreased. Her TCO$_2$ is significantly decreased and suggestive of a pathologic process. While renal tubular acidosis should be considered in this patient, her history of vomiting and diarrhea makes this diagnosis less likely.

References

Agrawal S, Zaritsky JJ, Fornoni A, Smoyer WE. Dyslipidaemia in nephrotic syndrome: mechanisms and treatment. Nat Rev Nephrol. 2018;14(1):57–70.

Al Balushi A, Mackie AS. Protein-losing enteropathy following Fontan palliation. Can J Cardiol. 2019;35(12):1857–60.

Alexander RT, Bitzan M. Renal tubular acidosis. Pediatr Clin N Am. 2019;66(1):135–57.

Alharbi FM. Update in vitamin D and multiple sclerosis. Neurosciences (Riyadh). 2015;20(4):329–35.

Andolino TP, Reid-Adam J. Nephrotic syndrome. Pediatr Rev. 2015;36(3):117–25. quiz 26, 29

Ayala-Lopez N, Harb R. Interpreting anion gap values in adult and pediatric patients: examining the reference interval. J Appl Lab Med. 2020;5(1):126–35.

Bak M, Serdaroglu E, Guclu R. Prophylactic calcium and vitamin D treatments in steroid-treated children with nephrotic syndrome. Pediatr Nephrol. 2006;21(3):350–4.

Banerjee S, Basu S, Akhtar S, Sinha R, Sen A, Sengupta J. Free vitamin D levels in steroid-sensitive nephrotic syndrome and healthy controls. Pediatr Nephrol. 2020;35(3):447–54.

Banerjee S, Basu S, Sen A, Sengupta J. The effect of vitamin D and calcium supplementation in pediatric steroid-sensitive nephrotic syndrome. Pediatr Nephrol. 2017;32(11):2063–70.

Banerjee S, Basu S, Sengupta J. Vitamin D in nephrotic syndrome remission: a case-control study. Pediatr Nephrol. 2013;28(10):1983–9.

Baum M. Pediatric glomerular diseases. Curr Opin Pediatr. 2008;20(2):137–9.

Baum M, Quigley R. Ontogeny of proximal tubule acidification. Kidney Int. 1995;48(6):1697–704.

Berend K. Review of the diagnostic evaluation of normal anion gap metabolic acidosis. Kidney Dis (Basel). 2017;3(4):149–59.

Bianchetti MG, Simonetti GD, Lava SAG, Bettinelli A. Differential diagnosis and management of Fluid, electrolyte, and acid-base disorders. In: Geary DF, Schaefer F, editors. Pediatric kidney disease. Berlin, Heidelberg: Springer Berlin/Heidelberg; 2017. p. 825–82.

Bikle DD, Malmstroem S, Schwartz J. Current controversies: are free vitamin metabolite levels a more accurate assessment of vitamin D status than total levels? Endocrinol Metab Clin N Am. 2017;46(4):901–18.

Biyikli NK, Emre S, Sirin A, Bilge I. Biochemical bone markers in nephrotic children. Pediatr Nephrol. 2004;19(8):869–73.

Brown DD, Reidy KJ. Approach to the child with Hematuria. Pediatr Clin N Am. 2019;66(1):15–30.

Chan JCM, Scheinman JI, Roth KS. Consultation with the specialist: renal tubular acidosis. Pediatr Rev. 2001;22(8):277.

Chaudhari PP, Monuteaux MC, Bachur RG. Urine concentration and pyuria for identifying UTI in infants. Pediatrics. 2016;138(5):e20162370.

Chen Y, Wan JX, Jiang DW, Fu BB, Cui J, Li GF, et al. Efficacy of calcitriol in treating glucocorticoid induced osteoporosis in patients with nephrotic syndrome: an open-label, randomized controlled study. Clin Nephrol. 2015;84(5):262–9.

Cobbaert CM, Baadenhuijsen H, Weykamp CW. Prime time for enzymatic creatinine methods in pediatrics. Clin Chem. 2009;55(3):549–58.

Colantonio DA, Kyriakopoulou L, Chan MK, Daly CH, Brinc D, Venner AA, et al. Closing the gaps in pediatric laboratory reference intervals: a CALIPER database of 40 biochemical markers in a healthy and multiethnic population of children. Clin Chem. 2012;58(5):854–68.

Costa A, Curro G, Pellegrino S, Lucanto MC, Tuccari G, Ieni A, Visalli G, Magazzu G, Santoro D. Case report on pathogenetic link between gluten and IgA nephropathy. BMC Gastroenterol. 2018;18(1):64.

Counahan R, Chantler C, Ghazali S, Kirkwood B, Rose F, Barratt TM. Estimation of glomerular filtration rate from plasma creatinine concentration in children. Arch Dis Child. 1976;51(11):875–8.

Cyriac J, Holden K, Tullus K. How to use urine dipsticks. Arch Dis Child Educ Pract Ed. 2017;102(3):148–54.

Daly K, Farrington E. Hypokalemia and hyperkalemia in infants and children: pathophysiology and treatment. J Pediatr Health Care. 2013;27(6):486–96. quiz 97-8

Davenport M, Mach KE, Shortliffe LMD, Banaei N, Wang TH, Liao JC. New and developing diagnostic technologies for urinary tract infections. Nat Rev Urol. 2017;14(5):296–310.

de la Guía-Galipienso F, Martínez-Ferran M, Vallecillo N, Lavie CJ, Sanchis-Gomar F, Pareja-Galeano H. Vitamin D and cardiovascular health. Clin Nutr. 2020;29:S0261-5614(20)30700-7.

Delanaye P, Cavalier E, Pottel H. Serum creatinine: not so simple! Nephron. 2017;136(4):302–8.

Delanghe JR, Speeckaert MM. Preanalytics in urinalysis. Clin Biochem. 2016;49(18):1346–50.

Desai DJ, Gilbert B, McBride CA. Paediatric urinary tract infections: diagnosis and treatment. Aust Fam Physician. 2016;45(8):558–63.

Ding WY, Saleem MA. Current concepts of the podocyte in nephrotic syndrome. Kidney Res Clin Pract. 2012;31(2):87–93.

Doern CD, Richardson SE. Diagnosis of urinary tract infections in children. J Clin Microbiol. 2016;54(9):2233–42.

Dong JY, Zhang WG, Chen JJ, Zhang ZL, Han SF, Qin LQ. Vitamin D intake and risk of type 1 diabetes: a meta-analysis of observational studies. Nutrients. 2013;5(9):3551–62.

Eneman B, Levtchenko E, van den Heuvel B, Van Geet C, Freson K. Platelet abnormalities in nephrotic syndrome. Pediatr Nephrol. 2016;31(8):1267–79.

Evans DC, Corkins MR, Malone A, Miller S, Mogensen KM, Guenter P, et al. The use of visceral proteins as nutrition markers: an ASPEN position paper. Nutr Clin Pract. 2020;

Facchini L, Venturini E, Galli L, de Martino M, Chiappini E. Vitamin D and tuberculosis: a review on a hot topic. J Chemother. 2015;27(3):128–38.

Filice CE, Green JC, Rosenthal MS, Ross JS. Pediatric screening urinalysis: a difference-in-differences analysis of how a 2007 change in guidelines impacted use. BMC Pediatr. 2014;14:260.

Finer G, Landau D. Clinical approach to proximal renal tubular acidosis in children. Adv Chronic Kidney Dis. 2018;25(4):351–7.

Flynn JTKD, Baker-Smith CM, et al. Subcommittee on Screening and Management of High Blood Pressure in Children. Clinical Practice Guideline for Screening and Management of High Blood Pressure in Children and Adolescents. Pediatrics. 2018;142(3).

Foreman JW. Fanconi syndrome. Pediatr Clin N Am. 2019;66(1):159–67.

Freundlich M, Bourgoignie JJ, Zilleruelo G, Abitbol C, Canterbury JM, Strauss J. Calcium and vitamin D metabolism in children with nephrotic syndrome. J Pediatr. 1986;108(3):383–7.

Fritzenwanker M, Imirzalioglu C, Chakraborty T, Wagenlehner FM. Modern diagnostic methods for urinary tract infections. Expert Rev Anti Infect Ther. 2016;14(11):1047–63.

Gabay C, Kushner I. Acute-phase proteins and other systemic responses to inflammation. N Engl J Med. 1999;340(6):448–54.

Gipson DS, Massengill SF, Yao L, Nagaraj S, Smoyer WE, Mahan JD, et al. Management of childhood onset nephrotic syndrome. Pediatrics. 2009;124(2):747–57.

Glatstein M, Carbell G, Boddu SK, Bernardini A, Scolnik D. The changing clinical presentation of hypertrophic pyloric stenosis: the experience of a large, tertiary care pediatric hospital. Clin Pediatr. 2011;50(3):192–5.

Golden NH, Carey DE. Vitamin D in Health and Disease in Adolescents: When to Screen, Whom to Treat, and How to Treat. Adolesc Med State Art Rev. 2016;27(1):125–39.

Greenbaum LA. Electrolyte and acid-base disorders. In: Kleigman RM, St Geme JW, Blum NJ, Shah SS, Tasker RC, Wilson KM, editors. Nelson textbook of pediatrics. Philadelphia, PA: Elsevier; 2020. p. 389–425.e1.

Greenbaum LA, Benndorf R, Smoyer WE. Childhood nephrotic syndrome—current and future therapies. Nat Rev Nephrol. 2012;8(8):445–58.

Guh JY. Proteinuria versus albuminuria in chronic kidney disease. Nephrology (Carlton). 2010;15(Suppl 2):53–6.

Gulati K, McAddo SP. Anti-glomerular basement membrane disease. Rheum Dis Clin N Am. 2018;44(4):651–73.

Gulati S, Sharma RK, Gulati K, Singh U, Srivastava A. Longitudinal follow-up of bone mineral density in children with nephrotic syndrome and the role of calcium and vitamin D supplements. Nephrol Dial Transplant. 2005;20(8):1598–603.

Hanudel MR, Salusky IB. Treatment of pediatric chronic kidney disease-mineral and bone disorder. Curr Osteoporos Rep. 2017;15(3):198–206.

Hari P, Khandelwal P, Smoyer WE. Dyslipidemia and cardiovascular health in childhood nephrotic syndrome. Pediatr Nephrol. 2020;35(9):1601–19.

Heath AK, Hodge AM, Ebeling PR, Eyles DW, Kvaskoff D, Buchanan DD, et al. Circulating 25-Hydroxyvitamin D concentration and risk of breast, prostate, and colorectal cancers: the Melbourne Collaborative Cohort Study. Cancer Epidemiol Biomark Prev. 2019;28(5):900–8.

Hechanova LA. Renal tubular acidosis. 2020. retrieved from https://www.merckmanuals.com/professional/genitourinary-disorders/renal-transport-abnormalities/renal-tubular-acidosis

Heilbron DC, Holliday MA, al-Dahwi A, Kogan BA. Expressing glomerular filtration rate in children. Pediatr Nephrol. 1991;5(1):5–11.

Herrmann M, Farrell C-JL, Pusceddu I, Fabregat-Cabello N, Cavalier E. Assessment of vitamin D status—a changing landscape. Clin Chem Lab Med (CCLM). 2017;55(1):3–26.

Hewitt I, Montini G. Vesicoureteral reflux is it important to find? Pediatr Nephrol. 2021;36(4):1011–7.

Hoxha TF, Azemi M, Avdiu M, Ismaili-Jaha V, Grajqevci V, Petrela E. The usefulness of clinical and laboratory parameters for predicting severity of dehydration in children with acute gastroenteritis. Med Arch. 2014;68(5):304–7.

Huang JP, Bai KM, Wang BL. Vitamin D and calcium metabolism in children with nephrotic syndrome of normal renal function. Chin Med J. 1992;105(10):828–32.

Iorember F, Aviles D. Anemia in nephrotic syndrome: approach to evaluation and treatment. Pediatr Nephrol. 2017;32(8):1323–30.

Joyce E, Glasner P, Ranganathan S, Swiatecka-Urban A. Tubulointerstitial nephritis: diagnosis, treatment, and monitoring. Pediatr Nephrol. 2017;32(4):577–87.

KDOQI. K/DOQI clinical practice guidelines for bone metabolism and disease in chronic kidney disease. Am J Kidney Dis. 2003;42(4 Suppl 3):S1–201.

Kamińska J, Dymicka-Piekarska V, Tomaszewska J, Matowicka-Karna J, Koper-Lenkiewicz OM. Diagnostic utility of protein to creatinine ratio (P/C ratio) in spot urine sample within routine clinical practice. Crit Rev Clin Lab Sci. 2020;57(5):345–64.

Kaplan BS, Pradhan M. Urinalysis interpretation for pediatricians. Pediatr Ann. 2013;42(3):45–51.

Karavanaki KA, Soldatou A, Koufadaki AM, Tsentidis C, Haliotis FA, Stefanidis CJ. Delayed treatment of the first febrile urinary tract infection in early childhood increased the risk of renal scarring. Acta Paediatr. 2017;106(1):149–54.

Kaufman J, Temple-Smith M, Sanci L. Urinary tract infections in children: an overview of diagnosis and management. BMJ Paediatr Open. 2019;3(1):e000487.

KDIGO. KDIGO clinical practice guideline for the diagnosis, evaluation, prevention, and treatment of chronic kidney disease-mineral and bone disorder (CKD-MBD). Kidney Int Suppl. 2009;113: S1–130.

KDIGO. KDIGO 2012 clinical practice guideline for the evaluation and management of chronic kidney disease. Kidney Int Suppl. 2013;3(1):1–150.

KDIGO. KDIGO 2017 Clinical Practice Guideline Update for the Diagnosis, Evaluation, Prevention, and Treatment of Chronic Kidney Disease-Mineral and Bone Disorder (CKD-MBD). Kidney Int Suppl (2011). 2017;7(1):1–59.

Klemm KM, Klein MJ. Biochemical markers of bone metabolism. In: McPherson RA, Pincus MR, editors. Henry's clinical diagnosis and management by laboratory medicine. 23rd ed. St. Louis, Missouri: Elsevier; 2017. p. 188–204.e2.

Kraut JA, Madias NE. Re-evaluation of the normal range of serum total CO_2 concentration. Clin J Am Soc Nephrol. 2018;13(2):343–7.

Kraut JA, Nagami GT. The serum anion gap in the evaluation of acid-base disorders: what are its limitations, and can its effectiveness be improved? Clin J Am Soc Nephrol. 2013;8(11):2018–24.

Ladenhauf HN, Stundner O, Spreitzhofer F, Deluggi S. Severe hyperphosphatemia after administration of sodium-phosphate containing laxatives in children: case series and systematic review of literature. Pediatr Surg Int. 2012;28(8):805–14.

Lai H-C, Chang S-N, Lin H-C, Hsu Y-L, Wei H-M, Kuo C-C, et al. Association between urine pH and common uropathogens in children with urinary tract infections. J Microbiol Immunol Infect. 2019;

Larcombe J. Urinary tract infection in children: recurrent infections. BMJ Clin Evid. 2015;2015:0306.

Lee YM, Baek SY, Kim JH, Kim DS, Lee JS, Kim PK. Analysis of renal biopsies performed in children with abnormal findings in urinary mass screening. Acta Paediatr. 2006;95(7):849–53.

Lehnhardt A, Kemper MJ. Pathogenesis, diagnosis and management of hyperkalemia. Pediatr Nephrol. 2011;26(3):377–84.

Leite HP, Rodrigues da Silva AV, de Oliveira Iglesias SB, Koch Nogueira PC. Serum albumin is an independent predictor of clinical outcomes in critically ill children. Pediatr Crit Care Med. 2016;17(2):e50–7.

Leung AK, Wong AH. Proteinuria in children. Am Fam Physician. 2010;82(6):645–51.

Leung AK, Wong AH, Barg SS. Proteinuria in children: evaluation and differential diagnosis. Am Fam Physician. 2017;95(4):248–54.

Leung AKC, Wong AHC, Leung AAM, Hon KL. Urinary tract infection in children. Recent Patents Inflamm Allergy Drug Discov. 2019;13(1):2–18.

Levey AS. Selecting the right estimated glomerular filtration rate. In: Essentials of chronic kidney disease [internet]. New York, NY: Nova Science; 2015. [11-6].

Liamis G, Liberopoulos E, Barkas F, Elisaf M. Spurious electrolyte disorders: a diagnostic challenge for clinicians. Am J Nephrol. 2013;38(1):50–7.

Lietman SA, Germain-Lee EL, Levine MA. Hypercalcemia in children and adolescents. Curr Opin Pediatr. 2010;22(4):508–15.

Lo S. Reference intervals for laboratory tests and procedures. In: Kleigman RM, St Geme JW, Blum NJ, Shah SS, Tasker RC, Wilson KM, editors. Nelson textbook of pediatrics. Philadelphia, PA: Elsevier; 2020. p. e5–e14.

Loh TP, Metz MP. Trends and physiology of common serum biochemistries in children aged 0-18 years. Pathology. 2015;47(5):452–61.

Lombel RM, Gipson DS, Hodson EM. Treatment of steroid-sensitive nephrotic syndrome: new guidelines from KDIGO. Pediatr Nephrol. 2013;28(3):415–26.

Lopez-Garcia SC, Emma F, Walsh SB, Fila M, Hooman N, Zaniew M, et al. Treatment and long-term outcome in primary distal renal tubular acidosis. Nephrol Dial Transplant. 2019;34(6):981–91.

Lozano P, Henrikson NB, Morrison CC, Dunn J, Nguyen M, Blasi P, et al. U.S. Preventive Services Task Force Evidence Syntheses, Formerly Systematic Evidence Reviews. Lipid screening in childhood for detection of multifactorial dyslipidemia: a systematic evidence review for the US preventive services task force. Rockville (MD): Agency for Healthcare Research and Quality (US); 2016.

Mambatta AK, Jayarajan J, Rashme VL, Harini S, Menon S, Kuppusamy J. Reliability of dipstick assay in predicting urinary tract infection. J Family Med Prim Care. 2015;4(2):265–8.

Marra G, Taroni F, Berrettini A, Montanari E, Manzoni G, Montini G. Pediatric nephrolithiasis: a systematic approach from diagnosis to treatment. J Nephrol. 2019;32(2):199–210.

Mazaheri M, Assadi F. Simplified algorithm for evaluation of proteinuria in clinical practice: how should a clinician approach? Int J Prev Med. 2019;10:35.

McIntyre NJ, Taal MW. How to measure proteinuria? Curr Opin Nephrol Hypertens. 2008;17(6):600–3.

McPherson RA. Specific proteins. In: McPherson RA, editor. Henry's clinical diagnosis and management by laboratory methods. 23rd ed. St. Louis, Missouri: Elsevier; 2017. p. 253–66.e2.

Meyrier A, Niaudet P. Acute kidney injury complicating nephrotic syndrome of minimal change disease. Kidney Int. 2018;94(5):861–9.

Mian AN, Schwartz GJ. Measurement and estimation of glomerular filtration rate in children. Adv Chronic Kidney Dis. 2017;24(6):348–56.

Misra M, Pacaud D, Petryk A, Collett-Solberg PF, Kappy M. Vitamin D deficiency in children and its management: review of current knowledge and recommendations. Pediatrics. 2008;122(2):398–417.

Montini G, Tullus K, Hewitt I. Febrile urinary tract infections in children. N Engl J Med. 2011;365:239–50.

Munns CF, Shaw N, Kiely M, Specker BL, Thacher TD, Ozono K, et al. Global consensus recommendations on prevention and management of nutritional rickets. J Clin Endocrinol Metab. 2016;101(2):394–415.

Mutlu EA, Keshavarzian A, Mutlu GM. Hyperalbuminemia and elevated transaminases associated with high-protein diet. Scand J Gastroenterol. 2006;41(6):759–60.

Nadar R, Shaw N. Investigation and management of hypocalcaemia. Arch Dis Child. 2020;105(4):399.

Nagami GT. Hyperchloremia—why and how. Nefrologia. 2016;36(4):347–53.

Nielsen CA, Jensen JE, Cortes D. Vitamin D status is insufficient in the majority of children at diagnosis of nephrotic syndrome. Dan Med J. 2015;62(2):A5017.

Nitu M, Montgomery G, Eigen H. Acid-base disorders. Pediatr Rev. 2011;32(6):240–51.

Noone D, Langlois V. Laboratory evaluation of renal disease in childhood. In: Geary DF, Schaefer F, editors. Pediatric kidney disease. Berlin, Heidelberg: Springer Berlin / Heidelberg; 2017. p. 77–105.

Oh MS, Briefel G. Evaluation of renal function, water, electrolytes, and acid-base balance. In: Henry's clinical diagnosis and management by laboratory methods [internet], vol. 23. St. Louis, Missouri: Elsevier; 2017. p. 162–87.e5.

Panteghini M, IFCC Scientific Division. Enzymatic assays for creatinine: time for action. Clin Chem Lab Med. 2008;46(4):567–72.

Park SJ, Shin JI. Complications of nephrotic syndrome. Korean J Pediatr. 2011;54(8):322–8.

Parker JL, Kirmiz S, Noyes SL, Davis AT, Babitz SK, Alter D, et al. Reliability of urinalysis for identification of proteinuria is reduced in the presence of other abnormalities including high specific gravity and hematuria. Urol Oncol Semin Original Invest. 2020;38(11):853.e9–.e15.

Pasala S, Carmody JB. How to use serum creatinine, cystatin C and GFR. Arch Dis Child Educ Pract Ed. 2017;102(1):37–43.

Pincus MR, Bock JL, Rossi R, Cai D. Chemical basis of analyte assays and common interferences. In: McPherson RA, Pincus MR, editors. Henry's clinical diagnosis and management by laboratory methods. St. Louis, Missouri: Elsevier; 2017. p. 428–40.e1.

Plumb LA, Oni L, Marks SD, Tullus K. Paediatric antineutrophil cytoplasmic antibody (ANCA)-associated vasculitis: an update on renal management. Pediatr Nephrol. 2018;33(1):25–39.

Pomeranz AJ, Sabnis S, Busey SL, Kliegman RM. Edema. In: Pomeranz AJ, editor. Pediatric decision-making strategies. Philadelphia, PA: Elsevier-Saunders; 2016a. p. 126–9.

Pomeranz AJ, Sabnis S, Busey SL, Kliegman RM. Proteinuria. In: Pomeranz AJ, editor. Pediatric decision-making strategies. Philadelphia, PA: Elsevier/Saunders; 2016b. p. 124–5.

Pomeranz AJ, Sabnis S, Busey SL, Kliegman RM. Red urine and hematuria. In: Pomeranz AJ, editor. Pediatric decision-making strategies. Philadelphia, PA: Elsevier/Saunders; 2016c. p. 120–3.

Poowuttikul P, Thomas R, Hart B, Secord E. Vitamin D insufficiency/deficiency in HIV-infected inner-city youth. J Int Assoc Providers AIDS Care (JIAPAC). 2013;13(5):438–42.

Primack W. AAP does not recommend routine urinalysis for asymptomatic youths. AAP News. 2010;31(12):16.

Quigley R. Evaluation of hematuria and proteinuria: how should a pediatrician proceed? Curr Opin Pediatr. 2008;20(2):140–4.

Quigley R. Developmental changes in renal function. Curr Opin Pediatr. 2012;24(2):184–90.

Ranch D. Proteinuria in children. Pediatr Ann. 2020;49(6):e268–e72.

Robinson JL, Venner AA, Seiden-Long I. Urine protein detection by dipstick: no interference from alkalinity or specific gravity. Clin Biochem. 2019;71:77–80.

Santos F, Gil-Pena H, Alvarez-Alvarez S. Renal tubular acidosis. Curr Opin Pediatr. 2017;29(2):206–10.

Santos F, Ordonez FA, Claramunt-Taberner D, Gil-Pena H. Clinical and laboratory approaches in the diagnosis of renal tubular acidosis. Pediatr Nephrol. 2015;30:2099–107.

Schlager TA. Urinary tract infections in infants and children. Microbiol Spectr. 2016;4:5.

Schmidt B, Copp HL. Work-up of Pediatric urinary tract infection. Urol Clin North Am. 2015;42(4):519–26.

Schwartz GJ, Haycock GB, Edelmann CM Jr, Spitzer A. A simple estimate of glomerular filtration rate in children derived from body length and plasma creatinine. Pediatrics. 1976;58(2):259–63.

Schwartz GJ, Muñoz A, Schneider MF, Mak RH, Kaskel F, Warady BA, et al. New equations to estimate GFR in children with CKD. J Am Soc Nephrol. 2009;20(3):629–37.

Schwartz JB, Gallagher JC, Jorde R, Berg V, Walsh J, Eastell R, et al. Determination of free 25(OH)D concentrations and their relationships to total 25(OH)D in multiple clinical populations. J Clin Endocrinol Metab. 2018;103(9):3278–88.

Shaoul R, Okev N, Tamir A, Lanir A, Jaffe M. Value of laboratory studies in assessment of dehydration in children. Ann Clin Biochem. 2004;41(Pt 3):192–6.

Sharma S, Gupta A, Saxena S. Comprehensive clinical approach to renal tubular acidosis. Clin Exp Nephrol. 2015;19(4):556–61.

Signorelli GC, Bianchetti MG, Jermini LMM, Agostoni C, Milani GP, Simonetti GD, Lava SAG. Dietary chloride deficiency syndrome: pathophysiology, history, and systematic literature review. Nutrients. 2020;12(11):3436–46.

Simerville JA, Maxted WC, Pahira JJ. Urinalysis: a comprehensive review. Am Fam Physician. 2005;71(6):1153–62.

Simões E Silva AC, Oliveira EA, Mak RH. Urinary tract infection in pediatrics: an overview. J Pediatr. 2020;96(Suppl 1):65–79.

Staples A, LeBlond R, Watkins S, Wong C, Brandt J. Validation of the revised Schwartz estimating equation in a predominantly non-CKD population. Pediatr Nephrol. 2010;25(11):2321–6.

Stenson EK, Cvijanovich NZ, Anas N, Allen GL, Thomas NJ, Bigham MT, Weiss SL, Fitzgerald JC, Checchia PA, Meyer K, Quasney M, Hall M, Gedeit R, Freishtat RJ, Nowak J, Raj SS, Gertz S, Grunwell JR, Wong HR. Hyperchloremia is associated with complicated course and mortality in pediatric patients with septic shock. Pediatr Crit Care Med. 2018;19(2):155–60.

Subcommittee On Urinary Tract Infection. Reaffirmation of AAP clinical practice guideline: the diagnosis and management of the initial urinary tract infection in febrile infants and young children 2-24 months of age. Pediatrics. 2016;138(6):e20163026.

Taib F, Jamal B. Diagnostic accuracy on the management of acute paediatric urinary tract infection in a general paediatric unit. J Acute Dis. 2015;4(1):54–8.

Thurman JM. Complement in kidney disease: core curriculum 2015. Am J Kidney Dis. 2015;65(1):156–68.

Touma E, Bisharat N. Trends in admission serum albumin and mortality in patients with hospital readmission. Int J Clin Pract. 2019;73(6):e13314.

Tutay GJ, Capraro G, Spirko B, Garb J, Smithline H. Electrolyte profile of pediatric patients with hypertrophic pyloric stenosis. Pediatr Emerg Care. 2013;29(4):465–8.

Utsch B, Klaus G. Urinalysis in children and adolescents. Dtsch Arztebl Int. 2014;111(37):617–25. quiz 26

Vaziri ND. Disorders of lipid metabolism in nephrotic syndrome: mechanisms and consequences. Kidney Int. 2016;90(1):41–52.

Verliat-Guinaud J, Blanc P, Garnier F, Gajdos V, Guigonis V. A midstream urine collector is not a good alternative to a sterile collection method during the diagnosis of urinary tract infection. Acta Paediatr. 2015;104(9):e395–400.

Vitale DS, Hornung L, Lin TK, Nathan JD, Prasad S, Thompson T, et al. Blood urea nitrogen elevation is a marker for pediatric severe acute pancreatitis. Pancreas. 2019;48(3):363–6.

Viteri B, Reid-Adam J. Hematuria and proteinuria in children. Pediatr Rev. 2018;39(12):573–87.

Wang C-s, Greenbaum LA. Nephrotic syndrome. Pediatr Clin N Am. 2019;66(1):73–85.

Weng FL, Shults J, Herskovitz RM, Zemel BS, Leonard MB. Vitamin D insufficiency in steroid-sensitive nephrotic syndrome in remission. Pediatr Nephrol. 2005;20(1):56–63.

Yates M, Watts R. ANCA-associated vasculitis. Clin Med (Lond). 2017;17(1):60–4.

Yaxley J, Pirrone C. Review of the diagnostic evaluation of renal tubular acidosis. Ochsner J. 2016;16(4):525–30.

Care of the Child with a Pediatric Endocrine Disorder

11

Rebecca Crespi, Leigh Pughe, and Amy Dowd

Learning Objectives

After completing the chapter, the learner should be able to:

1. Understand the basic physiology of the endocrine system.
2. Be able to explain different methods of endocrine lab evaluation.
3. Be able to evaluate basic thyroid dysfunction labs.
4. Evaluate the basic endocrine lab evaluation for growth disorders.
5. Recognize a variety of common pubertal disorders as well as the basic endocrine lab evaluations associated with each disorder.
6. Utilize knowledge of different laboratory tests used in the assessment for type 1 and type 2 diabetes.

11.1 Introduction

Endocrine glands secrete hormones into the bloodstream, which travel long distances to their target organs, where they exert their effects. The

endocrine system affects many other systems, and therefore it is important to understand their actions. In a clinical setting, the patient with hypothyroidism may present with fatigue, change in mood, tingling in an extremity, hair loss, cold hands and feet, and weight gain. The clinical presentation can mimic neurological and rheumatological diseases, so it is important to understand the variety of presentations and the results of endocrine diagnostic labs. This chapter will help you understand the significance of diagnostic laboratory results in evaluating patients with a possible endocrine problem.

11.2 Physiology of the Endocrine System

The pituitary gland sits in the middle of the brain in a protective bony structure called the sella turcica and is connected to the hypothalamus by the infundibular stalk. The pituitary gland is divided into the anterior and posterior pituitary gland. The posterior pituitary gland typically acts as a storage area for the pre-synthesized hormones antidiuretic hormone (ADH/vasopressin) and oxytocin. Oxytocin is synthesized in the hypothalamus and secreted into the bloodstream by the posterior pituitary. It is best known for its actions during lactation and parturition and is beyond the scope of this chapter since it is rarely ordered for a pediatric endocrine evaluation. The

Special acknowledgment: Thank you to Dr. Liane Eng for her assistance with this chapter.

R. Crespi (✉) · L. Pughe · A. Dowd
Department of Pediatric Endocrinology and Diabetes, The Children's Hospital at Montefiore, Bronx, NY, USA

Table 11.1 Overview of common pediatric pituitary hormones and their downstream effects

Pituitary hormone	End organ	Hormone produced	Effect on the body
Anterior pituitary hormones			
TSH	Thyroid gland	Thyroxine	Metabolism, growth, development
GH	Liver (and others)	Insulin-like growth factor 1 (IGF-1)	Growth, development
LH and FSH	Ovary/testicle	Estrogen/testosterone	Secondary sexual characteristics and ability to reproduce
ACTH	The adrenal cortex of the adrenal gland	Adrenal hormone cascade (i.e., cortisol, testosterone)	Secondary sexual characteristics, glucose homeostasis, sodium, blood pressure homeostasis
Prolactin	Breast	n/a	Stimulates mammary gland growth and milk production
Posterior pituitary			
ADH/vasopressin	Kidney	n/a	Fluid balance
Oxytocin	Uterus/breast	n/a	Parturition, lactation

Adapted from Styne (2016), Rosenbloom and Connor (2007)

Table 11.2 Endocrine hormones outside the pituitary gland

Hormone	Organ-producing hormone	Effect on the body
Insulin (beta cells)	Pancreas	Glucose homeostasis
Glucagon (alpha cells)	Pancreas	Glucose homeostasis
Parathyroid hormone (PTH)	Parathyroid gland	Calcium homeostasis

Adapted from Styne (2016)

anterior pituitary hormones communicate with specific end organs within the body, causing the release of other hormones (except for prolactin). The anterior pituitary gland secretes thyroid-stimulating hormone (TSH), growth hormone (GH), luteinizing hormone (LH), follicle-stimulating hormone (FSH), adrenocorticotropic hormone (ACTH), and prolactin (Styne 2016; Rosenbloom and Connor 2007). Table 11.1 is an overview of the pituitary hormones.

The endocrine system also involves hormones produced from organs in the body aside from the pituitary gland. Table 11.2 is an overview of other hormones.

11.3 Endocrine Diagnostic Laboratory Testing

Understanding which type of assays to order when evaluating a pediatric patient for a potential endocrine disorder can be confusing. As many

hormones have similar structures, similar testing procedures are used for different hormones.

11.3.1 Immunoassays and Endocrine Diagnostic Laboratory Testing

Immunoassays are used to measure many endocrine hormones and are currently one of the most commonly used methods (Haddad et al. 2019). Some immunoassays measure large-sized hormone molecules (noncompetitive), and some measure smaller-sized hormone molecules (competitive). All immunoassays involve binding an antibody to its antigen, also known as the "target analyte." The sensitivity of immunoassays is adequate, but there are concerns about immunoassay specificity for certain hormones (Kushnir et al. 2010; Rauh 2009). Immunoassays are rapid and relatively easy to run and require a small sample size; however, results tend to be inconsistent and not standardized, giving lower accuracy and decreased specificity than newer methods, especially if concentrations are normal or low (Rauh 2009).

11.3.1.1 Competitive Immunoassay

When a hormone molecule is being measured with a competitive assay, a labeled antibody, called a capture antibody (Ab), is added to the patient's sample and is attached to a solid substrate. A known amount of a labeled antigen is added to the sample and "competes" with the target analyte or serum hormone to bind to the capture Ab. The more target analyte present in the sample, the more binding to the capture Ab and the less signal response from the labeled analyte will be measured (Haddad et al. 2019; Luong and Vashist 2019). Therefore, the weaker the signal, the higher the concentration of endogenous hormone present (Haddad et al. 2019). The most commonly used competitive immunoassay is the radioimmunoassay (RIA). Other examples (based on the type of labeled antibody) include enzyme immunoassay (EIA) or fluorescence immunoassay (FIA) (Chandler et al. 2014).

11.3.1.2 Noncompetitive (Immunometric) Immunoassay

Similar to competitive assays, the noncompetitive or "sandwich" assay involves a capture Ab connected to a solid substrate. Additionally, in sandwich immunoassays, there is another Ab called the "detection" Ab, which is labeled with a molecule to provide a signal response (Luong and Vashist 2019). When the patient sample is added, the target analyte binds to the capture Ab, and then the labeled detection Ab binds to another site on the target analyte, forming a "sandwich." The remaining liquid is discarded, leaving the "sandwiches." Therefore, the stronger the signal from the capture antibody-hormone-detection antibody complex, the higher the endogenous hormone present (Haddad et al. 2019). As with the competitive immunoassays, there are different types of labeled antibodies. Examples include immunoradiometric (IRMA), enzyme-linked immunosorbent assay (ELISA), and immunochemiluminometric (ICMA) (Chandler et al. 2014). Table 11.3 reviews the method used for each of the commonly ordered hormones.

11.3.1.3 Liquid Chromatography-Tandem Mass Spectrometry (LC-MS/MS)

Liquid chromatography-tandem mass spectrometry (LC-MS/MS) is frequently the method of choice when evaluating endocrine

Table 11.3 Frequently used immunoassays for certain endocrine tests

Competitive immunoassays	Immunometric immunoassays
Adrenal cortisol	ACTH
DHEA-S	FSH
Total testosterone	LH
	Prolactin
	TSH
	Free T3
	Free thyroxine (free T4)
	Sex hormone-binding globulin (SHBG)

Adapted from Luong and Vashist (2019)

Table 11.4 Generalized comparison between immunoassay and LC-MS/MS

Immunoassays	LC-MS/MS
Measures one sample at a time	Measures multiple samples at a time
Easily automated	Not automated
More sensitive than LC-MS/MS	Enhanced specificity for steroid hormones
Reference intervals must be made for each test	Reference intervals must be made for each test
A larger volume of sample needed	A smaller volume of sample needed
Less expensive and more rapid testing	More expensive requires specialized technical experience
	It can also be used for enzyme activity assays (steroid converting enzymes) and samples other than blood/serum (saliva and hair)

Adapted from Rauh (2009)

hormones. It is more specific than other techniques used to measure hormone concentrations (Kushnir et al. 2010; Rauh 2009). Mass spectrometry is a method that uses mass and charge to separate ions (Chandler et al. 2014). The advantages of LC-MS/MS include the low volume of the sample, the ability to detect low hormone levels, measuring multiple hormones simultaneously, and providing high specificity (Rauh 2009). However, it is more expensive to obtain the equipment, more technical to run, and may vary from lab to lab (Pugeat et al. 2018). Table 11.4 is a comparison of immunoassays and LC-MS/MS.

11.4 Pitfalls of Endocrine Lab Tests

11.4.1 Biotin Interference with Immunoassays Utilizing Biotin-Streptavidin Chemistry

Biotin (vitamin B7) has been increasingly used as a dietary supplement for its potential benefits for the hair, skin, and nail health. Recently, elevated serum biotin has become a well-known interfering molecule in assays that utilize the biotin-streptavidin detection method. Many commercial laboratories employ biotin-streptavidin chemistry as their immunoassay platform (Luong and Vashist 2019). Streptavidin is a biotin-binding protein used to adhere the capture Ab to a solid surface. Capture antibodies in both the competitive and noncompetitive assays are labeled with biotin (biotinylated antibody). Competitive immunoassays are very susceptible to biotin interference because free serum biotin will compete to bind to the biotinylated antibody. In noncompetitive immunoassays, excess biotin in the serum has a higher affinity for the streptavidin magnetic particles and prevents the binding of the detection antibody, therefore preventing the "sandwich" from being formed, leading to falsely low results (Luong and Vashist 2019; Haddad et al. 2019). In competitive immunoassays, high concentrations of biotin bind to the biotinylated capture Ab instead of the serum hormone, causing a lower signal response, which is interpreted as a higher hormone value (Haddad et al. 2019).

Biotin doses of 5–100 mg (5000–100,000 mcg) per day are enough to cause interference (Luong and Vashist 2019). The general recommendation to diminish the biotin interference is to discontinue oral biotin for at least 48 h before testing. Endocrine hormones that may be affected include TSH, free T4, cortisol, DHEAS, total testosterone, SHBG, LH, FSH, prolactin, and ACTH (Luong and Vashist 2019).

11.4.2 High-Dose Hook Effect in Immunoassays

When there is an extremely high dose of endogenous hormone present in a sample or there are very low amounts of labeled antibodies in the kit from commercial manufacturers, the endogenous hormone may saturate the capture Ab and detection Ab, preventing the antibody-antigen-antibody complex. Thus, few "sandwiches" are left when the liquid component is discarded, hence a low signal suggesting low or mildly elevated serum hormone (Haddad et al. 2019). This hook effect used to describe the shape of the binding curve commonly occurs with very high concentrations of serum analyte, which are typically associated with large hormone-secreting tumors (Haddad et al. 2019). The hook effect has also been seen with thyroglobulin in patients with thyroid cancer and beta-human chorionic gonadotropin (hCG). It can also occur with prolactin levels. The hook effect can cause a falsely low result. If the clinician has suspicion for false low results due to the hook effect, serial dilutions can be used to evaluate further (Haddad et al. 2019).

11.4.3 Cross-Reactivity of Steroid Hormone Immunoassays

Many hormones have similar molecular structures and may cross-react in competitive immunoassays. Cross-reactivity can be seen when measuring testosterone and estradiol if other structurally similar molecules are present in the serum. Additionally, prednisolone can cross-react with cortisol assays (Haddad et al. 2019). If cross-reactivity is suspected, using LC-MS/MS may be beneficial since it can provide a more accurate measurement (Haddad et al. 2019).

Key Learning about Evaluating Hormones

- Selection of the type of assay is important to ensure that lab results are as accurate as possible.
- Understanding the pitfalls of certain laboratory tests is essential for proper diagnoses.
- If there is an abnormal lab result that is not consistent with the clinical presentation, consider possible laboratory interference.

11.5 Thyroid Disorders

Thyroid function tests should be evaluated when signs or symptoms of thyroid dysfunction are deduced from the history or physical exam. In terms of history, changes in stooling patterns, growth concerns, changes in energy level or mood, skin changes, and menstrual irregularities should prompt a thyroid evaluation. However, symptoms of thyroid dysfunction can be nonspecific and commonly seen in other pediatric conditions. Identifying which thyroid test to order is important. If baseline thyroid function tests are abnormal, the primary care clinician may refer to a pediatric endocrine specialist to further evaluate the etiology of hypothyroidism or hyperthyroidism. Sometimes the cause of the thyroid dysfunction will not alter treatment (i.e., Hashimoto's hypothyroidism), but sometimes it will (i.e., Graves' disease vs. a hyperfunctioning nodule).

11.5.1 Physiology of Thyroid Function

A basic understanding of thyroid physiology is integral when choosing which thyroid function test to evaluate. The hypothalamic-pituitary-thyroid axis is responsible for the control of thyroid hormone at the tissue and cellular level. The thyroid hormone production from the thyroid gland is regulated by thyrotropin-releasing hormone (TRH) from the hypothalamus, which stimulates the pituitary gland to release TSH. TSH stimulates the thyroid gland to secrete T4 and triiodothyronine (T3) through a complicated process of iodine uptake and enzymatic reactions. The thyroid gland secretes more T4 (85–90%) than T3 (10–15%), and both hormones are heavily bound to proteins (>99%), including albumin, transthyretin, and thyroid-binding globulin (TBG). The T4 and T3 that are not bound are called free T4 and free T3 and bind to specific cellular receptors. Free T3 is the active form of thyroid hormone but is found in much smaller quantities in the blood. T4 is converted to T3 through a group of enzymes called deiodinases (Koulouri et al. 2013; Sheehan 2016). Both free T4 and free T3 negatively feedback to the hypothalamus and pituitary gland to suppress the secretion of TRH and TSH, respectively. The inverse relationship between free T4, free T3, and TSH is log-linear, as opposed to linear, and is important to understand since small changes in free T4 result in large changes in TSH. In contrast, small changes in TSH result in insignificant changes in free T3 and free T4. Of note, TSH changes occur more slowly than changes in total and free T4 (Ross et al. 2016; Sheehan 2016; Soh and Aw 2019). This inverse log-linear relationship supports that, with an intact hypothalamic-pituitary axis, TSH is a more sensitive laboratory evaluation for thyroid status and is recommended as an initial screen for many thyroid disorders (Ross et al. 2016; Koulouri et al. 2013; Soh and Aw 2019). However, making a diagnosis on TSH alone is difficult. Evaluating TSH as it relates to free T4 helps provide a more accurate diagnosis and will determine the need for a pediatric endocrine evaluation.

11.5.2 Hypothyroidism

Subclinical hypothyroidism is diagnosed when the TSH level is elevated with a normal free T4

(Crisafulli et al. 2019; Bona et al. 2013). Patients are typically asymptomatic, and the process is usually benign, and self resolves over time, with few children progressing to overt hypothyroidism (Bona et al. 2013). When subclinical hypothyroidism is caused by thyroglobulin (TG) and/or thyroid peroxidase (TPO) antibodies (Hashimoto's disease), the chances of overt hypothyroidism are greater than if the subclinical hypothyroidism is idiopathic (Crisafulli et al. 2019; Wasniewska et al. 2015). The treatment of subclinical hypothyroidism should be based on the severity of the elevation of TSH (>10mIU/L), if the subclinical hypothyroidism is associated with antibodies and other chronic illnesses or conditions and if signs or symptoms of thyroid dysfunction are present (Bona et al. 2013; Crisafulli et al. 2019). In the National Health and Nutrition Examination Survey III, which evaluated TSH in a "disease-free" population of greater than 13,000 subjects aged 12 years and older, it was noted that 4.6% of the population studied had hypothyroidism, with 4.3% of the total hypothyroidism being subclinical hypothyroidism, and therefore only a small percentage of the population with overt hypothyroidism (Hollowell et al. 2002).

Children with Turner syndrome and Down syndrome who have subclinical hypothyroidism have an increased risk of developing overt hypothyroidism (Crisafulli et al. 2019).

Obesity has been associated with hypothyroidism. However, checking thyroid function tests should not be part of routine screening for obesity unless the clinician has other concerns that suggest hypothyroidism, such as growth failure or irregular menses (Styne et al. 2017).

It is well known that the thyroid plays an important role in basal, lipid, and glucose metabolism (Longhi and Radetti 2013) and that hypothyroidism may be associated with weight gain. Mildly elevated TSH levels may be noted and of no clinical significance in obese patients. Studies have noted elevated TSH levels or TSH levels at the upper end of normal in obese children and adolescents and elevated T3 levels (Biondi 2010; Longhi and Radetti 2013; Giannakopoulos et al. 2019). Reinehr, de Sousa, and Andler (2006) noted an elevation in TSH with normal free T4 in obese

children and a reduction in TSH with weight loss. Ghergherehchi and Hazhir (2015) also noted that TSH and total T4 were elevated in overweight and obese children, but free T4 and free T3 levels were not elevated. These studies suggested that an elevated TSH may be a consequence and not a result of increased weight. The pathophysiology of elevated TSH in obesity is unclear, and many mechanisms have been postulated.

- TSH may increase as a compensatory mechanism for decreased responsiveness of adipocytes to TSH in obese individuals.
- Leptin may also cause a role in increasing TSH in obese patients by increasing thyroid-releasing hormone from the hypothalamus, thus increasing TSH (Sanyal and Raychaudhuri 2016).
- Some studies have also discussed an increase of T4 to T3 conversion due to increased deiodinase activity, which may be adaptive to increase metabolic rate in children with obesity (Giannakopoulos et al. 2019).

Because obesity is associated with elevated TSH, clinicians must be careful before placing a diagnosis of subclinical hypothyroidism on an obese or overweight child.

11.5.3 Central Hypothyroidism

In central hypothyroidism, there is dysfunction at the level of the pituitary gland. TSH may appear normal but is low in relation to free or total T4. Although central hypothyroidism is rare (1:80,000–1:120,000), the primary care clinician should remember this in the differential diagnosis of thyroid disorders if the patient presents with other symptoms concerning for pituitary dysfunction (Gupta and Lee 2011).

11.5.4 Real-Life Examples

A 12-year 1-month-old male was referred to a pediatric endocrine clinic for obesity and risk of diabetes. Screening labs showed a mildly elevated TSH of 5.43uU/mL (0.3–4.2) and normal free T4 of 1.36 ng/dL (0.6–1.5). He was encouraged to focus on healthy lifestyle changes to reduce the risks of obesity-related complications. At the 6-month follow-up visit, the patient had lost 12 pounds. The TSH improved to 3.89 uU/mL (0.3–4.2), and the free T4 remained normal 1.4 ng/dL (0.6–1.5).

A 4-year 5-month-old female presented to her primary care clinician for her annual healthcare maintenance and noted poor growth and falling height percentiles. Thyroid function tests were completed which noted TSH 1.34uU/mL (0.4–4.6) and free T4 0.57 ng/dL (0.8–2.0). Although the TSH is within the normal range, it did not respond as expected to the low free T4. Further testing revealed an undetectable IGF-1, <25 ng/mL (57–260). A brain MRI revealed a craniopharyngioma. This patient was treated with surgery and is now being treated for postsurgical panhypopituitarism.

11.5.5 Congenital Hypothyroidism (CH)

Congenital hypothyroidism (CH) occurs in 1 out of 2000 births and must be diagnosed and treated early to avoid growth and brain development disturbances, leading to neurocognitive defects (van Trotsenburg et al. 2021; Kilberg et al. 2018). It is the most common endocrine disorder on newborn screening (Diaz and Lipman Diaz 2014), and thyroid dysgenesis is the most common reason for congenital hypothyroidism (Wassner 2018). Screening programs across the United States vary; some screening programs test a primary TSH followed by a T4, some test both TSH and T4 at the same time, and some screening programs complete a primary T4 screening, followed by TSH (van Trotsenburg et al. 2021; Kilberg et al. 2018). Some screening programs require a repeat newborn screening at 2–4 weeks of life, and others do not. All screening programs measure the TSH and have a specific level (varies by state) which prompts referral to a pediatric endocrine specialty center and requires a serum TSH for diagnosis (van Trotsenburg et al. 2021; Kilberg et al. 2018). Clinicians must consider that 10% of newborns with congenital hypothy-

roidism have other congenital anomalies, with cardiac anomalies being the most common anomaly (Wassner 2018).

11.5.5.1 TSH in the Newborn

TSH surges immediately after birth. Due to this surge, newborn screen testing is recommended between 48 and 72 h of life (van Trotsenburg et al. 2021; Kilberg et al. 2018). However, if the newborn screen is obtained within the first 24 h of life, there is an increased rate of false-positive results, especially with the screens for TSH only (van Trotsenburg et al. 2021).

Conversely, false-negative results are more common in preterm, LBW, and critically ill infants since they may not have a TSH surge (Diaz and Lipman Diaz 2014).

The clinician should consider a second screen or serum TSH and FT4 testing in the group of infants seen in Box 11.1. Some state programs perform second screens for some portion of the newborn screen or all of the newborn screen.

Box 11.1 Newborns Who May Need Second Screen at 10–14 Days for Congenital Hypothyroidism

Patients at risk of false-negative screening

- Preterm and low-birth-weight infants.
- Critically ill infants.
- Same-sex twins.
- When the first screen was done in the first 24 hours of life.
- Newborns with trisomy 21.
- Newborns at risk for iodine deficiency or excess.

Adapted from van Trotsenburg et al. (2021)

When the TSH-only method is used, it may pick up mild CH cases where there is an elevated TSH with normal FT4. This method does not detect patients with central hypothyroidism where the TSH and the T4 are low. A FT4-based screening will detect a benign X-linked congenital deficiency of TBG, which causes low levels of total T4, normal FT4, and TSH (Wassner 2018).

11.5.5.2 Pitfalls of Newborn Hypothyroidism Screening

The newborn hypothyroidism screen has high sensitivity, but the false-negative rate may be as high as 10% (Wassner 2018). There are several reasons for the false-negative rate outlined in Box 11.2.

Box 11.2 Reasons for False-Negative Rate in Primary Congenital Hypothyroidism

- A delay in the serum TSH—more common in preterm or infants with birth weight < 1500 g (delayed TSH increase occurs in as many as 1 in 85 infants with a birth weight of <1500 g).
- Infants in the neonatal intensive care units as a result of illness or treated with medications such as dopamine or glucocorticoids.
- Monozygotic twins—if they share the placental circulation, the normal twin will compensate for the twin with hypothyroidism.
- Technical or human errors in screening.

11.5.6 Hyperthyroidism

Hyperthyroidism can be subclinical with a low TSH and normal free T4 or overt with a low TSH and high free and/or total T4 and total T3. Overt hyperthyroidism may cause tachycardia, palpitations, growth acceleration, irregular menses, weight loss, diarrhea, emotional lability, and sleep disturbance. The most common cause of hyperthyroidism in children is Graves' disease, an autoimmune disorder caused by the stimulation of the TSH receptor by thyroid receptor antibodies, specifically thyroid-stimulating immunoglobulins (TSI) (Srinivasan and Misra 2015; Ross et al. 2016). Other less common causes of hyperthyroidism in children include a toxic adenoma or toxic multinodular goiter. Transient hyperthyroidism may be caused by the thyrotoxic phase of Hashimoto's disease, termed Hashitoxicosis. In Hashitoxicosis, TPO and/or TG antibodies are present, and preformed thyroid hormone is released before becoming hypothyroid. Amiodarone and excess iodine (secondary to increased use of iodine for medical procedures or by ingestion) can also cause hyperthyroidism.

The clinician should also be alert to signs and symptoms of hyperthyroidism in children who are being treated for hypothyroidism with levothyroxine, as increased intake of levothyroxine can cause hyperthyroidism. Symptomatic patients with hyperthyroidism may progress to thyroid storm and require an urgent referral to a pediatric endocrinologist (Srinivasan and Misra 2015; Ross et al. 2016).

11.5.7 Real-Life Example

A 3-year 4-month-old boy with congenital hypothyroidism presented for routine follow-up care to a pediatric endocrinology clinic. The mother reported some diarrhea for the past few days. Labs noted TSH 0.208 uU/mL (0.4–4.6), free T4 7.77 ng/dL (0.8–1.7), and total T4 24.5 ug/dL (5–12). Upon further investigation, the mother noted that some of the levothyroxine tablets were missing, and it was determined that the patient ingested the levothyroxine. Medication was held, and labs were repeated weekly. By 13 days postingestion, TSH increased to 13.5 uU/mL (0.4–4.6), free T4 decreased to 0.66 ng/dL (0.8–1.7), total T4 decreased to 3.78 ug/dL (5–12), and the patient was back to a hypothyroid state. Levothyroxine was restarted, and there were no long-term sequelae from the levothyroxine overdose.

11.5.8 Thyroid Diagnostic Laboratory Tests

As previously discussed, the clinician must know the normal ranges of the individual thyroid tests for the child's age and understand the differences between different types of tests. Understanding that obese children may have a slightly elevated

Table 11.5 Common thyroid dysfunction labs and associated thyroid state

TSH	Free T4	Diagnosis
Normal	Normal	Euthyroid
High	Low	Overt hypothyroid
High	Normal	Subclinical hypothyroid
Low	High	Overt hyperthyroid
Low	Normal	Subclinical hyperthyroid

Adapted from Styne (2016), Koulouri et al. (2013)

TSH and that TSH should not be routinely completed as part of the evaluation for the child with obesity can help avoid excessive worry and expense (Styne et al. 2017). Table 11.5 reviews the definitions of thyroid dysfunction based on TSH and free T4.

11.5.8.1   TSH

Thyroid-stimulating hormone is a protein with an alpha chain and beta-subunit. The alpha chain in TSH is similar to the alpha chains in hCG, FSH, and LH (Soh and Aw 2019). TSH is known to be the most sensitive first-line screening test for thyroid dysfunction. Still, because many factors can affect TSH values, clinicians should be cautious when using TSH as the only test in evaluating subclinical hypothyroidism or hyperthyroidism and secondary hypothyroidism (central hypothyroidism) and when evaluating a patient soon after treatment for hypothyroidism and hyperthyroidism.

TSH reference ranges continue to be debated and are known to increase with aging beyond the pediatric population (Vadiveloo et al. 2013). TSH is also known to be affected by ethnicity. The National Health and Nutrition Examination Survey III evaluated TSH and found it to be higher in females and non-Hispanic White and Mexican American subjects compared to non-Hispanic Black subjects. They found that the upper limit of normal for TSH was 4.5 mIU/L (Hollowell et al. 2002). However, other groups studying similar populations of people with no thyroid antibodies and no known thyroid dysfunction found that the upper limit of normal TSH was 4.12 mIU/L (Esfandiari and Papaleontiou 2017; Soh and Aw 2019; Sheehan 2016).

It is also important to remember that TSH changes are slower than thyroid hormone changes. Therefore, an improvement in thyroid hormone

levels may not be concordant with improvement in TSH levels. For example, a change in free T4 can be seen within days after the treatment of hypothyroidism with levothyroxine, but TSH levels may not show improvement for a few weeks. Therefore, additional testing of total T4 or free T4 may help assess thyroid status. Additionally, if thyrotoxicosis is suspected, diagnostic accuracy improves when TSH is measured along with free T4 and total T3 (Ross et al. 2016; Soh and Aw 2019).

Pitfalls of TSH testing. Although reference ranges for TSH are based on an intact hypothalamic-pituitary-thyroid axis, TSH can be affected by dysfunction of the hypothalamic-pituitary axis, age, pregnancy, adherence to medication treatment for hyperthyroidism and/or hypothyroidism, pituitary microadenoma, interference with TSH assays, non-thyroidal illness (NTI), and medications (Esfandiari and Papaleontiou 2017; Sheehan 2016; Biondi 2010).

It is important to remember that infants have a TSH surge during the first 24 h of life and TSH levels are higher during the first month of life and decline with age, though they are relatively constant in childhood (Kapelari et al. 2008). In pregnancy, TSH decreases but is rarely suppressed during the first trimester. Since hCG is structurally similar to TSH, it can act at the TSH receptor, causing a low TSH. Therefore, clinicians assessing thyroid function in girls of childbearing age should consider pregnancy tests in those with TSH levels below normal and with normal or slightly elevated total and free T4 (McNeil and Stanford 2015).

In patients with NTI, the hypothalamic function may be impaired, causing TSH to be normal or low during acute illness but rarely suppressed. As patients recover from a non-thyroidal illness, TSH may increase above normal levels, though rarely above 10 mIU/mL (Sheehan 2016; DeGroot 2015). Primary care clinicians should be cautious when evaluating patients with recent hospitalization or those with eating disorders. These patients may have a euthyroid sick syndrome and have a low TSH (Esfandiari and Papaleontiou 2017; DeGroot 2015), normal or low T4, and/or low T3 (Hornberger, Lane, AAP Committee on Adolescent 2021).

Primary care clinicians should always take a thorough history, including a comprehensive

Table 11.6 Medications that affect TSH and T4

Medication	Mechanism of action
Lithium	Inhibits thyroid hormone secretion
Iodide	Inhibits thyroid hormone secretion
Amiodarone	Inhibits thyroid hormone secretion
Methimazole	Inhibits thyroid hormone production
Propylthiouracil	Inhibits thyroid hormone production
Glucocorticoids	Suppresses TSH and decreases TBG
Dopamine agonist	Suppresses TSH
Somatostatin analogs	Suppresses TSH
Androgens	Decreases TBG
Estrogen	Increases TBG

Adapted from Haugen (2009)

medication history. Medications that can affect TSH at the level of the hypothalamus, and can suppress TSH, include glucocorticoids, dopamine agonists, and somatostatin analogs (Haugen 2009). Table 11.6 is a list of medications affecting TSH.

Assay interference can be caused by biotin, as discussed previously. Additionally, autoimmune anti-TSH antibodies and rheumatoid factor may interfere with assays causing falsely elevated TSH (Esfandiari and Papaleontiou 2017). Box 11.3 reviews factors affecting TSH.

Box 11.3 Factors Affecting TSH
- Age (i.e., neonatal period and TSH surge).
- Non-thyroidal illness (euthyroid sick syndrome).
  - Poor nutrition/starvation.
  - Chronic liver or renal disease.
  - Malabsorption syndromes.
- Pregnancy.
- Treatment with levothyroxine and adherence to treatment.
- Assay interference (i.e., biotin).

11.5.8.2 T4

Thyroid hormone is produced in the thyroid gland's follicular cells and secreted in abundance into the circulation. Most thyroid hormone in circulation is bound to proteins, most specifically, thyroid-binding globulin (TBG). The liver synthesizes TBG and secretes it into circulation to bind T4 and T3. Total T4 is the total amount of bound and unbound T4. Free T4 is the amount of T4 that is not bound to a protein. Second to TSH, free T4 is the most abundantly ordered thyroid test (Sheehan 2016) and the most widely ordered free hormone test (Faix 2013). Previously, free T4 was estimated based on the total T4 and TBG and was a unitless number called the free thyroxine index (FTI). Due to its limitations, FTI has been replaced by more direct measurements of free T4, such as immunoassay or LC-MS/MS (Faix 2013). Currently, most labs use immunoassays when assessing free T4; however, the gold standard for evaluation remains free T4 by equilibrium dialysis, which is rarely available but typically used by endocrinologists when the need arises (Faix 2013; Koulouri et al. 2013; Soh and Aw 2019). Measuring free T4 is helpful in certain situations when TSH alone will not be accurate. For example, after treatment of hyperthyroidism with radioactive iodine for hyperthyroidism, measuring free T4 to monitor for hypothyroidism and to make medication adjustments is important since it may take weeks to months for TSH to normalize. Since a low free T4 indicates hypothyroidism, measuring free T4 with TSH will help determine if the hypothyroidism is central (low or normal TSH) or primary (elevated TSH).

Pitfalls of T4 Testing. Like TSH, T4 can be affected by age, ethnicity, pregnancy, medications, and type of assay used. Kapelari et al. (2008) studied reference ranges of thyroid hormone in pediatric patients and noted that free T4 and free T3 decreased with age. Hollowell et al. (2002) reported that median T4 was higher in Mexican Americans than in White or Black subjects.

In pregnancy, total T4, free T4, and free T3 may be increased in the first trimester due to estrogen-induced increases in TBG (McNeil and Stanford 2015). Medications that can affect T4 secretion include lithium, amiodarone, and excess iodide and cause thyroid dysfunction. Table 11.6 lists medications that can affect T4. Additionally, as previously discussed, biotin can interfere with immunoassays that measure free T4.

11.5.8.3 Triiodothyronine (T3)

Triiodothyronine is the active form of thyroid hormone, but the total and free T3 concentration is less than that of total and free T4 in circulation. Therefore, difficulties remain in measuring such small amounts of the hormone. In hypothyroidism, measuring T3 has limited clinical significance since it is usually normal and does not add to the diagnosis or management of hypothyroidism. However, since T3 is thought to mediate the symptoms of hyperthyroidism, T3 is measured in addition to T4 in this clinical scenario. Immunoassays for free T3 are not as readily available as they are for free T4 and continue to need validation (Faix 2013; Ross et al. 2016; Esfandiari and Papaleontiou 2017).

11.5.8.4 Thyroid-Binding Globulin

As previously discussed, TBG is produced by the liver and is the most abundant binding protein for T4 and T3. It is not a useful screening test for thyroid dysfunction because its main role is to bind T4 and T3. Anything that affects TBG could also cause abnormal T4 or T3 levels. TBG levels are increased in pregnancy and by estrogen-containing medications (oral contraceptive pills) and are decreased with liver disease and medications like glucocorticoids and androgens (Haugen 2009; Koulouri et al. 2013; Soh and Aw 2019).

TBG is typically evaluated when there is a discrepancy between total T4 and free T4. For example, if the total T4 is elevated and the free T4 is normal, the endocrinologist may order a TBG level. TBG excess or TBG deficiency has been found incidentally during neonatal hypothyroidism screening and does not require treatment (Jin 2016).

11.5.8.5 Thyroglobulin

Thyroglobulin (TG) should not be confused with thyroid-binding globulin (TBG). TG is produced by the follicular cells in the thyroid gland and is essential in the synthesis of T4 and T3. TG is primarily used as a tumor marker after treatment for thyroid cancer. It may also be increased in patients with goiter, and the size of the goiter may correlate with the elevation in TG. The clinical usefulness of TG measurement is typically to monitor patients after treatment for thyroid cancer (Esfandiari and Papaleontiou 2017; Soh and Aw 2019). Patients being monitored during and after treatment for thyroid cancer should be referred to an endocrinologist.

11.5.8.6 Thyroglobulin (TG) and Thyroid Peroxidase (TPO) Antibodies

Both TG antibodies and TPO antibodies are markers of thyroid autoimmunity and are more common in females than males. They frequently occur in the general population and are diagnostic of Hashimoto's disease but may also be positive in Graves' disease. A patient may have positive TG and TPO antibodies and normal thyroid function, but the presence of TG and TPO antibodies puts a patient at risk for future thyroid dysfunction (Esfandiari and Papaleontiou 2017; Soh and Aw 2019; Sheehan 2016). Therefore, these patients should be monitored every 6–12 months with TSH and free T4, but sooner if they have symptoms of overt hypothyroidism.

In overt hypothyroidism, assessing TG and TPO antibodies may not add clinical significance and will not change the treatment of hypothyroidism. However, in patients with a family history of autoimmunity or other autoimmune conditions, like type 1 diabetes mellitus or Addison's disease, assessing thyroid antibody status may help predict which patients will develop thyroid dysfunction and which will not. In cases of subclinical hypothyroidism with mildly elevated TSH and normal free T4, knowing thyroid antibody status may provide more evidence to treat the subclinical hypothyroidism if the patient has TPO antibodies and, therefore, an increased risk of overt hypothyroidism in the future (Esfandiari and Papaleontiou 2017; Soh and Aw 2019; Sheehan 2016).

The National Health and Nutrition Examination Survey III (Hollowell et al. 2002; Spencer et al. 2007) examined nonpregnant people ages 12 and older without thyroid dysfunction to evaluate the influence of demographics on thyroid antibodies. It was found that 12.5% of the total population had either TPO or TG antibodies, and the prevalence of TPO and TG antibodies was greater in females than males and increased with age. Non-Hispanic White subjects had an increased percentage of both antibodies compared to non-Hispanic Black subjects and Mexican Americans. The study also noted that TG antibodies alone were not significantly associated with thyroid disease. When both antibodies were present, patients had the highest risk of developing hypothyroidism, but the risk of overt hypothyroidism was greater than the risk of subclinical hypothyroidism. It was also shown that the prevalence of TPO antibodies increased as TSH increased to >2 mIU/L (Spencer et al. 2007).

11.5.8.7 Thyroid Receptor Antibodies (TRab)

Both thyroid-stimulating immunoglobulin (TSI) and thyroid-binding inhibitory immunoglobulin (TBII) are thyroid receptor antibodies. TSI is secreted by B lymphocytes in Graves' disease and mimics the action of TSH, therefore causing increased secretion of T4 and T3 from the thyroid gland.

TBII blocks the action of TSH. TRab testing is most widely used to aid in the etiology of hyper-thyroidism in conjunction with radioactive iodine uptake and scan (Sheehan 2016; Ross et al. 2016). Measuring TRabs can also be useful before discontinuing treatment for Graves' disease when the patient is in a euthyroid state (Esfandiari and Papaleontiou 2017; Ross et al. 2016). A pediatric endocrinologist will typically recommend when medication for Graves' disease can be safely discontinued. Table 11.7 reviews the differential diagnosis based on common thyroid function test results.

11.5.9 Real-Life Examples

An 18-year-old female presented to her primary care clinician with a neck mass and 30 lb. weight loss. She also had intermittent palpitations, heat intolerance, and mild periorbital swelling. At the clinician's office, she was hypertensive and tachycardic to 130 beats/min. Laboratory tests

Table 11.7 Common thyroid function test results and associated diagnoses

Diagnosis	TSH	Free T4	Total T4	T3	Thyroglobulin Ab and TPO Ab	TRab
Hashimoto's hypothyroidism	↑	↓ or →	↓ or →	Rarely measured	Positive (either)	Negative (rarely measured)
Acquired hypothyroidism	↑	↓ or →	↓ or →	Rarely measured	Negative (both)	Negative (rarely measured)
Central hypothyroidism	↓ or →	↓ or →	↓ or →	Rarely measured	Negative	Negative
Iodine deficiency or excess[a]	↑	↓	↓	↓	Negative	Negative
Hashitoxicosis	↓	↑	↑	↑	Positive	Negative
Graves' disease	↓	↑	↑	↑	Negative or positive	Positive TSI
Hyperfunctioning nodule	↓	↑	↑	↑	Negative	Negative
Nonadherence to levothyroxine	↑	→ or ↓	→	n/a	n/a	n/a
Nonadherence to hyperthyroid medications	↓	↑	↑	↑	n/a	n/a
TBG deficiency	→	→	↑	n/a	n/a	n/a
Non-thyroidal illness	Depends on the stage of illness	Depends on the stage of illness	Depends on the stage of illness	Depends on the stage of illness	Negative	Negative (rarely measured)

Adapted from Koulouri et al. (2013), Soh and Aw (2019)
[a]The Wolff-Chaikoff effect occurs when the thyroid gland inhibits the synthesis of T4 in response to large amounts of iodine, irrespective of TSH level

were consistent with hyperthyroidism: TSH <0.05 uU/mL (0.4–4.6), FT4 > 6 ng/dL (0.8–1.7), T3 > 651 ng/dL (80–200), TG antibody 84.1 IU/mL, TPO 807.7 IU/mL (<5), and TSI 438% (<140%). She was diagnosed with Graves' disease and started on methimazole 10 mg BID and atenolol for HR >100 bpm. One month later, her thyroid function tests improved but was still not completely normal. She was feeling better. Her laboratory results were as follows: TSH <0.05uU/mL (0.4–4.6), FT4 1.8 ng/dL (0.8–1.7), and T3 237ng/dL (80–200). Due to difficulty controlling her Graves' disease with medication, the patient had a total thyroidectomy about 6 months later and is now on a stable dose of levothyroxine for postsurgical hypothyroidism.

A 16-year-old female with known congenital hypothyroidism, on treatment with levothyroxine, presented to her primary care provider for her annual health assessment. Due to her history, thyroid function tests were completed, and she noted an elevated total T4 20.5 mcg/dL (4.7–13.3) and normal TSH 2.050 uU/mL (0.45–3.98). The primary care provider repeated the labs and noted the same pattern of elevated total T4 14.9 mcg/dL (4.7–13.3) and normal TSH 1.62 uU/mL (0.45–3.98). The patient was asymptomatic and referred to pediatric endocrinology. Repeat lab testing with the pediatric endocrinologist revealed elevated total T4 13.28mcg/dL (5–12), normal free T4 1.46 ng/dL (0.8–1.7), normal TSH 4.04 uU/mL (0.4–4.6), elevated TBG 42.2 mcg/mL (10–23.8), normal T3 150 ng/dL (81–199), and normal TSI 41% (<140). The patient was diagnosed with TBG excess, which causes the total T4 (bound and unbound) to appear elevated. She was instructed to ask future providers to draw free T4 instead of total T4 when evaluating her thyroid.

A 6-year 2-month-old female was referred to pediatric endocrinology due to concerns of obesity and slowed growth. Thyroid function tests were normal (TSH 3.27 uU/mL (0.400–4.60) and free T4 1.18 ng/dL (0.80–1.70)), but the patient had positive TPO antibodies. Repeat studies 4 months later showed normal TSH and free T4 with positive TPO and thyroglobulin antibodies. Because of the positive antibodies, TSH and free T4 were monitored. The patient was lost to follow-up for 16 months. When she returned to the pediatric endocrine clinic, the TSH was elevated to 11.1 uU/mL (0.400–4.60), and the patient was started on treatment for subclinical hypothyroidism caused by Hashimoto's thyroiditis.

Key Learning about Thyroid Function

- TSH and free T4 are the most widely used thyroid function tests.
- TSH evaluation alone may not be sufficient to screen for thyroid dysfunction in children.
- Obesity without other signs/symptoms of hypothyroidism is not an indication for thyroid function tests.
- A low TSH and elevated free T4 (suggestive of untreated hyperthyroidism) warrants an immediate referral to a pediatric endocrinologist.
- A mildly elevated TSH and normal free T4 may be repeated with thyroid antibodies before referral to a pediatric endocrinologist.
- The absorption of levothyroxine is affected by the following:
  - Soy.
  - Calcium.
  - Fiber.
  - Iron.
- Remember that patients taking levothyroxine should take it on an empty stomach or at least 30–60 min before eating foods that contain those listed above.

11.6 Growth Disorders

In pediatrics, monitoring growth is a key part of well-child care. Height, weight, and body mass index (BMI) are plotted on every child over 2 years of age, while the length, weight for length, and head circumference are part of routine well-child care for the child under 3 years of age. BMI is not evaluated on a child under 2 years; rather, plotting weight for length is key in the younger pediatric patient. Electronic health records now plot growth parameters for clinicians, but the clinician needs to note any upward or downward trends. A growth disorder should be considered if a child is plotting along with a growth percentile and starts to trend upward or downward, crossing two percentiles.

11.6.1 Physiology of Growth

Growth hormone (GH) is produced by somatotroph cells within the anterior pituitary gland. The release of GH is regulated by stimulatory growth hormone-releasing hormone (GHRH) and inhibitory somatostatin from the hypothalamus leading to a pulsatile pattern of secretion. GH has various functions in different parts of the body. Specifically related to growth, GH acts on cells in the liver to produce insulin-like growth factors and binding proteins (including IGF-1 and IGF-BP3). Independent of stature, GH acts on adipose tissue by increasing lipolysis and decreasing lipogenesis. GH also acts on the muscles by increasing lean tissue and increasing energy expenditure (Backeljauw et al. 2014).

Growth hormone secretion is influenced by other hormones, including thyroxine, glucocorticoids, estrogens, and androgens. Various circumstances, including sleep, nutritional state, stress, exercise, hypoglycemia, and hemorrhage, also influence the secretion of GH. As far as growth, GH stimulates epiphyseal growth, stimulates osteoblast activity, stimulates osteoclast activity and differentiation, and promotes endochondral bone formation, thereby increasing bone mass. Because of GH's actions on bone mass, muscles, and lipolysis, people with true growth hormone deficiency may benefit from GH treatment as adults even when linear growth is complete (Backeljauw et al. 2014).

Short stature and tall stature are both considered to be forms of growth disorders. Referrals for short stature or growth failure are far more common than tall stature or growth excess, and therefore the focus on this section will mainly focus on short stature and growth failure. Short stature is defined as a height that is more than two standard deviations (SDs) below the mean for age, sex, and population, which would be below the third percentile on the growth curve (Cohen 2014). A child with a projected height that is more than 2 SDs below the calculated midparental height or has a poor growth velocity should be evaluated for growth failure (Barstow and Rerucha 2015).

11.6.2 Short Stature, Normal Variants of Growth, and Growth Failure

Causes of short stature can be subdivided into normal variants of growth and pathological causes of growth. It is important to distinguish whether the patient should be referred to endocrinology or if close monitoring is appropriate.

11.6.3 Familial Short Stature

Children with familial short stature typically have a height that plots at the low end of the growth curve and may fall below the third percentile. Their biological parents are often below the tenth percentile on the growth curves (Rogol and Hayden 2014). These children typically have a birth weight and birth length that are appropriate for gestational age. Their growth rate begins to decrease between 6 and 18 months of age, but they will establish their growth curve between 2 and 3 years of age. The bone age typically coincides with their chronological age (Rogol and Hayden 2014).

11.6.4 Constitutional Delay of Growth and Puberty (CDGP)

Constitutional delay of growth and puberty is the most common cause of short stature (Grimberg et al. 2016; Grimberg and Lifshitz 2007). These children are considered the "late bloomers." They tend to have family members who had later pubertal development. They are born with weights and lengths appropriate for gestational age. They tend to have a growth deceleration in the first 2 years of life and may have a slower growth velocity until 5 years. They establish a growth curve at or below the fifth percentile but growing at a normal growth velocity in the prepubertal years. They typically have a delayed bone age. Since they will start puberty later, they will demonstrate catch-up growth during the pubertal years, but their growth spurts may occur later than their peers (Rogol and Hayden 2014).

11.6.5 Idiopathic Short Stature

Idiopathic short stature (ISS) is defined as a height of −2 SDs below the mean for age and sex without any clear evidence of an endocrine, nutritional, systemic, or chromosomal cause (Cohen 2014). Children with ISS are typically born with a normal birth weight. They have normal screening labs, including IGF-1 levels and normal growth hormone response to a growth hormone stimulation test. It is, therefore, a diagnosis of exclusion (Rogol and Hayden 2014). Treatment with growth hormone therapy for ISS is approved by the United States Food and Drug Administration (FDA) when the height is ≤−2.25 SDs below the mean for age and sex without evidence of any other underlying cause and the child is unlikely to reach a height within the normal adult range, and no other underlying cause has been determined. A height that is ≤−2.25 SDs below the mean for age and sex corresponds to a height that is ≤1.2nd percentile on the growth curve, which is equivalent to an adult height of 63 inches (160 cm) for men and 59 inches (150 cm) for women (Grimberg et al. 2016).

11.6.5.1 Pathologic Causes of Short Stature

Short stature and poor growth can be due to various conditions and require a thorough history and physical exam. Evaluation of the growth curves for both height and weight can also give clues into the differential diagnosis (Rogol and Hayden 2014). There are endocrine and nonendocrine causes of short stature, some of which are treated with growth hormone.

Endocrine causes of short stature include hypothyroidism, Cushing's syndrome, and growth hormone deficiency. Lab testing related to hypothyroidism and Cushing's syndrome are discussed in other sections. Hypothyroidism is more prevalent than growth hormone deficiency or Cushing's syndrome. Therefore, it is essential to evaluate thyroid function tests in the initial poor growth evaluation (Styne 2016).

Growth hormone deficiency. Growth hormone deficiency can be congenital or acquired. In congenital growth hormone deficiency (GHD), a neonate may present with hypoglycemia or congenital midline defects (such as septo-optic dysplasia). GHD can be isolated or seen in combination with other pituitary deficiencies. Isolated idiopathic GHD is the most common cause of hypopituitarism (Di Iorgi et al. 2016). Acquired growth hormone deficiency may include head trauma, tumors near the pituitary gland such as craniopharyngiomas, or postcranial radiation treatment. Patients with congenital midline defects or conditions associated with acquired growth hormone deficiency should be screened routinely for pituitary deficiencies by a pediatric endocrinology team (Rosenbloom and Connor 2007).

The diagnosis of GHD can be challenging. Therefore, it is based on a combination of factors that includes appropriate growth measurements, bone age X-rays, IGF-1 and IGF-BP3 levels, growth hormone stimulation tests, brain MRI, and occasionally genetic testing (Stanley 2012).

Nonendocrine causes. Nonendocrine causes of short stature or growth failure may include chronic disease, malnutrition, skeletal dysplasia, and certain genetic conditions. Chronic systemic conditions that can cause short stature typically are not treated with growth hormone therapy, and the growth can improve if the systemic condition is treated. For example, a patient with celiac disease may present with short stature, and once the patient is following a gluten-free diet, the growth rate typically improves. Certain genetic conditions are treated with growth hormone, specifically Turner syndrome, Noonan syndrome, SHOX deficiency, and Prader-Willi syndrome (with precautions due to concern for obstructive sleep apnea) (Deal et al. 2013). These genetic conditions should be evaluated if the clinician has suspicion (Rogol and Hayden 2014; Powell et al. 1967). Psychosocial short stature may also occur (Styne 2016). Some studies associated severe emotional deprivation with poor growth. Reversal of the emotional stressors typically allows for catch-up growth (Rogol 2020; Styne 2016). Therefore, clinicians should ensure that a psychosocial history is included in a growth evaluation. Box 11.4 reviews the indications for growth hormone therapy.

Box 11.4 FDA Indications for Treatment with Growth Hormone Therapy

- Growth hormone deficiency.
- Small for gestational age (with failure to catch up in growth by 2–4 years old).
- Turner syndrome (including mosaic Turner syndrome).
- Noonan syndrome.
- Idiopathic short stature and at least −2.25 SD on the growth curve.
- Chronic kidney disease.
- Prader-Willi syndrome.

Adapted from Wilson et al. (2003), Romano (2019)

11.6.6 Short Stature and Growth Failure Evaluation

A thorough history, physical exam, imaging, and screening labs can help to narrow down the differential diagnosis and where to refer a patient.

The evaluation of short stature begins with making sure that a child is measured correctly. A child under 2 years old should be measured laying down using an Infantometer, and measurement should be plotted using the WHO standardized growth curves. For children 2–3 years of age, it is advised to do both a length and a standing height and plot the point on the WHO and CDC standardized charts. Any child 3 years old and older should be measured using a standing height. Growth charts provide a visualization for when there is a deviation in normal growth velocity. Growth velocity is most rapid during birth to 12 months of age and during puberty. Between 5 years of age and puberty, a

child's growth velocity should be at least 5 cm (~2 inches) per year (Barstow and Rerucha 2015).

Birth history is also important to guide growth evaluation. It is important to know if a child's birth length and/or birth weight were considered small for gestational age (SGA). Most children born SGA catch up to the growth curve by 2 years of age, but 10% of children do not (Barstow and Rerucha 2015). Preterm children born SGA may take up to 4 years to catch up to the growth curve. Children identified as SGA at birth and who have not caught up to the growth curve by 2–4 years old are unlikely to catch up. Therefore, a referral to pediatric endocrinology is warranted. SGA without catch-up growth is an approved indication for growth hormone therapy (Houk and Lee 2012).

Another key component of the history is the height of the biological parents. A clinician can estimate the patient's target height based on the calculated midparental height, and the formula is in Box 11.5. Midparental height is used to see if the child is growing within the genetic potential of the family. The pubertal timing of the biological parents may also provide valuable information, for example, if a parent was a "late bloomer." Box 11.6 is an overview of considerations for those who may need short stature evaluation.

Box 11.5 Calculation for Midparental Height

Girls: ([father's height cm − 13 cm] + mother's height cm)/2.

Boys: ([mother's height cm + 13 cm] + father's height cm)/2.

+/− 8.5 cm (is considered within normal range of the child's genetic potential).

Of note, various sources list the range to be different. Depending on the source, anywhere from +/−6.5 cm to +/− 10 cm is considered "within the normal range."

Adapted from Backeljauw et al. (2014), Barstow and Rerucha (2015), Cohen (2014), Cohen et al. (2008), Rogol and Hayden (2014)

Box 11.6 When to Consider Short Stature Evaluation

- Children born SGA who fail to catch up to the growth curve by 2 years of age.
- Any child over 3 years old who is below the third percentile on the growth curve.
- Signs of growth failure: downward crossing of percentiles on the height-for-age curve or slowed growth velocity.
- The child's predicted height is more than 2 SDs (~10 cm or 3–4 inches) below the child's calculated midparental height.

Adapted from Barstow and Rerucha (2015), Cohen (2014), Cohen et al. (2008), Rogol and Hayden 2014

11.6.6.1 Bone Age X-Ray

A bone age is based on an X-ray of the left hand and wrist. The hand and wrist have been used as a standard for bone ages because these bones and epiphyses have been shown to progress and mature to fusion in a relatively consistent manner (De Sanctis et al. 2014). The purpose of the bone age is to compare a patient's stage in skeletal maturation with chronological age. This can help give a better height prediction, but it can also help determine possible pathology. For example, children with true growth hormone deficiency almost always have a delayed bone age (Barstow and Rerucha 2015; Styne 2016). It is more difficult to evaluate the maturity of the hand and wrist bones in children less than 3 years old, and bone ages are less useful (Creo and Schwenk 2nd 2017). Over time, the epiphyseal plates of the ulna, radius, and phalanges fuse with the metaphysis. The most common method used to determine bone age is the Greulich-Pyle method. With this method, the patient's visual appearance and wrist will be compared to standard X-ray images of the left hand and wrist for various ages. There are different standards for males and females. The Tanner-Whitehouse (TW) is another method used

to determine bone age and calculates a score for each bone in the hand. In the United States, the Greulich-Pyle method is the most commonly used (Creo and Schwenk 2nd 2017).

There are some limitations to a bone age evaluation. The standard references used for both the Greulich-Pyle and the Tanner-Whitehouse methods are based on a primarily Caucasian population. There also can be inter-provider variability in the bone age reading as it is relatively subjective. A pediatric radiologist and/or pediatric endocrine clinician trained in reading bone ages should interpret the bone age. An automated bone age rating, BoneXpert, was developed and released by the Denmark company Visiana in 2008. This software can calculate the Greulich-Pyle and Tanner-Whitehouse scores (Creo and Schwenk 2nd 2017). It has not yet become widely adopted in practice which may be partially due to the cost. The BoneXpert system also does not evaluate the carpal bones. There are times when there are discrepancies in skeletal maturation between the carpal bones and phalanges which would be missed utilizing this system (De Sanctis et al. 2014).

11.6.6.2 IGF-1 and IGF-BP3

Insulin-like growth factors (IGF) are peptides that are structurally related to insulin. The liver produces IGF in response to GH; though it is believed that IGF-1 has actions independent of GH, this is not well defined. There are two IGFs: IGF-1 and IGF-2. Serum concentrations of IGF-1 are much more GH-dependent than IGF-2, and therefore, IGF-1 levels are typically used in clinical practice for monitoring purposes (Backeljauw et al. 2014). Over 99% of IGF-1 is bound to IGF-binding proteins (IGFBPs) (Faix 2013). There are six different IGF-binding proteins, the most prevalent being IGF-BP3. IGF-BP3 helps transport IGF-1 to target cell surface receptors (Varma Shrivastav et al. 2020).

Because IGF-1 binds so strongly to IGF-BP3, assays need to be used that can disassociate the IGF-BP3. This disassociation process can lead to variability between assays (Chinoy and Murray 2016). Double-antibody sandwich assays such as ELISA are frequently used, but the most advanced method used today is liquid chromatography followed by tandem mass spectrometry (Backeljauw et al. 2014).

IGF-1 levels also vary with age, sex, and pubertal status, so it is important to use specific reference ranges when making clinical decisions. IGF-1 shows less diurnal variation than GH and is the preferred screening test for evaluating children for short stature before testing GH (Guzzetti et al. 2016). It has been suggested that IGF-1 levels have a specificity of >90% and low levels of IGF-1 are very predictive of GHD but a sensitivity of 50–70%, particularly in children younger than 5 years of age, so a normal level does not rule out GHD (Chinoy and Murray 2016).

In clinical practice, IGF-1 is considered a better marker of growth hormone status than IGF-BP3. However, IGF-BP3 is a better marker of growth hormone status in children younger than 3 years of age since IGF-1 levels tend to be lower in that age range (Cohen et al. 2008).

When IGF-1 and/or IGF-BP3 levels are below −2 SD, it suggests that there could be an abnormality in the growth hormone axis, and it warrants further evaluation.

IGF-1/IGF-BP3 testing is affected by poorly controlled diabetes, cirrhosis, renal failure, malnutrition, hypothyroidism, and oral estrogen medication (Clemmons 2011). In general, there is less variability in IGF values compared to GH levels. Studies have shown that IGF-1 levels are lower in patients with BMIs <20 kg/m^2 or > 40 kg/m^2, though these studies were in adults (Junnila et al. 2015). IGF-BP3 is less affected by nutritional status (Chinoy and Murray 2016; Cohen 2014). When interpreting the IGF-1 level, it is important to remember that for patients who have a constitutional delay of growth and development, a normal IGF-1 level will correlate with the bone age and may not correlate with the chronological age (Styne 2016).

11.6.6.3 Growth Hormone (GH)

As discussed, growth hormone is released from the anterior pituitary in a pulsatile fashion. Therefore, a single GH sample is not adequate to diagnose GH deficiency and therefore is of no clinical value to the primary clinician or pediatric endocrinologist (Guzzetti et al. 2016; Junnila

et al. 2015; Grimberg et al. 2016). In conjunction with a pediatric endocrinologist, provocative growth hormone stimulation tests must be performed to assess peak growth hormone levels. These tests are performed by administering a choice of agents, including arginine, clonidine, glucagon, insulin, or L-dopa, following an overnight fast to stimulate the pituitary gland to release GH. A peak GH level of <10 μg/L is currently used as the cutoff value to support a diagnosis of GH deficiency in conjunction with auxological and clinical criteria (Growth Hormone Research Society 2000). Box 11.7 reviews the initial lab workup for a child with short stature.

Although there is a traditional cutoff level for peak growth hormone levels of <10 μg/L, this is still considered arbitrary. For example, some countries use a cutoff of <6 μg/L (Stanley 2012). Because GH levels are affected by various day-to-day factors, GH levels tend to be poorly reproducible. Factors that can affect growth hormone levels include weight and nutritional status. Obesity can blunt GH levels and causes faster GH clearance rates (Junnila et al. 2015). Alternatively, individuals with lower BMI levels may have higher peak GH levels (Stanley 2012). GH secretion is increased in females than males (Junnila et al. 2015; Veldhuis et al. 2000). Age and pubertal status are also important factors as GH levels peak during late adolescence. During puberty, the higher level of sex steroid hormones is thought to increase GH and IGF-1 levels. Children with delayed puberty tend to have low GH levels on GH stimulation testing when they are prepubertal but often have a normal GH response after puberty. The change has led to the debate on sex steroid priming in prepubertal children before GH stimulation testing to prevent false positives (Chinoy and Murray 2016). To "fail" the growth hormone stimulation test, the child should have an inadequate peak growth hormone level in response to two different provocative tests (either two different agents simultaneously or the same agent performed on different days). Stimulation testing should be performed in the morning and a fasting state. It is also important to remember that hypothyroidism can cause a diminished response to GH stimulation testing (Styne 2016).

Large discrepancies can be seen between various growth hormone assays. Initially, the normal values for GH were based on polyclonal radioimmunoassay and purified pituitary standards. Today, the growth hormone assays are performed with monoclonal antibodies and recombinant standards, which have higher specificities but question if the peak growth hormone concentration cutoff values should be lowered (Growth Hormone Research Society 2000; Grimberg et al. 2016). Assay variability may affect GH testing and interpretation of results. GH stimulation tests have low reproducibility, specificity, and sensitivity (Guzzetti et al. 2016). There is also minimal data about GH concentration comparisons between the various provocative agents that are used. A study by Zadik et al. (1990), for example, found that GH peak levels in normally growing children were similar between insulin and arginine agents, but the GH levels were higher when using clonidine (Grimberg et al. 2016; Zadik et al. 1990).

Due to the variability of GH testing, it is recommended that the diagnosis of growth hormone deficiency is based not only on growth hormone stimulation testing but with consideration of the history, growth measurements, additional lab testing (including a low IGF-1), and radiological evidence. Table 11.8 provides an overview of factors affecting growth hormone measurements, and Table 11.9 reviews common differential diagnoses for short stature.

Box 11.7 Routine Screening Labs for Short Stature
- IGF-1 and IGF-BP3.
- Complete blood count.
- Basic metabolic panel.
- Liver function tests.
- Celiac panel.
- TSH, free T4.
- Inflammatory markers (ESR, CRP).
- Urinalysis.
- Karyotype (any girl with short stature).

Adapted from Barstow and Rerucha (2015), Rogol and Hayden (2014)

Table 11.8 Factors affecting growth hormone levels

Factors	How is GH affected
Age	GH peaks during late adolescence
Gender	Females have higher average GH levels than males
BMI	– Obesity causes lower GH secretion and faster GH clearance – GH levels are higher in those with lower BMI on provocative testing
Food intake before GH testing	Peak GH levels highest after short-term fasting
Pubertal status	GH levels on provocative testing may be lower in children with delayed puberty
Time of day	GH is secreted in a pulsatile manner, with the most GH secreted in the early morning

Adapted from Junnila et al. (2015), Stanley (2012)

11.6.7 Real-Life Example

A 4-year-old boy was seen for the first time by the primary care clinician. The child's height was below the third percentile. The father was noted to be 60 inches tall, and the mother was 62 inches. The family was told that the child's short stature was a result of the paternal height. A complete history and physical exam failed to raise suspicion of another differential diagnosis. A workup for growth hormone deficiency was initiated and ultimately revealed that the child had inherited a genetic growth hormone deficiency from the father. The father was never diagnosed until his son's condition was correctly diagnosed. The initiation of growth hormone dramatically improved the child's stature. He ultimately followed the 75th percentile.

11.6.8 Real-Life Example

A 12-year 3-month-old male presented to the endocrine clinic for complaints of short stature and being the shortest in his class. He was born full-term, BW 9lbs. Past medical history was significant for psoriasis. The midparental target height (MPTH) was 69.5 inches. At presentation, his height was at the 0.7 percentile (−2.46 SDs below the mean), and his weight was at the 39th

Table 11.9 Common differential diagnoses of short stature

Diagnosis	IGF-1	IGF-BP3	Bone age
Familial short stature	Normal	Normal	Normal
CDGP	Normal	Normal	Delayed
ISS	Normal	Normal	Normal
SGA	Normal	Normal	Normal/advanced
GHD	Low	Normal/low	Delayed/normal
Hypothyroidism	Normal	Normal	Normal Delayed if significant hypothyroidism
Cushing's syndrome	Normal	Normal	Normal/advanced
Chronic illness	Low	Low/normal	Delayed/normal
Malnutrition	Low	Low/normal	Delayed/normal
Psychosocial dwarfism	Low	Low	Delayed/normal
Skeletal dysplasia	Normal	Normal	Variable
Genetic syndrome	Variable	Variable	Variable

Adapted from Styne (2016), Backeljauw et al. (2014), Rosenbloom and Connor (2007)

percentile. He was in very-early puberty with testes measuring 4 mL bilaterally. He was lost to follow-up for 7 months and had not completed his initial screening tests. At follow-up, his growth velocity was 3.6 cm/year. Screening tests noted normal TSH, free T4, LFTs, BMP, CBC, IGF-1 96 ng/dL (Tanner stage (TS) or sexual maturity rating (SMR) stage II: 192–689 ng/mL), and IGF-BP3 5.7 mg/L (TS or T II 2.3–6.3 mg/L). A bone age was completed and read as 10 years, at chronological age 12 years and 3 months (delayed bone age). Due to his poor growth velocity, short stature noted on the growth curve, low IGF-1, and delayed bone age, a GH stimulation test was completed. His GH peak was 4.3 µg/L. His brain MRI showed a normal pituitary. The patient was given a diagnosis of GHD and started GH treatment. After 4 years of GH treatment, his final adult height was 68.3 inches (33.7 percentile) within 2 inches of his MPTH.

Key Learning about Growth Disorders and Diagnostic Testing

- A random GH level is not helpful in the diagnosis of short or tall stature disorders.
- IGF-1 shows less diurnal variation compared to GH and is the preferred screening test used in the evaluation of children for short stature.
- Accurate measurements and growth charts are integral for any growth evaluation.
- A bone age evaluation is a helpful non-invasive tool to screen for growth concerns.
- If a parent has significant short stature - 2SD below the growth curve, consider that the parent could have a pathological cause of short stature that was missed and may be present in the child.
- A child who presents with short stature but has a normal height velocity, a normal bone age, and a normal IGF-1/IGF-BP3 is unlikely to have a growth hormone deficiency. Other causes of short stature should be evaluated.
- Growth concerns should prompt a referral to a pediatric endocrinologist since earlier treatment may improve final adult height.

11.6.9 Tall Stature

Tall stature is defined as a height that is 2 SDs or more above the mean for age, sex, and population or above the 97th percentile on the growth curve

(Rogol and Hayden 2014). Tall stature can also be defined as a projected height of more than 2 SDs above the midparental target height. Tall stature may be due to familial tall stature (Styne 2016). Obese children often have tall stature in the prepubertal years, but they tend to start puberty earlier and ultimately reach a near-normal adult height (Styne 2016). Precocious puberty will lead to tall stature and more rapid growth at an earlier age; however, these children tend to be within their genetic potential or shorter due to earlier fusion of the growth plates. Hyperthyroidism can also lead to excess growth and early fusion of the growth plates. Genetic syndromes associated with tall stature include Klinefelter syndrome, Beckwith-Wiedemann syndrome, Soto syndrome, and other rare disorders (Barstow and Rerucha 2015).

Acromegaly is a result of the pituitary gland producing excess GH. IGF-1 and IGF-BP3 levels can be used to screen for growth hormone excess. It is more common in adults, but it can lead to gigantism if it presents in childhood. An oral glucose tolerance test is used as the standard test for growth hormone excess as glucose will suppress growth hormone levels (<1 μg/L) (Katznelson et al. 2014; Junnila et al. 2015).

11.7 Pubertal Disorders

There are many different kinds of disorders related to puberty. They include premature adrenarche, premature thelarche, precocious puberty, delayed puberty, and abnormal menses. The clinician needs to evaluate the history, physical exam, and order diagnostic laboratory tests judiciously based on a knowledge of puberty physiology.

11.7.1 Puberty Physiology

GnRH (gonadotropin-releasing hormone) is released from the hypothalamus, and in the prepubertal state, it is released at a low amplitude and frequency. The timing of puberty is considered normal if a girl starts puberty no earlier than 8 years of age and a boy starts puberty no earlier than 9 years of age (Klein et al. 2017). When puberty begins, the pulsed releases of GnRH increase in amplitude and frequency, starting in the nighttime hours (Bozzola et al. 2018; Rosenfeld et al. 2014). GnRH then stimulates the release of LH and FSH from the anterior pituitary. LH acts on the ovaries in females, which produce estradiol, stimulating breast development, pubertal growth velocity, and changes in the vaginal mucosa (red indicating no estrogen exposure; pink indicating exposure to estrogen) (Klein et al. 2017), and acts on the testes in males which produce testosterone, stimulating penile growth and pubic hair and indirectly stimulates the pubertal growth spurt via testosterone conversion to estradiol (Kaplowitz and Bloch 2016).

When evaluating a patient for a potential pubertal disorder, it is important to include a thorough physical exam which should include growth velocity, assessment of breast tissue or testicular volume, acne, adult body odor, axillary, and/or pubic hair. Additionally, skin exam findings (i.e., acne or hyperpigmentation) may provide diagnostic information. In addition to a complete physical exam, it is important to include a pubertal history, including the timing of onset and speed of progression and potential concerning neurologic signs/symptoms (i.e., vision changes) and potential exposure to exogenous hormones (i.e., testosterone or estrogen). Finally, a family history may reveal precocious puberty or other pubertal disorders, which may be helpful in the evaluation (Latronico et al. 2016). Many pubertal conditions (including primary and secondary amenorrhea, oligomenorrhea, delayed puberty) can be caused by non-endocrine conditions, such as medications, systemic illness, or stress; therefore, a thorough history and physical exam are important in addition to the endocrine considerations mentioned in this chapter.

Adrenarche (adrenal androgen production) is a separate process from gonadarche (gonadal sex hormone production) (Klein et al. 2017). During adrenarche, the zona reticularis of the adrenal gland develops further and produces the precursors to adrenal androgens (DHEA and androstenedione) (Novello and Speiser 2018).

Normal variants of puberty include premature thelarche and premature adrenarche (Kaplowitz and Bloch 2016). Suppose a patient has a normal variant of puberty. In that case, it may be appropriate for the primary care clinician to monitor the patient and then refer to pediatric endocrinology if the progression of puberty or other signs of puberty emerge.

Abnormal variants include various other disorders that may be central (from the pituitary gland) or peripheral (from other endocrine glands) in origin. The adrenal glands produce pubertal hormones. Therefore, an adrenal source for disorders of puberty must be considered when evaluating a patient for pubertal concerns. For abnormal variants of puberty, patients should be referred to pediatric endocrinology for further evaluation; however, as discussed in this section, screening labs may be completed by the primary care clinician to begin the evaluation. When monitoring puberty in the primary care setting, it is important to assess the TS or SMR staging of pubic hair and the testicular volume (using a Prader orchidometer) in males and the staging of breast development in females.

11.7.2 Premature Adrenarche

Premature adrenarche is a diagnosis of exclusion (Voutilainen and Jääskeläinen 2015). Premature adrenarche occurs when there is an early increase in adrenal androgens and is considered a normal variant (Fuqua 2013; Oberfield et al. 2011). In girls, this is considered before 8 years of age and in boys, before 9 years of age. Premature adrenarche occurs in the absence of central puberty when the HPG axis is not activated; therefore, the pubertal hormones (LH, FSH, estradiol) will typically remain low (Kaplowitz and Bloch 2016; Klein et al. 2017). The patient may have all or some of the following signs: axillary hair, pubic hair, body

odor, and acne (Kaplowitz and Bloch 2016). There is no breast development or clitoromegaly in girls or testicular enlargement in boys (Klein et al. 2017). It is important to ensure that the patient has benign premature adrenarche instead of other conditions (see under "hyperandrogenism"). Premature adrenarche is considered benign once the clinician has ruled out excess androgen disorders.

Concern for a pathologic cause of premature adrenarche is stronger when there is a clitoral or penile enlargement or increased growth velocity (Kaplowitz and Bloch 2016) or advancing bone age (Oberfield et al. 2011). The primary care clinician may consider ordering a bone age X-ray, and if advanced, the patient should be referred to a pediatric endocrinologist; however, the primary care clinician can also refer before bone age X-ray, as the evaluation of a bone age can be difficult to interpret as previously discussed. Of note, the frequency is much higher in females, with the female-to-male ratio of 9:1 (Novello and Speiser 2018; Oberfield et al. 2011).

11.7.3 Premature Thelarche

Premature thelarche is considered a normal variant and can be seen in females under 2 years of age who have glandular breast tissue without growth acceleration or other signs of puberty (Kaplowitz and Bloch 2016; Rosenfeld et al. 2014). There is no progression, and frequently, the breast tissue regresses. If the primary care clinician is comfortable that the patient presents with only premature thelarche, it may be appropriate to monitor in the primary care setting (Kaplowitz and Bloch 2016).

11.7.4 Precocious Puberty

Precocious puberty is when girls have an onset of puberty before the age of 8 years of age and when boys have the onset of puberty before 9 years of age (Kaplowitz and Bloch 2016). Recently, it has been thought that puberty may be considered normal in White females as early as 7 years old or as early as 6 years old in African American females (Kaplowitz and Oberfield 1999).

In girls, the first sign of puberty is breast development (thelarche; TS or SMR stage 2), whereas, for boys, the first sign of puberty is testicular enlargement (gonadarche; testicular volume 4 mL) (Fuqua 2013). Puberty is often associated with acceleration in growth. It is important to distinguish between lipomastia (fatty tissue) and true breast tissue; this may be difficult to ascertain on physical exam in the setting of obesity, but with lipomastia, girls will not have glandular tissue or stimulated (darkened) areola and nipples (Kaplowitz and Bloch 2016).

A useful tool for evaluating a patient for precocious puberty is the bone age X-ray (see further detail, bone age in Sect. 11.6.6.1). This noninvasive test may provide valuable information to guide toward a diagnosis. Normal bone age should not prevent further evaluation (Latronico et al. 2016), but an advanced bone age is concerning and suggests that the patient has been exposed to estrogen or testosterone (Rosenfeld et al. 2014; Oberfield et al. 2011).

Precocious puberty can be characterized as central precocious puberty (HPG axis activation; GnRH-dependent) or peripheral precocious puberty (initiated independently from HPG axis; GnRH-independent). Since GnRH levels fluctuate throughout the day, a GnRH level is not routinely measured.

11.7.4.1 Laboratory Workup for Precocious Puberty

Baseline laboratory testing for evaluation of precocious puberty typically starts with LH, FSH, and estradiol (female) or testosterone (male) (Kaplowitz and Bloch 2016). These tests are discussed in detail in Sections 11.7.8.1–11.7.8.4. Baseline LH levels above 0.3 IU/L create a high suspicion for central precocious puberty. If the baseline LH level is low (<0.3 IU/L) (Kaplowitz and Bloch 2016; Klein et al. 2017) and baseline

estradiol level or testosterone level is low, but the clinician still has suspicion for puberty, the next step is the gonadotropin-releasing hormone stimulation test (also known as GnRH stimulation test or LHRH stimulation test). The stimulation test is considered the "gold standard" for the evaluation of central precocious puberty (Kletter et al. 2015) and is typically performed in conjunction with a pediatric endocrine team.

If central precocious puberty is confirmed, a brain MRI is indicated to rule out pathology. Specifically, in males with central precocious puberty, there is a high prevalence of CNS pathology (Kletter et al. 2015). Overall, the general concern surrounding precocious puberty is ruling out pathology (including CNS lesion or androgen producing tumor), ensuring puberty is at an appropriate time for emotional age and compared to peers, and ensuring adequate final adult height. Treatment is discussed in conjunction with a pediatric endocrinologist.

Peripheral precocious puberty is GnRH independent. It can be caused by genetic disorders (i.e., McCune-Albright syndrome) or acquired disorders such as a tumor that secretes pubertal hormones (i.e., ovarian tumor or hypothalamic hamartoma). Exposure to exogenous hormones and other substances (i.e., lavender, tea tree oil) can also cause peripheral precocious puberty (Klein et al. 2017). Baseline and stimulated LH and FSH levels are typically suppressed, but estradiol (female) or testosterone (male) levels are elevated. Patients with suspected peripheral precocious puberty should be referred to a pediatric endocrinologist for confirmatory testing and management discussion.

11.7.5 Delayed Puberty

Delayed puberty is considered when a girl has not started breast development by 13 years of age or has not had menarche by 15 years of age (primary amenorrhea) (Klein and Poth 2013) or by 3 years after thelarche, or a boy has not started testicular enlargement by 14 years of age (Bozzola et al. 2018; Rosenfeld et al. 2014). Evaluation for delayed puberty is similar to that of precocious puberty, including LH, FSH, and estradiol (females) or testosterone (males). The most common form of delayed puberty is a constitutional delay of growth and puberty (see "short stature") (Bozzola et al. 2018). Baseline labs will help distinguish between constitutional delay, hypogonadotropic hypogonadism (low LH and FSH with low estradiol or testosterone), or hypergonadotropic hypogonadism (elevated LH and FSH with low estradiol or testosterone). Referral to a pediatric endocrinologist should be initiated for the latter two suspicions. At the same time, it may be appropriate to monitor for progression if the patient is suspected of having a constitutional delay and then referring if no pubertal progression is noted after 1–3 months (Klein et al. 2017).

When the clinician has suspicion of delayed puberty, it is important to obtain a thorough medical history such as the history of chemotherapy, radiation, or CNS trauma. Prolactin is another hormone associated with amenorrhea (Klein and Poth 2013; Wei et al. 2017). It is important to remember that aside from endocrine conditions, there are genetic and structural causes of delayed puberty. In females, this includes Turner syndrome or an outflow tract obstruction, and in males, it may be Klinefelter syndrome or Kallmann syndrome (Klein and Poth 2013). Systemic illnesses such as celiac disease and anorexia nervosa can also cause delayed puberty (Bozzola et al. 2018).

11.7.6 Abnormal Menses

Primary amenorrhea occurs when a child has not started to menstruate by age 15 years or 3 years post thelarche and has normal pubertal progression and normal growth. Factors to consider when evaluating a child for primary amenorrhea include anatomical abnormalities, hypothalamic/pituitary disease, gonadal dysgenesis, outflow tract disorders, receptor abnormalities, enzyme insufficiencies, and hormonal excesses or deficiencies. The patient who has not had any menses should have a careful history and physical exam completed, including identifying a normal outflow tract.

Secondary amenorrhea is considered when a female has not had menses for 3 months after previously established regular menses or 6 months if menses have been irregular (Klein and Poth 2013). Oligomenorrhea is considered when a female does not have menses for longer than 3 months between cycles or longer than 45 days apart (from the first day of one period to the first day of the next period). Common causes include polycystic ovarian syndrome (PCOS), hyperprolactinemia, and non-classic congenital adrenal hyperplasia (NCCAH).

The initial evaluation generally consists of LH, FSH, estradiol, prolactin, TSH, and a pregnancy test (Gordon et al. 2017). Additional labs may be considered if there is suspicion for hyperandrogenism (see "hyperandrogenism") (Klein and Poth 2013). Hyperprolactinemia and thyroid disorders can cause amenorrhea or irregular menses. As with delayed puberty, secondary amenorrhea can be caused by systemic illness.

11.7.7 Hyperandrogenism

Hyperandrogenism in females can be suspected when there is hirsutism, acne, or male pattern hair loss on physical exam, or biochemically with elevated testosterone or other androgens. Hirsutism is excessive terminal male pattern hair growth in a female due to androgen excess (Mihailidis et al. 2017). Hirsutism can be evaluated using the Ferriman-Gallwey hirsutism scoring system, which evaluates hair growth in areas including chin, upper lip, chest, upper and lower abdomen, upper back, thighs, upper arms, and buttocks (Hatch et al. 1981). For a female with an abnormal hirsutism score (greater than or equal to 8), the primary care clinician should evaluate for an elevated androgen level (Rosenfield 2005).

Physical exam findings such as clitoromegaly may also lead the clinician toward a potential diagnosis. Common differential diagnoses for hirsutism include polycystic ovarian syndrome (PCOS) (about 70–80% of women with hirsutism), idiopathic hirsutism (5–20% of women with hirsutism), NCCAH (4.2% of women with hirsutism), or other excess androgen production such as androgen-secreting tumors (0.2% of women with hirsutism) or Cushing's syndrome (Martin et al. 2018). The degree of hirsutism in females may not be represented by the degree of elevation of the androgen levels (Rosenfield 2005; Martin et al. 2018). PCOS is a common form of hyperandrogenism and is a diagnosis of exclusion (must rule NCCAH) and other causes of hyperandrogenism) (Martin et al. 2018). Criteria for PCOS diagnosis can be based either on the Rotterdam criteria or the National Institutes of Health-based criteria (Rosenfield 2015). In general, patients have hyperandrogenism and ovulatory dysfunction and may or may not have polycystic ovarian morphology (McCartney and Marshall 2016).

For the primary care clinician, the most important labs that can be obtained are free and total testosterone levels (Martin et al. 2018; Rosenfield 2005). Free testosterone is more sensitive for hyperandrogenemia than total testosterone (Rosenfield 2005).

If the total or free testosterone level is elevated, additional androgen evaluation should be performed in conjunction with a pediatric endocrinologist to determine the cause of androgen excess. Additional androgens that can be assessed include androstenedione, DHEA-S, and early-morning 17-OHP (17-hydroxyprogesterone). In females, testosterone values above 200 ng/dL raise concern for a virilizing tumor (Hunter and Carek 2003; Rosenfield 2015). It is also important to consider a karyotype to rule out a disorder of sexual development (Rosenfield 2015).

11.7.8   Pubertal Disorders and/or Hyperandrogenism Diagnostic Laboratory Tests

This section will review important points about each of the laboratory tests mentioned above. It will detail the hormone level and possible pitfalls. Each section has outlined diagnostic testing to be considered in the workup of a child with a pubertal disorder.

11.7.8.1   Luteinizing Hormone (LH)

LH is a gonadotropin produced by the anterior pituitary gland when stimulated by gonadotropin-releasing hormone (GnRH) from the hypothalamus. LH stimulates the theca cells in the female's ovary to release ovarian sex steroids and stimulates the Leydig cells in the testes in the male to release androgens (particularly testosterone). LH is released in a pulsatile fashion and has a short half-life. Therefore, a random level is challenging to interpret. LH is affected by circadian rhythm, with LH levels typically higher in the morning (Lee and Chung 2019). The most sensitive assay is immunoradiometric, specifically third-generation ultrasensitive (Fisher 2007; Rosenfeld et al. 2014). In prepubertal children, LH levels are very low. Therefore, the assay used in pediatrics must have the ability to detect such levels (Carel et al. 2009).

LH testing is affected by when the specimen is drawn. An early morning baseline LH level is ideal (Lee and Chung 2019). A later-day random LH level may show pubertal value if the child is in puberty; however, a low LH level later in the day does not confirm prepubertal status. Use caution if testing LH in infants under 6 months of age (up to 2 years in females), as increased LH can be normal in minipuberty of infancy (Becker and Hesse 2020).

In some LH assays (competitive assays), there may be cross-reactivity between other pituitary hormones such as TSH, FSH, or hCG (Fisher 2007). LH assays are composed of two subunits (α-subunit and ß-subunit), and the α-subunit is consistent between them (Wei et al. 2017; Rosenfeld et al. 2014).

11.7.8.2   Follicle-Stimulating Hormone (FSH)

FSH, also a gonadotropin produced by the anterior pituitary gland when stimulated by GnRH, stimulates follicular growth in the ovary in the female and stimulates Sertoli cells in the testes, which stimulate testicular growth and spermatogenesis in the male. FSH is not as useful as LH in pediatric pubertal evaluation, especially when evaluating central precocious puberty (Latronico et al. 2016) because there is no significant response of FSH to GnRH compared to LH. The LH rises higher in relation to the FSH (Rosenfeld et al. 2014). However, FSH is frequently ordered in conjunction with LH. If FSH is significantly elevated, it can be a useful indicator of gonadal failure (Wei et al. 2017). FSH is typically measured with an immunometric assay (specifically ELISA) (Styne 2016).

In patients with precocious puberty, it is important to evaluate TSH and free T4 (Pant et al. 2019). A small number of children with significantly elevated TSH have activated FSH receptors (Wei et al. 2017), stimulating GnRH-independent precocious puberty. Suppose there is a slow growth velocity instead of an expected increase in growth velocity with puberty. In that case, the clinician should be suspicious of this syndrome, known as Van Wyk-Grumbach syndrome.

11.7.8.3 Estrogens

The most widely used estrogen in pediatrics is estradiol (E_2). In females, the primary production of estradiol is from the ovaries, and in males, testosterone from the testes is aromatized to estradiol. Estradiol is best measured via LC/MS-MS assay due to its improved sensitivity and specificity (Fisher 2007). Other methods, such as immunoassay, may not determine between prepubertal or early pubertal values due to the decreased specificity. As with LH levels, estradiol levels fluctuate throughout the day as well as throughout the menstrual cycle. Estradiol levels are highest in the early morning. In the menstrual cycle, the lowest estradiol levels are noted in the early follicular phase, and then the highest are commonly about 2–3 days before ovulation. In both females and males, estrone (E1) is produced from androstenedione (produced by the adrenal gland) and aromatized peripherally. Estrone is sometimes, but not routinely, measured during the workup for gynecomastia (Swerdloff and Ng 2019). Estriol (E_3) is not frequently used in pediatrics as it is mainly relevant to pregnancy (Fisher 2007).

Estradiol levels can be affected by SHBG levels since estrogens are highly bound to carrier proteins, which is SHBG (this is discussed in further detail later in this chapter). If estradiol is measured via LC/MS-MS, conjugated estrogens and synthetic estrogens (including ethinyl estradiol) do not cross-react; however, transdermal estradiol can cross-react, measuring a higher level of estradiol. If measured using immunoassay, there is a higher risk for cross-reactivity (Fisher 2007). Estradiol and estrone can have decreased clearance if the patient has liver disease.

11.7.8.4 Testosterone

Testosterone is an androgenic hormone. Testosterone is produced by the Leydig cells of the male testes and the Theca cells of the female ovaries (Styne 2016) and, to a significantly lesser degree in both sexes, by the adrenal glands. Therefore, if an elevated testosterone level is noted, it is important to evaluate both the pubertal axis and the adrenal gland to determine the origin. Testosterone levels are categorized into total testosterone and free testosterone. The majority of testosterone is bound to protein, most frequently to SHBG. About 40% of testosterone is bound to SHBG in men and about 80% in women (Faix 2013). A small fraction (1–3%) of testosterone is free (not bound) (Rosner et al. 2007). There is also a small fraction of testosterone that is weakly bound, to albumin. Both free and weakly bound testosterone are bioavailable.

Total testosterone measures all testosterone, while free testosterone measures only the small fraction that is not bound to proteins. The most significant testosterone level is free testosterone.

If a patient is in a state with elevated SHBG (see "SHBG"), testosterone levels will be elevated. Use caution in the evaluation of elevated testosterone in these patients to avoid unnecessary additional testing or inaccurate diagnoses (Aydın and Winters 2016).

For optimal accuracy, especially in pediatrics, testosterone should be measured by LC/MS-MS or, if unavailable, via extraction/chromatography RIA. This recommendation is supported by the recommendation of the Endocrine Society (Rosner et al. 2007). Immunoassay measurements for testosterone are completed via antibody with the testosterone molecule structure; however, that structure is close to other androgens' structure; therefore, specificity may be compromised. This specificity can be improved using an extraction technique after the competitive immunoassay (Pugeat et al. 2018). Analysis via immunoassay is not recommended for pediatric or female patients because of the lower levels of the hormone; however, immunoassay is frequently used for measuring total testosterone levels (Rosner et al. 2007).

One of the pitfalls of testosterone assays is that results vary from lab to lab; therefore, when evaluating testosterone results, be sure to use the reference interval, which is specific to the laboratory that ran the test (Rosenfield 2005). It is important to use reference values based on TS or SMR stage, gender, and age.

Testosterone is affected by diurnal variation (Martin et al. 2018), with peak levels occurring between 0530 h and 0800 h (Brambilla et al. 2009). Therefore, if a random baseline testosterone level is low, but the clinician has concerns regarding hyperandrogenism, early-morning testosterone (free and total) is important to obtain. Testosterone levels do vary during the menstrual cycle, but the changes in levels are relatively insignificant; therefore, a testosterone level at any time during the menstrual cycle is sufficient for evaluation (Pugeat et al. 2018). The degree of hirsutism in females may not be represented by elevated testosterone levels (Azziz et al. 2000; Martin et al. 2018).

11.7.8.5   Sex Hormone-Binding Globulin (SHBG)

SHBG is a glycoprotein that transports sex steroids in the blood to target tissues. It is produced in the liver. It has a high affinity for testosterone and dihydrotestosterone (not reviewed in this chapter) and a lesser degree for estrogen. Women have higher SHBG than men (Faix 2013). SHBG is evaluated most frequently during the workup for PCOS. Women with PCOS typically have low SHBG. Table 11.10 is a list of other conditions that can affect SHBG levels.

11.7.8.6   17-Hydroxyprogesterone (17-OHP)

17-OHP is a hormone produced by the adrenal glands. 17-OHP is measured if a patient presents

Table 11.10 Conditions that interfere with SHBG levels

Conditions that can cause low SHBG levels	Conditions that can cause high SHBG levels
Obesity	Estrogens (including oral contraceptive therapy)
Type 2 diabetes	Pregnancy
Polycystic ovarian syndrome	Growth hormone deficiency
Hypothyroidism	Hyperthyroidism
Congenital adrenal hyperplasia	
Glucocorticoid treatment	
Liver disease (notably in pediatrics, nonalcoholic fatty liver disease)	
Cushing's syndrome	
Androgens	

Adapted from Martin et al. (2018), Honour (2014), Rosenfeld et al. (2014), Aydın and Winters (2016)

with hyperandrogenism and is used for evaluation of congenital adrenal hyperplasia. 17-OHP should be evaluated via LC/MS-MS assay (Speiser et al. 2018; Honour 2014). It is also frequently measured via immunoassay (IA). The LC/MS-MS assay can differentiate 17-OHP and other steroids in the same pathway, thus avoiding potential cross-reactivity. If measured by IA, it can have cross-reactivity with 11-deoxycortisol or other steroids and can cause false-positive results (Speiser et al. 2018). Some assays can only measure up to 100 nmol/L; therefore, if the level is higher, the sample must be diluted (Honour 2014). Levels above 200 ng/dL prompt consideration of NCCAH (Rosenfield 2015; Trapp and Oberfield 2012); however, it is important to note that normal values do not rule out NCCAH (Honour 2014). If the clinician has concern for NCCAH, it is optimal to consult a pediatric endocrinologist who will likely perform an ACTH (cosyntropin) stimulation test. The ACTH stimulation test is the gold standard for evaluating congenital adrenal hyperplasia (Rosenfield 2015).

As with the hormones mentioned above in this pubertal disorder section, the 17-OHP level varies by time of day, typically highest in the morning. Ideally, the 17-OHP level should be drawn before 8 am (Speiser et al. 2018; Trapp and Oberfield 2012).

11.7.8.7 Dehydroepiandrosterone Sulfate (DHEA-S)

DHEA-S is the principal form of dehydroepian-drosterone (DHEA), a hormone produced by the zona reticularis in the adrenal glands (Oberfield et al. 2011). It is a precursor to the production of testosterone. The evaluation of DHEA-S is useful when evaluating excess adrenal androgen pro-duction, including congenital adrenal hyperpla-sia, adrenal tumors, or PCOS evaluation (Rosenfeld et al. 2014). Levels of DHEA-S do not vary throughout the day. It is robustly bound to albumin and has a long half-life (about 17 h) (Pugeat et al. 2018). DHEA-S is measured by immunoassay (Pugeat et al. 2018). A mildly ele-vated level of DHEA-S may not represent pathol-ogy; however, if the level is significantly elevated, it is important to consider an androgen-secreting tumor (adrenal or gonadal) (Rosenfield 2005) or a form of congenital adrenal hyperplasia (Rosenfeld et al. 2014).

The results must be evaluated according to specific reference ranges, including gender and TS or SMR stage, to avoid errors in the interpre-tation of DHEA-S (Styne 2016).

11.7.8.8 Androstenedione

Androstenedione is an androgen produced by the adrenal glands and the gonads. It is used in the evaluation of both males and females with hyper-androgenism. If the level is significantly elevated, as with DHEA-S, it is important to consider an androgen-secreting tumor (Rosenfeld et al. 2014). As with many endocrine hormones, the optimal technique for measurement is LC-MS/MS; if that technique is not available, RAI may be used to measure androstenedione (Rauh 2009).

It is important to evaluate androstenedione levels via specific reference ranges, including gender and TS or SMR stage (Styne 2016).

11.7.8.9 Prolactin

Prolactin is a hormone produced by the anterior pituitary gland released during pregnancy and after childbirth to stimulate breast milk produc-tion. In the realm of pediatric endocrinology, pro-lactin levels are measured in the evaluation of oligomenorrhea, amenorrhea, and galactorrhea. Baseline prolactin levels should be obtained in a non-stress environment and in the morning (ide-ally 2 h after waking) to avoid false elevations (Matalliotakis et al. 2019). The prolactin level can be falsely elevated if drawn nonfasting or if there is significant stress with the blood draw. Suppose a level is elevated (>20 ng/mL). In that case, a second measurement must be obtained on a separate day to confirm hyperprolactinemia unless the prolactin is exceptionally elevated (>100 ng/mL) or the patient has symptomatic hyperprolactinemia (Matalliotakis et al. 2019).

A prolactin level > 500 ug/L is clinically diag-nostic for a macroprolactinoma (Melmed et al. 2011). If a patient is managed on a medication that can cause elevated prolactin levels, the level may be above 200 ug/L without an adenoma being the cause (Melmed et al. 2011). Kidney function must also be obtained, and thyroid func-tion tests must be done because both renal failure and primary hypothyroidism can cause an eleva-tion in prolactin levels (Matalliotakis et al. 2019). Elevations in prolactin can also be caused by nipple stimulation, marijuana use, pregnancy, and stress/illness, among others (Matalliotakis et al. 2019; Vilar et al. 2019). If the prolactin level is significantly elevated, a brain MRI may be indicated (Vilar et al. 2019).

Prolactin is found in the serum in three differ-ent forms based on molecular weight, including monomeric (most common), dimeric (second most common), and macroprolactin (least com-mon) (Haddad et al. 2019). The smallest prolac-tin molecule (monomeric), discussed above, is typically the most abundant in the circulation. The dimeric prolactin molecule is rarely mea-sured. The largest, macroprolactin, is biologi-cally inactive. It is best measured by gel filtration chromatography (Haddad et al. 2019).

Macroprolactinemia is the state during which a patient has elevated levels of macroprolactin (Melmed et al. 2011; Haddad et al. 2019). A patient with elevated serum prolactin levels but no signs or symptoms of hyperprolactinemia, no radiologic evidence of a pituitary mass, and is not taking any medications that may increase

Table 11.11 Common differential diagnoses for pubertal disorders with expected diagnostic labs

	LH	FSH	Estradiol	Testosterone	17-OHP	DHEA-S	Androstenedione	Prolactin
Central precocious puberty	↑	→ or ↑	↑ (female)	↑ (male)	→	→ or ↑	→ or ↑	N/A
Peripheral precocious puberty	→	→	↑ (female)	↑ (male)	→	→	↑	N/A
Benign premature thelarche	→	→	→ (female)	→ (male)	→	↑[a]	→	N/A
Premature adrenarche	→	→	N/A	↑ (male and female)	→	→ or ↑[b]	→	N/A
Constitutional delay	→	→	→ (female)	→ (male)	→	→	→	N/A
Gonadal failure	↑	↑	↓ (female)	↓ (male)	→	→	→	→
PCOS (female)	→	→	→	↑	→	→	→	→
NCCAH	→	→	→ (female)	↑ (male and female)	↑	↑	↑	N/A
Ovarian tumor (female)	→ or ↓	→ or ↓	→ or ↑	↑↑	→	↑↑	↑	→ or ↑
Adrenal tumor	→ or ↓	→ or ↓	→ or ↑ (female)	↑↑ (male and female)	→	↑↑	↑	→

Adapted from Styne (2016), Oberfield et al. (2011)
[a]Increased for age
[b]Increased for age but in line with bone age

prolactin may have macroprolactinemia due to the biologically inactive macroprolactin. It is important to know this to avoid misdiagnosis (Haddad et al. 2019).

The hook effect occurs when the prolactin hormone concentration is very high or if there is a small amount of antibody in the assay from the manufacturer. If the clinician suspects an elevated prolactin level, but the lab result is normal, the patient should be referred to a pediatric endocrinologist. Specifically, Haddad et al. (2019) suggested that if there is a pituitary mass above 4 cm that is concerning for adenoma, the hook effect should be ruled out. Table 11.11 reviews the differential diagnoses and laboratory findings in disorders of pubert.

11.7.8.10   Cortisol

Cortisol is a steroid hormone that is produced in the zona fasciculata of the adrenal glands. Some conditions can cause too little cortisol (hypocortisolism, such as adrenal insufficiency) and too much cortisol (hypercortisolism). The adrenal gland releases cortisol in a diurnal pattern. LC-MS/MS is the optimal assay for cortisol (Rauh 2009), especially if a patient is on pred-

nisolone, as prednisolone can cause cross-reactivity if an immunoassay is used (Haddad et al. 2019). Clinicians concerned with a patient with hypocortisolism should urgently refer the patient to a pediatric endocrinologist, as patients can become severely ill without treatment (Bornstein et al. 2016). Patients who are suspected of hypercortisolism should also be referred to a pediatric endocrinologist for further evaluation. When evaluating for hypocortisolism, an 8-am cortisol level can be assessed, as the body's cortisol level peaks around that time (Miller and Flück 2014); however, even if the early-morning cortisol level is adequate, the optimal test for the evaluation of hypocortisolism is a corticotropin stimulation test (ACTH stimulation test), typically performed by a pediatric endocrinologist.

Hypercortisolism may be caused by Cushing's disease (excess ACTH production by pituitary adenoma causing excess cortisol production) or other sources of excess cortisol, known as Cushing's syndrome (Lodish et al. 2018). Pediatric patients with Cushing's syndrome typically have weight gain with poor growth, hypertension, and may have buffalo hump or abdominal striae (Lodish et al. 2018; Nieman et al. 2008). If there is a concern for hypercortisolism, including Cushing's syndrome, a 24 h urine cortisol level, midnight cortisol blood or saliva level, or a dexamethasone suppression test can be used (Honour 2014; Nieman et al. 2008). It is important to note that one test is not adequate for diagnosis; the tests are not fully accurate, and results can vary (Lodish et al. 2018; Nieman et al. 2008). Therefore, a normal result cannot be fully reassuring against pathology. Patients with suspected Cushing's syndrome should be referred to a pediatric endocrinologist for further evaluation and management. Box 11.8 reviews common reasons for immediate referrals.

Box 11.8 Common Reasons for Urgent Referrals
- Signs of precocious puberty with neurologic signs and symptoms (r/o CNS pathology—importance of vision exam).
- Estradiol or testosterone significantly elevated (r/o tumor, CNS pathology).
- Significantly elevated prolactin level (r/o CNS lesion).
- Concern for hypocortisolism/adrenal insufficiency.

11.7.9 Newborn Screening for Congenital Adrenal Hyperplasia (CAH)

The Endocrine Society recommends that congenital adrenal hyperplasia due to 21-OH deficiency is included in all newborn screening programs (Speiser et al. 2018). Early diagnosis and management of CAH can significantly decrease morbidity and mortality. There are two tiers to the analysis of CAH in the newborn screen. It is important to understand the types of screenings.

The initial screen (first-tier) is a 17-OHP level analyzed using immunoassay from the dried blood spot on the routine newborn screen filter paper card. It is recommended that the 17-OHP level is assessed based on norms for gestational age. The accuracy of first-tier 17-OHP results on the newborn screen may be affected by certain factors such as the following:

- Timing of the specimen: If taken in the first 2 days of life, the result may show a false low 17-OHP level if the baby has CAH (levels rise after birth) or a falsely high level if the baby is healthy (levels are naturally higher at birth and then decrease over days).
- Gender: 17-OHP levels are lower in females.
- Clinical status: 17-OHP levels can be raised if the baby is stressed by illness or is premature, thus possibly causing a false-positive result.
- Type of test: Immunoassays can be associated with low specificity.
- Antenatal steroids: Potentially reduce 17-OHP levels, causing a false-negative result.

The second-tier screen should be using LC-MS/MS. If LC-MS/MS is unavailable, a cosyntropin stimulation test should be used to verify diagnosis before treatment.

A positive CAH newborn screen should be referred to a pediatric endocrinologist, and a cosyntropin stimulation test (after 24–48 h of life) is typically used for further diagnostic purposes. Serum electrolytes should also be measured for babies with elevated 17-OHP levels (Speiser et al. 2018).

11.7.10 Real-Life Examples

A 14-year-old female with morbid obesity is referred to pediatric endocrinology for evaluation of irregular menses and prediabetes. On physical exam, she had hirsutism, acanthosis nigricans, and no clitoromegaly. Her labs reveal a total testosterone of 62 ng/dL (<40), free testosterone of 15.3 pg/mL (0.5–3.9), DHEA-S of

219 (35–430ug/dL), FSH of 4.7mIU/mL (3.1–17.7), LH of 8.10mIU/mL (0.04–10.80), prolactin of 8.0 (4.9–23.2 ng/mL), androstenedione of 139 mg/dL (22–225), hCG of <6mIU/mL (<6), A1c of 6.2%, TSH of 2.29mIU/L (0.5–4.3), T4 of 6.49 ng/dL (0.8–1.4), and 17-OH progesterone of 31 ng/dL (16–283). She was diagnosed with polycystic ovarian syndrome and was encouraged to work on healthy lifestyle changes prior to discussing medical treatment.

A 7-year-old Caucasian female is brought and presented to the primary care clinician because her mother noticed that she is growing pubic hair, and she is concerned that she will be getting her period soon. She has TS or SMR 1 breast development, no acne or apocrine body odor, and TS or SMR 2 pubic hair on exam. She has not had any vaginal bleeding or discharge, and there is no clitoromegaly. You decide to order a quick, non-invasive bone age X-ray, which returns with a reading of 8 years. You diagnose her with premature adrenarche and decide to monitor her. She develops TS or SMR stage II breasts at 10 years of age and has menarche at 12 years of age. As she gets older, she progresses through puberty appropriately and reaches her genetic potential for adult height.

A 7-year 8-month-old male is seen in the primary care office for an annual health assessment. His pubertal exam reveals a testicular volume of 4 cc bilaterally. He has no concerning neurologic symptoms. He has no acne, pubic hair or axillary hair, or adult body odor, but his parents say that he has developed "teenage-like behavior." His growth percentile jumped from 25 percentile last year to 45 percentile this year, with parents both around the 25 percentile for height. Baseline morning LH is noted at 0.3 IU/L and FSH 0.8 IU/L with free testosterone 0.8 pg/mL and total testosterone 2.6 pg/dL. He is referred to pediatric endocrinology, where he undergoes a GnRH stimulation test which confirms central precocious puberty. He has a brain MRI to rule out pathology, which is normal, and he was started on GnRH agonist therapy.

Key Learning about Pubertal Disorders

- Premature thelarche is considered a normal variant and can be seen in females under 2 years of age who have glandular breast tissue without growth acceleration or other signs of puberty.
- When monitoring puberty in the primary care setting, it is important to assess the TS or SMR staging of pubic hair along with the testicular volume (using a Prader orchidometer) in males and breast development staging in females.
- A complete pubertal physical exam, including testicular volume or breast development staging, is critical for any pubertal evaluation instead of only relying on pubic hair staging.
- Evaluating precocious puberty should occur if pubertal signs occur before 8 years of age in girls and 9 years of age in boys.
- Evaluation of delayed puberty should occur if girls do not develop breast development by 13 years of age or menarche by 15 years of age, or if boys do not develop testicular enlargement to at least 4 ccs by 14 years of age.
- Secondary amenorrhea is considered when a female has not had menses for 3 months after previously established regular menses or 6 months if menses have been irregular.
- There may not be a correlation between the degree of hirsutism and the elevation of androgens.

11.8 Disorders of Water Balance

This section will review the hormonal control of water balance. While rare, disorders of water balance can present with polyuria and polydipsia and needs to be differentiated from diabetes mellitus.

11.8.1 Diabetes Insipidus

The primary care clinician will rarely evaluate arginine vasopressin (AVP) or antidiuretic hormone (ADH) levels; however, diabetes insipidus (DI) needs to be ruled out when a patient complains of polyuria and polydipsia. Although rare, DI could lead to dehydration and hypernatremia unless patients have an intact thirst mechanism and can drink as needed. DI should be distinguished from primary polydipsia (excess water intake), which may present in patients with developmental delay or psychiatric illness.

DI can be central due to an AVP deficiency or nephrogenic due to an inadequate response to AVP at the V2 receptor in the kidney's collecting duct (Weiner and Vuguin 2020; Bankir et al. 2017). Primary polydipsia may also cause the suppression of AVP secretion over time due to excessive fluid intake, making diagnosis difficult. Central DI can be secondary to head trauma or post neurosurgery. It can also be caused by brain tumors, disorders of the pituitary gland, infections, autoimmune disease, medications, and genetic mutations (Wolfram syndrome). Nephrogenic DI can be caused by medications, kidney disease, genetic mutations, and electrolyte imbalances (Weiner and Vuguin 2020).

Patients presenting to the clinician with complaints of new-onset enuresis or polyuria must be evaluated for DI. Polyuria is defined as urine output greater than 4–5 mL/kg/h (Weiner and Vuguin 2020). A prompt evaluation is necessary if patients with polyuria also present with signs or symptoms suggestive of pituitary dysfunction like short stature or delayed puberty.

11.8.2 Diagnostic Laboratory Evaluation for the Child with Suspected Diabetes Insipidus

The patient with new-onset enuresis or polyuria should have a basic initial evaluation. If the clinician notes short stature or delayed puberty, the evaluation should be started immediately. Any abnormality should be discussed with the endocrine provider so that a sooner evaluation can be obtained.

11.8.2.1 Urinalysis

A urinalysis is an inexpensive screening tool to assess for urine-specific gravity in the primary care office. Information about a basic urinalysis can be found in Chapter 10, Sect. 10.2.1.1. Suppose the urine specific gravity is low (and no glucose is present in the urine—see section on diabetes) and the patient has polyuria. In that case, labs for simultaneous urine and serum osmolality and serum electrolytes should be obtained. The pediatric endocrinologist will complete a water deprivation test to confirm a diagnosis of DI, if necessary.

11.8.2.2 Serum Osmolality, Sodium Level, and Urine Osmolality

Simultaneous serum osmolality and sodium level and a urine osmolality and specific gravity are important diagnostic tools. DI is diagnosed when the serum osmolality is >300 mOsm/kg and the urine osmolality is <300 mOsm/kg. Serum sodium will likely be elevated (>145 mEq/mL), and urine-specific gravity will be low, <1.010 (Weiner and Vuguin 2020). Even when patients with DI are deprived of water, they are still unable to concentrate their urine. In patients with primary polydipsia, the urine osmolality is usually normal, even when water is deprived (Weiner and Vuguin 2020). Table 11.12 reviews the urine and serum findings in patients with DI vs. primary polydipsia. If the clinician is concerned about a diagnosis of DI, prompt referral to a pediatric endocrinologist is necessary.

11.8.2.3 AVP

AVP is synthesized in the hypothalamus and travels to the posterior pituitary via the infundibular stalk, where it is stored until it is released into the bloodstream in response to dehydration and rising serum osmolality (Bankir et al. 2017). AVP may also be released in response to increasing sodium levels and decreased blood volume or stress. Increased water intake will decrease AVP secretion. AVP acts at the distal convoluted tubule in the kidney to increase water reabsorption,

Table 11.12 Diagnostic laboratory tests in patients with disorders of water balance

	Urine SG	Serum sodium mEq/L	Urine osmolality mOsm/kg	Serum osmolality mOsm/kg
Normal	1.010–1.030	135–145	50–1400	275–295
DI	↓	↑*	↓	↑
Primary polydipsia	→ or ↓	→ or ↓	↓	↓

*Serum Sodium may be normal in patients with an intact thirst mechanism
Adapted from Weiner and Vuguin (2020), Styne (2016)

decreasing serum osmolality and increasing urine osmolality. AVP has a very short half-life, and the serum level of AVP is so low that it is too difficult for current immunoassays to quantify (Bankir et al. 2017). Therefore, measuring AVP is not clinically useful. Instead, urine osmolality, specific gravity, serum sodium, and serum osmolality are better markers of water balance. AVP must also be drawn in a specific tube that is at a low temperature. The sample must be transported in a specific method (iced and then refrigerated and then frozen). Therefore, not all labs will be able to obtain the specimen properly. If mishandled, results may not be accurate (Styne 2016). Box 11.9 reviews the common urinalysis findings in patients with polyuria.

Box 11.9 Common Urinalysis Findings and Considerations Related to Polyuria

Urinalysis findings	Considerations for diagnosis and further testing
Glucosuria	Diabetes mellitus and check fingerstick and/or HbA1c
SG <1.010	Diabetes insipidus and check urine and serum osmolality
Normal	Hypercalcemia and check serum calcium and PTH or primary polydipsia

---

11.8.3 Real-Life Example

A 13 ½-year-old female presented to the pediatric endocrinologist for concerns of short stature. Further history revealed that the patient was thirsty all of the time, was urinating almost every hour, and was waking at night to urinate. Initial screening tests showed a urine SG 1.006, urine

osmolality 36 mOsm/kg, serum osmolality 290 mOsm/kg, and serum sodium 143 mEq/L. These labs were suggestive of DI, and her intact thirst mechanism likely enabled her to maintain a normal serum osmolality. A water deprivation test was completed and confirmed the diagnosis of DI. The patient was deprived of water all night, and when she arrived at the clinic, repeat labs were assessed, which showed urine osmolality 136 mOsm/kg, serum osmolality 310 mOsm/kg, and serum sodium 156 mEq/L. She was treated with subcutaneous DDAVP. Repeat labs 60 mins later noted urine osmolality 210 mOsm/kg, serum sodium 140 mEq/L, and serum osmolality 271 mOsm/kg. She was diagnosed with central DI. Brain imaging revealed a germinoma. The patient had surgery to remove the tumor and was treated with chemotherapy and radiation. She was also noted to have GHD. She was treated with GH and has attained an acceptable adult height, and she remains with central DI.

11.9 Diabetes Mellitus

Diabetes mellitus (DM) is a term used to describe a group of disorders associated with abnormal glucose homeostasis. DM is further classified based on how glucose homeostasis is altered. The two main types of diabetes seen in the pediatric population are type 1 DM and type 2 DM (Styne 2016).

Type 1 DM is a result of insulin deficiency caused by an autoimmune response. This autoimmune response results in the destruction of the beta cells in the pancreas that release insulin (Styne 2016).

Type 2 DM results from a state of insulin resistance. Typically, the patient starts with insulin resistance, during which time endogenous insulin production may be elevated; however, it may progress to an insulin-deficient state. Type 2 DM was previously labeled adult-onset diabetes, but it is now evident that the prevalence of type 2 DM in youth has increased (Nadeau et al. 2016).

A group of monogenic disorders, including neonatal diabetes and maturity-onset diabetes of the young (MODY), are due to a genetic mutation that affects the formation or release of insulin and does not cause beta cell destruction. These forms of diabetes are rare but often misdiagnosed as type 1 DM or type 2 DM. Additionally, diabetes can be caused by medications (including steroids or posttransplant drugs) or exocrine pancreas dysfunction (such as cystic fibrosis) (ADA 2021).

As a primary care clinician, lab testing to evaluate for DM would be done either for a patient presenting with symptoms of diabetes (including polyuria, nocturia, new-onset enuresis, polydipsia, polyphagia, weight loss) or if a patient is asymptomatic but meets the criteria for routine screening (see Box 11.10). Pediatric patients with type 1 DM often present in diabetic ketoacidosis (DKA); however, it is important to remember that patients with type 2 DM may also present in DKA (ADA 2021). Symptoms of DKA include nausea, vomiting, abdominal pain, fatigue, fruity breath, shortness of breath, and confusion (Styne 2016). Due to the rapid progression to DKA in patients with type 1 DM, a pediatric endocrinologist should urgently be consulted if there is suspicion for type 1 diabetes.

In the year 2000, the American Diabetes Association (ADA) and the American Academy of Pediatrics recommended screening for type 2 diabetes and prediabetes in asymptomatic children 10 years and older or after the onset of puberty who were overweight and with at least two risk factors. The recommendation came as the prevalence of diabetes in the adult population was increasing, and various reports, including the Third National Health and Nutrition Examination Survey (NHANES III), were noting an increase in the prevalence of type 2 DM in the pediatric population (ADA 2000; Wallace et al. 2020).

Box 11.10 Criteria for Screening for Prediabetes and Type 2 DM in Pediatrics

- Patients who have started puberty or ≥ 10 years old (whichever comes first) who meet criteria for overweight status (BMI ≥85th percentile) or obese status (BMI ≥95th percentile) *and who have one or more of the following risk factors*.

  - The patient's mother has a history of diabetes during pregnancy or gestational diabetes during the pregnancy.
  - There is a family history of type 2 DM in a first- or second-degree relative.
  - The patient is of Native American, African American, Latino, Asian American, or Pacific Islander descent.
  - Signs of insulin resistance on the exam (acanthosis nigricans) or has a condition that is associated with insulin resistance (small-for-gestational age at birth, hypertension, dyslipidemia, or polycystic ovary syndrome).

Adapted from ADA 2021

11.9.1 Diabetes Diagnostic Laboratory Tests

According to the ADA (2021), the diagnosis of prediabetes and diabetes can be made based on hemoglobin A1C (HbA1C), fasting plasma glucose levels, or a 2-h plasma glucose following a 75-gram glucose load. DM can also be diagnosed with an elevated random plasma glucose in the presence of classic symptoms of hyperglycemia. The 2-h plasma glucose level during a 75-g oral glucose tolerance test (OGTT) is considered the "gold standard." It will diagnose more people with prediabetes and diabetes than either HbA1C or fasting glucose (Brar 2019). However, due to the convenience of the HbA1C test, which does not require fasting and the fact that it gives a measure

Table 11.13 Diagnostic criteria for diabetes

	HbA1c	FPG	2 h glucose on OGTT
Diabetes	≥6.5%	≥126 mg/dL	≥200 mg/dL
Prediabetes	5.7–6.4%	100–125 mg/dL	140–199 mg/dL

Adapted from ADA (2021)

of glycemic control over the past 3 months rather than a single data point, it has now been recognized as a diagnostic tool (ADA 2021). The cutoff values for diabetes are based on clinical studies and the risk for developing complications from diabetes. In contrast, the cutoffs for prediabetes levels are based on studies indicating a relative increase in risk for developing diabetes mellitus in the next 5 years (ADA 2021, Lee et al. 2011). Unless there is significant hyperglycemia, the patient should have at least two positive results to confirm the diagnosis of DM: either two positive results on the same blood sample (i.e., an elevated fasting plasma glucose and an elevated HbA1C) or two positive results on different samples (an elevated HbA1C on two different samples).

The cutoff values for HbA1C and glucose levels for both diabetes mellitus and prediabetes were based on studies on adult populations but extrapolated to the pediatric population. Table 11.13 reviews the diagnostic criteria for diabetes.

11.9.1.1 Hemoglobin A1C

Hemoglobin is a protein in the red blood cells that transports oxygen to the body's organs and tissues. The hemoglobin molecule is composed of two alpha-globin chains made up of the globin genes HbA1 and HbA2. A1c is a minor hemoglobin component that is a posttranslational modification of HbA and accounts for 70–90% of hemoglobin A1. Hemoglobin A1C (HbA1c) is formed by the combination of glucose molecules with the N-terminal proline amino acid groups of the hemoglobin B chain (Radin 2014). This modification of hemoglobin with glucose is termed glycosylation. The process of glycosylation will occur over the lifespan of an erythrocyte which is typically 120 days. Therefore, HbA1C is a good marker of overall glycemic control over the past 120 days (Guo et al. 2014). HbA1C was first used as a clinical marker to monitor glycemic control,

but the ADA added HbA1C as a diagnostic marker for diabetes in 2010 (Radin 2014).

The Diabetes Control and Complications Trial (DCCT), the UK prospective Diabetes Study (UKPDS), and the Epidemiology of Diabetes Interventions and Complications (EDIC) study concluded that the risks of diabetes-related complications are directly related to glycemic control as measured by the HbA1C value. In the past, HbA1C assays were not standardized and led to a wide variability. The lack of standardization led to the creation of the National Glycohemoglobin Standardization Program (NGSP) in 1996 (Radin 2014). The goal was for HbA1C levels to be standardized to the HbA1C levels of the DCCT and UKPDS trials. All NGSP-certified laboratories use the ion-exchange high-performance liquid chromatography (HLPC), which was the same method used in the DCCT and UKPD trials. HbA1C is measured using whole blood in a lavender-top tube (Radin 2014). There are methods of checking a point-of-care HbA1C which will yield a result within minutes. A venous sample must be used for diagnostic purposes as the quality concept typically used for lab testing of HbA1C is not used with point of care (Weykamp 2013).

Hemoglobin A1C evaluation. HbA1C is not a direct measure of glycemia and may be affected by various factors independent of glycemia. Hemoglobin A1C is part of a red blood cell. Therefore, any condition that affects red blood cell turnover can alter the HbA1C level and make it a less reliable indicator of glycemic control. If the life of an erythrocyte is longer, it will result in decreased red cell turnover, which will, in turn, expose the cell to glucose for longer periods resulting in higher HbA1C levels. On the contrary, HbA1C may be falsely lowered in patients who have a condition with increased red cell turnover (Radin 2014).

HbA1C levels can also be altered by certain hemoglobinopathies, including hemoglobins S, C, D, and E. Whether or not the HbA1C level may be altered in a person with a specific hemoglobinopathy is dependent on the specific HbA1C assay used. The NGSP provides written guidance on which assays will affect HbA1C levels for each hemoglobinopathy (Vajravelu and Lee 2018; Radin 2014). HbA1C can also be falsely lowered or increased due to the mechanisms of certain medications or vitamins (Vajravelu and Lee 2018; Radin 2014). Race and ethnicity can also impact HbA1C levels (ADA 2021). The Diabetes Prevention Program found that African Americans had HbA1C levels about 0.4% higher than Caucasians for the same average glucose levels. Differences in HbA1C were also seen in Asians, Hispanics, and American Indians (Herman et al. 2007; Vajravelu and Lee 2018). HbA1C has also been shown to increase with increasing age regardless of diabetes status (Brar 2019). As regards to age, the ADA diagnostic cutoff values, including for HbA1C, are based on adult epidemiologic studies. HbA1C has been found to have a lower sensitivity for detecting prediabetes in adolescents in comparison to adults though more research is needed to better evaluate the sensitivity of HbA1C in the diagnosis of diabetes in the pediatric population (Vajravelu and Lee 2018; Lee et al. 2011). Box 11.11 is a list of conditions that may falsely elevate or lower HbA1c.

Box 11.11 Conditions that May Falsely Affect HbA1C

Conditions that may falsely elevate HbA1C	Conditions that may falsely lower HbA1C
• Iron deficiency anemia	• Chronic blood loss
• Anemia caused by folate or vitamin B12 deficiency	• Recent blood transfusion
• Asplenia	• Hemolytic anemia (including sickle cell anemia and G6PD deficiency)
• Severe hypertriglyceridemia (concentrations >1750 mg/dL)	• End-stage renal disease
	• Cystic fibrosis
• Severe hyperbilirubinemia (concentrations >20 mg/dL)	• Pregnancy
	• Vitamin E (dosages higher than 600 mg)
• Lead poisoning	• Vitamin C (in high dosages)
• Chronic alcohol consumption	• Ribavirin
• Chronic salicylate ingestion	• Interferon alpha
	• HIV antiretroviral medication
• Chronic opioid ingestion	• Dapsone
	• Hydroxyurea

Adapted from Radin (2014); Vajravelu and Lee (2018), Kim et al. (2009); ADA (2021)).

11.9.1.2 Fasting Plasma Glucose and 2-Hour Plasma Glucose on OGTT

Until 2010, the diagnosis of diabetes was based only on glucose levels, not on HbA1C (Radin 2014). Diagnosing prediabetes and diabetes in children and adults can still be based on either fasting plasma glucose levels, a 2-h plasma glucose, or a random plasma glucose level accompanied by symptoms of hyperglycemia. Fasting is defined as no caloric intake for 8 h. The 2-h OGTT with a 75-g glucose load will detect diabetes in more patients than either fasting glucose or HbA1C. During the 2-h OGTT, a fasting glucose level is obtained, and then patients are given a 75-g glucose drink, and a blood glucose level is drawn 120 min later (ADA 2021). The glucose cutoff values for diagnosis of diabetes were updated by the International Expert Committee on the Diagnosis and Classification of Diabetes in 1997. At that time, the cutoff value for diagnosing diabetes with fasting glucose levels was lowered from 140 to 126 mg/dL. The cutoff value was lowered due to data that demonstrated an increase in the prevalence of diabetic retinopathy from the National Health and Nutritional Epidemiologic Survey (NHANES III) (Expert Committee on the Diagnosis and Classification of Diabetes Mellitus 2003; Mayfield 1998). Epidemiological data also demonstrated that people with a 2-h plasma glucose level of ≥200 mg/dL following a 75-g glucose load had a higher risk of developing eye and kidney disease (Gerstein 2001). This data was based on adult populations and has been extrapolated to the pediatric population (ADA 2021; Brar 2019).

Hemoglobin A1C, fasting plasma glucose levels, and 2-h oral glucose tolerance levels may be discordant and may not be reproducible. For example, a patient may have a normal HbA1C but an abnormal fasting glucose level. Typically, hyperglycemia is seen in postprandial glucose levels before hyperglycemia in fasting glucose levels; therefore, it is possible to miss a diagnosis of diabetes if only fasting glucose levels are evaluated (Gerstein 2001). If there is a high index of suspicion that the patient has diabetes, the 2-h

OGTT, considered the "gold standard," should be performed (ADA 2021).

Evaluation of fasting plasma glucose and 2-hour plasma glucose on OGTT. Performing a fasting plasma glucose and a 2-hour plasma glucose level following a glucose load is more labor-intensive than the HbA1C. A fasting plasma glucose requires an overnight fast of 8 h. Therefore, the test often needs to be done in the morning, which may not be convenient for the patient. It may also be challenging for a child to tolerate the 75-g glucose drink required for the 2-h glucose level. After drinking the 75-g glucose drink, it is also important that the patient does not eat or exercise, which can affect the 2-h glucose level.

Plasma glucose levels can be altered if the sample remains at room temperature for too long and is not centrifuged correctly (ADA 2021). Glucose levels can be affected by stress/illness, leading to individual variability in glucose levels (Brar 2019). Table 11.14 points out the advantages and disadvantages of diagnostic testing for diabetes.

11.9.1.3 Pancreatic Islet Cell Autoantibodies

Several autoantibodies have been found to bind to specific proteins in the islet cells of the pancreas (Winter and Schatz 2011). They are primarily tested in a patient diagnosed with DM to confirm a diagnosis of autoimmune type 1 DM. The autoantibodies typically appear in the blood months to years before symptoms actually present (Schmidt et al. 2005). Children genetically predisposed to develop type 1 DM frequently have seroconversion of autoantibodies between 6 months and 3 years of age and another peak in puberty (Williams and Long 2019). It is still unclear what triggers the initial autoimmune response (Winter and Schatz 2011).

Autoantibodies include antibodies to the 65-kDa isoform of glutamate decarboxylase (GAD65), insulin autoantibodies (IAA), islet cell antibodies (ICA), insulinoma-associated antigen-2A (IA-2) antibodies, and zinc transporter eight (ZnT8) antibodies. Additional autoantibodies have been documented, but they are either difficult to

Table 11.14 Advantages and disadvantages of diagnostic testing for diabetes

Diagnostic test	Advantages	Disadvantages
Hemoglobin A1C	• Does not require fasting • Less day-to-day variability due to stress, illness, or diet • Greater preanalytical stability (does not require centrifuge) • Good for monitoring trends in glycemic control (120-day average)	• Higher cost • Levels can be affected by various conditions affecting red blood cell turnover, medications, race/ethnicity, and age (see Box 11.11) • Lower sensitivity at cutoff value of 6.5%
Fasting plasma glucose	• Only one blood sample	• Requires 8 h of fasting • Stress/illness/diet can affect variability leading to poor reproducibility • Less preanalytical stability (needs to be kept at the correct temperature and centrifuged promptly)
2-hour glucose on OGTT	• Diagnoses more people with prediabetes and diabetes • Considered the gold standard	• Requires 8 h of fasting before the test • Long test • Some patients have difficulty drinking a 75-g glucose load • Stress/illness/diet can affect variability leading to poor reproducibility • Less preanalytical stability (needs to be kept at the correct temperature and centrifuged promptly)

Adapted from ADA (2021), Brar (2019), Radin (2014)

measure or do not have adequate sensitivity or specificity levels. They are therefore not used routinely in the clinical setting (Winter and Schatz 2011). IAA is more commonly seen in younger children diagnosed with new-onset Type 1 Diabetes Mellitus (typically, the IAA is the first to be seen, followed by GAD-65 antibodies). The prevalence of IAA has been found to decrease at older ages. The administration of exogenous insulin can cause the body to make insulin antibodies that cannot be distinguished from insulin autoantibodies on lab testing. Therefore, if a patient has already been given exogenous insulin for treatment, the insulin antibody test is less reliable as a positive result could indicate insulin antibodies due to administration of insulin and/or insulin autoantibodies (Winter and Schatz 2011). GAD-65 antibodies and ICA antibodies are seen in ~70–80% of patients diagnosed with new-onset T1DM. However, the positive ICA tends to decrease over time, so someone who has had diabetes for over 10 years may no longer have a positive ICA.

In contrast, the GAD-65 remains positive for longer (Winter and Schatz 2011).

The zinc transporter 8 (ZnT8) antibody is currently the newest of the islet autoantibodies to be recognized. It is highly specific to the pancreatic beta cells and localized in the insulin secretory granules (Williams and Long 2019). As this antibody was first described in 2007, patients diagnosed with antibody-negative insulin-dependent diabetes before 2007 should have a ZnT8 antibody tested (Wenzlau et al. 2007). ZnT8 is more commonly positive in older children at diagnosis than IAA, which is more common in younger children (Winter and Schatz 2011). The gold standard for measuring all islet autoantibodies is by radioimmunoassay (Williams and Long 2019).

There have been multiple research studies evaluating autoantibodies seen in first-degree relatives of patients with type 1 diabetes and the risk of progression to diabetes. The Colorado Diabetes Autoimmunity Study in the Young (DAISY), the Finnish Type 1 Diabetes Prediction and Prevention (DIPP) study, the German BABYDIAB and BABYDIET, Diabetes Prevention Trial (DPT-1), and TrialNet are monitoring islet autoantibodies in first-degree relatives of those with T1DM to better understand the rate of progression to diabetes from the time that autoantibodies first develop (Ziegler et al. 2013). In the DPT-1 study, 98% of first-degree relatives of patients with type 1 DM who developed T1DM had one or more autoantibodies (Verge et al. 1996; Pihoker et al. 2005). Following the DPT-1 study came the Type 1 Diabetes TrialNet. TrialNet is an ongoing, international study monitoring the presence of autoantibodies in first-degree relatives of patients with type 1 DM to prevent or slow the development of disease progression through various clinical trials (Bingley et al. 2018).

It is not recommended for the primary care clinician to perform routine screening of autoantibodies in asymptomatic first-degree relatives of a patient with type 1 DM (ADA 2021). Some autoantibodies are not disease-specific (Bonifacio and Achenbach 2019). For example, GAD-65 autoantibodies can be seen in neurological conditions such as Stiff-Man syndrome or cerebellar ataxia (Schmidt et al. 2005; Winter and Schatz 2011). First-degree relatives of those with T1DM can be referred to TrialNet for screening and risk assessment (www.trialnet.org).

11.9.1.4 C-Peptide

Connecting peptide, also known as C-peptide, is a measure of beta cell function. When a proinsulin molecule is cleaved, C-peptide and insulin are released in equivalent amounts. C-peptide has a longer half-life than insulin which makes it a more stable marker of endogenous insulin secretion. The additional benefit is that C-peptide levels are not affected by exogenous insulin administration, but serum insulin levels will measure both endogenous and exogenous insulin (Leighton et al. 2017). C-peptide levels are therefore used to assist in distinguishing the type of diabetes a patient may have. Typically, a patient with type 1 DM is characterized by endogenous insulin deficiency (low C-peptide). However, depending on when a patient is diagnosed with type 1 DM, the C-peptide may still be measurable due to functioning beta cells (VanBuecken and Greenbaum 2014). Patients with type 2 DM present with insulin resistance and hyperinsulinemia which will lead to elevated C-peptide levels. About 6% of pediatric patients aged 10–19 years old with type 2 DM present in DKA will have lower C-peptide levels at diagnosis (ADA 2021).

C-peptide may also help a clinician decide if a patient should be tested for MODY. Some forms of MODY may present like type 1 DM, but the cause of diabetes is due to a genetic mutation that affects the formation or release of insulin and does not cause beta cell destruction. Therefore, a patient with MODY may be on relatively low doses of exogenous insulin and continues producing some endogenous insulin. Therefore, the C-peptide will be measurable (Leighton et al. 2017; Levitt Katz 2015).

11.9.1.5 Insulin Levels

An insulin level in a patient with type 2 DM may not give useful clinical information since patients with type 2 DM may have variable insulin levels based on the stage of the disease progression due to insulin resistance and possible insulin deficiency (ADA 2021). Furthermore, the routine screening of insulin levels in children or adolescents with obesity is not recommended as it offers little diagnostic value.

11.9.1.6 Urinalysis

In the primary care setting, clinicians often check a urinalysis to screen for glucosuria. It is important to note that glucosuria will only be seen if the plasma glucose is elevated and above the renal threshold when the urine sample is given (Styne 2016). If the clinician is suspicious that a patient has diabetes mellitus and there is no glucosuria on urinalysis, further testing should be done with serum glucose levels or HbA1C.

11.9.2 Real-Life Example

A 13-year-old male with obesity and acanthosis nigricans was referred to the pediatric diabetes clinic due to an HbA1c of 6.6% noted by the primary care clinician. He was asymptomatic. The patient completed a 2-hour OGTT. The fasting glucose was 91 mg/dL, and the 2-hour glucose was 156 mg/dL. At this time, he was diagnosed with prediabetes. This patient was monitored and made lifestyle changes, and 3 months later, HbA1c was 5.9%.

Key Learning about Diabetes

- Remember to ask about polyuria, polydipsia, and polyphagia in any pediatric patient who presents with vomiting, particularly when there are no known sick contacts. DKA can be mistaken for acute gastroenteritis.
- It can be difficult to distinguish between the diagnosis of type 1 DM and type 2 DM in the pediatric population, given the current obesity epidemic. A child can be obese and have type 1 DM. Therefore, the ADA recommends the testing of islet autoantibodies in children and adolescents diagnosed with diabetes regardless of weight status.
- All patients who complain of polyuria and polydipsia should have a urinalysis.
- There is no utility to check an insulin level routinely on a patient with type 1 DM since it is an insulin-deficient state.

Questions

1. A 10-month-old baby with congenital hypothyroidism comes for his routine follow-up appointment. The mother states that she gives him the levothyroxine every day with his morning bottle of soy formula. The labs show TSH 10.69 mIU/mL (0.80–8.20 mIU/L) and free T4 1.0 ng/mL (0.9–1.4 ng/dL). What is your next step?
   (a) Increase the dose of levothyroxine.
   (b) Decrease the dose of levothyroxine.
   (c) Repeat the thyroid function test because maybe there was assay interference.
   (d) Ask the mother to give the levothyroxine with a small amount of water and repeat the thyroid function tests in 6–8 weeks.
2. Bobby is a 12-year-old boy who is in puberty. He does not play organized sports and loves his video games. His height is 62 inches (152 cm), and his weight is 165lbs (75 kg). His BMI is >95th percentile. His mother wants you to check his thyroid to see if that's the cause of his weight gain. He denies

constipation, diarrhea, dry skin, or fatigue. How do you counsel the mother?

(a) Check the thyroid function tests to make her happy.

(b) Explain that it is important for children to exercise daily and make goals with Bobby to improve his physical activities.

(c) Explain that current guidelines do not recommend checking TSH when evaluating obesity and that obesity may cause an elevated TSH, which typically does not require treatment.

(d) Both b and c.

3. An 18-year-old female patient complains about irregular menses and fatigue. She is stressed out about getting into college and having to help care for her young brother with type 1 diabetes. She thinks that her hair has been thinning, so she has been trying to take supplements to feel better. You do a screening test and note an elevated TSH of 9.7mIU/L. What is not in her differential diagnosis?

(a) Hashimoto's hypothyroidism.

(b) Assay interference.

(c) Subclinical hypothyroidism.

(d) TSH-secreting adenoma.

(e) Graves' disease.

4. A mother brings an 8-year-old male into your office because he has started to develop pubic hair, and she thinks he is too young for that. On physical exam, he has TS or SMR 2 pubic hair, no acne, and no apocrine body odor. He has a normal growth velocity. What initial evaluation may be appropriate for you to order and may avoid referral to pediatric endocrinology (in favor of monitoring) if normal?

(a) 17-OHP

(b) TSH and free T4.

(c) Bone age X-ray.

(d) Testosterone.

5. Brian is a 15-year-old male, and he comes to your office because he is worried that he is not developing like his friends are. He has no other medical history and no surgical history. On exam, he has SMR stage V pubic hair.

Testes are 4 cc b/l. You decide to draw labs and refer to pediatric endocrinology. What initial tests would be helpful to have for the referral?

(a) 17-OHP

(b) LH, FSH, and testosterone.

(c) Testosterone only.

(d) Morning cortisol.

6. Tina is a 16-year-old female who comes to you because she isn't getting her periods regularly. She also has been dealing with acne, and it is bothering her. She has excessive hair on her chin and chest, which she shaves. Which test listed below is not a recommended first-line evaluation?

(a) LH, FSH, and estradiol.

(b) Testosterone.

(c) Pelvic ultrasound.

(d) DHEA-S.

7. Sam is a 13-year-old male who presents to your office because his mother is concerned that he is shorter than the rest of the kids in his class. His midparental height is around the 25th percentile, but his height is currently at the 5th percentile for age and he has an appropriate prepubertal growth velocity. His mother notes that she got her period when she was 14 years old, and she thinks that Sam's father was growing when he was in college. Sam is prepubertal on the exam. What would be an appropriate first-line evaluation?

(a) LH, FSH, and testosterone.

(b) IGF-1 and IGF-BP3.

(c) Growth hormone.

(d) Bone age X-ray.

8. Lauren is a 5-year-old female who presents to your office for her annual healthcare maintenance exam. Her only pertinent medical history is that she was born small for gestational age; otherwise, she has no other medical conditions and is a healthy weight with a BMI at the 40th percentile. You notice that she has been consistently at the 2nd percentile for height and is not falling off the growth curve, but her midparental height is on the 25th percentile. What do you tell her parents when they ask if she will improve her growth?

(a) "Her growth velocity is steady, so don't worry; she will make it to the 25th percentile eventually."

(b) "She might have a growth hormone deficiency, so we will do some screening labs today."

(c) "She was born small for gestational age and has not exhibited catch-up growth; therefore, let's refer her to pediatric endocrinology to discuss possible evaluation and treatment."

(d) "She should gain some weight, and that will help her grow faster."

9. John is a 12-year-old male who presents to your office because his parents are concerned about his weight loss, and they feel he is shorter than the rest of his peers. You notice that his growth percentiles dropped from the 40th percentile about 2 years ago to the 25th percentile currently and his weight has dropped from the 30th percentile to the 10th percentile. What are some screening tests that you could consider for further evaluation?

(a) Celiac screen.

(b) CBC.

(c) ESR and CRP.

(d) All of the above.

10. Steven is a 14-year-old male who presents to your office with 2 weeks of excessive urination and thirst. He has lost 12lbs, but his BMI is still above the 90th percentile. He has mild acanthosis on the back of his neck, and he has TS or SMR stage III pubic hair, and his testes are 10 cc bilaterally. His father and maternal grandmother both have type 2 DM. You perform a urinalysis in the office and notice glucose in his urine. A random finger stick shows blood glucose of 266 mg/dL. Which of the following is the best response to the parents?

(a) "Steven has diabetes. You should go home and cut out sugary drinks and candy and eat a low-carb diet."

(b) "Steven has type 2 DM because he is obese, and you have a strong family history of type 2 DM."

(c) "Steven's symptoms and glucosuria and elevated blood sugar suggest that he has diabetes. I will refer you to the pediatric endocrinologist emergently for further evaluation."

(d) "I'm glad Steven lost weight. He was obese. Please continue healthy eating and incorporate exercise into his daily routine so he can continue with weight loss. We will re-evaluate him in 1 month."

11. You just determined that Steven (Question 10) has diabetes. What blood tests will the endocrinologist complete to determine if Steven has type 1 DM and type 2 DM?

(a) HbA1c.

(b) C-peptide and insulin.

(c) 2-hour OGTT

(d) Autoantibodies (GAD-65, IAA, ICA, IA-2, ZnT8).

12. Sarah is a 17-year-old female who presents to your office for her annual visit before heading to college. Since her last visit, she has gained a lot of weight, and her BMI has increased from the 82nd percentile to the 90th percentile. She has a family history of type 2 DM in her maternal and paternal grandparents. You perform annual fasting screening labs. The glucose on the complete metabolic panel is 137 mg/dL. You call Sarah back because you are worried that she might have diabetes. You ask more questions about diabetes. She denies polyuria, polydipsia, and nocturia. You have her come back for an HbA1c and OGTT. The HbA1c is 6%. The fasting blood glucose on the OGTT is 121 mg/dL, and the 2-hour blood glucose is 167 mg/dL. How do you counsel Sarah?

(a) "You have diabetes and need to start medication immediately."

(b) "You have prediabetes and should focus on healthy eating and exercise and healthy weight loss to prevent progression to diabetes."

(c) "You have prediabetes. If you begin to have increased thirst or urination or start waking at night to urinate or drink, you should seek medical attention. These could be signs that your prediabetes is progressing to diabetes."

(d) "You have diabetes, and if you're not careful, you will end up blind."

(e) Both b and c.

13. Charlie is a 10-year-old boy who presents to your office with new-onset nocturnal enuresis over the past month. You learn during the history that he is not doing well in school because he is missing class to use the bathroom. His weight has been stable. What findings on his urinalysis would make you suspect diabetes insipidus?

(a) Specific gravity: 1.005.

(b) Color: clear.

(c) Glucose: 2+.

(d) Ketones: 1+.

(e) Both a and b.

Rationale

1. Answer: d

Levothyroxine should be given on an empty stomach, and iron, fiber, calcium, and soy can affect the absorption of levothyroxine. Waiting to repeat the TSH for 6–8 weeks is important because TSH changes slowly in response to small changes in free T4. Increasing the dose of levothyroxine before changing the way the baby gets the levothyroxine could cause the baby to become hyperthyroid if the mother suddenly starts to give the levothyroxine the correct way. Decreasing the dose of levothyroxine does not make sense because, based on the elevated TSH, the baby needs more levothyroxine. There could be an assay interference, but the clinician should take the first step to ensure that the baby is getting the levothyroxine on an empty stomach, free from soy, fiber, calcium, or iron.

2. Answer: d, both b and c

It is important to remember that current guidelines do not suggest checking thyroid function tests in obese children. The TSH is elevated in children with obesity and has also been found to improve with weight loss, suggesting that the elevated TSH seen in obesity may be a consequence and not a cause of obesity. Since obesity can have other long-term effects on children, counseling Bobby to improve his diet and physical activity should be part of all visit types.

3. Answer: e

An elevated TSH is seen in Hashimoto's thyroiditis, subclinical hypothyroidism (which can be caused by Hashimoto's thyroiditis), and TSH-secreting adenomas (though the TSH would likely be higher). Immunoassays can be affected by biotin. In Graves' disease, the clinician should expect to see a low TSH.

4. Answer: c

Suppose the clinician has concerns regarding non-classic congenital adrenal hyperplasia. In that case, a baseline 17-OHP may be appropriate, but given the patient's mild premature adrenarche, the clinician may not have to jump to a 17-OHP. Thyroid function tests would not be routinely evaluated in the case of premature adrenarche. A bone age X-ray is helpful. If it is mildly advanced, then monitoring may be appropriate; if significantly advanced, a referral to pediatric endocrinology is warranted to rule out pathologic causes of premature adrenarche. Testosterone is not elevated in benign premature adrenarche. A testosterone level could be helpful for reassurance. Still, if it is normal and there is a concern for the pathologic cause of premature adrenarche, additional adrenal hormone testing should be considered.

5. Answer: b

17-OHP is typically used when concerned for non-classic congenital adrenal hyperplasia; this patient has delayed puberty; therefore, 17-OHP would not be a first-line evaluation. LH, FSH, and testosterone levels may be helpful. If LH and FSH are elevated, it can be indicative of gonadal failure. If LH and FSH are low, there may be a pituitary concern. Morning cortisol can be monitored if there is a concern for hypocortisolism.

6. Answer: c

The pelvic ultrasound is not recommended as a first-line evaluation for hyperandrogenism and oligomenorrhea, even if the patient likely has PCOS. LH, FSH, estradiol, testosterone, and DHEA-S are appropriate evaluations.

7. Answer: d

Sam likely has a constitutional delay of growth and development since both his parents seem to have puberty on the later end of normal. Sam's bone age would likely reveal a delayed bone age.

8. Answer: c

Children born small for gestational age and who fail to exhibit catch-up growth are approved by the FDA for growth hormone therapy. She may not "catch up" on her own to her midparental height. The child should be referred to a pediatric endocrinologist for further evaluation and discussion about treatment. Growth hormone deficiency is lower on the differential since she has not had a slow growth velocity. Her BMI is adequate and should not be expected to cause poor growth.

9. Answer: d

Due to his weight loss, John's height velocity decrease could be due to a non-endocrine cause. Therefore, screening for celiac disease, an inflammatory condition (i.e., Crohn's disease), and a hematologic process should be ruled out.

10. Answer: c

Steven definitely has diabetes due to his symptoms of polyuria, polydipsia and weight loss and his glucosuria and elevated random blood sugar. Steven could have type 2 DM based on his weight and family history of type 2 DM and his acanthosis nigricans. However, obese children can still have type 1 DM, and you cannot definitively tell the parents which type of diabetes Steven has without further testing. Regardless of diabetes, Steven should cut out sugary drinks, eat a low-carb diet, and incorporate exercise into his daily routine to prevent future obesity-related complications. Any child with signs and symptoms of diabetes requires an urgent referral to a pediatric endocrinologist.

11. Answer: d

Autoantibodies are the only way to determine if a patient has T1DM or T2DM. An HbA1c will tell you the average blood sugar for the past 2–3 months and will likely be elevated in Steven's case. A C-peptide and insulin level may be helpful but will not determine the type of diabetes that Steven has. C-peptide and insulin levels may be high in patients with type 2 DM. However, C-peptide and insulin levels can also be low when a person presents acutely with type 2 DM. A 2-hour OGTT is not useful for a patient presenting with signs and symptoms of diabetes and will not provide any additional information on the type of diabetes that Steven has.

12. Answer: e, both b and c

Sarah has prediabetes based on the results of her OGTT (neither blood glucose is in the diabetes range) and her A1c of 6%. She is obese and at risk for type 2 DM based on her family history. She should focus on weight loss in a healthy way and should monitor for symptoms of diabetes like increased thirst or urination. If she notices symptoms of diabetes, she should seek care immediately.

13. Answer: e, both a and b

A patient with diabetes insipidus would have a low specific gravity and clear urine. A patient should not have glycosuria or ketonuria with diabetes insipidus.

References

American Diabetes Association. Type 2 diabetes in children and adolescents. Pediatrics. 2000;105(3 Pt 1):671–80.

American Diabetes Association. Standards of diabetes care in 2021. Diabetes Care. 2021;44(Suppl):1.

Aydın B, Winters SJ. Sex hormone-binding globulin in children and adolescents. J Clin Res Pediatr Endocrinol. 2016;8(1):1–12.

Azziz R, Carmina E, Sawaya ME. Idiopathic hirsutism. Endocr Rev. 2000;21(4):347–62.

Backeljauw PF, Dattani MT, Cohen P, Rosenfeld RG. Chapter 10: disorders of growth hormone/insulin-like growth factor secretion and action. In: Sperling MS, editor. Pediatric endocrinology. 4th ed. Saunders/Elsevier; 2014. p. 291–404.

Bankir L, Bichet DG, Morgenthaler NG. Vasopressin: physiology, assessment and osmosensation. J Intern Med. 2017;282(4):284–97.

Barstow C, Rerucha C. Evaluation of short and tall stature in children. Am Fam Physician. 2015;92(1):43–50.

Becker M, Hesse V. Minipuberty: why does it happen? Horm Res Paediatr. 2020;93(2):76–84.

Bingley PJ, Wherrett DK, Shultz A, Rafkin LE, Atkinson MA, Greenbaum CJ. Type 1 diabetes TrialNet: a multifaceted approach to bringing disease-modifying therapy to clinical use in type 1 diabetes. Diabetes Care. 2018;41(4):653–61.

Biondi B. Thyroid and obesity: an intriguing relationship. J Clin Endocrinol Metab. 2010;95(8):3614–7.

Bona G, Prodam F, Monzani A. Subclinical hypothyroidism in children: natural history and when to treat. J Clin Res Pediatr Endocrinol. 2013;5(Suppl 1):23–8.

Bonifacio E, Achenbach P. Birth and coming of age of islet autoantibodies. Clin Exp Immunol. 2019;198(3):294–305.

Bornstein SR, Allolio B, Arlt W, Barthel A, Don-Wauchope A, Hammer GD, et al. Diagnosis and treatment of primary adrenal insufficiency: an Endocrine Society Clinical Practice Guideline. J Clin Endocrinol Metab. 2016;101(2):364–89.

Bozzola M, Bozzola E, Montalbano C, Stamati FA, Ferrara P, Villani A. Delayed puberty versus hypogonadism: a challenge for the pediatrician. Ann Pediatr Endocrinol Metab. 2018;23(2):57–61.

Brambilla DJ, Matsumoto AM, Araujo AB, McKinlay JB. The effect of diurnal variation on clinical measurement of serum testosterone and other sex hormone levels in men. J Clin Endocrinol Metab. 2009;94(3):907–13.

Brar PC. Update on the current modalities used to screen high risk youth for prediabetes and/or type 2 diabetes mellitus. Ann Pediatr Endocrinol Metab. 2019;24(2):71–7.

Carel JC, Eugster EA, Rogol A, Ghizzoni L, Palmert MR, ESPE-LWPES GnRH Analogs Consensus Conference Group, et al. Consensus statement on the use of gonadotropin-releasing hormone analogs in children. Pediatrics. 2009;123(4):e752–62.

Chandler DW, Chia DJ, Nakamoto J, Chun KY, Pepkowitz SH, Rapaport R. Chapter 4: laboratory methods in pediatric endocrinology. In: Sperling MS, editor. Pediatric endocrinology. 4th ed. Saunders/Elsevier; 2014. p. 90–106.

Chinoy A, Murray PG. Diagnosis of growth hormone deficiency in the paediatric and transitional age. Best Pract Res Clin Endocrinol Metab. 2016;30(6):737–47.

Clemmons DR. Consensus statement on the standardization and evaluation of growth hormone and insulin-like growth factor assays. Clin Chem. 2011;57(4):555–9.

Cohen LE. Idiopathic short stature: a clinical review. JAMA. 2014;311(17):1787–96.

Cohen P, Rogol AD, Deal CL, Saenger P, Reiter EO, Ross JL, et al. Consensus statement on the diagnosis and treatment of children with idiopathic short

stature: a summary of the growth hormone research society, the Lawson Wilkins Pediatric Endocrine Society, and the European Society for Paediatric Endocrinology Workshop. J Clin Endocrinol Metab. 2008;93(11):4210–7.

Creo AL, Schwenk WF 2nd. Bone age: a handy tool for pediatric providers. Pediatrics. 2017;140(6):e20171486.

Crisafulli G, Aversa T, Zirilli G, Pajno GB, Corica D, De Luca F, et al. Subclinical hypothyroidism in children: when a replacement hormonal treatment might be advisable. Front Endocrinol (Lausanne). 2019;10:109.

De Sanctis V, Di Maio S, Soliman AT, Raiola G, Elalaily R, Millimaggi G. Hand X-ray in pediatric endocrinology: skeletal age assessment and beyond. Indian J Endocrinol Metab. 2014;18(Suppl 1):S63–71.

Deal CL, Tony M, Höybye C, Allen DB, Tauber M, Christiansen JS. Growth hormone research society workshop summary: consensus guidelines for recombinant human growth hormone therapy in Prader-Willi syndrome. J Clin Endocrinol Metab. 2013;98(6):E1072–87.

DeGroot LJ. The non-thyroidal illness syndrome. In: Feingold KR, Anawalt B, Boyce A, et al., editors. Endotext. South Dartmouth (MA): MDText.com, Inc.; 2015.

Di Iorgi N, Morana G, Allegri AE, Napoli F, Gastaldi R, Calcagno A, et al. Classical and non-classical causes of GH deficiency in the paediatric age. Best Pract Res Clin Endocrinol Metab. 2016;30(6):705–36.

Diaz A, Lipman Diaz EG. Hypothyroidism. Pediatr Rev. 2014;35(8):336–47.

Esfandiari NH, Papaleontiou M. Biochemical testing in thyroid disorders. Endocrinol Metab Clin N Am. 2017;46(3):631–48.

Expert Committee on the Diagnosis and Classification of Diabetes Mellitus. Report of the expert committee on the diagnosis and classification of diabetes mellitus. Diabetes Care. 2003;26(Suppl 1):S5–S20.

Faix JD. Principles and pitfalls of free hormone measurements. Best Pract Res Clin Endocrinol Metab. 2013;27(5):631–45.

Fisher. Quest Diagnostics Manual: Endocrinology test selection and interpretation. In: Fisher DA, ed. 4th ed. Quest Diagnostics Nichols Institute; 2007.

Fuqua JS. Treatment and outcomes of precocious puberty: an update. J Clin Endocrinol Metab. 2013;98(6):2198–207.

Gerstein HC. Fasting versus post-load glucose levels: why the controversy? Diabetes Care. 2001;24(11):1855–7.

Ghergherehchi R, Hazhir N. Thyroid hormonal status among children with obesity. Ther Adv Endocrinol Metab. 2015;6(2):51–5.

Giannakopoulos A, Lazopoulou N, Pervanidou P, Kanaka-Gantenbein C. The impact of adiposity and puberty on thyroid function in children and adolescents. Child Obes. 2019;15(6):411–5.

Gordon CM, Ackerman KE, Berga SL, Kaplan JR, Mastorakos G, Misra M, et al. Functional hypothalamic amenorrhea: an Endocrine Society Clinical

Practice Guideline. J Clin Endocrinol Metab. 2017;102(5):1413–39.

Grimberg A, DiVall SA, Polychronakos C, Allen DB, Cohen LE, Quintos JB, et al. Guidelines for growth hormone and insulin-like growth factor-I treatment in children and adolescents: growth hormone deficiency, idiopathic short stature, and primary insulin-like growth factor-I deficiency. Horm Res Paediatr. 2016;86(6):361–97.

Grimberg A, Lifshitz F. Chapter 1: worrisome growth. In: Lifshitz F, editor. Pediatric endocrinology, volume 2: growth, adrenal, sexual, thyroid, calcium, and fluid balance disorders. 5th ed. Informa Healthcare; 2007. p. 1–50.

Growth Hormone Research Society. Consensus guidelines for the diagnosis and treatment of growth hormone (GH) deficiency in childhood and adolescence: summary statement of the GH research society. GH research society. J Clin Endocrinol Metab. 2000;85(11):3990–3.

Guo F, Moellering DR, Garvey WT. Use of HbA1c for diagnoses of diabetes and prediabetes: comparison with diagnoses based on fasting and 2-hr glucose values and effects of gender, race, and age. Metab Syndr Relat Disord. 2014;12(5):258–68.

Gupta V, Lee M. Central hypothyroidism. Indian J Endocrinol Metab. 2011;15(Suppl 2):S99–S106.

Guzzetti C, Ibba A, Pilia S, Beltrami N, Di Iorgi N, Rollo A, et al. Cut-off limits of the peak GH response to stimulation tests for the diagnosis of GH deficiency in children and adolescents: study in patients with organic GHD. Eur J Endocrinol. 2016;175(1):41–7.

Haddad RA, Giacherio D, Barkan L. Interpretation of common endocrine laboratory tests: technical pitfalls, their mechanisms and practical considerations. Clin Diabetes Endocrinol. 2019;5:12.

Hatch R, Rosenfield RL, Kim MH, Tredway D. Hirsutism: implications, etiology, and management. Am J Obstet Gynecol. 1981;140(7):815–30.

Haugen BR. Drugs that suppress TSH or cause central hypothyroidism. Best Pract Res Clin Endocrinol Metab. 2009;23(6):793–800.

Herman WH, Ma Y, Uwaifo G, Haffner S, Kahn SE, Horton ES, et al. Differences in A1C by race and ethnicity among patients with impaired glucose tolerance in the Diabetes Prevention Program. Diabetes Care. 2007;30(10):2453–7.

Hollowell JG, Staehling NW, Flanders WD, Hannon WH, Gunter EW, Spencer CA, et al. Serum TSH, T (4), and thyroid antibodies in the United States population (1988 to 1994): National Health and Nutrition Examination Survey (NHANES III). J Clin Endocrinol Metab. 2002;87(2):489–99.

Honour JW. 17-Hydroxyprogesterone in children, adolescents and adults. Ann Clin Biochem. 2014;51(Pt 4):424–40.

Hornberger LL, Lane MA, AAP Committee on Adolescent. Identification and management of eating disorders in children and adolescents. Pediatrics. 2021;147(1):e2020040279.

Houk CP, Lee PA. Early diagnosis and treatment referral of children born small for gestational age without catch-up growth are critical for optimal growth outcomes. Int J Pediatr Endocrinol. 2012;2012(1):11.

Hunter MH, Carek PJ. Evaluation and treatment of women with hirsutism. Am Fam Physician. 2003;67(12):2565–72.

Jin HY. Thyroxine binding globulin excess detected by neonatal screening. Ann Pediatr Endocrinol Metab. 2016;21(2):105–8.

Junnila RK, Strasburger CJ, Bidlingmaier M. Pitfalls of insulin-like growth factor-i and growth hormone assays. Endocrinol Metab Clin N Am. 2015;44(1):27–34.

Kapelari K, Kirchlechner C, Högler W, Schweitzer K, Virgolini I, Moncayo R. Pediatric reference intervals for thyroid hormone levels from birth to adulthood: a retrospective study. BMC Endocr Disord. 2008;8:15.

Kaplowitz P, Bloch C. Section on Endocrinology, American Academy of Pediatrics. Evaluation and referral of children with signs of early puberty. Pediatrics. 2016;137:1. https://doi.org/10.1542/peds.2015-3732.

Kaplowitz PB, Oberfield SE. Reexamination of the age limit for defining when puberty is precocious in girls in the United States: implications for evaluation and treatment. Drug and Therapeutics and Executive Committees of the Lawson Wilkins Pediatric Endocrine Society. Pediatrics. 1999;104(4 Pt 1):936–41.

Katznelson L, Laws ER Jr, Melmed S, Molitch ME, Murad MH, Utz A, et al. Acromegaly: an endocrine society clinical practice guideline. J Clin Endocrinol Metab. 2014;99(11):3933–51.

Kilberg MJ, Rasooly IR, LaFranchi SH, Bauer AJ, Hawkes CP. Newborn screening in the US may miss mild persistent hypothyroidism. J Pediatr. 2018;192:204–8.

Kim PS, Woods C, Georgoff P, Crum D, Rosenberg A, Smith M, et al. A1C underestimates glycemia in HIV infection. Diabetes Care. 2009;32(9):1591–3.

Klein DA, Emerick JE, Sylvester JE, Vogt KS. Disorders of puberty: an approach to diagnosis and management. Am Fam Physician. 2017;96(9):590–9.

Klein DA, Poth MA. Amenorrhea: an approach to diagnosis and management. Am Fam Physician. 2013;87(11):781–8.

Kletter GB, Klein KO, Wong YY. A pediatrician's guide to central precocious puberty. Clin Pediatr (Phila). 2015;54(5):414–24.

Koulouri O, Moran C, Halsall D, Chatterjee K, Gurnell M. Pitfalls in the measurement and interpretation of thyroid function tests. Best Pract Res Clin Endocrinol Metab. 2013;27(6):745–62.

Kushnir MM, Rockwood AL, Bergquist J. Liquid chromatography-tandem mass spectrometry applications in endocrinology. Mass Spectrom Rev. 2010;29(3):480–502.

Latronico AC, Brito VN, Carel JC. Causes, diagnosis, and treatment of central precocious puberty. Lancet Diabetes Endocrinol. 2016;4(3):265–74.

Lee DM, Chung IH. Morning basal luteinizing hormone, a good screening tool for diagnosing central precocious puberty. Ann Pediatr Endocrinol Metab. 2019;24(1):27–33.

Lee JM, Wu EL, Tarini B, Herman WH, Yoon E. Diagnosis of diabetes using hemoglobin A1c: should recommendations in adults be extrapolated to adolescents? J Pediatr. 2011;158(6):947–952.e9523.

Leighton E, Sainsbury CA, Jones GC. A practical review of C-peptide testing in diabetes. Diabetes Ther. 2017;8(3):475–87.

Levitt Katz LE. C-peptide and 24-hour urinary C-peptide as markers to help classify types of childhood diabetes. Horm Res Paediatr. 2015;84(1):62–4.

Lodish MB, Keil MF, Stratakis CA. Cushing's syndrome in pediatrics: an update. Endocrinol Metab Clin N Am. 2018;47(2):451–62.

Longhi S, Radetti G. Thyroid function and obesity. J Clin Res Pediatr Endocrinol. 2013;5(Suppl 1):40–4.

Luong JHT, Vashist SK. Chemistry of biotin-streptavidin and the growing concern of an emerging biotin interference in clinical immunoassays. ACS Omega. 2019;5(1):10–8. Published 2019 Dec 18

Martin KA, Anderson RR, Chang RJ, Ehrmann DA, Lobo RA, Murad MH, et al. Evaluation and treatment of hirsutism in premenopausal women: an Endocrine Society Clinical Practice Guideline. J Clin Endocrinol Metab. 2018;103(4):1233–57.

Matalliotakis M, Koliarakis I, Matalliotaki C, Trivli A, Hatzidaki E. Clinical manifestations, evaluation and management of hyperprolactinemia in adolescent and young girls: a brief review. Acta Biomed. 2019;90(1):149–57.

Mayfield J. Diagnosis and classification of diabetes mellitus: new criteria. Am Fam Physician. 1998;58(6):1355–70.

McCartney CR, Marshall JC. Clinical practice. Polycystic ovary syndrome. N Engl J Med. 2016;375(1):54–64.

McNeil AR, Stanford PE. Reporting thyroid function tests in pregnancy. Clin Biochem Rev. 2015;36(4):109–26.

Melmed S, Casanueva FF, Hoffman AR, Kleinberg DL, Montori VM, Schlechte JA, et al. Diagnosis and treatment of hyperprolactinemia: an Endocrine Society clinical practice guideline. J Clin Endocrinol Metab. 2011;96(2):273–88.

Mihailidis J, Dermesropian R, Taxel P, Luthra P, Grant-Kels JM. Endocrine evaluation of hirsutism. Int J Womens Dermatol. 2017;3(1 Suppl):S6–S10.

Miller WL, Flück CE. Chapter 13: adrenal cortex and its disorders. In: Sperling MS, editor. Pediatric endocrinology. 4th ed. Saunders/Elsevier; 2014. p. 471–532.

Nadeau KJ, Anderson BJ, Berg EG, Chiang JL, Chou H, Copeland KC, et al. Youth-onset type 2 diabetes consensus report: current status, challenges, and priorities. Diabetes Care. 2016;39(9):1635–42.

Nieman LK, Biller BM, Findling JW, Newell-Price J, Savage MO, Stewart PM, et al. The diagnosis of Cushing's syndrome: an Endocrine Society clinical practice guideline. J Clin Endocrinol Metab. 2008;93(5):1526–40.

Novello L, Speiser PW. Premature adrenarche. Pediatr Ann. 2018;47(1):e7–e11.

Oberfield SE, Sopher AB, Gerken AT. Approach to the girl with early onset of pubic hair. J Clin Endocrinol Metab. 2011;96(6):1610–22.

Pant V, Baral S, Van Wyk. Grumbach syndrome with precocious puberty and ovarian cysts: value of thyroid function tests. JPS Case Rep. 2019;43:32–43.

Pihoker C, Gilliam LK, Hampe CS, Lernmark A. Autoantibodies in diabetes. Diabetes. 2005;54(Suppl 2):S52–61.

Powell GF, Brasel JA, Blizzard RM. Emotional deprivation and growth retardation simulating idiopathic hypopituitarism. I. Clinical evaluation of the syndrome. N Engl J Med. 1967;276(23):1271–8.

Pugeat M, Plotton I, de la Perrière AB, Raverot G, Déchaud H. Raverot management of endocrine disease, Hyperandrogenic states in women: pitfalls in laboratory diagnosis. Eur J Endocrinol. 2018;178(4):R141–54.

Radin MS. Pitfalls in hemoglobin A1c measurement: when results may be misleading. J Gen Intern Med. 2014;29(2):388–94.

Rauh M. Steroid measurement with LC-MS/MS in pediatric endocrinology. Mol Cell Endocrinol. 2009;301(1–2):272–81.

Reinehr T, de Sousa G, Andler W. Hyperthyrotropinemia in obese children is reversible after weight loss and is not related to lipids. J Clin Endocrinol Metab. 2006;91(8):3088–91.

Rogol AD. Emotional deprivation in children: growth faltering and reversible hypopituitarism. Front Endocrinol (Lausanne). 2020;11:596144.

Rogol AD, Hayden GF. Etiologies and early diagnosis of short stature and growth failure in children and adolescents. J Pediatr. 2014;164(5 Suppl):S1–14.e6.

Romano AA. Growth and growth hormone treatment in Noonan syndrome. Pediatr Endocrinol Rev. 2019;16(Suppl 2):459–64.

Rosenbloom AL, Connor EL. Chapter 3: hypopituitarism and other disorders of the growth hormone-insulin-like growth factor-1 axis. In: Lifshitz F, editor. Pediatric endocrinology, volume 2: growth, adrenal, sexual, thyroid, calcium, and fluid balance disorders. 5th ed. Informa Healthcare; 2007. p. 65–99.

Rosenfeld RL, Cooke DW, Radovick S. Chapter 15: puberty and its disorders in the female. In: Sperling MS, editor. Pediatric endocrinology. 4th ed. Saunders/Elsevier; 2014. p. 569–663.

Rosenfield RL. Clinical practice: hirsutism. N Engl J Med. 2005;353(24):2578–88.

Rosenfield RL. The diagnosis of polycystic ovary syndrome in adolescents. Pediatrics. 2015;136(6):1154–65.

Rosner W, Auchus RJ, Azziz R, Sluss PM, Raff H. Position statement: utility, limitations, and pitfalls in measuring testosterone: an Endocrine Society position statement. J Clin Endocrinol Metab. 2007;92(2):405–13.

Ross DS, Burch HB, Cooper DS, Greenlee MC, Laurberg P, Maia AL, et al. 2016 American Thyroid Association Guidelines for diagnosis and management of hyperthyroidism and other causes of thyrotoxicosis. [published correction appears in Thyroid. 2017 Nov;27(11):1462]. Thyroid. 2016;26(10): 1343–421.

Sanyal D, Raychaudhuri M. Hypothyroidism and obesity: an intriguing link. Indian J Endocrinol Metab. 2016;20(4):554–7.

Schmidt KD, Valeri C, Leslie RD. Autoantibodies in type 1 diabetes. Clin Chim Acta. 2005;354(1–2): 35–40.

Sheehan MT. Biochemical testing of the thyroid: TSH is the best and, oftentimes, only test needed—a review for primary care. Clin Med Res. 2016;14(2):83–92.

Soh SB, Aw TC. Laboratory testing in thyroid conditions - pitfalls and clinical utility. Ann Lab Med. 2019;39(1):3–14.

Speiser PW, Arlt W, Auchus RJ, Baskin LS, Conway GS, Merke DP, et al. Congenital adrenal hyperplasia due to steroid 21-hydroxylase deficiency: an Endocrine Society Clinical Practice Guideline. [published correction appears in J Clin Endocrinol Metab. 2019 Jan 1;104(1):39–40]. J Clin Endocrinol Metab. 2018;103(11):4043–88.

Spencer CA, Hollowell JG, Kazarosyan M, Braverman LE. National health and nutrition examination survey III thyroid-stimulating hormone (TSH)-thyroperoxidase antibody relationships demonstrate that TSH upper reference limits may be skewed by occult thyroid dysfunction. J Clin Endocrinol Metab. 2007;92(11):4236–40.

Srinivasan S, Misra M. Hyperthyroidism in children. Pediatr Rev. 2015;36(6):239–48.

Stanley T. Diagnosis of growth hormone deficiency in childhood. Curr Opin Endocrinol Diabetes Obes. 2012;19(1):47–52.

Styne DM. Pediatric endocrinology: a clinical handbook. Springer; 2016.

Styne DM, Arslanian SA, Connor EL, Farooqi IS, Murad MH, Silverstein JH, et al. Pediatric obesity-assessment, treatment, and prevention: an Endocrine Society clinical practice guideline. J Clin Endocrinol Metab. 2017;102(3):709–57.

Swerdloff RS, Ng CM. Gynecomastia: etiology, diagnosis, and treatment. In: Feingold KR, Anawalt B, Boyce A, et al., editors. Endotext. South Dartmouth (MA): MDText.com, Inc.; 2019.

Trapp CM, Oberfield SE. Recommendations for treatment of nonclassic congenital adrenal hyperplasia (NCCAH): an update. Steroids. 2012;77(4):342–6.

Vadiveloo T, Donnan PT, Murphy MJ, Leese GP. Age- and gender-specific TSH reference intervals in people with no obvious thyroid disease in Tayside, Scotland: the Thyroid Epidemiology, Audit, and Research Study (TEARS). J Clin Endocrinol Metab. 2013;98(3):1147–53.

Vajravelu ME, Lee JM. Identifying prediabetes and type 2 diabetes in asymptomatic youth: should HbA1c be used as a diagnostic approach? Curr Diab Rep. 2018;18(7):43. Published 2018 Jun 4

van Trotsenburg P, Stoupa A, Léger J, Rohrer T, Peters C, Fugazzola L, et al. Congenital hypothyroidism: a 2020-2021 Consensus Guidelines Update-An ENDO-European Reference Network Initiative Endorsed by the European Society for Pediatric Endocrinology and the European Society for Endocrinology. Thyroid. 2021;31(3):387–419.

VanBuecken DE, Greenbaum CJ. Residual C-peptide in type 1 diabetes: what do we really know? Pediatr Diabetes. 2014;15(2):84–90.

Varma Shrivastav S, Bhardwaj A, Pathak KA, Shrivastav A. Insulin-like growth factor binding protein-3 (IGFBP-3): unraveling the role in mediating IGF-independent effects within the cell. Front Cell Dev Biol. 2020;8:286.

Veldhuis JD, Roemmich JN, Rogol AD. Gender and sexual maturation-dependent contrasts in the neuroregulation of growth hormone secretion in prepubertal and late adolescent males and females--a general clinical research center-based study. J Clin Endocrinol Metab. 2000;85(7):2385–94.

Verge CF, Gianani R, Kawasaki E, Yu L, Pietropaolo M, Jackson RA, et al. Prediction of type I diabetes in first-degree relatives using a combination of insulin, GAD, and ICA512bdc/IA-2 autoantibodies. Diabetes. 1996;45(7):926–33.

Vilar L, Vilar CF, Lyra R, Freitas MDC. Pitfalls in the diagnostic evaluation of hyperprolactinemia. Neuroendocrinology. 2019;109(1):7–19.

Voutilainen R, Jääskeläinen J. Premature adrenarche: etiology, clinical findings, and consequences. J Steroid Biochem Mol Biol. 2015;145:226–36.

Wallace AS, Wang D, Shin JI, Selvin E. Screening and diagnosis of prediabetes and diabetes in US children and adolescents. Pediatrics. 2020;146(3): e20200265.

Wasniewska M, Aversa T, Salerno M, Corrias A, Messina MF, Mussa A, et al. Five-year prospective evaluation of thyroid function in girls with subclinical mild hypothyroidism of different etiology. Eur J Endocrinol. 2015;173(6):801–8.

Wassner AJ. Congenital hypothyroidism. Clin Perinatol. 2018;45(1):1–18.

Wei C, Davis N, Honour J, Crowne E. The investigation of children and adolescents with abnormalities of pubertal timing. Ann Clin Biochem. 2017;54(1): 20–32.

Weiner A, Vuguin P. Diabetes insipidus. Pediatr Rev. 2020;41(2):96–9.

Wenzlau JM, Juhl K, Yu L, Moua O, Sarkar SA, Gottlieb P, et al. The cation efflux transporter ZnT8 (Slc30A8) is a major autoantigen in human type 1 diabetes. Proc Natl Acad Sci U S A. 2007;104(43): 17040–5.

Weykamp C. HbA1c: a review of analytical and clinical aspects. Ann Lab Med. 2013;33(6):393–400.

Williams CL, Long AE. What has zinc transporter 8 autoimmunity taught us about type 1 diabetes? Diabetologia. 2019;62(11):1969–76.

Wilson TA, Rose SR, Cohen P, Rogol AD, Backeljauw P, Brown R, et al. Update of guidelines for the use of growth hormone in children: the Lawson Wilkins Pediatric endocrinology society drug and therapeutics committee. J Pediatr. 2003;143(4):415–21.

Winter WE, Schatz DA. Autoimmune markers in diabetes. Clin Chem. 2011;57(2):168–75.

Zadik Z, Chalew SA, Kowarski A. Assessment of growth hormone secretion in normal stature children using 24-hour integrated concentration of GH and pharmacological stimulation. J Clin Endocrinol Metab. 1990;71(4):932–6.

Ziegler AG, Rewers M, Simell O, Simell T, Lempainen J, Steck A, et al. Seroconversion to multiple islet autoantibodies and risk of progression to diabetes in children. JAMA. 2013;309(23):2473–9.

Care of the Child with a Possible Rheumatological Disorder

12

Rita Marie John and Kathleen Kenney-Riley

Learning Objectives

After completing the chapter, the learner should be able to:

1. Develop a diagnostic workup for a child presenting with a possible rheumatological problem.
2. Interpret common laboratory studies to evaluate the child with possible rheumatological diseases.
3. Identify the pitfalls of the laboratory studies used in pediatric rheumatological diseases.
4. Understand the diagnostic laboratory tests used in patients with rheumatological complaints.

Evaluate a child for possible juvenile idiopathic arthritis, systemic lupus erythematosus and possible vasculitis.

12.1 Introduction

Rheumatology labs are challenging to understand and interpret in the pediatric population. When seeing children with rheumatologic-type complaints, clinicians often inappropriately order lab tests (Suresh 2019). Children and adolescents often have complaints similar to those seen in rheumatologic disorders and are also seen in common pediatric conditions. A recent review of primary care pediatricians demonstrated several rheumatological laboratory tests are ordered incorrectly despite guidelines for testing (Correll et al. 2016). It is important to consider the history and physical exam findings and carefully order rheumatological diagnostic testing.

12.2 Evaluation of the Child with Possible Rheumatological Complaints

The child who presents with vague complaints of fatigue or lack of energy with arthralgia must be fully evaluated with a careful history and physical exam before any diagnostic laboratory tests are ordered. The importance of doing a history and physical exam cannot be understated as laboratory tests may not be diagnostic. There is no gold standard test for common rheumatological diseases in children. While arthralgia is the most common presenting complaint of rheumatological

R. M. John (✉)
Columbia University School of Nursing,
New York, NY, USA
e-mail: rmj4@cumc.columbia.edu

K. Kenney-Riley
School of Health and Natural Sciences, Mercy
College, New York, NY, USA

diseases in children (Ventura et al. 2018), younger children may not be able to verbalize these complaints. They may present with a behavior change, difficulty in moving in the morning or general irritability. The clinician should start with a complete history and physical exam and should not randomly order a rheumatology panel. The diagnostic criteria for many pediatric rheumatological diseases are based on the clinical history and physical exam rather than laboratory tests (Correll et al. 2016).

12.2.1 Patient History

Musculoskeletal (MSK) pain without any other signs of rheumatological disease such as joint swelling, skin rashes, or gait abnormality is rarely the result of an inflammatory condition (Correll et al. 2016). Abnormality in laboratory tests should not be the only reason for referring a child to a rheumatologist. A complete history that includes routine questioning regarding nutrition, elimination, i.e., development, and sleep/sexual activity in older children (NEEDS) should be obtained.

Nonspecific symptoms such as fatigue, fever, night sweats, or weight loss can occur with rheumatological disease, infections, and oncological diseases. Autoinflammatory syndromes are generally genetic and can cause recurrent periodic fever in pediatric patients.

The clinician should elicit a history of dry mouth by asking about the need for frequent sips of water, difficulty swallowing dry foods, tooth decay, or gingivitis. In addition, a history of mouth ulcers more than once a month should raise clinical concern for a rheumatological or autoimmune problem (Ventura et al. 2018). Behcet's disease is characterized by recurrent mouth or genital ulcers and may be associated with folliculitis, pustular eruptions, and inflammatory eye diseases.

A history of white, blue, or grey color changes in the digits, when exposed to cold weather or under stress, is important to elicit. The older child may complain of pain or numbness associated with the color changes. These color changes may occur in the face of relatively minor temperature changes such as exposure to air conditioning or a freezer. Alopecia may not only be the sign of autoimmune thyroid disease but can be found in discoid lupus, vitiligo, morphea, and other skin conditions. A positive pull test occurs with true alopecia and is done by pulling approximately 40 hairs. The test is positive when six or more hairs come out in the examiner's hands (Ventura et al. 2018).

The skin manifestation of rheumatological diseases includes the classic butterfly or malar rash of SLE. Discoid lesions are usually found on the neck up in patients with discoid lupus. Cutaneous sclerosis is an area of thickening and lightning of the skin and can be primary or evolve into secondary sclerosis. Morphea is confined to the skin and subcutaneous areas with loss of hair follicles and sweat glands. A linear pattern is more common in children. It is not a marker for systemic sclerosis.

In patients with dermatomyositis, Gottron papules are pathognomonic, and the lesions are violaceous or wine-colored. They are generally found on the elbow, knees, and medial malleoli and in children, when are found on larger joints are called the Gottron sign (Ventura et al. 2018). Livedo reticularis with digital microinfarct and ulcerations can be found in more severe dermatomyositis. A heliotropic rash is found around the eyes with violaceous color changes of the upper eyelid and is considered pathognomonic for dermatomyositis. Calcinosis cutis or dystrophic calcification of the skin are more common in children. The child will report that the areas are painful.

Complaints such as arthralgias, muscle pain, fatigue, muscle aches, mouth ulcers, and rashes can be the chief complaint. A more specific history regarding arthralgia is included in Table 12.1.

12.2.2 Physical Exam

A complete physical exam is key to making the correct diagnosis. The clinician must carefully evaluate each joint to see if the pain is actually in the articular or periarticular structures. It is

Table 12.1 Questions to include when taking a history for arthralgia for a child with a possible rheumatological complaint

Questions	What it could mean
1. Ask about the character of the joint pain. Is there a temporal pattern to the pain?	• Inflammatory joint pain peaks in the morning, and it lasts longer than 30 min and can take about 2 h to improve, but it does not completely disappear with rest (Suresh 2019)
• What joints are involved? What is the progression of the pain?	• The pattern of small joint disease is important as JIA tends to affect the proximal interphalangeal joint (PIP), metacarpophalangeal joints (MCP), and wrist joints (Ventura et al. 2018; Suresh 2019)
• How long has the child had the pain?	• Symptoms of less than 6 weeks may be post-viral or postinfectious (Ventura et al. 2018)
• Does the patient have extraarticular symptoms such as muscle weakness, skin rashes, sicca symptoms, Raynaud's phenomena, breathlessness, pleuritic chest pain, or oral ulcers?	• Symptoms involving the skin, oral mucosa, or other organ systems with severe constitutional symptoms such as fatigue point to an autoimmune process. Oral ulcers and a butterfly skin rash may point to systemic lupus erythematosus (SLE). In contrast, muscle weakness, heliotrope, Gottron papules, dysphonia, dysphagia, and periungual erythema with capillaropathy may point to juvenile dermatomyositis (JDM) (Benham and Wright 2021a)
• Is it made worse by weight-bearing? Does it improve with rest?	• Noninflammatory joint pain improves with rest and is made worse with activities involving the joint such as weight-bearing
• Is this an inflammatory process or a mechanical one?	• The inflammatory process generally means that the joint pain and stiffness lasts more than 30 min

Adapted from Benham and Wright (2021a), Suresh (2019), Ventura et al. (2018)

important to look at the joint, feel it, and lastly, move it (Ventura et al. 2018). Soft tissue swelling surrounding a joint is a sign of an effusion. The eye should be examined for ciliary injection, which would indicate uveitis.

Testing for hypermobility using the Brighton scale should be done to evaluate for hypermobility which can cause arthralgias.

12.2.3 Diagnostic Laboratory Tests for Rheumatological Diseases

Additional challenges occur when interpreting the lab results related to pediatric rheumatologic conditions. Clinicians should be prudent when ordering rheumatologic labs and appropriately interpret them. All too often, labs are ordered to "open pandora's box", resulting in unnecessary stress, worry, and expensive workups. Ahrari et al. (2020) reported that at least 50% of laboratory tests, including ANA, RF, anti-dsDNA, and ENA, were inappropriately ordered. Further, many pediatric rheumatologic conditions are not diagnosed on lab tests alone; rather, specific clinical findings must be used in conjunction with test results to make the diagnosis (Agarwal and Sawhney 2010; Shojania 2000). Finally, clinicians must recognize that some common rheumatologic labs may be positive in healthy children; therefore, a comprehensive history and exam must be completed before ordering any labs.

Among the most common reasons for a referral of a child to a pediatric rheumatologist is for abnormal lab results. The most common abnormal labs resulting in referrals include elevated inflammatory markers, positive ANA, and/or positive rheumatoid factors (Jarvis 2008). Yet, positive results for these labs are not diagnostic for most pediatric rheumatologic diseases. Autoantibody testing is important in the workup of children presenting with rheumatologic complaints, but autoantibodies are often not diagnostic of most pediatric rheumatologic conditions (Saikia et al. 2016). For example, it has been found that between 3% and 15% of healthy people have a positive antinuclear antibody test (ANA), with no evidence of an actual rheumatologic condition (ACR, 2019). Research has demonstrated that while clinicians often order rheumatologic labs on children, the reasons for ordering them are not congruent with recommendations from experts for these tests. Lab tests are responsible for only 5% of the rheumatologic diagnosis, with history and clinical exam accounting for the other 95% of the diagnosis (Agarwal and Sawhney 2010). Therefore, lab tests should help support making the diagnosis, monitoring the disease, and assessing the efficacy of treatments. Clinicians need to remember that positive autoantibodies do not mean autoimmune disease. These labs must be used in relation to clinical signs and symptoms (Saikia et al. 2016; Shojania 2000). The following laboratory tests are nonspecific for rheumatological disease and should be considered part of the workup for rheumatological disorders.

12.2.3.1 CBC

A complete blood count (CBC) is commonly ordered in pediatric patients with rheumatologic complaints such as joint pain, fatigue, rashes, recurrent fevers, and/or weight loss. The CBC can offer some insight into potential rheumatologic diagnoses to consider. The CBC in pediatric rheumatology should assist in diagnosing, disease acuity evaluation, and medication monitoring. The NP should consider these lab values in relationship to the patient's history, exam, and diagnosis.

White cell count. The white blood cell (WBC) count can be elevated in patients with active or new-onset systemic juvenile idiopathic arthritis (SJIA) or Kawasaki's disease. Lymphocytopenias may be seen in patients with SLE, reflecting active disease or a side effect of some medications used to treat rheumatologic conditions (Agarwal and Sawhney 2010). Lymphopenia and neutropenia may be seen in systemic lupus erythematosus (SLE) at presentation and/or during flares (Mehta 2012). Leukocytosis can also occur from medications used to treat specific pediatric rheumatologic conditions. It is important to recognize that the WBC count can be affected by many other conditions such as infection, stress, and diseases such as cancers. Thus, the provider must consider the rest of the history and clinical picture when making diagnoses or treatment plans.

Red cell count and hemoglobin. Like the WBC, hemoglobin is affected in many conditions, including rheumatologic diseases; thus, care must be taken when considering the hemoglobin in the clinical picture. Anemia may be present in many pediatric rheumatologic conditions. Anemias in these patients may be due to ongoing inflammation as well as due to the disease itself. SLE, mixed connective tissue disease (MCTD), and SS may cause hemolytic anemia. Anemia may be seen in up to 50% of children with SLE due to anemia of chronic disease, iron deficiency, and/or hemolysis. Children with systemic-onset juvenile idiopathic arthritis (SoJIA) may also present with significant anemia during the acute phases of the disease.

Platelet count. The platelet count is another common inflammatory maker useful for assessing ongoing inflammation in rheumatologic conditions. Thrombocytosis can be seen in Kawasaki's disease and systemic onset JIA (SJIA) as an acute-phase reaction. Conversely, thrombocytopenia can be seen in SLE and antiphospholipid syndrome (APL) as well as in malignancies (Mehta 2012). The clinician should use the platelet count in relation to the history, physical exam, and other lab tests to determine its significance regarding diagnosis and treatment options.

12.2.3.2 Urinalysis

A urinalysis can help evaluate the child with a possible rheumatological problem. Renal involvement can occur as a primary manifestation of Henoch-Schonlein purpura (HSP), SLE with nephritis, antineutrophil cytoplasmic antibody (ANCA)-associated vasculitis, and SoJIA with secondary amyloidosis (Pilania and Singh 2019). Microscopic hematuria, urinary cellular casts, and proteinuria can be a sign of SLE nephritis (Mehta 2012). HSP or immunoglobulin A vasculitis is a small blood vessel vasculitis and tends only to have renal involvement in children >7 years. Since the renal involvement in HSP may not be present initially, follow-up is recommended weekly for the first months and every 2–4 weeks for 6 months (Pilania and Singh

2019). Kawasaki's disease (KD) can cause pyuria.

12.2.4 Acute-Phase Reactants

Acute-phase reactant values change by more than 25% during any inflammatory state and are thus not specific to rheumatologic conditions alone (Agarwal and Sawhney 2010). Acute-phase reactants commonly used in pediatric rheumatology include ESR, CRP, and ferritin.

12.2.4.1 Erythrocyte Sedimentation Rate (ESR)

The erythrocyte sedimentation rate (ESR) is an indirect measure of inflammation due to proteins that occur with inflammation. The ESR can be affected by many things, including anemia, obesity, polycythemia, hypo, or afibrinogenemia. Thus, providers should be cautious in interpreting these results (Litao and Kamat 2014; Mehta 2012). The ESR can assist in evaluating patients with possible rheumatologic issues and/or be used to monitor disease activity and treatment responses in JIA but should not be used as a diagnostic indicator (Agarwal and Sawhney 2010).

12.2.4.2 C-Reactive Protein

The C-reactive protein (CRP) is a more sensitive indicator of current inflammation than ESR. The CRP rises early in the inflammatory process and normalizes more quickly. Finally, it is not impacted by conditions such as anemia or obesity. When using the CRP in children with rheumatologic diagnoses, the clinician should know that this lab test is not a sensitive measure of inflammation in patients with SLE. An elevated CRP in patients with SLE is more commonly associated with bacterial infections with these patients. Thus, the provider should be concerned about infection when noting an elevated CRP with SLE patients (Mehta 2012). In evaluating children with rheumatologic conditions, the ESR should be utilized to assess for chronic inflammation. In contrast, the CRP should assess acute inflammation and infection in patients with SLE.

12.2.4.3 Serum Ferritin

Serum ferritin increases in the setting of ongoing inflammation and can be used to assess disease status in patients with SoJIA and SLE. Ferritin is more commonly used in assessing the child with SoJIA to assess disease activity level. During times of acute inflammation and active disease with SoJIA, the serum ferritin will be elevated. While increases in ferritin may be seen during active SLE flares, it is not a common lab used for routine monitoring (Mehta 2012).

12.2.4.4 Serum Calprotectin

Serum calprotectin is a heterodimer formed by two proteins found in the cytosolic protein content of monocytes and neutrophils (Ometto et al. 2017). Most of the results reflect the activity of neutrophils (Jarlborg et al. 2020). It is not yet available to use but may be a marker for rheumatological disease activity. A recent adult study found that elevation of calprotectin reflected higher disease activity in both RA and axial spondyloarthritis but not in psoriatic arthritis (Jarlborg et al. 2020). More studies are needed in children to determine the usefulness of the serum calprotectin.

12.2.4.5 Complements: C3 and C4

Complements are a group of proteins that are part of the immune system, which help to clear foreign invaders. When autoimmune diseases occur as part of the immune response, complements may decrease due to consumption during the autoimmune attack. Thus, during active autoimmune diseases such as active SLE, the patient may have low complements. Complements are not used for diagnoses but can be used to assess for disease activity in SLE.

Decreased levels can also occur from other immunocomplex disorders (i.e., vasculitis, some types of glomerulonephritis, and inherited complement deficiencies). More information on complement deficiencies is found in Sect. 6.8.2.5.

The pediatric rheumatologist would most often order complements during the management and ongoing disease activity assessment of children with SLE. The use of them in screening in primary care is limited but may be done in areas where there is limited access to a pediatric subspecialist.

12.2.5 Real-Life Example

An 11-year-old female presented with joint pain, predominantly located on the knees, hips, and elbows. The pain was present for the last 4 weeks and was worse after she did cheerleading practice on Monday through Friday. The child denied any history of fever, swelling, night waking, or limitation of motion. She reported that she is one of the best cheerleaders on the squad since she can do splits in both directions and do backflips, handstands, and cartwheels. This was her first year doing cheerleading, and she was very excited about making the squad. There was no family history of sudden death or aortic dissection. The mother reports that the 44-year-old father and his 78-year-old mother have some hypermobility.

A careful physical exam revealed no swelling, no effusions, and no redness on any of the joints. There was no murmur, lymphadenopathy, splenomegaly, or hepatomegaly. The positive physical exam finding was marked hypermobility of all joints. A Brighton score system was done, which assesses joint hypermobility on the knuckle of both little, fifth, and pinky fingers; the base of both thumbs; elbows; knees; and spine. The scale is a nine-point scale, and the child scored nine points. The possibility of Ehlers-Danlos syndrome versus a benign hypermobility syndrome was considered. The mother was very worried that she had arthritis and demanded diagnostic laboratory tests done. Once a CBC and CRP were normal, she accepted a genetics referral. The genetic testing was normal, and benign joint hypermobility syndrome (BJHS) was confirmed as the source of her joint pain. BJHS is one of the most common causes of amplified pain syndrome. It is a heritable disorder of connective tissue which presents with musculoskeletal pain, joint hypermobility, and joint laxity and increased risk of injury (Weiss and Stinson 2018).

The family was counseled about the increased risk of dislocation and the reason for the child's joint pain. Using shared decision-making, the clinician and family discussed the options. The final decision was to keep the child in cheerleading.

Key Learning about the Evaluation of the Child with Possible Rheumatological Complaints

- A complete history and physical exam guide the use of laboratory tests.
- A CBC is nonspecific in rheumatological disorders, but the WBC can be elevated in patients with active or new-onset systemic juvenile idiopathic arthritis (SJIA) or Kawasaki's disease.
- Lymphocytopenias may be seen in patients with SLE.
- Anemia may be present in rheumatologic conditions and results from either chronic illness or inflammation.
- The CRP is more sensitive to current inflammation than ESR. It rises early in the inflammatory process, normalizes more quickly, and is not impacted by conditions such as anemia or obesity.
- Serum ferritin increases with inflammation and is also used to assess disease status in patients with SoJIA and SLE.
- A urinalysis can help diagnose HSP, SLE, ANCA-associated vasculitis, and amyloidosis.

12.3 Juvenile Idiopathic Arthritis (JIA)

Juvenile arthritis is a common childhood chronic disease, with a prevalence estimated at 1 per 1000 children (Ringold et al. 2019). Juvenile idiopathic arthritis (JIA) is a group of diseases characterized by pain in either one or multiple joints before 16 years of age and lasts at least 6 weeks. Other synovitis causes must be excluded

Table 12.2 Types of JIA

Subtypes of JIA	Characteristics of the subtype
Systemic JIA	• Affects about 10% of children with JIA • Affects the whole body • Constitutional symptoms include daily fever for 2 weeks with at least one of the following—Evanescent rash, lymphadenopathy, hepatosplenomegaly, serositis • Has arthritis in one or more joints
Oligoarthritis	• The most common form of JIA with 25% of children having this form of JIA • Typical onset between 1 and 3 years • The most typical joints are the ankles, knees, and elbows • One to four joints with arthritis in the first 6 months of disease ○ Persistent but no more than four joints in the first 6 months ○ Extended greater than four joints after 6 months
Polyarticular arthritis (polyJIA), rheumatoid factor (RF) negative	• About 20% of children have the RF negative polyJIA with a typical onset of either 1–3 years or early adolescence • Often affects the joints on both sides of the body (i.e., both knees, both elbows) • RF test is negative • Has involvement of five or more joints in the first 6 months of the disease
PolyJIA, RF positive	• 5% of children have RF-positive polyJIA with a typical onset of 9–11 years • RF test is positive twice 3 months apart • Has involvement of five or more joints in the first 6 months of the disease
Psoriatic arthritis	• Skin symptoms do not have to be present before the joint symptoms. It can occur after the joint symptoms • Psoriasis and arthritis or arthritis only with two of the following: ○ A first-degree relative with a history of dactylitis, nail pitting, and history of psoriasis

Table 12.2 (continued)

Subtypes of JIA	Characteristics of the subtype
Enthesitis-related arthritis, also known as spondyloarthritis	• Affects where the muscles, ligaments, or tendons attach to the bone (entheses) • The hips, knees, and feet are commonly affected but can also cause pain in the elbows, chest, fingers, pelvis, digestive tract (Crohn's disease or ulcerative colitis), and lower back (ankylosing spondylitis) • Boys are more affected, and the usual age is between 8 and 15 years • Arthritis with enthesis or has at least two of the following: ○ Sacroiliac tenderness and/or inflammatory lumbosacral pain ○ +HLA-B27 ○ Onset in boys older than 6 years ○ A first-degree relative with a history of ankylosing spondylitis, enthesis-related arthritis, IBD, Reiter syndrome, an acute anterior uveitis
Undifferentiated arthritis	Arthritis fails to fulfill the criteria in the categories above, but inflammation is present in two or more joints

Adapted from Benham and Wright (2021b); Crayne and Beukelman (2018)

as a cause of joint pain (Ringold et al. 2019). JIA is divided into several subtypes that reflect the number of involved joints and considers other axial involvement such as fever, rash, organ involvement, and constitutional symptoms. The seven different types of JIA are seen in Table 12.2.

A diagnosis of JIA is usually made as a result of a history and physical examination. Joint stiffness gets worse with inactivity and is worse in the am when the child walks like an older adult. The child may play quietly or prefer a stroll to walking, especially in the morning (Crayne and Beukelman 2018). When the pain is severe or there is associated joint erythema, septic arthritis, rheumatic fever, or other infectious causes should be considered (Benham and Wright 2021b). A child with JIA may have joint effusion, warmth, swelling, tenderness, and pain along with a

Table 12.3 JIA types putting a child at high risk for uveitis

JIA type	Screen for uveitis
High-risk children	
• Oligoarthritis and antinuclear antibody (ANA) positive • PolyJIA (rheumatoid factor negative) but ANA positive • Psoriatic arthritis but ANA positive • Undifferentiated arthritis who are ANA positive • Age under 7 years of age at JIA onset • Duration of JIA of 4 years or less	• Screen every 3 months
Low- or moderate-risk children	
• Those with high-risk JIA categories but who are ANA negative • Age 7 years or older at JIA onset • JIA duration of more than 4 years • Systemic JIA, polyarthritis (rheumatoid factor positive), and enthesitis-related arthritis	• Screen every 6–12 months

Adapted from Angeles-Han et al. (2019)

decreased range of motion (Crayne and Beukelman 2018).

The most common extraarticular manifestation is uveitis, which occurs in 10–20% of children. The external exam of the eye is normal, and there is no evidence of inflammation, making it an asymptomatic disease. It is advised to screen the child every 3 months if they are at high risk for uveitis (Angeles-Han et al. 2019). Table 12.3 lists the conditions that place a child at high risk for uveitis.

12.3.1 Diagnostic Laboratory Tests Used in JIA

While JIA diagnosis is made by history and physical exam, the nonspecific diagnostic labs in Sects. 12.2.3 and 12.2.4 are used as a baseline and to monitor treatment response. Testing for Lyme disease should be done on any patient presenting with pain out of proportion to the swelling. Information about this test can be found in Sect. 6.5.1. The ANA is used to determine the need for uveitis follow-up (see Table 12.3). The

rheumatoid factor (RF) and the anti-cyclic citrullinated peptide antibodies (anti-CCP) may be positive, and RF is used to classify the disease in polyJIA.

12.3.1.1 Antinuclear Antibodies (ANA)

The antinuclear antibody (ANA) is a measure of antibodies in the blood that can be seen in a variety of pediatric rheumatologic conditions, including systemic lupus erythematosus (SLE), juvenile idiopathic arthritis (JIA), SS, mixed connective tissue disease (MCTD), and juvenile dermatomyositis (JDM). While this test can be positive in these conditions, it is not diagnostic, and up to 30% of the general population can have a positive ANA with no disease.

This test assesses antibodies against nuclear antigens and is reported using a titer. Any patient having a titer of 1:20 or higher will be reported as having a positive ANA, but a titer of 1:160 or higher is more suggestive of rheumatologic conditions including SLE, scleroderma, SS, and JDM (Agarwal and Sawhney 2010; Ali 2018).

The ANA does not help make or exclude JIA as a diagnosis in children presenting with arthritis. This test is used to assess the risk of developing uveitis and helps determine guidelines for ophthalmological exam timing. Children diagnosed with JIA should also have an ANA drawn during the diagnostic workup by pediatric rheumatology to assess the child's risk for developing uveitis. Children with JIA with the highest frequency of ANA are younger onset, female, and have oligo-disease (Agarwal and Sawhney 2010). Children diagnosed with JIA with a positive ANA are at the highest risk for the development of uveitis. They require frequent close ophthalmologic assessment, regardless of the level of arthritis activity (Angeles-Han et al. 2019; Crayne and Beukelman 2018).

12.3.1.2 Rheumatoid Factor (RF)

The RF is a highly confusing test for clinicians. Often RF testing is used to determine if a child presenting with joint pain has juvenile idiopathic arthritis (JIA), formerly known as juvenile rheumatoid arthritis (JRA). The RF has a sensitivity of 69% in diagnosing rheumatoid arthritis and a specificity of 85% (Suresh 2019). Only 3% of children with JIA have a positive RF; thus, most children presenting with joint complaints will have a negative RF (Correll et al. 2016). A positive RF can be seen in other conditions, including TB, bacterial endocarditis and SS, systemic sclerosis, MCTD, vasculitis, sarcoid, syphilis, HIV, liver cirrhosis, mixed cryoglobulinemia, hepatitis, and parasitic diseases. Additionally, between 5% and 25% of the healthy population can have a positive RF with no systemic disease (Agarwal and Sawhney 2010; Suresh 2019; Ali 2018).

It is important to note a negative RF does not mean a child does not have JIA. When providers mistake a negative RF as criteria to say a child does not have JIA, the result can be delays in diagnosis and treatment for these children, putting them at risk for permanent joint damage. Positive RF titers are not common in children younger than 7 years of age. Current guidelines do not recommend routine testing for RF unless there are actual clinical findings of active arthritis; musculoskeletal pain alone is not enough to justify this test.

Children with polyJIA are mostly likely to have a positive RF, but this only reflects 3% of children with JIA (Correll et al. 2016). The JIA subgroup more likely to be associated with elevated RF titers are those who present at a later age, have a polyJIA (>5 joints), and have evidence of joint destruction. The International League of Associations for Rheumatology (ILAR) requires two positive RFs performed at least 3 months apart in a child with polyJIA within the first 6 months of presenting with the disease to classify a child as having RF-positive polyJIA. The test should be repeated since it may be transiently elevated due to the immune system's response to infection (Crayne and Beukelman 2018). Children with RF-positive polyJIA are more likely to have poor prognoses and a more aggressive and prolonged disease course (Saikia et al. 2016). The higher the titer, the more likely they are to have a poorer prognosis and erosive disease over time (Ali 2018).

12.3.1.3 Anti-Cyclic Citrullinated Peptide Antibodies (Anti-CCP)

Anti-CCP is more specific for RF-positive JIA but, again, is not diagnostic. In adults, the sensitivity of anti-CCP antibodies is 67%, and specificity in the presence of a positive RF is 99–100% (Suheir et al. 2013). The sensitivity and specificity of anti-CCP antibodies in children are less established. The anti-CCP is almost exclusively seen in polyJIA (Saikia et al. 2016). Children with JIA who are RF positive and CCP positive usually have a more aggressive course of their disease and more joint damage (Agarwal and Sawhney 2010; Suresh 2019; Saikia et al. 2016).

Although it is not recommended to routinely test children with musculoskeletal complaints with no clinical evidence of arthritis, it is important to note that a positive RF may be present before symptoms present. The risk for developing arthritis when seeing a child with a positive RF with no symptoms depends upon their titter level, family history, and co-presence of a positive anti-CCP. Providers who happen to order these tests and find a child with a positive RF and anti-CCP should carefully observe the child over time to develop any signs or symptoms of arthritis.

Children presenting with active arthritis in multiple joints and/or those diagnosed with JIA can classify the JIA category and guide treatment. When caring for the child with suspected new-onset JIA, the RF should be tested twice at least 3 months apart during the first 6 months of symptoms. Children who are found to have polyJIA and a positive RF should have an anti-CCP ordered to assist with categorizing the subtype of JIA, prognosis, and treatment decisions.

12.3.1.4 Synovial Fluid Analysis

Synovial fluid is found in the joint in small quantities. The testing includes protein, glucose, total leukocyte count, and differential. The synovial fluid leukocyte count in active JIA can be as high as 100,000/mm^3 with a neutrophil predominance. The glucose is low, and the protein count is high. The CD4+:CD8 = T-cell ratio is reversed, and

Table 12.4 Specific laboratory tests used in JIA

Test	Disease	Comments
ANA in JIA	PolyJIA with a positive JIA	Important for determining follow-up for uveitis
RF	PolyJIA *Other conditions* SS SLE Vasculitis Tuberculosis Bacterial endocarditis Hepatitis C Systemic sclerosis MCTD Sarcoid Syphilis HIV Parasitic diseases	Helpful in making treatment decisions and prognosis Need two positive tests 3 months apart during the first 6 months of disease for classification as RF+ polyJIA RF has a sensitivity of 69% in diagnosing rheumatoid arthritis and a specificity of 85% (Suresh 2019)
Anti-CCP	PolyJIA Psoriatic arthritis *Other conditions* SS SLE Hepatitis C infection	Associated with more aggressive disease in children with JIA Most commonly seen in polyJIA May assist in determining treatments for JIA Sensitivity and specificity in children are less clear

Adapted from Pilania and Singh (2019), Pincus and Sokka (2009), Suresh (2019)

there is an increase in interleukin (IL) 18 levels in the synovial fluid when JIA is active (Pilania and Singh 2019). Table 12.4 is a summary of the specific laboratory tests used in diagnosing JIA.

12.3.2 Real-Life Example

A 15-year-old presented with a 2-month history of left knee pain and swelling. The child states that the pain is worse in the am and improves as the day progresses, but she still misses school since it is hard for her to get out of bed and move around. She reports missing 10 days of school over the past 2 months. She describes her gait as painful and stiff. The exam is remarkable for a swollen left knee with effusion, effusions on three PIPs on the left hand, and effusions on all MCPs on the right hand. When you question her about pain when she uses her hands, she confirms that her hands are also painful in the am. She admits that she does not want to complain.

You are practicing in a rural area without any pediatric or adult rheumatologist for 100 miles. You order a CBC with differential, sedimentation rate, CRP, ANA, RF, and Anti-CCP. Her CBC shows mild anemia with a HCT of 31% and a mild leukopenia of 3.9 with an ANC of 1560. Her CRP is elevated at 25 (normal 0.1–1.7) and her RF and ANA (1:160). The anti-CCP was elevated. The results were reviewed with the mother, and the need for subspecialty care from a pediatric rheumatologist and an ophthalmologist was discussed. The mother decided to go to a children's hospital for subspecialty care.

Key Learning for JIA

- History and physical exam are key to making the diagnosis of JIA.
- There are seven types of JIA, and appropriate diagnostic laboratory testing is needed to determine the need for the type and frequency of subspecialty care.
- An ANA is done when JIA is suspected to determine the risk for uveitis.
- An RF is not usually positive in JIA but should be done to classify the type of JIA.
- Up to 30% of ANAs are false positive.
- A synovial fluid analysis in JIA will show a significant elevation of leukocytes with a neutrophil predominance. The protein is elevated, but the glucose is low in synovial fluid analysis in a child with suspected JIA.

12.4 Systemic Lupus Erythematosus (SLE)

SLE is an autoimmune disease that can affect any organ system in the body. Several mechanisms contribute to the pathophysiology, including genetic factors, abnormal exposure to autoantigens, high B-cell stimulatory cytokines, hormonal factors, complement activation, and a failure to eliminate apoptotic bodies (Aragón et al. 2020; Smith et al. 2019). A study showed that among genetically identical twins, the rate of SLE is between 25% and 40% (Rahman and Isenberg 2008). A recent publication cited several genes implicated in SLE development (Charras et al. 2021).

Around 20% of the time, SLE is diagnosed in children less than 16 years. The child with SLE will have a higher degree of SLE activity based on the SLE Disease Activity Index (Benham and Wright 2021a). In pediatrics, the gender distribution is approximately equal in children <5 years of age but does increase in females by adolescence (Smith et al. 2019). A child less than 5 years of age may have an atypical presentation of SLE (i.e., lack of autoantibodies) with a severe disease course and, ultimately, a poor prognosis. The nonspecific symptoms include oral ulcers, arthralgias, headache, fever 38.2 °C, and weight loss. The kidney is the most common organ involved in children and can affect up to 80% of children with SLE. Mucocutaneous manifestations include nonscarring alopecia, oral ulcers, photosensitivity, a photosensitive rash, malar rash, and mucocutaneous rash. Childhood SLE has a greater risk of nephritis, hemolytic anemia, and facial malar rash. The anti-double-stranded DNA (anti-dsDNA) antibodies are more likely to be positive in childhood-onset SLE (Tarvin and O'Neil 2018).

Diagnostic laboratory tests may show a positive ANA >1:80 or positive tests for extractable nuclear antigens, antiphospholipid antibodies, or 24-h urine for protein with >0.5 g/24 h (Aringer et al. 2019). Neuropsychiatric involvement with psychosis is more common in children than adults with SLE. CNS dysfunction includes seizures and delirium. Hematological involvement presents as hemolytic anemia, lymphopenia, and thrombocytopenia. In children, there is a higher incidence of renal, cardiovascular, and neuropsychiatric involvement (Charras et al. 2021). Premature death is related to premature atherosclerosis, malignancy, infection, and renal disease.

Neonatal lupus occurs when there is the passage of anti-SSA and/or anti-SSB antibodies via the placenta, resulting in cardiac conduction abnormalities in the fetus or a photosensitive annular rash in the newborn when the newborn is exposed to ultraviolet light (Noaiseh and Baer 2020).

12.4.1 Diagnostic Laboratory Tests for SLE

Tarvin and O'Neil (2018) recommend a CBC with differential, a comprehensive metabolic profile, complement studies of C3 and C4, an antinuclear antibody titer, and an anti-dsDNA antibody titer. The evaluation of a child with proteinuria and the associated diagnostic laboratory tests are discussed in Sect. 10.3 and include protein/creatinine ratio in spot urine and the 24-h urine proteinuria/creatinine clearance. Several urinary biomarkers are being explored to evaluate for lupus nephritis, and they are still in the research phase (Aragón et al. 2020).

12.4.1.1 Antinuclear Antibodies (ANA)

In children with suspected jSLE, a high ANA titer is almost always present (Universal (Wichainun et al. 2013). The ANA is also reported according to patterns based on the staining of the cell nucleus in the lab. Common patterns that will be reported include homogeneous or diffuse, speckled, nucleolar and peripheral, or rim patterns. While these patterns are not specific for any one illness, they can help differentiate which autoimmune disease to consider: homogeneous, peripheral patterns are seen with SLE, speckled patterning is seen in SS, a nucleolar pattern is seen with scleroderma, and a centromere pattern is seen with CREST syndrome (limited scleroderma) (Ali 2018). The recent classification and criteria for SLE pointed out that an ANA titer >1:80 had a sensitivity of 98% associated with a lower limit of the 95% confidence interval at 97%. Low-titer ANAs (<1:80) should be considered with caution as research has found that people with low-titer ANAs of less than 01.% have SLE (Bossuyt et al. 2020). A positive ANA can be seen in numerous other conditions such as autoimmune thyroid disease, myasthenia gravis, cancers, and certain drugs, including hydralazine, procainamide, and minocycline.

While the ANA is not diagnostic of SLE, it contributes to making the diagnosis. A negative ANA result can almost always rule out SLE, but a positive ANA has a poor predictive value for diagnosing SLE (Saikia et al. 2016; Suresh 2019). The presence of other clinical and laboratory findings is required to make the diagnosis of SLE. When it is ordered in the setting of history and clinical findings and other abnormal labs, it is much more predictive. Most patients with SLE will have a positive ANA (sensitivity of 97%, specificity 96%), but a positive ANA should not be used to tell the patient they have SLE (Suresh 2019; Wichainun et al. 2013). Patients with a positive ANA and symptoms concerning SLE require further testing and evaluation by a pediatric rheumatologist. The ANA can have different patterns reported by the laboratory. A diffuse pattern is commonly seen in patients with SLE, especially those with nephritis or in drug-induced SLE. A speckled pattern is seen in a variety of rheumatological disorders, including SLE. A nucleolar ANA pattern is seen in scleroderma, and a cytoplasmic ANA pattern is seen in SLE and an overlap syndrome (Pilania and Singh 2019).

Clinicians should consider ordering an ANA in children who present with symptoms concerning SLE, while recognizing this is not diagnostic, it can rule SLE out.

12.4.1.2   Antibodies to DNA (dsDNA)

Antibodies to DNA (dsDNA) are used to diagnose SLE in children and monitor disease activity. This test is highly specific for SLE with a sensitivity of 70% and specificity of 95%; thus, they are helpful when determining if a patient has SLE (Correll et al. 2016; Ali 2018). dsDNA is also used to assess the level of disease activity in children with SLE (Agarwal and Sawhney 2010). While the dsDNA is specific to lupus, it can also be seen with SS and RA, although it is more commonly associated with SLE. When the anti-dsDNA antibody is high, the C3 and C4 or albumin is low, and an evaluation for lupus nephritis is warranted (Tarvin and O'Neil 2018).

The dsDNA should be ordered as part of the workup for children with a positive ANA and suspected SLE. Providers should not test dsDNA if there is a negative ANA.

12.4.2   ENAs—Extractable Nuclear Antigens (Anti-Ro, anti-La, Anti-RNP, Anti-Smith, AntiScl-70)

Antibodies to extractable nuclear antigens (ENAs) are more specific to help clinicians assess those children with positive ANAs. These tests can help with making the correct diagnosis and treatment plans.

12.4.2.1   Smith Antinuclear Antibodies

Anti-Sm antigens are highly specific for making the diagnosis of SLE (98.6%); therefore, they are very useful in the workup for SLE. Negative anti-SM antigens do not, however, rule out the diagnosis of SLE.

12.4.2.2   Anti-RNP Antibodies

High titers of anti-RNP antibodies in children are associated with mixed connective tissue disease (MCTD). These antibodies are part of the criteria to diagnose MCTD, with 95 to 100% of patients having high titers (Saikia et al. 2016).

12.4.2.3   AntiSCL-70

AntiSCL-70 is diagnostic of diffuse systemic scleroderma and is associated with increased morbidity and incidence of interstitial lung disease (Ali 2018). Another antibody, anti-centromere antibodies, is often found in limited cutaneous scleroderma, also known as CREST syndrome; they are not seen in systemic sclerosis.

Most of these tests would be ordered by the pediatric rheumatologist during the diagnostic workup of children with specific rheumatologic conditions. The use of them in screening in primary care is limited. The types of antiphospholipid antibodies will be discussed under APL. Table 12.5 reviews the tests that are used in the diagnosis of SLE.

Table 12.5 Diagnostic laboratory tests used in SLE

Test	Disease	Comments
ANA	Systemic lupus erythematosus (SLE) Juvenile idiopathic arthritis (JIA) *Other conditions* SS Mixed connective tissue disease (MCTD), juvenile dermatomyositis (JDM)	Should be drawn in the presence of symptoms of lupus Should be completed by a pediatric rheumatologist in the workup of children with JIA to evaluate the risk of uveitis
Anti-dsDNA	SLE Other conditions SS JIA	These labs should be ordered by a pediatric rheumatology and have limited value in primary care
ENAs—Extractable nuclear antigens (anti-Ro, anti-La, anti-RNP, anti-Smith, antiScl-70)		
Anti-RNP	Mixed connective tissue disease	These labs should be ordered by pediatric rheumatology and have limited value in primary care
Anti-Sm	SLE	These labs should be ordered by pediatric rheumatology and have limited value in primary care
AntiScl-70	Diffuse cutaneous systemic sclerosis	These labs should be ordered by pediatric rheumatology and have limited value in primary care

Adapted from Ali (2018), Saikia et al. (2016), Pilania and Singh (2019)

12.4.3 Real-Life Example

A 15-year-old African-American presented to the office with hearing voices for the last 48 h. Her other complaints included arthralgia for a 1-month duration. The arthralgia was not accompanied by any joint swelling or morning stiffness. The child did report a fever of 102 several times over the past month, which was relieved with acetaminophen. There was an increase in headache frequency to two to three times a week for the past month, not correlated with the fever. She also reported light sensitivity along with a rash on the cheeks after sunlight exposure. She had an unremarkable medical and psychiatric family history. She denies any family history of arthritis or any other rheumatological disease but reported that her mother had thyroid disease.

The diagnosis of SLE was considered due to the above history. The initial workup included a CBC with differential, sedimentation rate, CRP, and an ANA. Her CBC showed a mild leukopenia (3.6; normal for the age 4.5–13.0, mild anemia (HCT was 30; normal for age 37 to 41), and thrombocytopenia (platelet count 110,000; normal for age 150,000 to 450,000). Her sedimentation rate was 64 (normal 5–15), and her CRP was 11 (normal 0.1–1.3). The ANA revealed a high titer of 1:320 in a diffuse pattern. The child was referred to rheumatology for a same-day evaluation and possible admission.

The anti-double-stranded DNA (anti-dsDNA) antibodies were positive. Her rheumatoid factor, anti-Sjögren's syndrome B (La), anti-Sjögren's syndrome A (Ro), anti-Smith (Sm), anticardiolipin, and anti-b2 glycoprotein antibodies were all negative. The diagnosis of neuropsychiatric lupus was made. The child was subsequently managed successfully by rheumatology.

> **Key Learning for SLE**
>
> - SLE is a multisystem disease that can present with a wide variety of clinical presentations. The clinician must be careful not to order an ANA for nonspecific symptoms that do not indicate possible SLE.
> - The initial workup can include nonspecific tests such as a CBC and acutes phase reactants and an ANA.
> - An ANA titer >1:80 had a sensitivity of 98%, but low titers should be interpreted cautiously.
> - More specific tests for SLE should be ordered by rheumatology whenever a referral is possible.

12.5 Antiphospholipid Antibody Syndrome (APL)

APL is an autoimmune disease. The hallmark is thrombosis in venous or arterial thrombosis in small vessels and/or early pregnancy loss, fetal loss, or pregnancy morbidity. The adolescent will have persistent antiphospholipid antibodies (aPL). There are three main antibodies—lupus anticoagulant (LA), anticardiolipin, or anti-β2Glycoprotein I antibodies. The non-criteria-associated clinical findings include poorly healing cutaneous ulcerations (livedoid vasculopathy), livedo reticularis, nephropathy, valvular heart disease (valve thickening and vegetation mitral > aortic valve), pulmonary hypertension, pulmonary emboli, cognitive dysfunction, seizures, thrombocytopenia, and hemolytic anemia (Kokosi et al. 2019; Sammaritano 2020).

It is considered primary when there are no associated diseases and secondary when the patient has another autoimmune disease such as SLE (Whitaker 2017). At a minimum, the adolescent should meet one clinical criterion (pregnancy morbidity (≥ 1 fetal loss after 10 weeks of gestation, ≥ 3 early pregnancy losses at <10 weeks of gestation or preeclampsia/placental insufficiency at ≤ 34 weeks) or vascular thrombosis) and one laboratory criterion (LA, anticardiolipin IgG and IgM antibodies and anti-beta$_2$-glycoprotein 1 (anti-beta$_2$ GP1) IgG and IgM antibodies) to be diagnosed with APS (Gómez-Puerta and Cervera 2014). The antibody must be positive at two separate times, done with a minimum of 12 weeks apart. One positive test for antibodies can be the result of infection or lab error. This is usually not associated with clinical findings.

APL is an uncommon disease in children but can be found in older female adolescents 15 and over. The pathophysiology is the result of aPL binding to β2GP1 on the cell membrane. The binding causes activation of monocytes, endothelial cells, and platelets. This activation results in proinflammatory and prothrombotic phenotypes as well as complement activation. This activation causes thrombosis and the ability to interference with trophoblast and decidual cells.

12.5.1 Diagnostic Laboratory Tests for Antiphospholipid Antibody Syndrome

In the early 1990s, researchers discovered that antiphospholipid antibodies (aPL) mostly bind to a circulating plasma protein β2-glycoprotein 1 (β2GP1) attached to a phospholipid. The anti-β2GP1 antibody ELISA was added to the available diagnostic laboratory tests to detect the presence of aPL (Sammaritano 2020). Since there are considerable variations in laboratory and clinical findings, there is a risk of overdiagnosis and underdiagnosis (Sammaritano 2020). Classification criteria include three different antiphospholipid antibodies (LA, anticardiolipin, and anti-beta) and two glycoproteins I. aPL positivity can be present in up to 10% of the entire population, with anticardiolipin antibodies being the most common test to be positive and LA being the least common. If all three of the tests below are positive two times, there is a greater risk of thromboembolism. If the lupus anticoagulant is positive, and there is a moderate to a high titer of anticardiolipinanti-beta-2GP1; there is a moderate risk of thromboembolism (Suresh 2019).

However, it felt most false-positive results are related to an infection and are transient, or the positivity is on the low side of positive (Sammaritano 2020).

12.5.1.1 Anti-Beta 2 Glycoprotein 1 (GP1) Antibodies

The result for this test should be >99th percentile to be positive for APL, according to the APL criteria (Sammaritano 2020). The anti-beta 2 GP1 tests can be positive in 1–5% of healthy people (Suresh 2019). It is important to repeat this test after 12 weeks to confirm a positive titer.

12.5.1.2 Anticardiolipin Antibodies (IgG or IgM)

Anticardiolipin IgG, IgM is an aβ2GP1-dependent ELISA and a positive result is > 40 MPL or GPL units.

12.5.1.3 Lupus Anticoagulant (LA)

It is important to know which antibody test is positive, as LA is the most likely to be associated

Table 12.6 Summary of the criteria of the diagnostic laboratory tests for APL

Test	Criteria
Anti-beta2-GP1 IgG and IgM antibodies	> 99th percentile, based on two or more tests done with a minimum of 12 weeks apart using the standard ELISA test
IgG or IgM anticardiolipin antibodies	Medium or high titer (more than 40 GPL or MPL units or > 99th percentile), based on two or more tests done with a minimum of 12 weeks apart using the standard ELISA test
Lupus anticoagulant	A positive result on two or more tests done with a minimum of 12 weeks apart

Adapted from Sammaritano (2020), Suresh (2019)

with risk (Sammaritano 2020). Table 12.6 reviews the antibody testing for APL.

12.6 Juvenile Sjögren's Syndrome (jSS)

jSS is a systemic autoimmune disease that tends to be defined in terms of dry mouth and eyes; however, it is a multisystem disease (Noaiseh and Baer 2020). The average age of diagnosis is 10 years. The disease, while systemic, has few treatment options to exocrine glandular damage, internal organ involvement, and development of lymphoma. The monitoring for lymphoma includes persistent glandular enlargement, low C4 levels, IgM kappa monoclonal protein, and positive cryoglobulins, but this is rare in children with SS (Noaiseh and Baer 2020). The extraglandular manifestations are related to vasculitis, autoimmune epithelitis, and lymphoproliferation and affect up to 25% of patients. Children and late adolescents with jSS are more likely to have salivary gland enlargement, recurrent parotitis, and nephritis with less frequent sicca complaints (Noaiseh and Baer 2020). A child with jSS can have persistent lymphadenopathy and visible parotid gland enlargement (Tarvin and O'Neil 2018). jSS can be found in adolescents with other autoimmune diseases, with the most frequently associated diseases being autoimmune thyroid disease, JIA, and SLE (Anaya et al. 2016). jSS is primary if it is the only autoimmune disease or secondary when it is associated with another autoimmune disease (Parisis et al. 2020).

The pathophysiology is related to autoantibody production since B-cell activation is a constant abnormality of immunoregulatory (Jonsson et al. 2018). The trigger is likely by environmental factors such as viral infections in patients with a genetic predisposition, epigenetic factors, and the regulation of sex hormones (Parisis et al. 2020).

12.6.1 Diagnostic Laboratory Tests for jSS

The criteria for jSS are not defined by a single clinical feature, diagnostic laboratory test, radiological finding, or pathology result. There is no "gold standard" laboratory test for the diagnosis and classification of jSS as a result (Jonsson et al. 2018). The American College of Rheumatology (ACR) or European League Against Rheumatism (EULAR) established five criteria for primary SS. They include the following: (1) labial salivary gland with focal lymphocytic sialadenitis and focus score ≥ 1 + 3, (2) anti-SSA (Ro): +3, (3) ocular staining score ≥ 5 (or van Bijsterveld score ≥ 4 on at least one eye): +1, (4) Schirmer ≤5 mm/5 min on at least one eye: +1, and (5) unstimulated whole unstimulated saliva flow rate ≤ 0.1 ml/min: +1. The most studied antibodies in jSS patients are the antibodies against the autoantigens Ro/SSA and La/SSB (Parisis et al. 2020).

Laboratory abnormalities include the following: normochromic, normocytic anemia, leukopenia, lymphopenia, neutropenia, thrombocytopenia, elevated ESR, hypergammaglobulinemia, high levels of serum IgG, high levels of beta2-microglobulin, free light chains of immunoglobulins, serum monoclonal band, positive ANA, positive rheumatoid factor, anti-Ro antibodies, anti-La antibodies, hypocomplementemia, and cryoglobulins (Brito-Zerón et al. 2016). The levels of beta2 microglobulin and free light chains are available tests that will be higher in very active jSS disease and can monitor disease activity. Other antibodies associated with jSS are anti-centromere (see Sect. 12.4.2.3), anti-CCP (see Sect. 12.3.1.3), or anti-RNP (see Sect. 12.4.2.2) (Noaiseh and Baer 2020).

12.6.1.1 Anti-Ro/SS-A and Anti-La/SS-B

Anti-Ro/SS-A and anti-La/SS-B antibodies are associated with SS (prevalence, 60–80%) and with SLE (30–40%). They can also be found in patients with subcutaneous lupus, systemic sclerosis, rheumatoid arthritis, mixed connective tissue disorders, inflammatory myopathies, and polymyositis (Brito-Zerón et al. 2016). These markers are not specific for SS since they can be found in other diseases (Beckman et al. 2017).

Anti-Ro/SSA, when present in a pregnant female, is associated with neonatal lupus and congenital heart block. When infants are born with congenital heart block, the mother should have these tests done to assess the above conditions.

12.6.1.2 The SJO Test

This diagnostic test uses the four traditional biomarkers for SS—anti-SS–/Ro, anti-SSB/La, ANA, and RF. Three novel biomarkers, carbonic anhydrase VI (CA-6), salivary protein (SP-1), and parotid secretory protein (PSP), are also included in the test. The SP-1 has the greatest sensitivity and specificity for early SS disease (Beckman et al. 2017) (Table 12.7).

Table 12.7 Diagnostic laboratory tests used in SS

Test	Disease	Comments
Anti-Ro/SS-A and anti-La/SS-B	SLE SS *Other conditions*: Subcutaneous lupus Systemic sclerosis Rheumatoid arthritis Polymyositis Neonatal lupus erythematosus	These labs are generally done by pediatric rheumatology but may be ordered if the primary care provider has a strong index of suspision for Sjogrens and lack of access to pediatric rheumatologist

Adapted from Brito-Zerón et al. (2016), Beckman et al. (2017)

12.7 Spondyloarthritis (jSpA)

Juvenile spondyloarthritis (jSpA) refers to a set of heterogeneous conditions in children under 16 years. It is characterized by enthesis or tenderness at the insertion of ligaments and tendons, lower extremity arthritis, bowel inflammation, joint inflammation of the spine and sacroiliac joint, sausage digits or dactylitis, uveitis, and a positive human leukocyte antigen B27 (HLA-B 27) allele (Adrovic et al. 2016). Spondyloarthritis ranges from the more common childhood enthesitis-related arthritis (ERA) to ankylosing spondylitis, which is more common in adults (Adrovic et al. 2016). In children, axial involvement in jSpA is uncommon in the early disease course. The peripheral disease is more common in children. The RF is not positive, but the HLA-B27 is positive.

The symptoms in children include arthritis of the lower extremities, enthesitis or tenderness at insertion sites, inflammation of the bowel, sacroiliac joint inflammation, psoriasis, dactylitis, anterior uveitis, and spine joint involvement. Ultimately, jSpA can cause significant axial skeletal involvement, which leads to abnormal bone formation and, subsequently, spine ankylosis. In jSpA, the enthesitis is usually persistent, symmetrical, and involves three or more sites. The most common sites are the Achilles tendon attachment, superior patella quadriceps, and the superior patella quadriceps (Weiss and Colbert 2018). The arthritis is typically asymmetric and is an oligoarticular pattern. Axial involvement, likely sacroiliitis, is present in 28–37% of children (Weiss and Colbert 2018). Cardiac involvement is rare and usually is an asymptomatic aortic regurgitation. Children may have bowel inflammation either before or after joint involvement (Weiss and Colbert 2018).

The orthopedic differential diagnosis includes sever disease, Osgood-Schlatter disease (tibial tuberosity), and Sinding-Larsen-Johansson syndrome; other causes include osteomyelitis, amplified pain syndromes, infection, and tumor (Weiss and Colbert 2018).

12.7.1 Diagnostic Laboratory Tests for Spondyloarthritis

The diagnostic workup for a child with symptoms of jSpA is a CBC, acute-phase reactants, chemistry panel, urinalysis, and HLA-B27. The child with anemia and elevated acute-phase reactants with GI symptoms needs further workup for inflammatory bowel disease. HLA-B27 is encoded in the major histocompatibility complex (MHC), HLA is a significant genetic risk factor for jSpA occurring in 60 to 70% of patients (Pagnini et al. 2010), and in ankylosing spondylitis (AS), the HLA-B27 positivity is around 90% (Weiss, Colbert). BA-positive HLA-B27 with elevated inflammatory markers is usually present in children with spondyloarthritis. The laboratory characteristics include seronegative ANA and RF and seropositive HLA-B27 (Adrovic et al. 2016).

12.7.1.1 Human Leukocyte Antigen B27 (HLA-B27)

The HLA gene complex is found on the sixth chromosome and is categorized into three classes: 1, II, and III. A positive HLA-B27 means that the particular gene is found in the child (Suresh 2019). HLA-B27 are proteins located on the surface of white blood cells that cause an autoimmune response. HLA-B27 is associated with spondyloarthropathies. Up to 9% of the general population are HLA-B27 positive, with approximately 10–15% developing a spondyloarthropathy. Among patients diagnosed with ankylosing spondylitis, 90% will have a positive HLA-B27 (Colbert et al. 2017). They are also seen in children with enthesitis-related arthritis. They are present in 50–80% of patients with reactive arthritis, psoriatic arthritis with spondylitis, and IBD-associated arthritis (Agarwal and Sawhney 2010; Suresh 2019).

It is justifiable to order HLA-B27 in children with symptoms of inflammatory back pain (insidious onset, morning stiffness, jelling, relief with movement and NSAIDs), presence of arthritis, enthesitis, dactylitis, psoriasis, IBD, family history, or recurrent uveitis (Correll et al. 2016; Mehta 2012).

Test	Disease	Comments
HLA-B27	Ankylosing spondylitis Enthesitis-related arthritis Reactive arthritis Psoriatic arthritis with spondylitis IBD-associated arthritis	Should be drawn in children with enthesitis or inflammatory back pain, active uveitis, and/or sacroiliitis

Adapted from Weiss and Colbert (2018)

12.7.2 Real-Life Example

A 17-year-old female presented for a well visit. Her chief complaint was that she had had two miscarriages after 10 weeks of gestation. The child reported that she wants a baby. She is a senior in high school and plans on becoming a beautician. She loves makeup and hair. She reports having one sexual partner since ninth grade, and they are planning on getting married after her high school graduation. She reports that he is 20 and has a baby from another relationship. She reports he is faithful to her. She also reports that she was diagnosed with SLE when she was 15 but is presently doing well on Plaquenil. She discussed the possibility of congenital disabilities with her obstetrician, and he felt that this would be the best choice for her, given her desire to have a baby (Huybrechts et al. 2021). The family history is unremarkable, and she denies any relative with a developmental disability. There is no rheumatologist in the area, and the adolescent reports that the old rheumatologist left the practice. The diagnosis of APL was considered, and anticardiolipin antibodies, lupus anticoagulant, and anti-beta 2 glycoprotein 1 (GP1) antibodies were ordered. All three results meet the criteria for APL. The results were reviewed, but the adolescent was told that a repeat in 3 months was needed for diagnosis. The adolescent was told that Plaquenil is recommended for patients with suspected APL (Tarvin and O'Neil 2018). The child came in for her follow-up, and the result was positive. She agreed to see a rheumatologist located 50 miles from her home for management.

treatment. There are several kinds of vasculitis seen in Box 12.1.

Box 12.1 Types of Vasculitis
Henoch-Schönlein purpura.
   Kawasaki's disease.
   Takayasu arteritis.
   Childhood polyarteritis nodosa.
   Cutaneous polyarteritis.
   Microscopic polyangiitis.
   Isolated cutaneous leukocytoclastic vasculitis.
   Hypocomplementemic urticarial vasculitis.
   Granulomatosis with polyangiitis (GPA).
   Churg-Strauss syndrome.
   Behçet disease.
   Vasculitis secondary to infection, malignancy, drugs.
   Vasculitis associated with connective tissue disease.
   Isolated vasculitis of the central nervous system.
   Cogan syndrome.
   Unclassified.
   Adapted from Weiss (2012)

12.8 Vasculitis

Pediatric vasculitis is an inflammation in the blood vessel wall. The disease severity and phenotype will depend on the size of the vessel involved, the site of the vessel, the vascular injury, and the underlying pathology (Weiss 2012). The symptoms of vasculitis are vague with malaise, diffuse pain, and fever, and elevated acute-phase reactants can be the initial manifestations.

Henoch-Schönlein purpura (HSP) and Kawasaki's disease (KD) are the two most common vasculitis that when combined account for 72% of all pediatric vasculitis. These two diseases tend to be self-limited with appropriate

12.8.1 Diagnostic Laboratory Tests for Vasculitis

As more vessel damage occurs due to the disease process, more specific disease presentations evolve, including antineutrophil cytoplasmic antibodies (ANCAs) (Weiss 2012). The diagnostic lab workup for vasculitis should include a CBC and acute-phase reactants, significantly elevated. Liver transaminases, BUN, creatinine, and urinalysis detect hepatic and renal involvement. Specific antibody testing such as ANA, antineutrophilic cytoplasmic antibodies (ANCAs), and complements C3 and C4 can be part of the workup, depending on the type of vasculitis the clinician is under consideration.

12.8.1.1 Antineutrophilic Cytoplasmic Antibodies

ANCAs are a group of autoantibodies commonly detected in autoimmune disorders. They are most associated with certain systemic vasculitis: GPA (formerly Wegener's granulomatosis), microscopic polyangiitis vasculitis, and Churg-Strauss syndrome (Suresh 2019). Conditions that can be ANCA positive but are not related to vasculitis include IBD, autoimmune hepatitis, viral hepatitis, endocarditis, TB, malaria, RA, and SLE. Additionally, specific drugs may result in a positive ANCA, such as minocycline, hydralazine, and allopurinol.

ANCAs are ordered in children with the following clinical presentations: glomerulonephritis, chronic destructive lung disease, progressive, rapid renal failure, pulmonary hemorrhage, prolonged sinusitis or prolonged otitis, retro-orbital mass, or with cutaneous vasculitis and systemic features (Ali 2018; Saikia et al. 2016; Suresh 2019). Testing for ANCA should be considered for a persistent fever of >2 weeks, multiple organ involvement, petechial or purpuric rash or diagnostic labs with an increase in acute-phase reactants, anemia of chronic disease, or thrombocytosis (Mehta 2012). Testing for ANCA should only be done when the pretest probability for an ANCA-associated vasculitis is high.

Two methods are used to measure ANCA—indirect immunofluorescence and ELISA. The ELISA is more specific, and the IF is more sensitive (Mehta 2012). The IF method has two staining patterns—cytoplasmic (c-ANCA) or perinuclear (p-ANCA). The ELISA method evaluates antibodies against MPO and PR3. C-ANCA stating correlates with an ELISA that is positive for PR3 seen to GPA. Current guidelines recommend using the antigen-specific assay for PR3 and MPO as the primary method for screening (Suresh 2019). This recommendation is a result of the large variability of the different IF methods. Damoiseaux et al. (2017) reported the specificity for PR3-ANCA was 98% to 99%, and specificity for MPO-ANCA was 96–99%.

Test	Disease	Comments
ANCA	Rheumatological diseases: • GPA • Microscopic polyangiitis, vasculitis • Churg-Strauss syndrome • SLE • JIA Other autoimmune diseases • Autoimmune hepatitis • Inflammatory bowel disease • Sclerosing cholangitis Other non-autoimmune diseases • Infections such as endocarditis, HIV, and malaria • Drug-induced such as minocycline and propylthiouracil	Should be ordered only in the presence of symptoms pointing to vasculitis

Adapted from Ali (2018), Mehta (2012), Saikia et al. (2016), Suresh (2019)

12.9 Kawasaki's Disease

KD accounts for 23% of all vasculitides and is the second common childhood vasculitis (Weiss 2012). KD's pathogenesis is unclear, but the current leading theory centers around an unknown stimulus causing an immune-mediated inflammatory cascade in a genetically susceptible child (Rife and Gedalia 2020). The highest incidence of KD is in children who are of East-Asian and Pacific-Islander descent (Rife and Gedalia 2020). The American Heart Association's diagnostic criteria for typical Kawasaki's disease must include fever for at least 5 days plus at least four of the following criteria: (1) bilateral conjunctival injection, (2) lip and oral cavity changes, (3) cervical lymphadenopathy, (4) polymorphous exanthem, and (5) changes found in the extremities or perineal area (Singh et al. 2018). Atypical or incomplete Kawasaki's disease does not have to meet all the criteria. The worst complication of KD and atypical KD is the development of coronary artery abnormality (Agarwal and Agrawal 2017).

The differential diagnosis includes measles, adenovirus, enterovirus, Epstein-Barr virus, scarlet fever, acute rheumatic fever, Rocky Mountain spotted fever, Leptospirosis, cervical lymphadenitis, toxin-mediated staphylococcal-scalded skin syndrome, toxic shock syndrome, hypersensitivity reactions, drug hypersensitivity reaction, Steven-Johnson syndrome, JIA, polyarteritis nodosa, reactive arthritis, acrodynia, and multisystem inflammatory syndrome in children (Rife and Gedalia 2020).

12.9.1 Diagnostic Laboratory Tests for Kawasaki's Disease

There is no specific diagnostic laboratory test for KD. Several nonspecific diagnostic laboratory test abnormalities including a high WBC count of 15,000 with neutrophil predominance and immature forms of neutrophils, anemia, and a high platelet count of >450,000/mm^3, which peaks during week 3. The common acute-phase reactants such as a sedimentation rate of >40 mm/h, a CRP of >3.0 g/dL, and elevated serum ferritin are also affected. The albumin is low (<3.0 g/dL), and the alanine aminotransferase (ALT) is elevated, as is the GGT will occur in up to 40–60% of patients (Agarwal and Agrawal 2017). The urine has sterile pyuria with urine WBCs >10 WBCs/HPF. If a spinal tap is done, the CSF will have mononuclear pleocytosis without hypoglycorrhachia and/or elevated protein (Rife and Gedalia 2020).

12.9.1.1 N-Terminal Pro-Brain Natriuretic Peptide (NT-pro-BNP)

NT-pro-BNP is a cardiac biomarker that can be elevated when a disease causes myocardial damage. The use of an NT-pro-BNP-based diagnostic algorithm has been proposed for use as part of the diagnostic criteria in the AHA algorithm for incomplete KD (Singh et al. 2018). NT-pro-BNP as an additional diagnostic marker

to help establish KD in children with prolonged fever is controversial. It is a nonspecific test without clear cut-point values for a positive result (Dahdah et al. 2009; Kwon et al. 2016; Lin et al. 2015). Some studies have suggested that it might be a useful marker for detecting early coronary artery disease in the hyperacute phase of KD (Jung et al. 2019; Rodriguez-Gonzalez et al. 2019).

12.10 Immunoglobulin A (IgA) Vasculitis (Formerly Henoch-Schonlein Purpura)

Immunoglobulin A vasculitis (IgAV) is a systemic small-vessel leukocytoclastic vasculitis with a clinical presentation that includes nonthrombocytopenic palpable purpura, arthritis, and abdominal pain (Reamy et al. 2020). It accounts for 49% of all childhood vasculitis. It typically has a limited course, but it can have a remitting-relapsing course. The most common complications are glomerulonephritis and gastrointestinal bleeding.

The diagnosis of IgAVs requires the presence of palpable purpura or petechiae involving lower limb predominance and without thrombocytopenia or coagulopathy with at least one of the following: (1) acute diffuse abdominal pain, (2) histopathology diagnosis of leukocytoclastic vasculitis or a kidney biopsy showing proliferative glomerulonephritis and a predominant IgA deposition, (3) acute arthritis or acute arthralgia, and (4) renal involvement with hematuria or proteinuria (Ozen et al. 2010).

12.10.1 Initial Diagnostic Laboratory Tests for IgAV

The initial diagnostic tests include a CBC with differential, coagulation profile, metabolic profile, urinalysis, and serum albumin. These tests are discussed in greater detail in Chaps. 7 and 8. The urinalysis will show hematuria with or without RBC casts. There may be no or mild proteinuria (Viteri and Reid-Adam 2018).

12.11   Juvenile Dermatomyositis (DM)

Dermatomyositis (DM) is considered an idiopathic inflammatory myopathy with systemic and cutaneous signs and symptoms resulting in the variability of childhood clinical presentations (Wolstencroft and Fiorentino 2018). DM can present with cutaneous signs, pulmonary disease, joint disease, muscle abnormalities, and malignancy.

12.11.1   Diagnostic Laboratory Tests for Juvenile Dermatomyositis

The child who presents with a possible inflammatory myopathy should have muscle enzymes done, including creatinine phosphokinase (CPK), LDH, aspartate aminotransferase (AST), alanine aminotransferase (ALT), and serum aldolase (Bellutti Enders et al. 2017). Muscle enzymes are used in rheumatology when an inflammatory myopathy is being considered. Up to 26% of children with JDM will have a normal value for one of the muscle enzymes (Mehta 2012).

The hematological tests include a CBC with differential and smear and acute-phase reactants. Renal (including urinalysis) and liver function tests and possible infectious causes for the weakness and dermatological findings should be done. Thyroid functions and vitamin D levels should be done. If there are atypical features and a lack of rash, metabolic and mitochondrial myopathies need to be included in the diagnostic laboratory tests (Bellutti Enders et al. 2017).

12.11.1.1   Myositis-Specific Antibodies

Myositis-specific autoantibodies (MSAs) are present in patients with idiopathic inflammatory myopathies. The idiopathic inflammatory myopathies include dermatomyositis, necrotizing myopathies, polymyositis, and inclusion body myositis (Wolstencroft and Fiorentino 2018). Anti-Mi2 is generally considered the prototype dermatomyositis autoantibody and is found in

children with DM at a low rate (4–10% of affected patients) (Li and Tansley 2019). Anti-MDA5 autoantibodies are present in children with less prominent muscle disease, but these children have a greater risk of developing interstitial lung disease, ulcerations, and arthritis. Patients with anti-NXP2 will have greater muscle involvement and a greater risk of ulcers, dysphagia, and gastrointestinal bleeding. The child with anti-TIF1γ autoantibody can have milder muscle involvement but have a severe cutaneous disease, including ulceration and lipodystrophy (Li and Tansley 2019).

12.11.1.2   Creatine Kinase

Creatine kinase (CK) is found in the muscle, heart, and brain. Sex, activity level, race, and muscle mass can influence CK levels. A mild elevation is <5 to 10 times the upper limit of normal, whereas a marked elevation is >20 times the upper limit of normal (Venance 2016). When the clinician notes an exaggerated lumbar lordosis, scapular winging, and Gower's maneuver or difficulty getting up from the floor, weakness should be considered, and a CK should be done.

Primary skeletal muscle disorder presents with a history of fatiguability, weakness, and pain and CK increases (Brancaccio, Lippi, Maffullis, 2010). CK is elevated in genetic diseases such as muscular dystrophies (marked elevation Duchenne muscular dystrophy/Becker muscular dystrophy as well as some types of limb-girdle muscular dystrophy), myotonic dystrophies (mild elevation), metabolic myopathies, and congenital myopathies. It also elevated in acquired myopathies due to myotoxic drugs, endocrine disorders (thyroid or hypoparathyroidism), and immune/inflammatory myopathies (Venance 2016). Muscular dystrophy will have the highest CK (Brancaccio et al. 2010). However, in the later stages of MD, the CK drops due to the fibrotic changes in the muscle tissue (Brancaccio et al. 2010). Excessive physical activity or a seizure can cause a mild elevation of CK, but it will be markedly elevated in rhabdomyolysis. The inflammatory myopathies such as JDM will have a marked elevation of the CK. It is the first enzyme to rise and the first to fall in JDM as disease activity increases and then decreases (Pilania and Singh 2019). The enzyme can rarely be normal in JDM but can be normal in some metabolic myopathies, facioscapulohumeral muscular dystrophy, and milder limb-girdle muscular dystrophies. With dilated cardiomyopathy and desmin-related myopathy, weakness and pain with mild muscle enzymes increase are seen (Brancaccio et al. 2010).

12.11.1.3 Liver Function Tests (FTs)

Liver function tests are discussed in detail in Sect. 9.4.3.2. LDH and AST are the best predictors of disease activity in inflammatory myopathies. Five isoenzymes (LDH1, LDH2, LDH3, LDH4, LDH5) are found in the body's cells. Serum LDH is a marker of cell damage, and, in nontraumatic rhabdomyolysis, the isoenzyme increase is helpful in diagnosis. AST and LDH can increase significantly after the exercise. The amount and duration of the exercise determine the degree of increase. For example, after a marathon, the LDH will double and remain elevated for 2 weeks (Brancaccio et al. 2010).

An increase in muscle enzymes occurs approximately 5–6 weeks before clinical changes in JDM (Pilania and Singh 2019). LFTs can also be elevated in neuromuscular diseases as well as inflammatory myopathies.

12.11.1.4 Serum Aldolase

The serum aldolase is found in both the cytoplasm and cell nucleus. There are three aldolase isoenzymes. Aldolase A is the muscle type; aldolase B is the liver type; and aldolase C is expressed in the nervous tissue, including the brain. In diseases like muscular dystrophy, polymyositis, and myotonic dystrophy, the serum aldolase is elevated, and it is aldolase A isoenzyme that is increased.

12.11.2 Real-Life Example

An 18-month-old Asian male presents with a 6-day history of fever, a polymorphous rash, cervical lymphadenopathy, bilateral conjunctivitis with sparing of the limbus, and red lips. A rapid strep test is negative, and KD is considered as a possible diagnosis. The child is mildly dehydrated as the mother reports the child is irritable and not drinking well. The child is admitted for hydration and possible KD. IVIG is given with marked improvement. An echocardiogram is normal, and the child is discharged after clinical improvement is seen.

A heart-healthy diet is reviewed along with cardiology follow-up. The child was followed for 3 years and discharged by cardiology. Since the child is at higher risk for coronary artery disease, continual reinforcement of a healthy diet is done at every well visit.

Key Learning for a Child with Dermatomyositis and Kawasaki's Disease

- There is no specific diagnostic laboratory test for KD.
- The use of NT-pro-BNP is not yet on any criteria for the diagnosis of KD, but it may be helpful in the early phase of KD.
- Total serum creatine kinase comes primarily from skeletal muscle, with a small amount from the cardiac muscle and a minimal amount from the brain.
- Muscle enzymes include CK, LDH, AST, ALT, and serum aldolase, and they may show an elevation in JDM.
- The highest elevation in CK occurs early in muscular dystrophy; since as the disease progresses, the muscle becomes fibrotic and no longer release CK.

Rheumatologic conditions in children can be challenging to evaluate. The most important aspects of rheumatologic lab evaluation in the pediatric client are history and physical exam findings. As discussed, most rheumatologic labs are most useful when ordered in the presence of signs and symptoms of rheumatologic conditions. Clinicians working in the primary care setting should assure a detailed history and physical exam have been completed to support the need for lab testing. Clinicians can complete an initial workup and refer children to a pediatric rheumatologist for more in-depth testing and evaluation.

Questions

1. What is the best test to order in a patient who presents with vague joint pain for 2 weeks, has a normal examination, and has a negative family history?
   (a) A CBC with differential, CRP, and erythrocyte sedimentation rate.
   (b) An ANA.
   (c) a and b.
   (d) Hold off doing diagnostic testing.
2. A 7-year-old female with systemic lupus has had two separate highly positive tests (>99th percentile) for anticardiolipin IgA/IgM/IgG along with a positive lupus anticoagulant. What condition is she at risk of having?
   (a) Meningitis.
   (b) Thromboembolism.
   (c) Intussusception.
   (d) Pericarditis.
3. A child has SLE. Which of the following would be the best test to evaluate her kidney function further?
   (a) Antinuclear antibody screen.
   (b) Check urine protein to creatinine ratio
   (c) C-reactive protein.
   (d) Renal ultrasound.
4. A 15-year-old presents with a history of hair loss, weakness, and fatigability. The physical exam is remarkable for Gottron's papules and a heliotrope rash. Her hair is also showing diffuse hair loss. What is the best test to order?
   (a) N-terminal pro-brain natriuretic peptide (NT-pro-BNP).
   (b) Antineutrophilic cytoplasmic antibodies.
   (c) Myositis-specific autoantibodies (MSA).
   (d) Human leukocyte antigen B27 (HLA-B27).
5. An 8-year-old has a clinical presentation that includes nonthrombocytopenic palpable pur-

pura, arthritis, and abdominal pain. Which are the best laboratory tests to order?
   (a) N-terminal pro-brain natriuretic peptide (NT-pro-BNP).
   (b) Antineutrophilic cytoplasmic antibodies.
   (c) CBC with differential, coagulation profile, metabolic profile, urinalysis, and serum albumin.
   (d) Human leukocyte antigen B27 (HLA-B27).
6. A 15-year-old who has SLE is complaining of the new onset of dry eyes and a dry mouth. She also has myalgias that have increased. Her pediatric rheumatologist manages her SLE. What is the best next step?
   (a) Refer her back to rheumatology and let them determine the workup.
   (b) Order a CBC with differential and acute-phase reactants.
   (c) Order an SJO test.
   (d) Reassure the patient.
7. A child has a 2-month history of knee pain. The child's knee is swollen out of proportion to the pain level she is reporting. What must be included in her laboratory workup?
   (a) Lyme titer.
   (b) Human leukocyte antigen B27.
   (c) CBC with differential, coagulation profile, metabolic profile, urinalysis, and serum albumin.
   (d) Acute-phase reactants.
8. A child has oligoarthritis and antinuclear antibody (ANA) positive. A pediatric rheumatologist follows her. What other referrals are needed for this patient?
   (a) Orthopedics once a month.
   (b) Ophthalmology every year.
   (c) Orthopedics once a year.
   (d) Ophthalmology every 3 months.
9. Which test, if positive, would make the diagnosis of JIA?
   (a) Antinuclear antibody.
   (b) Rheumatoid factor.
   (c) CBC with differential.
   (d) Acute-phase reactants, CRP, and sedimentation rate.
   (e) None of the above.

Rationale

1. Answer: d

   This child has a vague history and a normal examination. The likelihood that the child has a positive ANA but is healthy is 30%. An ANA is an expensive test and leads to increases in healthcare costs. If the pretest probability of a disease is high, then the ANA is indicated (Fritzler 2016). In this case, the pretest probability is low. Follow-up is indicated in this child.

2. Answer: b

   Given the child's positive testing, the diagnosis of APL is likely. Therefore, the child is at greater risk for thromboembolism.

3. Answer: b

   Of the choices given, the urine protein-to-creatinine ratio is the best way to evaluate the child's kidney function. A urinalysis would also be helpful.

4. Answer: c

   The choices are very specific. N-terminal pro-brain natriuretic peptide (NT-pro-BNP) might be ordered in a patient with prolonged fever, and the clinician is considering Kawasaki's disease. Antineutrophilic cytoplasmic antibodies (ANCAs) are a group of autoantibodies commonly detected in autoimmune disorders. They are most associated with certain systemic vasculitis: GPA (formerly Wegener's granulomatosis), microscopic polyangiitis vasculitis, and Churg-Strauss syndrome (Suresh 2019). Human leukocyte antigen B27 is a specific test for juvenile spondylarthritis (jSpA), a set of heterogeneous conditions in children under 16 years.

   Myositis-specific autoantibodies (MSA) is the correct answer as it might be very helpful in a patient that you are considering JDM.

5. Answer: c

   As noted above, the N-terminal pro-brain natriuretic peptide (NT-pro-BNP) might be ordered in a patient with prolonged fever, and the clinician is considering Kawasaki's disease. Antineutrophilic cytoplasmic antibodies (ANCAs) are a group of autoantibodies commonly detected in autoimmune disorders.

There is no specific test for immunoglobin A vasculitis (IgAV). IgAV is a systemic small-vessel leukocytoclastic vasculitis with a clinical presentation that includes nonthrombocytopenic palpable purpura, arthritis, and abdominal pain (Reamy et al. 2020). Myositis-specific autoantibodies (MSA) are specific for inflammatory myopathies.

6. Answer: a

   There is no "gold standard" laboratory test for the diagnosis and classification of jSS as a result (Jonsson et al. 2018). In this case, referral back to the rheumatologist is the best next step. You could order the SJO test for Sjogren's syndrome, but, since she already has a rheumatologist, a referral is the best next step.

7. Answer: a

   A Lyme titer should be ordered especially given the history of swelling out of proportion to the pain. While acute-phase reactants are not wrong, they are not the best choice as nonspecific tests. It would be important to remember that a Lyme titer should be done in patients with unilateral joint swelling.

8. Answer: d

   This child is at high risk for asymptomatic uveitis and needs to see ophthalmology every 3 months.

9. Answer: e

   The diagnosis of JIA is made by history, physical exam, and diagnostic laboratory tests. No one test will confirm the diagnosis. The ANA does not help make or exclude JIA as a diagnosis in children presenting with arthritis. It is important to note a negative RF does not mean a child does not have JIA. When providers mistake a negative RF as criteria to say a child does not have JIA, the result can be delays in diagnosis and treatment for these children, putting them at risk for permanent joint damage. A CBC with differential and acute-phase reactants are nonspecific tests.

References

Adrovic A, Barut K, Sahin S, Kasapcopur O. Juvenile spondyloarthropathies. Curr Rheumatol Rep. 2016;18(8):55.

Agarwal M, Sawhney S. Laboratory tests in pediatric rheumatology. Indian J Pediatr. 2010;77(9):1011–6.

Agarwal S, Agrawal DK. Kawasaki disease: etiopathogenesis and novel treatment strategies. Expert Rev Clin Immunol. 2017;13(3):247–58.

Ahrari A, Barrett SS, Basharat P, Rohekar S, Pope JE. Appropriateness of laboratory tests in the diagnosis of inflammatory rheumatic diseases among patients newly referred to rheumatologists. Joint Bone Spine. 2020;87(6):588–95.

Ali Y. Rheumatologic tests: a primer for family physicians. Am Fam Physician. 2018;98(3):164–70.

Anaya JM, Rojas-Villarraga A, Mantilla RD, Arcos-Burgos M, Sarmiento-Monroy JC. Polyautoimmunity in Sjogren syndrome. Rheum Dis Clin N Am. 2016;42(3):457e72.

Angeles-Han ST, Ringold S, Beukelman T, Lovell D, Cuello CA, Becker ML, et al. 2019 American College of Rheumatology/Arthritis Foundation Guideline for the screening, monitoring, and treatment of juvenile idiopathic arthritis-associated uveitis. Arthritis Care Res (Hoboken). 2019;71(6):703–16.

Aragón CC, Tafúr RA, Suárez-Avellaneda A, Martínez MT, Salas AL, Tobón GJ. Urinary biomarkers in lupus nephritis. J Transl Autoimmun. 2020;3:100042.

Aringer M, Costenbader K, Daikh D, Brinks R, Mosca M, Ramsey-Goldman R, et al. 2019 European League Against Rheumatism/American College of Rheumatology classification criteria for systemic lupus erythematosus. Ann Rheum Dis. 2019;78(9):1151–9.

Aringer M, Costenbader K, Daikh D et al. 2019 European League against Rheumatism/American College of rheumatology classification criteria for systemic lupus erythematosus. Arthritis Rheumatol. 2019;71:1400–12.

Beckman KA, Luchs J, Milner MS, Ambrus JL Jr. The potential role for early biomarker testing as part of a modern, multidisciplinary approach to Sjögren's syndrome diagnosis. Adv Ther. 2017;34(4):799–812.

Bellutti Enders F, Bader-Meunier B, Baildam E, Constantin T, Dolezalova P, Feldman BM, et al. Consensus-based recommendations for the management of juvenile dermatomyositis. Ann Rheum Dis. 2017;76(2):329–40.

Benham H, Wright TB. Overview of pediatric rheumatology: part two. Physician Assist Clinic. 2021a;6:193–207.

Benham H, Wright TB. Overview of pediatric rheumatology: part one. Physician Assist Clinic. 2021b;6:177–91.

Bossuyt X, De Langhe E, Borghi MO, Meroni PL. Understanding and interpreting antinuclear antibody tests in systemic rheumatic diseases. Nat Rev Rheumatol. 2020;16(12):715–26.

Brancaccio P, Lippi G, Maffulli N. Biochemical markers of muscular damage. Clin Chem Lab Med. 2010;48(6):757–67.

Brito-Zerón P, Theander E, Baldini C, Seror R, Retamozo S, Quartuccio L, et al. Eular Sjögren Syndrome Task Force. Early diagnosis of primary Sjögren's syndrome: EULAR-SS task force clinical recommendations. Expert Rev Clin Immunol. 2016;12(2):137–56.

Charras A, Smith E, Hedrich CM. Systemic lupus erythematosus in children and young people. Curr Rheumatol Rep. 2021;3:20.

Colbert RA, Navid F, Gill T. The role of HLA-B*27 in spondyloarthritis. Best Pract Res Clin Rheumatol. 2017;31(6):797–815.

Correll CK, Spector LG, Zhang L, Binstadt BA, Vehe RK. Use of rheumatology laboratory studies among primary pediatricians. Clin Pediatr (Phila). 2016;55(14):1279–88.

Crayne CB, Beukelman T. Juvenile idiopathic arthritis: oligoarthritis and polyarthritis. Pediatr Clin N Am. 2018;65(4):657–74.

Dahdah N, Siles A, Fournier A, Cousineau J, Delvin E, Saint-Cyr C, et al. Natriuretic peptide as an adjunctive diagnostic test in the acute phase of Kawasaki disease. Pediatr Cardiol. 2009;30(6):810–7.

Damoiseaux J, Csernok E, Rasmussen N, Moosig F, van Paassen P, Baslund B, et al. Detection of anti-neutrophil cytoplasmic antibodies (ANCAs): a multicentre European Vasculitis Study Group (EUVAS) evaluation of the value of indirect immunofluorescence (IIF) versus antigen-specific immunoassays. Ann Rheum Dis. 2017;76(4):647–53.

Fritzler MJ. Choosing wisely: review and commentary on anti-nuclear antibody (ANA) testing. Autoimmun Rev. 2016;15(3):272–80.

Gómez-Puerta JA, Cervera R. Diagnosis and classification of the antiphospholipid syndrome. J Autoimmun. 2014;48-49:20–5.

Huybrechts KF, Bateman BT, Zhu Y, Straub L, Mogun H, Kim SC, et al. Hydroxychloroquine early in pregnancy and risk of birth defects. Am J Obstet Gynecol. 2021;224(3):290.e1–290.e22.

Jarlborg M, Courvoisier DS, Lamacchia C, Martinez Prat L, Mahler M, Bentow C, et al. Physicians of the Swiss Clinical Quality Management (SCQM) registry. Serum calprotectin: a promising biomarker in rheumatoid arthritis and axial spondyloarthritis. Arthritis Res Ther. 2020;22(1):105.

Jarvis JN. Commentary—ordering lab tests for suspected rheumatic disease. Pediatr Rheumatol Online J. 2008;17(6):19.

Jonsson R, Brokstad KA, Jonsson MV, Delaleu N, Skarstein K. Current concepts on Sjögren's syndrome—classification criteria and biomarkers. Eur J Oral Sci. 2018;126(Suppl 1):37–48.

Jung JY, Ham EM, Kwon H, Kwak YH, Kim DK, Lee JH, Jung JH. N-terminal pro-brain natriuretic peptide and prediction of coronary artery dilatation in hyperacute phase of Kawasaki disease. Am J Emerg Med. 2019;37(3):468–71.

Kokosi M, Lams B, Agarwal S. Systemic lupus erythematosus and antiphospholipid antibody syndrome. Clin Chest Med. 2019;40(3):519–29.

Kwon H, Lee JH, Jung JY, Kwak YH, Kim DK, Jung JH, et al. N-terminal pro-brain natriuretic peptide can be an adjunctive diagnostic marker of hyperacute phase of Kawasaki disease. Eur J Pediatr. 2016;175(12):1997–2003.

Li D, Tansley SL. Juvenile dermatomyositis-clinical phenotypes. Curr Rheumatol Rep. 2019;21(12):74.

Lin KH, Chang SS, Yu CW, Lin SC, Liu SC, Chao HY, et al. Usefulness of natriuretic peptide for the diagnosis of Kawasaki disease: a systematic review and meta-analysis. BMJ Open. 2015;5(4):e00670.

Litao MK, Kamat D. Erythrocyte sedimentation rate and C-reactive protein: how best to use them in clinical practice. Pediatr Ann. 2014;43(10):417–20.

Mehta J. Laboratory testing in pediatric rheumatology. Pediatr Clin N Am. 2012;59(2):263–84.

Noaiseh G, Baer AN. Toward better outcomes in Sjögren's syndrome: the promise of a stratified medicine approach. Best Pract Res Clin Rheumatol. 2020;34(1):101475.

Ometto F, Friso L, Astorri D, Botsios C, Raffeiner B, Punzi L, Doria A. Calprotectin in rheumatic diseases. Exp Biol Med (Maywood). 2017;242(8):859–73.

Ozen S, Pistorio A, Iusan SM, Bakkaloglu A, Herlin T, Brik R, et al. EULAR/PRINTO/PRES criteria for Henoch-Schönlein purpura, childhood polyarteritis nodosa, childhood Wegener granulomatosis and childhood Takayasu arteritis: Ankara 2008. Part II: final classification criteria. Ann Rheum Dis. 2010;69(5):798–806.

Pagnini I, Savelli S, Matucci-Cerinic M, Fonda C, Cimaz R, Simonini G. Early predictors of juvenile sacroiliitis in enthesitis-related arthritis. J Rheumatol. 2010;37(11):2395–401.

Parisis D, Chivasso C, Perret J, Soyfoo MS, Delporte C. Current state of knowledge on primary Sjögren's syndrome, an autoimmune exocrinopathy. J Clin Med. 2020;9(7):2299.

Pilania RK, Singh S. Rheumatology panel in pediatric practice. Indian Pediatr. 2019;56(5):407–14.

Pincus T, Sokka T. Laboratory tests to assess patients with rheumatoid arthritis: advantages and limitations. Rheum Dis Clin N Am. 2009;35(4):731–4.

Rahman A, Isenberg DA. Systemic lupus erythematosus. N Engl J Med. 2008;358(9):929–39.

Reamy BV, Servey JT, Williams PM. Henoch-Schönlein purpura (IgA Vasculitis): rapid evidence review. Am Fam Physician. 2020;102(4):229–33.

Rife E, Gedalia A. Kawasaki disease: an update. Curr Rheumatol Rep. 2020;22(10):75.

Ringold S, Angeles-Han ST, Beukelman T, Lovell D, Cuello CA, Becker ML, et al. 2019 American College of Rheumatology/Arthritis Foundation guideline for the treatment of juvenile idiopathic arthritis: therapeutic approaches for non-systemic polyarthritis, sacroiliitis, and enthesitis. Arthritis Care Res (Hoboken). 2019;71(6):717–34.

Rodriguez-Gonzalez M, Perez-Reviriego AA, Castellano-Martinez A, Cascales-Poyatos HM. N-terminal pro-brain natriuretic peptide as biomarker for diagnosis of Kawasaki disease. Biomark Med. 2019;13(4):307–23.

Saikia B, Rawat A, Vignesh P. Autoantibodies and their judicious use in pediatric rheumatology practice. Indian J Pediatr. 2016;83(1):53–62.

Sammaritano LR. Antiphospholipid syndrome. Best Pract Res Clin Rheumatol. 2020;34(1):101463.

Shojania K. Rheumatology: 2. What laboratory tests are needed? Can Med Assoc J. 2000;162(8):1157–63. http://www.cmaj.ca/cgi/content/abstract/162/8/1157

Singh S, Jindal AK, Pilania RK. Diagnosis of Kawasaki disease. Int J Rheum Dis. 2018;21(1):36–44.

Smith EMD, Lythgoe H, Midgley A, Beresford MW, Hedrich CM. Juvenile-onset systemic lupus erythematosus: update on clinical presentation, pathophysiology and treatment options. Clin Immunol. 2019;209:108274.

Suheir A, Hasssan L, Khalil K. Sensitivity and specificity of anti-cyclic citrullinated peptide antibodies, compared to rheumatoid factor in Syrian rheumatoid arthritis patients. Int J Pharm Sci Rev Res. 2013;2(20):1–4.

Suresh E. Laboratory tests in rheumatology: a rational approach. Cleve Clin J Med. 2019;86(3):198–210.

Tarvin SE, O'Neil KM. Systemic lupus erythematosus, Sjögren syndrome, and mixed connective tissue disease in children and adolescents. Pediatr Clin N Am. 2018;65(4):711–37.

Venance SL. Approach to the patient with HyperCKemia. Continuum (Minneap Minn). 2016;22(6):1803–14.

Ventura I, Reid P, Jan R. Approach to patients with suspected rheumatic disease. Prim Care. 2018;45(2):169–80.

Viteri B, Reid-Adam J. Hematuria and proteinuria in children. Pediatr Rev. 2018;39(12):573–87.

Weiss JE, Stinson JN. Pediatric pain syndromes and noninflammatory musculoskeletal pain. Pediatr Clin N Am. 2018;65(4):801–26.

Weiss PF. Pediatric vasculitis. Pediatr Clin N Am. 2012;59(2):407–23.

Weiss PF, Colbert RA. Juvenile Spondyloarthritis: a distinct form of juvenile arthritis. Pediatr Clin N Am. 2018;65(4):675–90.

Whitaker KL. Antiphospholipid antibody syndrome: the difficulties of diagnosis. JAAPA. 2017;30(12):10–4.

Wichainun R, Kasitanon N, Wangkaew S, Hongsongkiat S, Sukitawut W, Louthrenoo W. Sensitivity and specificity of ANA and anti-dsDNA in the diagnosis of systemic lupus erythematosus: a comparison using control sera obtained from healthy individuals and patients with multiple medical problems. Asian Pac J Allergy Immunol. 2013;31(4):292–8.

Wolstencroft PW, Fiorentino DF. Dermatomyositis clinical and pathological phenotypes associated with myositis-specific autoantibodies. Curr Rheumatol Rep. 2018;20(5):28.

Printed in the United States
by Baker & Taylor Publisher Services